Handbook of Clinical Nutrition and Aging

NUTRITION ◊ AND ◊ HEALTH

Adrianne Bendich, Series Editor

HANDBOOK OF CLINICAL NUTRITION AND AGING

Edited by

CONNIE WATKINS BALES, PhD, RD, FACN

Durham VA Medical Center and
Duke University Medical Center,
Durham, NC

and

CHRISTINE SEEL RITCHIE, MD, MSPH

Louisville VA Medical Center and
University of Louisville Schools of Medicine and Public Health,
Louisville, KY

Foreword by

ROBERT M. RUSSELL, MD

Tufts University, Boston, MA

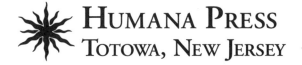

HUMANA PRESS
TOTOWA, NEW JERSEY

© 2004 Humana Press Inc.
999 Riverview Drive, Suite 208
Totowa, New Jersey 07512

www.humanapress.com

The content and opinions expressed in this book are the sole work of the authors and editors, who have warranted due diligence in the creation and issuance of their work. The publisher, editors, and authors are not responsible for errors or omissions or for any consequences arising from the information or opinions presented in this book and make no warranty, express or implied, with respect to its contents.

Due diligence has been taken by the publishers, editors, and authors of this book to assure the accuracy of the information published and to describe generally accepted practices. The contributors herein have carefully checked to ensure that the drug selections and dosages set forth in this text are accurate and in accord with the standards accepted at the time of publication. Notwithstanding, since new research, changes in government regulations, and knowledge from clinical experience relating to drug therapy and drug reactions constantly occur, the reader is advised to check the product information provided by the manufacturer of each drug for any change in dosages or for additional warnings and contraindications. This is of utmost importance when the recommended drug herein is a new or infrequently used drug. It is the responsibility of the treating physician to determine dosages and treatment strategies for individual patients. Further, it is the responsibility of the health care provider to ascertain the Food and Drug Administration status of each drug or device used in their clinical practice. The publishers, editors, and authors are not responsible for errors or omissions or for any consequences from the application of the information presented in this book and make no warranty, express or implied, with respect to the contents in this publication.

This publication is printed on acid-free paper. ∞
ANSI Z39.48-1984 (American Standards Institute) Permanence of Paper for Printed Library Materials.

Production Editor: Jessica Jannicelli.
Cover design by Patricia F. Cleary.

For additional copies, pricing for bulk purchases, and/or information about other Humana titles, contact Humana at the above address or at any of the following numbers: Tel.: 973-256-1699; Fax: 973-256-8341; E-mail: humana@humanapr.com; or visit our Website: www.humanapress.com

Printed in the United States of America. 10 9 8 7 6 5 4 3 2 1
E-ISBN: 1-59259-391-7
        Library of Congress Cataloging-in-Publication Data

Handbook of clinical nutrition and aging / edited by Connie W. Bales and
Christine Seel Ritchie.
    p. ; cm. -- (Nutrition and health)
Includes bibliographical references and index.
    ISBN 1-58829-055-7 (alk. paper)
  1. Aged--Diseases--Nutritional aspects--Handbooks, manuals, etc. 2.
Aged--Diseases--Diet therapy--Handbooks, manuals, etc. 3. Nutrition
disorders in old age--Handbooks, manuals, etc. 4.
Aged--Nutrition--Handbooks, manuals, etc.
    [DNLM: 1. Nutrition--Aged. 2. Aging. 3. Chronic
Disease--therapy--Aged. 4. Diet Therapy--Aged. WT 115 H236 2003] I.
Bales, Connie W. II. Ritchie, Christine Seel. III. Series: Nutrition and
health (Totowa, N.J.)
    RC952.5.H344 2003
    615.8'54'0846--dc21
                                        2003012862

DEDICATION

C. W. B. dedicates this book to her parents, Betty and Bud, in humble appreciation of their support, unconditional love, and life lessons about courage under fire.

C. S. R. dedicates this book to her husband Tim, and her children, Ivy and Ramsay, in gratitude for the support, love, and joy they give her each day.

Series Introduction

The overriding mission of the *Nutrition and Health* series of books is to provide health professionals with texts that are considered essential because each includes: (1) a synthesis of the state of the science; (2) timely, in-depth reviews by the leading researchers in their respective fields; (3) extensive, up-to-date fully annotated reference lists; (4) a detailed index; (5) relevant tables and figures; (6) identification of paradigm shifts and the consequences; (7) virtually no overlap of information between chapters, but targeted, interchapter referrals; (8) suggestions of areas for future research; and (9) balanced, data-driven answers to patient and/or health professionals' questions that are based on the totality of evidence rather than the findings of any single study.

The series volumes are not the outcome of a symposium. Rather, each editor has the potential to examine a chosen area with a broad perspective, both in subject matter as well as in the choice of chapter authors. The international perspective, especially with regard to public health initiatives, is emphasized where appropriate. The editors, whose trainings are both research and practice oriented, have the opportunity to develop a primary objective for their book, define the scope and focus, and then invite the leading authorities from around the world to be part of their initiative. The authors are encouraged to provide an overview of the field, discuss their own research, and relate the research findings to potential human health consequences. Because each book is developed *de novo*, the chapters are coordinated so that the resulting volume imparts greater knowledge than the sum of the information contained in the individual chapters.

Handbook of Clinical Nutrition and Aging, edited by Connie Bales and Christine Ritchie, clearly exemplifies the goals of the *Nutrition and Health* series. In fact, this is the first book in the series to be designated a handbook because it is clearly the most comprehensive volume available concerning the role of clinical nutrition in preserving the health of the elderly—especially those suffering from chronic disease. As the editors and chapter authors remind the reader, the fastest growing population in the United States as well as globally is the oldest-old. This important text provides practical, data-driven options to enhance this at-risk population's potential for optimal health and disease prevention with special emphasis on secondary disease prevention. The overarching goal of the editors is to provide fully referenced information to health professionals so they may enhance the nutritional welfare and overall health of older adults.

Bales and Ritchie have organized the volume into four major areas of focus: (1) epidemiological findings that point to significant trends in nutritional aspects of aging, (2) key fundamentals of geriatric nutrition, (3) the effects of aging on the senses and effects of chronic diseases of aging on overall patient health concerns that can be affected by nutrition—as well as nutrition's potential to reduce disease progression, and (4) broad clinical topics that include all of the major organ systems of the body in health and in disease. Unique areas of focus include legal and ethical aspects of end-of-life care, extensive review of herbal and nutritionally based dietary supplements, hearing and nutrition, and cardiac rehabilitation programs including exercise and nutritional guidance. Each chapter includes a discussion of the physiology of the condition, the effects of aging, chronic disease(s), pertinent drugs or other treatments, relevant treatment guidelines, and the consequences of malnutrition and/or dietary recommendations and/or supplemental sources of nutrients.

Handbook of Clinical Nutrition and Aging sets the benchmark for providing the most critical data on drug/nutrient interactions with specific emphasis on drugs that affect taste. This practical information is provided in extensive, well-organized tables that are now accessible in this valuable volume. Understanding the complexities of the aging process, drug use, physical debilities, and mental changes that also affect nutrient status certainly is no simple task; the standards used can often seem daunting. However, the authors are intent on assisting those unfamiliar with this field in understanding the critical issues and important new research findings that can impact their fields of interest. The editors have taken special care to use the same terms and abbreviations between chapters, and to provide clear reference to relevant material between chapters. Moreover, the Foreword by the well-acknowledged leader in the field, Dr. Robert Russell, provides a clear overview of the critical importance of this volume to the understanding of clinical nutrition and health of the aging population.

Drs. Bales and Ritchie have drawn from world renowned researchers to communicate the relevant role of clinical nutrition in the health of aging populations. The authors have worked hard to make their information accessible to health professionals who are interested in public health, geriatrics, nursing, pharmacy, and psychology, as well as nutrition-related health issues. The well-referenced tables and figures as well as the detailed references provide a great value to the reader. Many of the tables provide health professionals with guides to assessment in not only the nutritional status of the senior patient, but also help in evaluating activities of daily living, mental performance, multiple drug uses, and lists of other well-regarded resources. A very useful and unique component of virtually each chapter is a final section on "Recommendations for Clinicians."

In conclusion, *Handbook of Clinical Nutrition and Aging* provides health professionals in many areas of research and practice with the most up-to-date, well-referenced, and easy-to-understand volume on the importance of nutrition for optimal health during the senior years. This volume will serve the reader as the most authoritative resource in the field of clinical nutrition and aging to date and is a very welcome addition to the *Nutrition and Health* series.

Adrianne Bendich, PhD, FACN
Series Editor

FOREWORD

Handbook of Clinical Nutrition and Aging, edited by Connie Bales and Christine Ritchie, is a welcome addition to the *Nutrition and Health* series. The study of the role of nutrition in the aging process has indeed "come of age." Public interest on this subject is at its highest peak—in hope that specific nutrients alone (or in combination) might play a role in the prevention of chronic diseases of aging, and indeed of aging itself. In this light, the Recommended Dietary Allowances (RDA) have been redefined according to a new paradigm: instead of an RDA representing how much of a nutrient it may take to protect a population against the deficiency state, it is now defined as how much of a nutrient it takes to prevent a chronic disease or metabolic disorder from occurring. For example, calcium and vitamin D requirements, in part, have been set according to the amounts needed to prevent bone demineralization and osteoporosis.

It is amazing what the last 20 years have brought forth with regard to our knowledge of nutrition in aging. We knew very little on this subject 20 years ago. We knew that underfed rats lived longer than ad libitum fed rats, and we knew that severe obesity had many dire health consequences—but that was about all. Over the last 20 years, the importance of calcium and vitamin D in bone health has been defined, the importance of B vitamins in cardiovascular disease has been demonstrated, and the roles that nutrients play in the prevention of other age-related diseases, such as hypertension, cancer, eye disease, and diabetes, have been better determined. But this continues to be a dynamic area of research, as we are learning more each day, not only about new biochemical mechanisms, but also the interplay between nutrients and the gene. Nutrients not only control certain aspects of gene expression, but genetic endowment controls the response to nutrients and diet that the individual is eating.

Twenty years ago it was thought that elderly people malabsorbed most nutrients. In fact, we now know that this is not true, and that some nutrients may be superabsorbed with age (e.g., vitamin A). One cannot generalize about nutrient needs in aging, e.g., that all nutrients are needed in more or less amounts. The need is very specific and individualized for each nutrient. For example, the need for vitamin D is greater with aging as a result of decreased skin synthesis with ultraviolet light exposure, whereas iron requirements are lower in postmenopausal women because of a loss of menstrual periods. Whereas it was thought that riboflavin requirements would be lower with aging owing to decreased energy expenditure, it has been shown that requirements for riboflavin are, in fact, steady throughout the aging process.

All practitioners have a need to communicate with their patients, and increasingly this requires a working knowledge of the role of nutrition in aging and age-related diseases. The *Handbook of Clinical Nutrition and Aging* is an up-to-date reference that provides (1) the trends in nutrition and health in older adults, (2) the fundamentals of geriatric nutrition, (3) geriatric syndromes related to nutrition (e.g., loss of taste, smell, and other senses), and (4) specific clinical topics that are intimately related to nutritional status (vascular disorders, pulmonary disease, cancer, musculoskeletal disorders, and so forth). Physicians who wish to take an active role in educating their patients in the prevention of chronic diseases associated with aging will find this book invaluable. Indeed, I hope *Handbook of Clinical Nutrition and Aging* will appear on the bookshelves, not only of medical libraries, but of a wide range of health practitioners.

Robert M. Russell, MD
Tufts University, Boston, MA

PREFACE

The "successful aging" strategies of the 20th century, along with the reduced birth rates in the United States and throughout much of the world, now bring us into the new millennium with a unique challenge. The "graying" of the world population is recognized as a major demographic trend that will bring dramatic change to the nature of many societies. In the United States, the current proportion of the population age 65 and older is 13%, an all-time high and up by 22% since 1980. This segment of the population is expected to increase to 20% by 2030. Most striking will be the increase in the proportion of "oldest-old"; the number of US citizens age 85 and older is projected to triple in this same time period. These trends are the same in many parts of the world. The global average life span has increased from 49.5 yr in 1972 to more than 63 yr currently. And the Third World, although still somewhat youthful, is aging more quickly than the rest of the world. This is particularly troublesome in view of the economic constraints in these countries; loss of workforce-age citizens will complicate the accommodations needed for elderly populations.

The aging of our world has important social, political, and economic implications for the future. But the most profound effect, from the standpoint of public health, will be the fundamental changes it brings in the medical profile of much of the world's citizenry. Older adults have more complex health problems and use health care services at a greater rate than any other subgroup of the population. In the United States, older adults make an average of more than five outpatient physician visits annually and account for more than 38% of hospitalizations, although they constitute only 13% of the population. In addition, the elderly tend to spend more time in the hospital once admitted and are far more likely to be discharged to an intermediate care facility or nursing home than younger patients.

The importance of applying interventions to prevent or delay age-associated disease has never been more evident. The health concerns of older adults tend to be more serious and often occur in tandem with one or more other chronic conditions. Moreover, medical problems continue to escalate as individuals get older and result in "add-ons" for medical therapies. For example, 45% of older persons with diabetes mellitus were diagnosed at age 65 or later and 26% at or after age 75 yr. At age 75 and beyond, rates of use for five or more prescription drugs soar to 13.7% for men and 16.8% for women. These trends and the anticipated increase in numbers of elderly will almost certainly stress global medical and economic resources. We can expect increasing total health care expenditures, increased needs for long-term care services, and a demand for more focused health care services for older adults living at home as the mean age of the population continues to escalate.

The purpose of *Handbook of Clinical Nutrition and Aging* is to provide strategies for understanding and managing nutrition-related medical disorders in older adults. Good nutritional care will improve the short- and long-term courses of many illnesses that are common in older adults. Although primary prevention is the goal whenever possible, the foremost goal of this text is to provide expert advice on secondary prevention and offer appropriate nutritional therapies for older adults with established health problems. We offer this handbook as a guide to health care workers (including physicians, nurses, and dietitians) who provide care for this high-risk population.

Handbook of Clinical Nutrition and Aging provides a comprehensive overview of disorders that can seriously affect and be affected by nutrition and, wherever possible, presents specific recommendations for secondary prevention, management, and therapy. It is organized into parts, each of which contain related information on health and diseases that are major determinants of morbidity and mortality in older and elderly adults. Each chapter presents a discussion of the physiological basis of the disorder or concern, with special emphasis on interactions with nutrition, and concludes with a section on practical application and treatment guidelines (wherever applicable). It is our hope that the nutritional welfare and overall health of older adults will be enhanced through the use of the information contained here.

Connie Watkins Bales, PhD, RD, FACN
Christine Seel Ritchie, MD, MSPH

CONTENTS

CONTRIBUTORS

KENT J. ADAMS, PhD, FACSM, CSCS • *Exercise Physiology Laboratory, University of Louisville, Louisville, KY*

JOHN J. B. ANDERSON, PhD • *Department of Nutrition and Medicine, Schools of Public Health and Medicine, University of North Carolina, Chapel Hill, NC*

CONNIE WATKINS BALES, PhD, RD, FACN • *Geriatrics Research, Education and Clinical Center, Durham VA Medical Center and Division of Geriatric Medicine, Duke University Medical Center, Durham, NC*

SHIRISH BARVE, PhD • *Division of Gastroenterology/Hepatology, University of Louisville, Louisville, KY*

CHRISTOPHER J. BATES, MA, DPhil • *Medical Research Council, Human Nutrition Research, Cambridge, UK*

MELANIE BERG, MS, RD, LDN • *The Vanderbilt Center for Human Nutrition, Vanderbilt University Medical Center, Nashville, TN*

GIULIANO BRUNORI, MD • *Cattedra e Divisione di Nefrologia, Spedali Civili e Università degli Studi, Facoltà di Medicina e Chirurgia, Brescia, Italy*

MARIANNE CABLE, RD • *Audiology and Speech Pathology, Nutrition, and Radiology Services, Durham VA Medical Center, and Department of Medicine, Duke University Medical Center, Durham, NC*

PAUL M. COATES, PhD • *Office of Dietary Supplements, National Institutes of Health, Bethesda, MD*

REBECCA B. COSTELLO, PhD • *Office of Dietary Supplements, National Institutes of Health, Bethesda, MD*

DAVID CURTIS, MD • *Audiology and Speech Pathology, Nutrition, and Radiology Services, Durham VA Medical Center, and Department of Medicine, Duke University Medical Center, Durham, NC*

ALBERT R. DeCHICCHIS, PhD • *Department of Communication Sciences and Disorders, College of Education, University of Georgia, Athens, GA*

LISETTE C. P. G. M. DE GROOT, MSc, PhD • *Division of Human Nutrition and Epidemiology, Department of Agrotechnology and Food Sciences, Wageningen University, Wageningen, The Netherlands*

MARK H. DeLEGGE, MD • *Digestive Disease Center, Division of Gastroenterology, Medical University of South Carolina, Charleston, SC*

GERALD W. DRYDEN, MD • *Division of Gastroenterology/Hepatology, Department of Medicine, University of Louisville, Louisville, KY*

LINDA EVANKO, RD • *Audiology and Speech Pathology, Nutrition, and Radiology Services, Durham VA Medical Center, and Department of Medicine, Duke University Medical Center, Durham, NC*

DANIEL E. FORMAN, MD • *Section of Cardiology, Department of Medicine, Boston University School of Medicine, Boston, MA*

CHRISTIAN DAVIS FURMAN, MD • *Division of General Internal Medicine, Geriatrics and Health Policy Research, University of Louisville, Louisville, KY*

KATHERINE GRAY-DONALD, PhD • *School of Dietetics and Human Nutrition, McGill University, Montreal, Quebec, Canada*

CAROL SMITH HAMMOND, PhD • *Audiology and Speech Pathology, Nutrition, and Radiology Services, Durham VA Medical Center, and Department of Medicine, Duke University Medical Center, Durham, NC*

GORDON L. JENSEN, PhD, MD • *The Vanderbilt Center for Human Nutrition, Vanderbilt University Medical Center, Nashville, TN*

ELIZABETH J. JOHNSON, PhD • *Jean Mayer USDA Human Nutrition Research Center on Aging at Tufts University, Boston, MA*

MARY ANN JOHNSON, PhD • *Department of Foods and Nutrition, Faculty of Gerontology, University of Georgia, Athens, GA*

KAUMUDI JOSHIPURA, DDS, ScD • *Department of Oral Health Policy and Epidemiology, Harvard School of Dental Medicine, and Department of Epidemiology, Harvard School of Public Health, Boston, MA*

JUDY KINNALLY, MEd • *Audiology and Speech Pathology, Durham VA Medical Center, Durham, NC*

MAUREEN LESER, MS, RD • *Office of Dietary Supplements, National Institutes of Health, Bethesda, MD*

PAO-HWA LIN, PhD • *Department of Medicine, Sarah W. Stedman Center for Nutritional Studies, Duke University Medical Center, Durham, NC*

LISA W. MARKLEY, MS • *Audiology and Speech Pathology, Durham VA Medical Center, Durham, NC*

TIMOTHY E. MCALINDON, MD, MPH • *Division of Rheumatology, Tufts-New England Medical Center, Boston, MA*

CRAIG J. MCCLAIN, MD • *Division of Gastroenterology, Department of Medicine, University of Louisville, Louisville, KY*

STEPHEN A. MCCLAVE, MD • *Division of Gastroenterology, University of Louisville, Louisville, KY*

MARJI MCCULLOUGH, ScD, RD • *American Cancer Society, Atlanta, GA*

ROGER B. MCDONALD, PhD, MD • *Department of Nutrition, University of California, Davis, CA*

BARBARA E. MILLEN, DrPH, RD, FADA • *Department of Social and Behavioral Sciences and Sociomedical Sciences, Boston University Schools of Medicine and Public Health, Boston, MA*

SRI PRAKASH MOKSHAGUNDAM, MD • *Division of Endocrinology, Department of Medicine, University of Louisville, Louisville, KY*

JOHN E. MORLEY, MB, BCh • *Division of Geriatric Medicine, St. Louis University Health Sciences Center, St. Louis, MO*

PETER A. NAGI, MD • *Division of Gastrointestinal Surgery, UAB School of Medicine, University of Alabama at Birmingham Medical Center, Birmingham, AL*

C. ARIEL NASON, MA • *Boston University School of Medicine, Boston, MA*

ROBERT J. NOZZA, PhD • *Section of Audiology, Temple University School of Medicine, Philadelphia, PA*

DAVID A. ONTJES, MD • *Department of Medicine, School of Medicine, University of North Carolina, Chapel Hill, NC*

PAULA A. QUATROMONI, DSc, RD • *Department of Health Sciences, Sargent College of Health and Rehabilitation Sciences, Boston University, Boston, MA*

MICHAEL W. RICH, MD • *Cardiovascular Division, Washington University School of Medicine, St. Louis, MO*

CHRISTINE SEEL RITCHIE, MD, MSPH • *Louisville VA Medical Center, Division of General Internal Medicine, Geriatrics and Health Policy Research, Department of Medicine, University of Louisville, Louisville, KY*

MAMIE O. ROGERS • *Department of Psychiatry and Behavioral Sciences, Duke University Medical Center, Durham, NC*

RODNEY C. RUHE, PhD • *Department of Nutrition, University of California, Davis, CA*

ROBERT M. RUSSELL, MD • *Friedman School of Nutrition Science and Policy, Tufts University, Boston, MA*

DAVID A. SABOL, MD • *Digestive Disease Center, Division of Gastroenterology, Medical University of South Carolina, Charleston, SC*

HELGA SAUDNY-UNTERBERGER, MSc • *School of Dietetics and Human Nutrition, McGill University, Montreal, Quebec, Canada*

CANDICE HUDSON SCHARVER, MA • *Audiology and Speech Pathology, Durham VA Medical Center, Durham, NC*

SUSAN S. SCHIFFMAN, PhD • *Department of Psychiatry and Behavioral Sciences, Duke University Medical Center, Durham, NC*

KELLY J. SHEA-MILLER, PhD • *School of Graduate Medical Education, Seton Hall University, South Orange, NJ*

GIULIA L. SHEFTEL, MD • *Section of Cardiology, Department of Medicine, Boston University School of Medicine, Boston, MA*

DAVID A. SPAIN, MD • *Department of Surgery, Stanford University School of Medicine, Stanford, CA*

BARBARA STETSON, PhD • *Department of Psychological and Brain Sciences, University of Louisville, Louisville, KY*

LAURA P. SVETKEY, MD • *Duke Hypertension Center, Department of Medicine, and Sarah W. Stedman Center for Nutritional Studies, Duke University Medical Center, Durham, NC*

WIJA A. VAN STAVEREN, MSc, RD, PhD • *Division of Human Nutrition and Epidemiology, Department of Agrotechnology and Food Sciences, Wageningen University, Wageningen, The Netherlands*

DAVID R. THOMAS, MD, FACP, FAGS • *Division of Geriatric Medicine, St. Louis University Health Sciences Center, St. Louis, MO*

SELWYN M. VICKERS, MD • *Division of Gastrointestinal Surgery, UAB School of Medicine, University of Alabama at Birmingham Medical Center, Birmingham, AL*

YANFANG WANG, PhD, MD • *Geriatrics Research, Education and Clinical Center, Durham VA Medical Center and Center for the Study of Aging and Human Development, Duke University Medical Center, Durham, NC*

HEIDI K. WHITE, MD • *Division of Geriatric Medicine, Department of Medicine, Center for the Study of Aging and Human Development, Duke University Medical Center; and Geriatrics Research, Education and Clinical Center, Durham VA Medical Center, Durham, NC*

JAMES F. WILLOTT, PhD • *Department of Psychology, University of South Florida, Tampa, FL*

MARGARET-MARY G. WILSON, MB, BS • *Division of Geriatric Medicine, St. Louis University Health Sciences Center, St. Louis, MO*

JENNIFER ZERVAKIS, PhD • *Department of Psychiatry and Behavioral Sciences, Duke University Medical Center, Durham, NC*

I TRENDS IN NUTRITION AND HEALTH IN OLDER ADULTS

1

"Global Graying" and Nutritional Trends in the New Millennium

A Cross-Cultural Perspective

Connie Watkins Bales and Yanfang Wang

1. INTRODUCTION

Why are we leading off this book on clinical nutrition and aging discussing "global graying"? It is because we recognize that the population of the world is changing in a way that will dramatically alter health care, and therefore nutritional care, in the near future. During the first half of the 21st century, the proportion of the population that is older or elderly (65 yr and up) will reach an all-time high. This demographic shift toward an older population will inevitably create a greater demand for health care services, calling our attention to the application of nutritional prevention and intervention. As illustrated in subsequent chapters of this volume, health problems that are not thwarted by primary prevention strategies may eventually present themselves as diseases and disorders that require nutritional intervention later in life.

The present day world faces population age shifts toward "gray" that are completely unprecedented. In terms of health care policy, there is no model to follow or previous experience to serve as a guide. In fact, it is evident that the modern health care system will experience an increase in demand that could exceed its capacity unless careful planning for the future is implemented. This book reinforces the optimistic view that nutritional interventions have the potential to improve health care scenarios for the elderly, not only when implemented at an early stage, but also when applied during more advanced illness (secondary and tertiary prevention and intervention; *see* Table 1). When optimally implemented, these interventions could reduce health care needs and costs and enhance the quality of life *(1)* for the elder citizens of the world.

In the following sections, demographic projections for the future of the world's elderly population will be briefly reviewed, emphasizing specific implications for health and nutrition. The reader is also referred to Chapter 2, which provides additional detailed information on the demographics of aging. As an illustration of the potent interaction of aging trends with nutrition and public health, we then explore the implications of expected

From: *Handbook of Clinical Nutrition and Aging*
Edited by: C. W. Bales and C. S. Ritchie © Humana Press Inc., Totowa, NJ

Table 1
Levels of Preventive Health Care for Older Adults

Level	Health issues
Primary	Incident disease
Secondary	Prevalent and recurrent disease, geriatric syndromes
Tertiary	Disease, disability, health care needs, institutionalization, mortality

Source: Adapted from ref. 1.

demographic trends, using as an example, the country in which the most dramatic changes are expected—the Peoples' Republic of China. Because of restricted birth rates since the 1970s and increased life expectancies, China faces the most rapid "graying" of any population in the world, serving as a dramatic example of the challenges expected in many other countries. Finally, we will emphasize that the lessons learned in one culture can be beneficially applied in other settings and comment on the interplay of primary and secondary prevention with nutritional outcomes in the future.

2. POPULATION DEMOGRAPHICS IN THE NEW MILLENNIUM

The life expectancy of human beings has experienced a more or less steady increase over time, roughly tripling during human history. For most of recorded time, increases in life expectancy have resulted from improvements in standard of living and organized efforts to reduce infectious disease (2). Athough previous increases in life expectancy have been a result of the reduction of infectious diseases in the early years of life, in the future, this trend will be mainly attributed to increases in life expectancy at ages 65 and 85 yr (Fig. 1). As more and more of the world's citizenry survive to adulthood, the primary causes of death will shift to degenerative conditions, such as heart disease, cancer, and stroke. These chronic conditions are often amenable to prevention and treatment via lifestyle and medical interventions. In industrialized countries, the implementation of these interventions has resulted in a decline in the rates of death from cardiovascular disease and cancer (3). Therefore, during the latter half of the 20th century, the developed countries witnessed a decline in mortality rates at older ages. In fact, in many parts of the world, the elderly population is growing at a faster rate than the population as a whole.

2.1. The Developed and Developing Worlds

At the beginning of the 20th century, fewer than half of all Americans lived past 65 yr, now over 80% have this expectation. Presently, 13 of every 100 Americans are age 65 yr or older; this proportion will increase to 20 of every 100 by the year 2030 (4). In particular, the baby boom generation (i.e., persons born during 1945–1965) will "swell the ranks" of the elderly both in the US and other Western countries in the early part of the 21st century (5).

Worldwide, a "longevity revolution" is also in progress. Japan has the longest life expectancy in the world (82.9 and 76.4 yr for females and males, respectively). China and Korea lead the world in expected growth of their older populations. While lagging behind

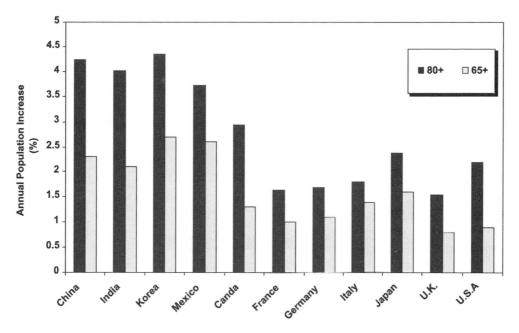

Fig. 1. International comparison of rates of average annual (percent) increases in elderly population for ≥65 and ≥80 yr. *Source*: ref. *21*.

the developed world, developing countries also anticipate important changes in their distribution of population age groups. Two-thirds of older persons live in developing countries, and that number is growing *(6)*. By the year 2030, it is estimated that 71% (686 million) of the world's elderly population will live in the developing world *(7)*. This will result from the combined effects of a sharp decline in early mortality from infections and other diseases and substantial reductions in fertility (e.g., improved availability of contraceptives in India and the "one-child-per-family" policy introduced in China in 1979). The implications of this population shift are complex, but include concerns about the effects that illiteracy, poverty, and poor social support may have on the ability of these countries to care for or support self-care for their older populations *(6)*. Nutritional status, both for prevention and treatment of chronic illness, will be growing concerns in many of these countries *(8–10)*.

2.2. Exceptional Increases in Numbers of the "Oldest-Old"

The fastest growing segment of the elderly population is the "oldest-old," persons age 85 yr and older (*see* Fig. 1). This is true in many countries of the world. Because rates of illness, disability, dementia and utilization of health care are all known to escalate sharply when persons enter this age group, this trend leads to serious concerns about increasing demands for expensive and highly intensive health care measures in the coming years (*see* Chapter 2).

2.3. The Predominance of Women in the Older Population

Today, and in the near future, in virtually all the elderly populations of the world, women do and will substantially outnumber men (*see* Fig. 2). This phenomenon has

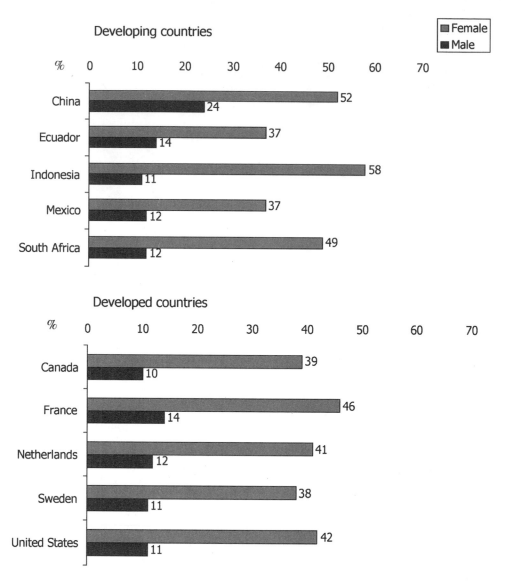

Fig. 2. Percent of female and male individuals widowed in selected developing and developed countries (circa 1990). *Source*: ref. *56*.

developed, for the most part, in the last 100 yr. Before that time, the number of females and males was roughly equal in many countries. In contrast, by the 1990s, the number of women per 100 men (aged 75+) ranged from 100 to 355 worldwide *(11)*. In particular, women predominate in the oldest-old segment; currently 7 of 10 persons aged ≥85 yr are female. This, along with the fact that at all ages after 65 yr, women are more likely to be disabled and have higher rates of nursing home residence than men, fosters a greater emphasis on women's health care in the years ahead. As noted in the next section, the low status of women in many developing countries may also be a serious barrier to their health in old age *(6)*.

2.4. Income and Ethnicity Will Influence Nutritional Concerns

It is well established that poverty, economic uncertainly, and food insufficiency or insecurity increases the likelihood of malnutrition. The percent of persons reporting fair or poor health is four times higher for persons living below the poverty level when compared with those families at least two times the poverty level *(5)*. When income is limited, the quantity and variety of food purchased and consumed is unavoidably curtailed. This is particularly true in high-risk populations like the elderly, who may also lack other resources and have poor social support. Food insufficiency prevalence, last reported for 1988–1994 in National Health and Nutrition Examination Survey (NHANES) III, was 1.7% in all persons over 60, but 5.9% in persons of low income in this same age group.

Worldwide, the gap between rich and poor is widening *(12)*. This is occurring both between developed and developing countries and, within individual countries over the past two decades. The "rich get richer" and "poor get poorer" scenario will only enhance many of the problems as limited food access is already seen in vulnerable subgroups of the aged population. Economic adversity affects mortality by reducing personal incomes and further burdening the medical sector; therefore, the health of the elderly in developing countries is particularly sensitive to periods of economic crisis *(6)*.

There are also differential expectations regarding population increases in elderly minority populations. In the United States, for example, the proportion of the population aged 65 yr grew more than five times as fast among Hispanics as among non-Hispanic persons in the period 1990–1997 *(5)*. There are differential patterns of health concerns in the elderly determined by ethnic origin. For example, the life expectancy for black males lags behind that of white males by 7.1 yr. Although differences in health and longevity associated with minority, race, or ethnicity may be determined in part by income and education, there are also genetic differences in the types and prevalences of certain age-related chronic diseases (e.g., hypertension and diabetes).

3. NUTRITIONAL CONCERNS OF THE AGING COMMUNITY

As more individuals are able to "achieve old age," they enter a period of increased susceptibility to age-related chronic diseases, including cardiovascular disease, cancer, and stroke. In the United States, these three conditions account for 60% of all deaths occurring in individuals older than 65 yr *(13)*. Other major contributors to mortality in old age are chronic obstructive pulmonary disease, diabetes, pneumonia, and influenza. In addition, overweight and obesity are now major contributors to morbidity and mortality in the older adults *(14)*. In the year 2000, the rates of obesity (body mass index >30) were 22.9% and 15.5% in US adults aged 60–69 and >70 yr, respectively *(15)*.

The shifts in population distribution towards progressively more older citizens will also produce new disease patterns for developing countries. By the year 2020, age-related chronic diseases, particularly, cardiovascular disease, cancer, and diabetes, will replace infectious disease and become the main burden of disease *(6)*.

Because of this international trend, nutritionists need to think broadly and creatively about the ways that nutrition may help to prevent or delay progression of these typically age-associated chronic diseases. This may be an uphill battle because even within developed countries, these are pockets of nutritionally "at risk" individuals in the elderly population.

4. STUDIES OF NUTRITIONAL STATUS

A number of national studies of nutritional status that include elderly subjects have been conducted in the United States. The best known are the NHANES, including the 1971–75 NHANES, the 1976–80 NHANES II, and the 1988–94 NHANES III. NHANES IV (1999–2003) is currently in the field. Other studies include the 1977–78, 1987–88 Nationwide Food Consumption Survey (NFCS) and the 1994–96, 1998 Continuing Survey of Food Intake by Individuals (CSFII). In 1991, NHANES became an ongoing survey, and in 2002, was merged with CSFII. The Baltimore Longitudinal Study *(16)* includes a strong emphasis on nutrition as do a number of other studies (*see* Chapter 2). In Europe, the Survey on Nutrition and the Elderly, a Concerted Action (SENECA) study (*see* Chapter 5) has surveyed elderly subjects in a number of cities, and in Chapter 6, Dr. Bates reviews nutritional concerns of the elderly in the United Kingdom.

In virtually every case, these studies find that although body weight rarely decreases until the eighth decade, total calorie intake gradually and progressively decreases with age. Although protein intake also decreases, it usually remains in the adequate range because protein intake tends to be high in the diets of Western countries. However, the reduced total consumption of food also decreases the total intake of vitamins and minerals unless careful food choices are made to adjust for the need for increased nutrient density. The result is that some micronutrients are often found to be at risk for inadequacy. The exact nutrients found to be in marginal dietary supply differ depending on the population surveyed, but often include vitamin E, vitamin B_6, calcium, and zinc. A variety of other vitamins and minerals are often reported to be consumed in amounts lower than recommended.

There is limited reliable information available concerning the present and projected nutritional status of elderly persons living in developing countries. Only a few of these countries have conducted national health surveys that include nutrition measures, and some government surveys are not published. Most published studies have been conducted in small populations that are not necessarily representative of the entire elderly population. Rather than review these studies one by one, we have picked one country, the Peoples' Republic of China, which is in transition from developing to developed, and one that expects a dramatic graying of its population in the coming years.

5. AGING IN CHINA: THE INTERACTION OF CULTURE WITH NUTRITION AND HEALTH

Although aging is an experience common to all societies, with consequences that are similar in social, economic, and health terms, significant differences across cultures are evident. Cross-cultural perspectives can benefit studies on population aging because the association between age and functional impairment, morbidity, and mortality is influenced by variations in the cultural, socioeconomic, and physical environments. The differences in health and nutritional status may be owing more to environmental and lifestyle factors that occur over the entire life span of the individual than to variations in the underlying physiological mechanisms associated with morbid and functional changes of advanced age *(17)*. This section describes the wave of rapid population aging in China, the transition in dietary habits and nutrition in recent years led by rapid economic development, the potential interaction of nutrition, health, and aging, the impact of population aging on the public health and social system, and the response of the country to its rapid

Table 2
Life Expectancy at Birth and the Number of Aged in China and the United States

	China	United States
Total population (million)	1295.3	235.3
Life expectancy at birth (year)		
1949	39	68
1989	68.6	71.8
2000	71	73.4
Population 65+ (million and as % of total)		
1990	63 (5.5%)	28 (12%)
2000	88 (6.96%)	35.3 (12.5%)
2030	232 (15.7%)	69.8 (20.6%)
2050	334 (22.6%)	75.8 (21.7%)

Sources: refs. 21,57–61.

aging. The goal of this chapter is to provide comparative information on aging and related issues beyond a single society, providing insights into the potential impact of societal structure and nutritional interventions on possible scenarios for the future of public health in the elderly.

5.1. Overview of Demographic Changes in China

Population aging represents a major demographic shift, not only in the developed countries, but also in the developing countries worldwide. China, a country that consists of more than two-fifths of the world's total population, has been experiencing an extraordinarily rapid age structure transition since the 1980s. Over the last 50 yr, the Chinese government's efforts toward improving public health and nutrition and reducing infant mortality have led to an increase in life expectancy for all age groups and a prolonged life span. The average life expectancy of the Chinese population has almost doubled since the early 1950s, yet it still varies between rural and urban areas, as well as among areas with delayed economic development. In particular, the implementation of family planning, especially the one-child policy, has largely slowed the population growth; the crude birth rate declined from 33.43 per thousand in 1970 to 22.28 per thousand in 1982 (18). This number has continuously decreased to 15.23 per thousand by 1999, as reported in the 2000 China Population Survey (19). Thus, the annual growth rate of the Chinese population declined from 25.83 per thousand in the 1970s to 11.87 per thousand in the 1980s (20). By the end of the 1990s, it had reached 8.77 per thousand (19). As a consequence of the slowing fertility rate, and the steady increase in life expectancy, China has begun to experience the effects of a "rapid graying" of its population on health, social, and economic concerns. Table 2 presents information on total population numbers and the life expectancies of the Chinese population in the years 1949, 1989, and 2000, in comparison with those in the United States at the same time points. Although it took the United States 90 yr (1900–1990) to triple the proportion of people 65 yr and older from 4.1% to 12.8%, this same proportionate increase will occur in approx 40 yr in China (5.5%–15.8%), reaching a total of more than 232 million people aged 65 yr and older by 2030 (21). Although China is considered a youthful country by Western standards, with its percentage of older persons only moderate, a population of 1.3 billion of which 7% is aged 65 and over, makes the elderly Chinese population more than 90 million people! China has the largest absolute number of elderly people in the world—more than that of all European countries combined *(22)*. For obvious reasons, the need to understand the health status of the aged, the underlying risk factors to their health, and the role of prevention and intervention in their care is receiving growing interest and is a leading public health issue for the new millennium *(1)*.

The rapid aging in China has very important policy implications for provision of care for elderly people, particularly in view of China's family planning policy. Traditionally, care of the elderly is the task of family members, primarily their children within the traditional family structure. This traditional Chinese approach to family care for elderly members is successful, but may become difficult in the future because of smaller family sizes and the disruption of migration. If family care continues to be viewed as the best option, there will be huge burdens on the one or two children in any family *(22)* and families without any child living nearby.

5.2. Transitions in Dietary Patterns and Potential Interaction with Disease

5.2.1. CHANGES IN DIET

As a developing nation transitions to a more "developed" status, industrialization, urbanization, economic development, and market globalization create rapid changes in diet and lifestyle that impact the nutritional status of the population. The processes of modernization and economic transition eventually result in an improved standard of living. However, there may also be significant negative consequences. In China, it has been the shifting of the dietary patterns from the traditional to a more Westernized diet. Since the early 1980s, economic reform and the new policy for agriculture have accelerated agricultural and industrial development, resulting in widespread food adequacy and increased per capita income *(23)*. As a consequence, there has been a remarkable diet and nutrition transition in the Chinese population. During the last two decades, the dietary pattern in China has shifted from the traditional low-fat, low-protein, plant-dominated diet toward that typical of the "affluent" diet of Western countries. Figure 3 shows total energy, protein, and fat intake from 1978 to 1986. Intake escalates from the low levels in the early 1970s, increasing consistently to the middle 1980s. Per capita total grain consumption and per capita vegetable consumption increased between 1978 and 1984, then reached a plateau *(24)*. However, the intake of animal food has steadily increased over the same period. The national food disappearance data shows that from 1978 to 1987, the consumption of meat, eggs, and cooking oil (fat and plant oil) has increased 2.0-, 2.8-, and 2.9-fold, respectively *(25)*. The comparisons of 1982 *(26)* and 1992 China National Nutrition Surveys *(27)* demonstrated that the national average intake of all food groups showed substantial increase over the 10-yr period with the exception of grain foods, which decreased consumption by 12%. Figure 4 illustrates the remarkable increase in consumption of animal foods, including milk, eggs, fish, cooking oil, and meat, demonstrating the clear decline in grain, vegetable, and starchy tuber intake. Thus, the national average intake of dietary fat has reached 22% of the total energy intake in 1992 compared with only 18% in 1982. However, in major metropolitan cities, such as Beijing and Shanghai, the percent of energy from fat has well exceeded 30% of the total energy intake *(28)*. There is still a wide gap in animal food/fat intake between urban and rural areas, and across regions with different levels of economic development. The survey in

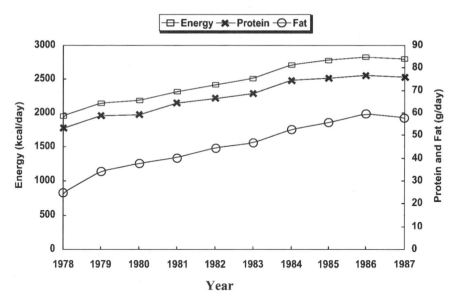

Fig. 3. Energy, protein and fat intake in Chinese adults from 1978 to 1987. *Source*: ref. *24*.

1992 *(27)* also shows that the national average fat intake contributed to 28% of total energy in urban populations and only 18% in rural peoples. Popkin et al. *(29)* found strong evidence from the China Health and Nutrition Survey that the dietary pattern of the Chinese population is rapidly changing to one similar to the typical high-fat, high-sugar diet of the West, also indicating that higher income levels, particularly in urban areas, are associated with consumption of a diet higher in fat and with the problem of obesity.

5.2.2. Changes in Disease Patterns

Diet-related diseases, including obesity, diabetes, cardiovascular disease, hypertension, stroke, and various forms of cancer, are increasingly significant causes of disability and premature death in both developing and newly developed countries *(23)*. Such diseases are replacing more traditional public health concerns, such as malnutrition and infectious disease, leading an impressive change in disease patterns in China. Although nutritional deficiency and infectious diseases have not been eradicated, these conditions are now largely confined to specific economic and age groups and particular regions of the country.

The overall mortality in China has declined from 20 per thousand in the early 1950s to 6.6 per thousand in the late 1990s *(30)*, largely by the reduction of infectious diseases. The health implication of these disease pattern changes is illustrated by the national health statistics of the ten leading disease causes of mortality in China in 1957 and 1999 (Table 3). Acute communicable diseases that caused approx 8% of deaths in 1957 have disappeared from the list of the top 10 leading causes of death in China. Cancer, cerebrovascular, and cardiovascular diseases now top the list of the leading causes of death. Figure 5 describes such disease pattern transitions in Shanghai, the largest city in China, from 1950 to 1985 *(31)*. Death from infectious diseases steadily declined during the 35-yr period, whereas cancer, cerebrovascular, and cardiovascular diseases increased at least four times over the same period.

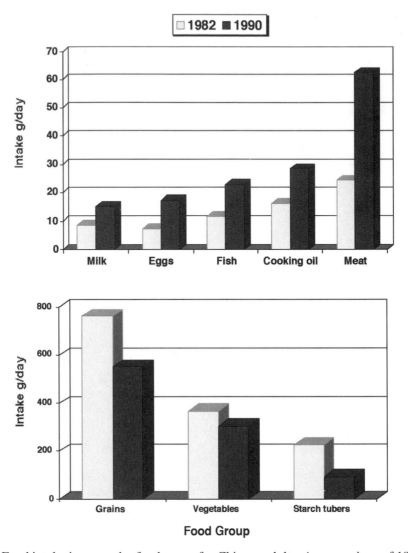

Fig. 4. Food intake in grams by food group for Chinese adults: A comparison of 1982 and 1992 data. *Source*: refs. *26* and *27*.

5.2.3. IMPLICATIONS OF DIET AND DISEASE PATTERN CHANGES

The previously noted changes in lifestyle and dietary patterns are likely to be major causes for the continuing increase in the prevalence of obesity, type 2 diabetes, and hypertension, which has been widely established in Western societies, and may be increasing in the developing countries *(32)*. A large-scale survey of diet and cancer carried out in rural China during the 1980s *(33)* has provided important evidence that the prevalence of chronic diseases is associated with high dietary fat consumption and other lifestyle factors. Figure 6 shows the prevalence of overweight and obesity in China in 1991, 1993, and 1997 (Zhai F, personal communication). Although the prevalences are still very low in China when compared with Western society and many other developing countries, they have increased by 34% and 22% for overweight and obesity, respectively.

Table 3
Ten Leading Causes of Mortality (per 100,000) and Percent of Total Death in China in 1957 and 1999

	1957[a]				1999[b]		
Rank	Disease	Mortality	% of death	Rank	Disease	Mortality	% of death
1	Respiratory system diseases	120.3	16.9	1	Cancer	140.5	23.9
2	Acute communicable diseases	56.6	7.9	2	Cerebrovascular diseases	127.2	21.6
3	Pulmonary tuberculosis	54.6	7.5	3	Cardiovascular diseases	98.9	16.8
4	Digestive system disease	52.1	7.3	4	Respiratory system diseases	81.7	13.9
5	Cardiovascular diseases	47.2	6.6	5	Trauma and intoxication	37	6.3
6	Cerebrovascular diseases	39	5.5	6	Digestive system disease	17.9	3
7	Cancer	36.9	5.2	7	Endocrinology diseases	16.9	2.8
8	Nervous system diseases	29.1	4.1	8	Urinary and reproductive system diseases	8.9	1.5
9	Trauma and intoxication	19	2.7	9	Psychosis	6.7	1.1
10	Other tuberculosis	14.1	2	10	Nervous system diseases	5.3	0.9

[a]Data from 13 cities of China, Ministry of Health, 1987.
[b]Data from 35 cities, Ministry of Health, 1999.

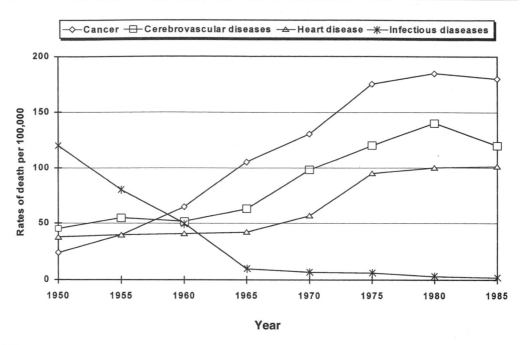

Fig. 5. Changes in rates of death due to infectious and selected chronic diseases in Shanghai, China, from 1950 to 1985. *Source*: ref. *31*.

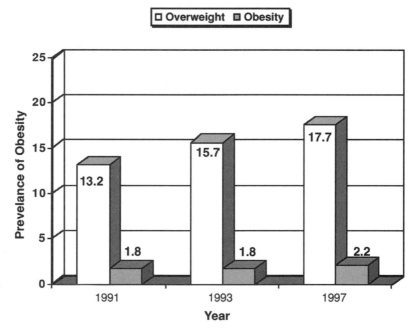

Fig. 6. Changes in the prevalence (percent) of overweight and obesity in Chinese adults between 1991 and 1997. *Source*: Zhai F, personal communication.

Studies have found that dietary energy and fat intakes are positively and significantly associated with the body mass index in the Chinese population. The changing dietary pattern and other behavior factors, together with a rising life expectancy of the population and increasing urbanization in the country, may have contributed to the emergence of dietary-related chronic diseases, such as obesity and coronary heart disease *(35–37)*. Meanwhile, stroke, which causes approx 22% of deaths each year *(64)*, and hypertension (the major risk factor of stroke in the Chinese population) are now important health problems *(38)*. The prevalence of hypertension has increased more than fourfold from 1959 to 1997, as shown in Fig. 7, nearly doubling during the 6-yr period between 1991 and 1997 *(see* Fig. 7). Considering the large population of the country, such an increase in the prevalence of hypertension could become a burden to public health, particularly in the older population. More recently, the prevalence of type 2 diabetes, that is closely associated with dietary behavior and prevalence of obesity and overweight, has spread nationwide, particularly in the urban population. Results from the 1995–1997 China National Diabetes Prevalence Study provides evidence that the overall prevalence of type 2 diabetes has reached 3.21% *(34)*. This represents a fivefold increase in approx 15 yr, compared with a threefold increase over 35 yr in the United States *(39)*. Thus, it appears that even a moderate change in lifestyle and dietary patterns can cause a significant shift in health outcomes in the Chinese population and have a tremendous influence on health and longevity.

5.3. Nutritional and Health Status of the Chinese Elderly

There have been limited studies focusing on general nutritional and health status in the elderly Chinese population. There are very few longitudinal studies on aging and national food consumption, and nutritional status data for the aging population is absent. The only available information is from isolated studies with small sample sizes. Therefore, it is difficult to predict the long-term effects of shifts in dietary patterns and nutrient intakes on the health of older Chinese individuals.

Studies of overall health generally indicate satisfactory status in urban elderly Chinese. In a cross-sectional study, Wang *(40)* examined the diet and health of 305 urban individuals aged 55–85 yr (Beijing area) and found that the majority reported that they were healthy and physically active. More than 80% of the study participants reported participating in daily physical exercise. A large percentage of elderly people lived with their adult children and were able to do some type of housework, such as daily vegetable shopping, cleaning, cooking, and taking care of their grandchildren. An epidemiological study *(41)* by the Center for Disease Control and Prevention (formally called the Chinese Academy of Preventive Medicine) (1986 to 1987) examined the general nutrition and health status of elderly in six different regions of the country and found that most older adults consumed adequate intakes of energy (mean = 2123 kcal/d) and protein (mean = 65 g/d), as well as other nutrients. Dietary intake of energy from fat was significantly higher for the urban elderly (30%) compared with their rural peers (17%).

The cross-sectional study conducted in Beijing *(40)* also found that average energy and protein intakes for elderly men and women were 2313 and 1820 Kcal/d and 74 and 59 g/d, respectively. Consistent with previous findings *(41)*, grain foods were a major source of energy and contributed to 48% of total energy intake. Also consistent with previous studies of the Chinese diet, calcium, and dairy food intake was very low in the population studied, particularly in individuals living in rural areas. The calcium intake in the Beijing elderly population was 476 and 420 mg/d in men and women, respectively. Dairy food contributed only 30% of total daily calcium intake, whereas vegetables,

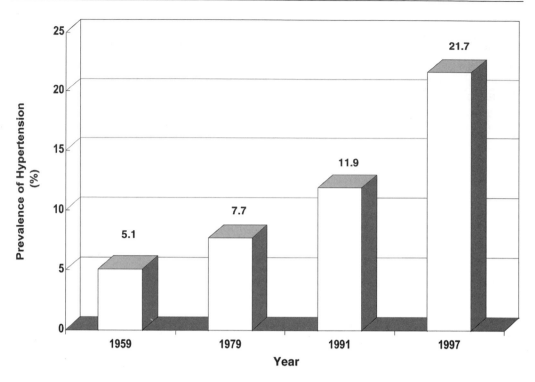

Fig. 7. Changes in the prevalence of hypertension (percent) in Chinese adults between 1959 and 1997. *Source*: ref. *34* and Chen J, personal communication.

grains, and legumes contributed 23%, 15%, and 11% of total daily calcium intake, respectively. Nuts and eggs contributed 4% and 3.5% of total daily calcium intake, respectively. Zhao et al. *(41)* reported very low intakes of dairy foods in rural areas, with an average intake of 0.4 g/d. Another study of two rural regions with 12,000 participants (Li M, personal communication) found that about 92% of people reported consuming no milk or milk products during the previous year.

In the study of Beijing elderly *(40)*, fat intakes averaged 87 and 72 g/d for men and women, respectively. The percent of energy from fat was 35% of the total energy intake, a higher proportion than the national average of 23%, reported from the 1992 National Nutrition Survey. Study *(27,28,40)* results showed that intakes of several nutrients indicated potential risk (mean intakes below national recommendations), including vitamin A and riboflavin; however, there was no sign of deficiency in the study population for either of these nutrients.

Age-related degenerative diseases, such as cardiovascular and cerebrovascular disease, hypertension, obesity, diabetes, osteoporosis, and cancer, are all potentially diet-affected, and this fact may be expected to influence health patterns in urban areas of China where diet pattern shifts are more predominant. He et al. *(42)* found from the 1992 Chinese National Nutrition Survey ($n = 15,684$, age range 45–80 yr) that the mean BMI of urban elderly was 24 kg/m^2, compared with 21.6 kg/m^2 for rural elderly individuals. The prevalence of overweight (BMI 25–29.9 kg/m^2) and obesity (BMI $\geq$ 30 kg/m^2) was 28.8% and 4.9% for urban elderly and 10.2% and 1.3% for rural elderly, respectively.

Being overweight and obese was much more prevalent in women than in men in both urban and rural areas.

In a longitudinal study, He et al. (43) followed 749 urban subjects over age 65 yr from 1979 to 1990 and found that the prevalence of cerebrovascular disease, cardiovascular disease, and diabetes had increased 8.5-, 2-, and 3.9-fold, respectively. Thus, the pattern of chronic diseases was already emerging in Chinese elderly living in urban areas. More recently, the in-depth analyses of the Chinese National Diabetes Survey data (Wang et al., personal communication) showed that among 8217 participants aged 55–74 from both urban and rural areas, approx 26% men and 31% women were overweight, and approx 2.9% men and 6.9% women were obese according to WHO criteria (44). In the same study, the prevalence of diabetes and hypertension was 8.9% and 45% in men and 11.6% and 48% in women, respectively. The prevalence of diabetes in the overall population has increased threefold since 1982, and this trend is unfortunately expected to continue. Figure 8 compares the prevalence of diabetes in the US population (45) and Chinese (Wang et al., personal communication) aged 50–74 yr and illustrates that the prevalence of diabetes in the older Chinese women is growing closer to that of American women. With the changes in dietary patterns and lifestyle, and the continued increase of obesity and overweight in young and middle-aged Chinese, the prevalence of diabetes in the older Chinese will be expected to be higher in the near future. In addition, it is likely that age-related health problems, such as arthritis, hearing loss, dental diseases, gastrointestinal conditions, liver disease, dementia, and various other disabilities, may affect or be affected by the need for dietary and other long-term care services in elderly Chinese individuals. Psychological changes, especially depression, may also affect nutritional status in this population, but these changes have not yet been adequately studied in this population.

5.3.1. TRADITIONAL POSITION OF AGING IN CHINA: A MODEL OF POSITIVE EFFECTS

The health- and nutrition-related issues of concern in China's aging population must be considered within the context of the traditional position held by the elderly in Chinese society. In contrast to Western culture, Chinese culture takes a positive view of the value and benefits of old age. Respect for older people is generally an ingrained, pervasive value in Chinese society. In the traditional Chinese family structure, age was a key determinant of authority, and the elderly held particularly high status (46). Although increases in education and modern technology in urban areas have given younger Chinese greater status, elderly citizens continue to command a high degree of respect. In addition, the traditional patterns of interdependence between generations have largely been maintained (47). The position of the aged is defined by the Constitution of 1982 (48): Children who have come of age have the duty to support and assist their parents. The newly updated Marriage Law of 2001 also incorporates this position again, going further to stipulate that when children fail to perform the duty of supporting their parents, parents who have lost the ability to work, or have difficulties providing for themselves, have the right to demand that their children pay for their support (49). Therefore, the Family Law is trying to make the tradition of family care obligatory. People who do not take care of their elderly parents might thus be criticized or even penalized (50).

In the present-day Chinese family, the elderly have very close relationships with their children; most elderly people are not living alone, especially in the rural areas. Many elderly Chinese depend on support from a spouse and/or their children for financial aid

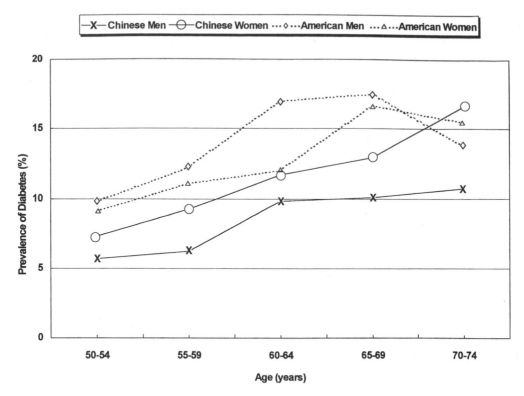

Fig. 8. The prevalence (percent) of diabetes in American and Chinese adults distributed by age. Data from American subjects is for 1989 and for Chinese subjects is 1995–1997. *Source*: refs. *34* and *45*.

and to support their emotional and physical needs *(21)*. Family or children are still principally responsible for their elderly parents.

Their position of being respected and their close family relations very likely has a positive impact on the health and nutritional status of Chinese elderly. Foreman et al. *(51)* studied the relationship between social support, which includes marriage, family size, proximity, relationship, as well as the use of health services in a group of Chinese elderly in Beijing, China. This study indicated that the "structural" social support of marriage and living with children demonstrates a variegated pattern: the availability of social support seems to increase physician use (by increasing access) while diminishing hospitalization. Feelings of self-worth and respect were thought to increase the access to and use of physician and hospital services. Functional social support, such as respect and harmony (filial piety), also contributed to better health care serve usage, whereas household harmony diminished the use of health services. Care from family members likely substituted for hospital care.

In the future, the Chinese tradition of family care for elderly will undoubtedly be altered. Changes of family context and structure that inevitably accompany fertility reduction and increasing life expectancy, along with the fact that more young people are choosing to seek a brighter future outside their impoverished hometowns, will contribute to this change. Thus, it is likely that more and more elderly people will be living alone without a child at home. Alternatively, when family care continues to be viewed as the "best option," there will be huge burdens on the single child in a family. This is an almost inevitable consequence of a strict population policy and increasing longevity in China. The country is facing the challenge of how to balance traditional family care of the elderly and the social support of modern society. The nutrition and health status of the Chinese elderly will also be challenged in the new millennium. Chinese health professionals and nutritionists are facing many questions about the influence of social/family support, and its changes on the health and nutritional status of the elderly. The shift toward a more Westernized treatment of the elderly is unlikely to be beneficial and may instead exacerbate the problems associated with population graying in China unless it can be averted or satisfactorily adapted to enhance rather than endanger health.

6. THE FUTURE OF SECONDARY PREVENTION AND NUTRITIONAL THERAPY

The example of China's shift toward an elderly population highlights the urgent need for preventing and managing the diseases of old age that may be modulated by nutrition. In developed, developing, and transitional countries, the proportion of the population that is elderly will grow to be a serious public health concern in the coming years. Therefore, the use of preventive health practices including nutrition to help "compress morbidity" *(52,53)* into the very last years of life becomes a critically important goal. This is because the extension of the length of life without a concomitant reduction of age-related diseases may only increase the number of years of illness and disability *(54)*. In addition to prolonging the number of years that health problems must be endured, this would greatly increase the burden and costs of medical care. The impact of this increased cost could have detrimental effects on health care availability for world citizens of all ages. Most would agree that unless the quality of life can be extended, there is little point in increasing its quantity.

Fortunately, disease and disability are not inevitable consequences of aging. Currently, available lifestyles interventions, particularly diet and exercise, have the potential to prevent or delay many chronic health problems. However, although primary preventive nutrition has rightfully received much attention, nutritional interventions that constitute secondary or tertiary prevention (*see* Table 1; *see also* Table 2 in Chapter 2) have not been adequately explored. These interventions have the potential to improve both quantity and quality of life and are the subject of this book. They are based on the premise that the second and third level preventive nutrition services, the reduction of risk factors, and the adoption of healthy lifestyle behaviors can all become major determinants of health in old age.

7. SUMMARY

Aging is accompanied by a variety of physiologic, psychologic, economic, and social changes that may compromise nutritional status. While not all changes occur in all individuals, many elderly people experience health and mobility changes with advancing age. Because the growth of elderly populations worldwide is certain to be accompanied by serious health concerns in the future, diet, exercise, and family/social support will also become increasingly important to help prolong good health to old age *(55)*. The idea that preventive nutrition (primary, secondary, and tertiary) has the potential to avert or delay diet-related disease is clearly illustrated when a population (e.g., urban dwellers in China) with relatively healthy eating patterns shifts to a less-healthy diet pattern, and subsequently experiences an increase in the occurrence of these chronic health problems. Hopefully, nutritionists and clinicians worldwide will learn from these examples and institute preventive practices that promote health and help delay disease until very near the end of life.

REFERENCES

1. Fried LP. Epidemiology of aging. Epi Rev 2000;22:95–106.
2. Wilmoth JR. Demography of longevity: past, present, and future trends. Exp Gerontol 2000;35: 1111–1129.
3. Sahyoun NR, Lentzner H, Hoyert D, Robinson KN. Trends in causes of death among the elderly. In: Trends in Health and Aging; no. 1. Hyattsville, MD.
4. Healthy Aging: Preventing Disease and Improving Quality of Life Among Older Americans, 2002. Dept. Health Human Services. www.cdc.gov/nccdphp. Accessed April 2, 2002.
5. Kramarow E, Lentzner H, Rooks R, Weeks T, Saydah S. Health and Aging Chartbook. Health, United States, 1999. National Center for Health Statistics, Hyattsville, MD, 1999.
6. Gutierrez-Robledo LM. Looking at the Future of Geriatric Care in Developing Countries. J Geron Med Sci 2002;57A:M162–M167.
7. Kinsella K, Velkoff VA. An Aging World: 2001. US Government Printing Office, U.S. Census Bureau, Washington DC, Ser P95/01–1, 2001.
8. Solomons NW. Demographic and nutritional trends among the elderly in developed and developing regions. Eur J Clin Nutr 2000;54:S2–S14.
9. Forrester T, Copper RS, Weatherall D. Emergence of Western diseases in the tropical world. The experience with chronic cardiovascular diseases. Br Med Bull 1998;54:463–473.
10. Popkin BM. Nutrition transition in low-income countries: an emerging crisis. Nutr Rev 1994;52: 285–298.
11. Guralnik JM, Balfour JL, Volpato S. The ratio of older women to men: historical perspectives and cross-national comparisons. Aging 2000;12:65–76.
12. Darnton-Hill I, Coyne ET. Feast and famine: socioeconomic disparities in global nutrition and health. Public Health Nutrition 1998;1:23–31.
13. Desai MM, Zhang P, Hennessy CH. Surveillance for Morbidity and Mortality Among Older Adults-United States, 1995–1996. MMWR CDC Surveillance Summaries. December 17, 1999/48(SS08), pp. 7–25.
14. Wilson PW, Kannel WB. Obesity, diabetes, and risk of cardiovascular disease in the elderly. Am J Geriatr Cardiol 2000;11:119–123.
15. Prevalence of Obesity Among U.S. Adults, by Characteristics. Behavioral Risk Factor Surveillance System (1991–2000); Self-reported data. National Center for Chronic Disease Prevention and Health Promotion. Accessed at www.cdc.gov/nccdphp/dnpa/obesity/trend/prevchar.h on April 3, 2002.
16. Elahi VK, Andres R, Tobin JD, Butler MG, Norris AH. A longitudinal study of nutritional intake in men. J Gerontol 1983;38:162–180.
17. Andrews CR. Cross-cultural studies: An important development in aging research. Am Geri Soc 1989;37:5–6.
18. Li Y, Rogers G. The graying of American and Chinese Societies: Young adults' attitudes toward the care of their elderly parents. Geri Nurs 1999;20:45–47.
19. Information Office of the State Council of the People's Republic of China. China's population and development in the 21st Century. Beijing Review, December, 2000.
20. Yu X. China's response to demographic pressures: the aging complex. DSE Publication 2000. Accessed at www.dse.de/ef/kop5/yu.htm on September 5, 2001.
21. Zeng, Y, George L. Extremely rapid ageing and the living arrangements of older persons: the case of China. Technical meeting on population aging and living arrangements of older persons: critical issues and policy responses. population: an English selection, 2001;13:95–116.
22. Bartlett H, Phillips D. Ageing and aged care in the People's Republic of China: national and local issues and perspectives. Health Place 1997;3:149–159.
23. Diet, nutrition, and the prevention of chronic diseases: Report of a WHO Study Group. WHO Tech Rep Ser #797, 1990.

24. Chen C. Dietary guideline for food and agricultural planning in China. In Proceedings of the international symposium on food, nutrition and social economic development. Publication House of Chinese Science and Technology. Beijing, China, 1991, pp. 40–48.

25. Chen J. Dietary changes and disease transition in China. Nutrition 1999;15:330–331.

26. Report on 1982 National Nutritional Survey. Institute of Nutrition and Food Hygiene, Chinese Academy of Preventive Medicine. Institute document, 1986.

27. Ge K. (ed.) The Dietary and Nutritional Status of Chinese Population: 1992 National Nutritional Survey. People's Medical Publishing House, Beijing, China, 1996.

28. Ge K. Dietary Pattern and physical development in China-based on the 1992 national nutrition survey. Asia Pacific J Clin Nutr 1995;4(Suppl 1):19–23.

29. Popkin BM, Ge K, Zhai F, Guo X, Ma H, Namvar Z. The nutrition transition in China: a cross-sectional analysis. Eur J Clin Nutr 1993;47:333–346.

30. Statistical Yearbook of China. State Statistic Bureau. China Statistical Publishing House, Beijing, China, 1997.

31. Zhao F, Guo J, Chen H. Studies on the relationship between dietary composition, health, and disease. Proceedings of International symposium on Food, Nutrition and social Economic Development. Publishing House of Science and Technology, Beijing, China, 1991.

32. Zimmet P. The pathogenesis and prevention of diabetes in adults. Diabetes Care 1995;18:1050–1064.

33. Chen J, Campbell TC, Li J, Peto R. Diet, Lifestyle and Mortality in China. A study of the Characteristics of 65 Chinese Rural Counties. Oxford University Press, Oxford, 1990.

34. Wang KA, Li T, Xiang H, et al. Study on the epidemiological characteristics of diabetes mellitus and IGT in China. Chinese J Epidemiol 1998;19:282–285.

35. Popkin BM, Paeratakul S, Ge K, Zhai F. Body weight patterns among the Chinese: results from the 1989 and 1991 China Health and Nutrition Surveys. American J Public Health 1995;85:690–1694.

36. USA PRC Collaborative Study of Cardiovascular and Cardiopulmonary Epidemiology. Data Preview. National Heart Lung and Blood Institute, Washington, DC, 1989, pp. 1–16.

37. Gu XY, Chen ML. Vital statistics, health services in Shangshai County. Am J Public Health 1982; 72:19–23.

38. People's Republic of China-United States Cardiovascular and Cardiopulmonary Epidemiology Research Group. An epidemiological study of cardiovascular and cardiopulmonary disease risk factors in four populations in the People's Republic of China. Circulation 1992;85:1083–1096.

39. Harris, MI. Summary. In Diabetes in America, 2nd edition. National Institute of Health, National Institute of Diabetes and Digestive and Kidney Diseases, (NIH Publication No. 95–1468), 1995.

40. Wang Y. A Cross-Sectional Study of Dietary Intake, Health and Socio-Demographic Characteristics of an Elderly Population in Beijing, China. Dissertation of Cornell University, 1994.

41. Zhao XH, Xue A, Wen Z, Bai J, Chen X. Dietary survey of the elderly in selected areas of China. Age Nutr 1992;3:78–81.

42. He Y, Lin H, Zhi F, Ge K. Analysis of Obesity and its Effective Factors in Elderly Chinese. Workshop on Obesity in China. International Life Sciences Institute Focal Point on China. Beijing, China, 2000.

43. He HD. A perspective study of health status of elderly in Beijing. In: (He, HD ed.) China Directory of Aging Research. Beijing Medical University Publishing House and Beijing Union Medical University Publishing House, Beijing, China, 1994.

44. World Health organization (WHO): Obesity: Preventing and Managing the Global Epidemic. Report of a WHO Consultation on Obesity, Geneva, June 3–5, 1997, #894.

45. Cowie CC, Eberhardt MS. Sociodemographic characteristics of persons with diabetes. In: Diabetes in America. 2nd ed.: National Institute of Diabetes and Digestive and Kidney Diseases, Bethesda, MD, (NIH publication no. 95–1468), 1995.

46. Yang CK (ed.). Chinese Communist Society: the Family and the Village. MIT Press, Cambridge, MA, 1965.

47. Davis-Friedmann D. Long Lives: Chinese Elderly and the Communist Revolution. Harvard University Press, Cambridge, MA, 1983.

48. Marriage Law: Chinese Government Document. National People's Congress, Beijing, China, 1983.

49. Marriage Law: Chinese Government Document. National People's Congress, Beijing, China, 2001.

50. Davis-Friedmann D. Long lives: Chinese Elderly and the Communist Revolution. Stanford University Press, Stanford, CA, 1991.

51. Foreman, SE, Earl JD, Lu L. Use of health services by Chinese elderly in Beijing. Medical Care 1998; 36:1265–1282.

52. Fries JF. Aging, natural death and the compression of morbidity. N Eng J Med 1980;313:407–428.
53. Fries JF. Compression of morbidity in the elderly. Vaccine 2000;18:1584–1589.
54. Vita AJ, Terry RB, Hubert HB, Fries JF. Aging, health risks, and cumulative disabiltiy. N Eng J Med 1998;338:1035–1041.
55. Rowe J, Kahn RL. Human aging: usual and successful. Science 1987;237:143–149.
56. Gist YJ, Gender VA. Aging: Demographic Dimensions. International Brief. US Department of Commerce, December, 1997.
57. Chen MZ, et al. (eds.). Public Health in the People's Republic of China, 1986. People's Medical Publishing House, Beijing, China, 1987.
58. Statistical Yearbook of China: State Statistic Bureau. China Statistical Information and Consultancy Service Center, Beijing, China, 1991.
59. Statistical Yearbook of China. State Statistic Bureau. China Statistical Information and Consultancy Service Center, Beijing, China, 2001.
60. National Center for Health Statistics. National Vital Statistics Report, vol. 47, no. 28, December 13, 1999.
61. US Department of Health and Human Services. Life expectancy hits new high in 2000; mortality declines for several leading causes of death. HHS News, October 10, 2001.

2

Creating a Continuum of Nutrition Services for the Older Population

Barbara E. Millen and C. Ariel Nason

1. INTRODUCTION

As a society, we are in the midst of a dramatic demographic transition that is resulting in the progressive aging of the US population. Today, 35 million or one in eight Americans is 65 yr of age or older. Average life expectancy at birth is currently 77 yr compared with 47 yr at the turn of the 20th century. Individuals who live to age 65 can expect to live an additional 18 yr and those who reach 85 yr of age will live 6–7 yr longer. By 2010, persons 65 yr and older will comprise 20% of the population; by 2030, the older population will double to 70 million *(1,2)*.

The primary contributors to the increasing population life expectancy are declining fertility rates, lower infant mortality rates, and the improved health status of children and middle-aged adults. Research indicates that recent improvements in the health status of older Americans are also contributing to the rising population life expectancy. Although health-related problems are more prevalent with advancing age, rates of disability appear to be declining. Based on an analysis of the 1984 and 1994 National Health Interview Survey Supplements on Aging, Liao et al. *(3)* concluded that the older US population in 1994 was healthier than its counterpart 10 yr earlier. In particular, older persons surveyed in 1994 were more likely to report being socially active and exercising regularly, whereas they were less likely to report functional limitations, confinement to bed or hospital admissions when compared to members of the earlier cohort.

The aging of the American population has important health policy implications. Despite improvements in health, older individuals who currently represent about 12% of the population account for about 30% of total health expenditures, which reached over $1.2 trillion in 1999 *(4)*. They also account for nearly 40% of all hospital admissions and almost half of total hospital days of care *(5)*. Additionally, in comparison to individuals under age 65, older persons have more than double the number of physician contacts *(5)*, utilize almost 72% of all home health care services, and represent the majority of nursing home admissions *(6,7)*.

Mechanisms to promote healthful aging and to reduce health care costs (including costly institutionalization and frequent episodic care) through the increased provision of

From: *Handbook of Clinical Nutrition and Aging*
Edited by: C. W. Bales and C. S. Ritchie © Humana Press Inc., Totowa, NJ

preventative services have been widely discussed *(8,9)*. Experts have recommended the increased delivery of a wide range of clinical preventive services, such as assessment of independent functioning in older adults, health promotion programs, blood pressure, cholesterol, and other diagnostic screening tests (clinical breast examinations, mammograms, Pap tests, fecal occult blood testing, proctosigmoidoscopy, and so on); routine reviews of cognitive, emotional, and behavioral functioning by primary care providers; immunizations for infectious diseases; and counseling services. Emphasis has been placed on improving access to and utilization of supportive social and primary health care services in the older population. Recent reports have also underscored the importance of medical nutrition therapies for older individuals, particularly nutritional assessment, counseling and education *(8,9)*.

Mounting scientific evidence indicates that nutritional status plays a prominent role in health, functional status and overall well-being in advancing age. Nutritional well-being and dietary factors are associated with the prevention of at least 4 of the 10 leading causes of death and disability in the older population, including coronary heart disease, certain cancers, cerebrovascular disease, and noninsulin-dependent diabetes mellitus *(9)*. Clinical research demonstrates that nutrition services play a key role in the treatment of and the reduction of costly complications associated with these causes of mortality, as well as other common conditions in the older population such as hypertension, dyslipidemia, obesity, and osteoporosis *(8,10–14)*. Nearly 90% of the older population has one or more conditions in which nutritional interventions may be beneficial *(8)*. Poor nutrition and lack of exercise are exceeded only by tobacco use as behavioral factors contributing to preventable death and disability *(15)*. Nutritional interventions and clinical nutrition therapies are therefore viewed by many experts as central components of the improved model for medical and health services management of the older population *(8)*.

In spite of recent evidence linking nutrition and health in advancing age, the major mechanism for financing health services for older Americans, in particular Medicare, has only limited coverage for nutrition services. This creates a significant barrier for many older Americans, preventing access to medical nutrition therapies within the traditional health care delivery system. As a result, this gap in service reimbursement contributes to high levels of nutritional risk in the older population *(8,16)*.

This chapter will demonstrate the importance of integrating appropriate nutrition services at all levels of the continuum of medical and related health care for the older population. It will also discuss current mechanisms to provide nutritional services to the older population and note the challenges that lie ahead to create a fully-integrated continuum of care.

2. HEALTH AND DEMOGRAPHIC TRENDS
IN THE OLDER POPULATION

The older population is most often defined as those individuals aged 65 yr and older, although this is an arbitrary assignment based more on social contexts than physiological changes associated with advancing age. Within this broad definition, some experts recommend further categorization based on specific age ranges. The "young-old" category includes persons 65–74 yr of age; the "old" category includes those who are 75–84 yr of age; and the "oldest-old" subgroup includes individuals who are aged 85 yr and older *(16)*. Within these age groups, there is considerable heterogeneity in terms of health status, gender, race and ethnicity, income, living situation, as well as health services access and utilization (1,5). While profiling the older population, these differences and their implications will be discussed.

The majority of older Americans perceive their health to be good to excellent (1), engage regularly in social activities, and are fully independent (3). In spite of relatively good health perceptions and functional independence, most older Americans have been diagnosed with at least one chronic disease and many experience multiple coexisting conditions (17,18). Heart disease, cancer, and cerebrovascular diseases account for 60% of deaths annually among those 65 yr of age and older (19).

In terms of functional capacity and well-being, about one-third of noninstitutionalized individuals aged 70 yr or older in a national survey in 1995 reported having difficulty performing at least 1 of 9 physical activities (e.g., walking a quarter of a mile without assistance, climbing a flight of stairs, or stooping, crouching or kneeling) and 20% reported being unable to perform at least one of them (18). In addition, 20% of this population reported having difficulty performing at least one activity of daily living (ADL) and 10% reported having difficulty performing at least one instrumental activity of daily living (IADL) without assistance. The conditions that contribute most to morbidity and loss of function in the older population are arthritis, visual impairments, hypertension, heart disease, cancer, diabetes, and stroke (18).

Certain segments of the older population are at greater risk for poor health status, most notably, those of advanced age, women, minorities, the poor, those living in particular geographic areas, and those who are institutionalized. The potential health policy ramifications are dramatic when considering the "oldest-old" age segment is expected to expand most rapidly in the next 50 yr (from 4 million today to 19 million in 2050); certain minority groups are also expected to increase, and women will continue to outnumber their male counterparts in all older age groups, continuing to do so even more disproportionately among individuals age 85 yr and older (1). This rapidly expanding population will place increasingly major demands on the US health care system.

In addition, the fact that older women and minorities are more likely to be poor and disabled than their younger, male, and nonminority counterparts will also have serious implications for our society and health care system. This is not only because projected growth rates are greatest for the oldest old, women, and minorities, but also because the adverse effects of income on health are strongest at the lowest levels of income (20,21).

As shown in Table 1, the costs associated with institutionalization are tremendous, including societal and personal financial expenditures, as well as personal loss of independence, compromised quality of life, and weakened community ties. Clearly, it is essential to improve mechanisms to prevent or delay costly institutionalization and reduce episodic health care and medical services for older persons. As noted by various expert groups, the successful integration of nutritional services and therapies along the continuum of health care is a critical component in these improvements (9,16,22).

3. NUTRITIONAL RISK IN THE OLDER POPULATION

Nutritional well-being is integrally related to the maintenance of health, independence, and quality of life of all older individuals (9,16,31–33). Proper nutrition plays a significant role in health promotion and the prevention of chronic diseases and their complications, improves the management of many acute and chronic conditions, delays

Table 1
Demographic Factors Related to Increased Risk of Disease, Disability, and Mortality in the Older Population

Advanced Age

- Compared with those 65–84 yr of age, persons 85 yr and older have poorer health status, report a higher number of disabilities and functional limitations, and utilize a greater number of health services *(1,3)*.

Gender

- Despite a greater life expectancy, compared to older men, older women have higher rates of certain diseases that are typically associated with disability and functional limitations, most prominently arthritis, osteoporosis, and hypertensive disease *(2,18)*.
- Consequently, women 70 yr of age and older are more likely than men to have functional limitations and to require assistance performing ADLs and IADLs *(18)*.

Race/Ethnicity

- Non-Hispanic black persons suffer from a substantially greater burden of chronic diseases such as hypertension, diabetes, and other cardiovascular diseases, with morbidity established at earlier ages than in non-Hispanic white Americans *(9,17)*.
- By age 75, more than half of the surviving non-Hispanic blacks suffer limitations compared with 40% of non-Hispanic whites *(23)*.
- One-third or more of non-Hispanic blacks who survive to age 75 experience extreme limitations (for example, limitations that affect their ability to go outside alone or to take care of his or her personal needs in the home such as bathing and dressing), compared with one-fifth to one-quarter of non-Hispanic whites of the same age *(23)*.
- Native American, Hispanic, and Asian/Pacific Islander elders appear to be at increased risk for obesity, diabetes, hypertension, and some cancers compared to white elders *(24)*.

Poverty

- Income plays a major role in improving overall health status by providing the opportunity to attain sufficient living conditions, improve access to quality medical and health services, and relieve acute and chronic stresses related to financial deprivation *(21,25)*.
- The inverse relationship between income or socioeconomic status and health is well-documented historically and is one of the strongest findings in social epidemiology *(20)*.
- The poverty rate remains higher for individuals aged 85 and older, older women, non-married older individuals and among elderly minority groups. In particular, the highest poverty rate in 1998 was for older African-American women living alone *(1)*.

Geographical Area of Residence

- Older Americans living in rural areas are often socially and geographically isolated, have limited access to health care, and reside in regions with highly variable health care services and resources *(26–28)*.
- Similarly, older Americans living in high poverty urban areas are also likely to be vulnerable.
  In fact, there is evidence that they experience higher levels of excess mortality than their rural counterparts and that, contrary to general national trends, their health status and excess mortality rates worsened between 1980 and 1990 and may still be climbing *(23,29)*.

Institutionalization

- Although the vast majority of older Americans live independently in noninstitutional community-based settings, about 4% of older Americans currently reside in skilled nursing facilities *(1)*, indicating a serious deterioration in health and a loss of independence for certain individuals.
- Fifty percent of nursing home residents in 1997 were 85 or older *(1)*.
- Women account for 75% of all nursing home residents *(1)*.
- Compared to nursing home residents in 1985, residents in 1997 were more functionally impaired and received more services *(7,30)*.
- In 1997, 53% of older nursing home residents had visual impairments, 46% had either partial or severe hearing impairments *(7)*, 79% required mobility assistance, while 65% were incontinent, 45% required eating assistance, and 36% required mobility and eatingassistance and were also incontinent *(1)*. About 22% of older nursing home residents received help with 1 or 2 ADLs, while 75% received helped with 3–5 ADLs *(7)*.
- Average annual health care expenditures for institutionalized older Americans in 1996 were $38,906, some $32,546 more than their counterparts living freely in the community *(1)*.

the onset of comorbidities; and reduces premature mortality *(8,31,34–36)*. Nutritional risk is used most often to describe either actual malnourishment, being at risk of malnourishment, or being at risk of health problems due to malnourishment. As Bales *(37)* points out, the multiple interpretations of "nutritional risk" can be confusing to other clinicians and detract from their understanding of the effects of poor nutrition on health outcomes. In our use of the term, we encompass the spectrum of both undernutrition and overnutrition. In this section, evidence of the prevalence of nutritional risk and of the relationship between nutrition and the common causes of morbidity and mortality in advancing age is presented.

An array of nutritional problems are present in the older population, ranging from undernutrition such as protein-energy malnutrition and nutrient deficiencies to nutrition-related chronic diseases and conditions of overnutrition like obesity *(38)*. Numerous risk factors for clinically-evident malnutrition have been identified, including inappropriate food intake, poverty, social isolation, dependence/disability, acute and chronic diseases or conditions, chronic medication use, and advanced age *(22)*. Elders appear to be at increased risk for malnutrition because they may experience many of these risk factors *(31)*. Of note, a recent study by Jensen et al. *(39)* demonstrates that community-living elders that were identified as having certain nutritional-related risk factors such as eating problems, weight loss, and consuming a therapeutic or "special" diet experienced an increased risk of hospitalization.

Although there have been few studies of nutritional status in nationally representative populations of older adults *(40)*, the findings of population-based research reveal serious problems with nutrition in the general older population, even if the population prevalence cannot be precisely determined. In addition, these studies document links between nutritional status, health status, and health care utilization. Studies of nutritional status examine a variety of indicators including dietary, clinical, anthropometric, and biochemical parameters or determine the presence of nutrition-related conditions and diseases *(34)*. There are comparatively more studies examining nutritional status using these indicators in acute and long-term care settings than in the community. This section mainly focuses on evidence of nutritional risk in community living elders.

3.1. Community-Based Studies of Compliance with Dietary Guidelines

This section presents findings from six studies of community-dwelling elders. Evidence of poor adherence to expert standards of dietary quality, including the Recommended Dietary Allowances (RDAs) and suggested intakes of macro and micronutrients in the older population, has been demonstrated using data derived from the third National Health and Nutrition Examination Survey (NHANES III), examinations of highly selected elder populations, and large population-based studies of community-living elders.

NHANES III analyses show mean dietary intakes of energy, protein, calcium, magnesium, zinc and vitamins A, E, and B_6 to be less than 100% of RDAs in older study participants *(41)*. These data further indicate lower than recommended fiber intakes in the older population *(42)*, but excess dietary intakes of total fat and saturated fat, particularly in older men *(43)*.

In a sample of 1154 community-living New England elders, 70 yr of age and older, Posner et al. *(35)* found that whereas group mean intake levels were adequate for all nutrients examined except for calcium, many individuals fell substantially below recommended intake levels for specific nutrients. These researchers defined "inadequate" or "low" intakes as those below 75% of the RDA. Some 58% of the sample had inadequate calcium intakes, and nearly 42% had low vitamin A intakes. In addition, 30% of the study population had low thiamin intakes and 20% were inadequate in vitamin C content. Protein intake was also found to be low in one-fifth of the study sample. Over one quarter (29%) of study participants had estimated intakes below the RDA standards for at least three nutrients.

In the same study, mean cholesterol intake (268 mg) was within the recommended range; however, mean carbohydrate intake (45.3% of total calories) was below recommended levels, and mean total and saturated fat (36.5% and 12.2% of total calories, respectively) were above recommended levels. Subjects 80 yr of age or older and those who smoked were more likely to have dietary lipid consumption levels that exceeded recommendations, yet they were also at risk for nutrient deficiencies. Subjects who lived with other persons in their home were also more likely to have high dietary lipid intakes, whereas those with lower levels of educational attainment and those with dental problems were more likely to have inadequate intakes of one or more of the nutrients examined (35).

A large study of 2886 semirural community-living elders in Maryland (44) reported a similarly high prevalence of dietary nutrient inadequacy. These researchers used the probability approach to estimate prevalence of inadequacy which takes into account the variability of nutrient requirements across individuals. The estimated prevalence of inadequacy was over 43% for zinc and over 30% for calcium and vitamins E and B-6. Inadequate nutrient intake was more prevalent among women than men, and among both black men and women when compared to their white counterparts. Prevalence estimates of nutrient intake inadequacy for black women were especially notable, with rates greater than 20% for protein, thiamin, riboflavin, niacin, and iron and greater than 40% for vitamins B_6 and E, and calcium and zinc (44).

In a study comparing the diets of 708 Hispanic and 490 non-Hispanic rural elders, Marshall et al. (45) found higher rates of inadequate consumption of dairy products, fruits, and vegetables in the Hispanic cohort. Nearly three-fourths of the entire sample reported consuming inadequate levels of dairy products, and 45% reported inadequate fruit intake. Similarly, Jensen et al. (46) found that over half of study subjects in a rural community reported consuming fewer daily servings of fruit, vegetables, milk, and grain products than the US Department of Agriculture's Food Guide Pyramid recommendations suggest.

A Boston study of 239 urban homebound elders demonstrated that all participants failed to meet recommended intake levels for one or more of the essential micronutrients or dietary components examined (47). The majority of study participants had dietary intakes that did not comply with recommended guidelines for 13 of the 24 dietary components examined. Moreover, greater than 80% failed to meet recommended standards for intake of fiber, vitamin D, folate, calcium, and magnesium. On the other hand, dietary levels of total and saturated fat and sodium were higher than recommended for over half of study participants.

These findings are of great concern. Low-nutrient intakes and dietary excesses place elders at risk for a myriad of health conditions and related complications. Poor nutrient intake in the form of inadequacy, imbalance, and/or excess may contribute to the development of clinical conditions, including serious nutrient deficiencies, weight loss, protein-energy malnutrition, and osteoporosis. Further, poor nutrition may contribute to the development of obesity, dyslipidemia, hypertension, diabetes, and heart disease as well as their health-related complications.

3.2. Community-Based Studies of Nutritional Status Using Anthropometric Indices

In addition to the high prevalence of poor dietary intake profiles, many elders are either under- or overweight by current standards as indicated by body mass index (BMI) and other anthropometric indices. In a study of free-living congregate and home-delivered meal program participants age 60 yr or older, Ponza et al. *(48)* found two-thirds of subjects had BMIs reflecting either underweight or overweight (below 22 kg/m^2 or above 27 kg/m^2, respectively). Of ambulatory participants, 19% were underweight and 42% were overweight. Of homebound participants, over one-third were underweight, and over one-third were overweight by these guidelines.

In an earlier publication, Posner et al. *(35)* reported that 16% of a study sample of non-institutionalized New England elders were underweight and 42% were overweight. Using identical BMI cutpoints to evaluate a large cohort of rural elders, Jensen et al. *(46)* identified few elders to be underweight (only 2.6%), but noted that over half were overweight. Millen et al. *(47)* found 5% of a sample of Boston homebound elders to have a BMI less than 18.5 kg/m^2, where nearly one-fourth had BMIs between 25 and 29.9 kg/m^2. These findings are consistent with national data from NHANES III, which indicate that 34% of older Americans (>60 yr) have BMIs greater than 27 kg/m^2 *(49)*.

Of further concern, the National Center for Health Statistics *(50)* estimates that 19% of men and 23% of women aged 65 yr or older are obese (BMI > 30 kg/m^2). Even higher prevalence rates of obesity in the older population were found in community-based studies of both rural and urban elders. Jensen et al. *(46)* reported that 33% of a rural cohort of elders were obese. Over one-third of the Boston homebound elders were obese, consistent with Jensen's observation in a rural cohort *(47)*.

Although it is assumed that being under and overweight are risk factors for increased morbidity and mortality, and obesity has been associated with increased morbidity and functional limitations *(51)*, few studies on the relationship between BMI and mortality in the elderly have been conducted. Moreover, the results of those found in the literature are inconsistent. Heiat et al. *(52)* reviewed 13 studies examining the relationship between BMI and mortality. These researchers concluded that the general association between BMI and mortality in the older population can be expressed as a U-shaped curve with a broad flat bottom and an increased slope, particularly at BMIs greater than 31 or 32. In many of the studies reviewed, weight loss and being underweight were stronger predictors of mortality in older adults than were higher BMIs. However, the low BMI level found to be associated with increased mortality differed across studies. Heiat and colleagues *(52)* did not present a conclusion as to a lower level cutpoint of BMI associated with high risk for mortality.

Weight and changes in weight have also been studied in relation to various health outcomes in older populations. For example, weight loss in white females *(53)* and white males *(54)* was found to be positively correlated with an increased risk for hip fracture. Langlois et al. *(53)* also found a decreased risk of hip fracture associated with a 10% weight gain in postmenopausal women. In a multivariate analysis of nutritional risk factors, functional status, and demographic variables, as predictors of health care costs in a large sample of enrollees in a single Medicare + Choice plan, a 10-pound weight loss in a 6-mo period and BMI > 27 were significant predictors of adverse outcomes, although BMI < 22 was not *(46)*. French et al. *(55)*, distinguished between involuntary and voluntary weight loss, finding involuntary weight loss to be a risk factor for increased morbidity and mortality in older women in the Iowa Women's Health Study, but not finding an increased risk with voluntary weight loss.

According to conventional wisdom and many available studies, deviations from ideal weight are associated with health-related problems. However, while there is strong evidence that obesity and being extremely underweight are related to increased mortality rates, the evidence of an effect of less extreme variation from recommended BMI standards is weaker. Furthermore, while being under- and overweight as measured by BMI have been associated with increased morbidity in the elderly, the causal mechanisms for the observed outcomes are not clear. For example, the prevalence of elevated low-density lipoprotein (LDL) levels, diabetes and hypertension in the older population, individually and in combination, increase with increasing BMI. The prevalence of having each condition or all three is greater in people with a BMI greater than 30. However, an estimated 81% of the older population with a BMI less than 25 have at least one of these nutrition-related cardiovascular conditions *(17)*. As noted previously, comparisons across research studies is problematic because the definitions of under- or overweight according to BMI vary across studies. Despite the limitations of existing research, the uncertainty about the implications of under- and overweight or the unproven efficacy of interventions for weight management in older populations, studies are consistent in reporting that many older Americans deviate from the currently recommended weight for height guidelines, particularly in the direction of being overweight.

3.3. Laboratory Evidence of Nutritional Risk

In addition to evidence of poor dietary intake and the high prevalence of unhealthy weights, analyses of various biochemical parameters also indicate poor nutritional status in the older population. Serum albumin level is the most commonly used parameter, although levels decrease in response to acute phase reactions and therefore nutritional interpretation of hypoalbuminemia remains in question. Researchers have found that among hospitalized elders *(56)* and geriatric rehabilitation unit patients *(57,58)*, hypoalbuminemia (defined as serum albumin less than 3.5 g/dL) is quite common. In community-living elders, this condition appears to be less prevalent. Analyses of data from the Established Populations for Epidemiologic Studies of the Elderly (EPESE), a large prospective study of free-living elders aged 71 yr and older, indicate only 3% of this cohort exhibit albumin levels less than 3.5 g/dL *(59)*. However, low serum albumin levels appear more commonly among the oldest-old, affecting 10% of subjects aged 90 yr and older in this cohort *(60)*.

Two separate studies targeting urban homebound elders found higher rates of hypoalbuminemia than population-based studies of the general older population such as EPESE. In a study in Alabama, Ritchie et al. *(61)* found low serum albumin levels (<3.5 g/dL) in 19% of their study sample. In a Boston study, Millen et al. *(47)* found that 18% of subjects had fasting serum albumin levels that were low to borderline low (≤3.8 g/dL). In the same cohort, 32% of subjects had low hemoglobin concentrations (≤11.9 g/dL), and nearly one-third had low absolute lymphocyte concentrations (≤1.5 K/µL), suggesting a fair number of individuals in this cohort of elders had evidence of compromised nutritional status *(47)*.

Overall, a small percentage (6%) of subjects in the Boston study had total cholesterol levels indicative of hypocholesterolemia (<160 mg/dL). However, 37% had high total cholesterol levels (≥240 mg/dL), and 12% of these urban homebound elders had high triglyceride concentrations (>200 mg/dL) *(47)*. In addition, nearly a third of the women in this sample had high levels of LDL cholesterol (≥160 mg/dL). These data are largely consistent with prevalence rates of dyslipidemia reported among a national sample of elders surveyed in NHANES III *(8)*.

Abnormal values of these biochemical parameters have been associated with many adverse clinical outcomes. For example, many researchers have found low and border-line-low serum albumin levels to be associated with adverse clinical outcomes in hospitalized elders including complications, prolonged hospital stays, greater likelihood of hospital readmission, and both in-hospital and postdischarge mortality *(57,58,62–66)*. The predictive value of hypoalbuminemia on mortality in community-living elders has also been shown *(59,67,68)*. The relationship of dyslipidemia or specific nutrient deficiencies to poor health is well documented.

Studies of nutritional status and hospital length of stay, discharge disposition, and health outcomes provide strong evidence of the complex interrelationship between nutrition and health and further underscore the importance of maintaining proper nutritional status for all elders. For example, in a prospective study of 173 hospitalized older patients, using BMI less than 75% of ideal body weight, low serum albumin, or an unintentional weight loss of 10% or more in the month preceding admission as criteria, Chima et al. *(69)* classified patients either at-risk or not-at-risk for malnutrition. Some 32% were classified as "at-risk." Compared to "not at-risk patients," at-risk patients had significantly longer lengths of stay, had higher hospitalization costs, were less likely to be discharged to home, and were more likely to require home health care services. In a study of 369 patients aged 70 yr and older admitted to a tertiary care hospital's general medical service, Covinsky et al. *(70)* reported 24% to be moderately malnourished and 16% to be severely malnourished as indicated by assessments, including weight loss and physical signs of malnutrition. Severely malnourished patients had higher 90-d and 1 yr mortality rates compared to moderately-malnourished and well-nourished patients. Even when controlling for acute illness severity, comorbidity, and functional status on admission, these researchers found well-nourished hospitalized patients had lower mortality rates, reduced functional recovery time, including less dependence in performing ADLs and lower rates of nursing home use following hospital discharge *(70)*. The next section provides an overview of expert panel reports on the nutritional status of the older population, which provide the basis for recommendations to create a continuum of nutritional services for promoting health and well-being among the elderly.

4. EXPERT RECOMMENDATIONS FOR NUTRITION SERVICES

Over the last few decades, mounting concern regarding the nutritional status of older Americans as well as the growing prevalence of nutrition-related chronic conditions and their associated impact on physical disability prompted the development of key public policy statements and recommendations to promote the health of the elderly population. The components of these initiatives that focus on nutrition-related health improvements and the importance of providing a continuum of appropriate nutrition services for the older population are reviewed here. Table 2 summarizes the elements of the nutrition services continuum, the focus of preventive intervention and treatment, and the settings in which nutrition services are likely to be provided. These details are presented across the four stages of prevention, including primordial, primary, secondary, and tertiary prevention intervention.

In 1979, the first Surgeon General's Report, "Healthy People: Health Promotion and Disease Prevention" was issued setting forth five national health goals. One specific goal was "to improve the health and quality of life for older adults and, by 1990, to reduce the average annual number of days of restricted activity due to acute and chronic conditions..." (71). This report recognized that many older Americans suffer from a variety of conditions that are often linked to other debilitating conditions and some individuals, such as those with diabetes, heart disease, or hypertension, may require therapeutic diets. Therefore, it was emphasized that older Americans require a range of integrated services, including dietary guidance, social assistance, and dental care in addition to routine medical care.

Nearly a decade later, the Surgeon General issued a report on nutrition and health (32), which specifically recognized the need for coordinated health and related services to maintain and improve the health and well-being of older Americans. This report went a step further than the previous one by not only acknowledging the importance of nutrition in health, but also by recommending strategies to improve older Americans' health, quality of life, and independence, with specific emphasis on the importance of nutritional services. Recommendations included implementing appropriate nutrition services for the entire older population, including homebound elders, within all health care settings across the continuum of health care services. Particular emphasis was placed on the need for routine nutritional assessment, counseling, education, therapeutic intervention, and referral to community services and food assistance programs as necessary, as well as continuous monitoring of nutritional well-being. In addition, the report advised that individualized nutrition counseling should be provided by credentialed nutrition professionals for older individuals with nutrition-related chronic diseases. Additionally, improved clinical nutrition education was advocated for all health professionals, emphasizing the inclusion of trained nutrition professionals in the provision of dietary counseling and nutrition services to all patient populations.

"Healthy People 2000", released in 1990, identified nutrition as one of 22 priority areas set forth to improve the nation's health, thus building on the earlier goals of the Surgeon General's Healthy People initiative. Primary attention was placed on dietary improvements to reduce total and saturated fat intake, lower sodium consumption and increase fruit, vegetable, and grain product consumption. Other objectives focused on decreasing the population prevalence of overweight, improving access for older Americans to food services, such as home-delivered meals and congregate dining, and increasing nutrition education, assessment, counseling, and referrals (36).

In response to the consistent recommendations to increase nutrition screening in older Americans set forth by the Surgeon General's report, the "Surgeon General's Workshop: Health Promotion and Aging" (72) and "Healthy People 2000" (36), the Nutrition Screening Initiative (NSI) was formed over a decade ago by a consortium of over 25 professional medical, health, and aging organizations in the United States *(73)*. The alliance is led by the American Academy of Family Physicians, the American Dietetic Association and the National Council on the Aging Inc. The NSI is devoted to improving older American's health through the promotion of routine nutritional screening and establishment of higher quality nutritional care within all aspects of our health care system. Toward this end, NSI developed several widely distributed screening tools designed to increase awareness of nutritional risk. NSI tools establish a nutritional risk score that serves to identify older persons who may be at risk and to guide these individuals to further nutritional assessment and into appropriate interventions if warranted.

In addition to the development of screening tools, the NSI developed a multitude of manuals, reports, and guides directed at older individuals, their families and physicians, and other health professionals caring for elders. These materials establish strategies to incorporate nutrition screening, interventions, and treatments into medical practice, Medicare health plans, managed care organizations, and home health care settings *(34,73–75)*. Recently, the NSI developed two new guides, "Nutrition Care Alerts for Nursing Facilities" and "Nutrition Care Alerts for Home Care," designed to assist health care providers and primary caregivers, respectively, in identifying warning signs of common nutrition-related conditions and actions recommended to address various problems, such as unintended weight loss, dehydration, pressure ulcers, and tube feeding complications *(76)*. A complete listing of NSI materials and additional information on the NSI is available online at the American Academy of Family Physicians' website (www.aafp.org/nsi).

In 1992, the Institute of Medicine *(77)* also recognized the importance of nutrition in the maintenance of health, quality of life and physical independence in older persons. Their report further acknowledged the complex interaction between disease and nutritional status, including the effects of certain disease states on nutritional status and the potential effects of diet and nutritional status on a variety of risk factors for disability among elders. Major recommendations included the need for the development of specific guidelines for nutritional screening and monitoring of asymptomatic older persons, the promotion of nonpharmacological treatments for elders who are physically inactive, and for elders with atherosclerosis, hypertension, diabetes, and osteoporosis. Participation in meal assistance programs such as home delivered meals and congregate meal programs for community-living elders was also encouraged in an effort to maintain independent functioning. The Institute of Medicine also recommended that federally-funded hospitals, nursing homes, and extended care facilities be required to implement functional assessments and nutritional care plans designed to maintain functional independence and nutritional status while decreasing polypharmacy and increasing physical activity *(77)*.

"Healthy People 2010" *(9)*, issued in 2000 by the US Department of Health and Human Services, is the most recent national health policy statement. This initiative provides new goals and guidelines to improve the nation's health and expands on goals and objectives set forth in earlier "Healthy People" initiatives but not yet achieved. Two general goals identified for the nation to achieve by 2010 are to increase the quality and years of healthy life and to eliminate health disparities. Nutrition and being overweight is one of 28 focus areas and the major goal in this category is to promote health and reduce chronic disease associated with diet and excess body weight. Several strategic actions were recognized as being necessary to achieve the objectives put forth in this focus area. These included

Table 2
The Continuum of Preventive Nutrition Services and Medical Nutrition Therapies for Older Individuals

Stages of prevention and treatment	Community and institutional care settings	Preventive intervention and treatment focus	Preventive nutrition services and medical nutrition therapy
Primordial prevention: policies and interventions designed to prevent health problems in relatively healthy populations.	State and area agencies on aging, senior centers, elderly nutrition programs, community health centers.	Population screening and monitoring. Population health promotion. Health communications campaigns.	Nutritional screening and monitoring. Nutrition-related health education. Nutrition-related health communications. Food stamps and congregate meals programs.
Primary prevention: programs and interventions designed to promote health before the manifestation of a health problem at the individual level.	Community social and health centers, ambulatory care centers, primary care provider practices, health maintenance organizations.	Individual health screening and risk assessment, immunization, blood pressure monitoring, smoking cessation, weight reduction, exercise programs, chronic disease risk reduction programs (obesity, diabetes, coronary heart disease, hypertension, stroke, cancer, etc.).	Nutritional assessment and monitoring at the individual, group or family/household levels. Nutrition education and counseling. Referral to food stamps and congregate meal programs.
Secondary prevention: interventions aims at early detection and treatment of diseases and disorders to reduce their severity or halt their progression and restore functioning of the individual.	Community social and health centers, primary care provider practices, ambulatory care centers, health maintenance centers, hospital day centers and programs.	Chronic disease risk management programs: obesity, diabetes, coronary heart disease, hypertension, cancer, chronic obstructive pulmonary disease, congestive heart failure, dementia, failure to thrive, osteoporosis, pneumonia, arthritis, etc.	Nutritional assessment and monitoring. Individual, group or family education and counseling. Congregate meal programs. Food stamps. Home-delivered meal services. Medical nutrition therapies: services related to treatment of established diseases and conditions. Nutrition services complementary to ongoing ambulatory or institutional care.
Tertiary prevention: interventions to reduce or limit disability in established disorders among individuals. Palliative and terminal care.	Adult day care centers, community social and health centers, hospices.	Rehabilitation related to conditions noted in secondary prevention); post-trauma counseling.	Medical nutrition therapies: services related to treatment of established diseases and conditions. Nutrition services complementary to ambulatory, institutional, supervised community or home care.

improving access for all population groups to healthy foods, nutrition information, education, counseling and related services across a wide range of settings. The role of primary care physicians as providers of preventive services, including nutrition screening and assessment and referrals to qualified nutrition professionals as necessary, was also emphasized. Further attention focused on the merits and effectiveness of nutrition services provided by registered dietitians and the key role nutrition services play in improved health outcomes for many diseases and conditions through nutrition screening, assessment, and primary and secondary prevention counseling (9).

Also in 2000, the Institute of Medicine released its report (8) to Congress: "The Role of Nutrition in Maintaining Health in the Nation's Elderly." This congressionally mandated report is the result of the Committee on Nutrition Services for Medicare Beneficiaries' comprehensive evaluation of the current coverage of nutrition services for Medicare beneficiaries across the continuum of health-related care. The Institute of Medicine's report presents the committee's findings and a set of compelling recommendations to improve coverage of nutrition services in the older population. The report delineates nutrition services into two "tiers." The first tier, basic nutrition education and advice, is recommended for continued delivery as currently provided accompanying other health services and routine medical care. They considered this service to be "...generally brief, informal, and typically not the focal reason for the health care encounter. More often than not, it's aim is to promote general health and/or the primary prevention of chronic diseases or conditions" (8). The committee determined that this tier of services can be effectively provided by most health professionals including physicians, nurses, and pharmacists under the current reimbursement mechanisms.

The second tier, nutrition therapy, encompasses

"...individualized assessment of nutritional status; evaluation of nutritional needs; intervention, which ranges from counseling on diet prescriptions to the provision of enteral (tube feeding) and parenteral (intravenous feeding) nutrition; and follow-up care as appropriate. Nutrition therapy generally addresses nutrition interventions specific to the management or treatment of certain existing conditions and is usually individualized to meet the food habits of the patient" (8).

The committee concluded that currently only registered dietitians are sufficiently educated and trained to provide this tier of nutrition services. Although they found sufficient evidence to recommend the provision of nutrition therapy by registered dietitians as an integral component of the treatment and management of only certain conditions (dyslipidemia, hypertension, heart failure, diabetes, and kidney failure), the committee made an even broader recommendation, concluding that nutrition therapy provided by a registered dietitian be a reimbursable benefit for Medicare beneficiaries for any condition contingent on a physician's referral.

The committee also recommended that the reimbursement systems and regulations currently in place for nutrition services be carefully examined in acute, ambulatory, and home care, skilled nursing facilities, and long-term care settings to ensure adequacy of services and improved continuity of nutrition care throughout the continuum of health and medical care. In order to address the major gap in coverage of nutrition services, including reimbursement for enteral and parenteral nutrition support, outside of acute care settings and skilled nursing facilities, they also called for major improvements of Medicare coverage and availability of comprehensive nutrition services provided and managed by nutrition professionals in ambulatory and home-health care settings. Additional emphasis was placed on the need for adequate staffing of registered dietitians in skilled nursing and long-term care facilities to educate other staff members about preventing, identifying, and treating nutrition problems, to oversee nutrition support and to improve nutritional care and feeding practices *(8)*.

Like the aforementioned organizations, the American Dietetic Association (ADA) also recognizes elders as a high-risk group for malnutrition. In 2000, the ADA released its position *(16)* on "Nutrition, aging and the continuum of care." In this statement, the ADA encouraged an array of strategies dietetic professionals should employ to provide continuity of food and nutrition services across all settings in the continuum of care. The ADA called upon dietetic professionals to use their expertise to develop effective methods to augment the range of food and nutrition services available to elders. Recommended strategies for dietetic professionals included collaborating with other health care professionals and professionally assisting caregivers in clinical and community settings, establishing professional relationships with various agencies at the community, state, and federal levels to develop new programs or enrich existing programs, and advocating for legislative changes. Emphasis was also placed on the need for creating and integrating curriculum on nutrition in aging for dietetic students and continuing education for dietitians and other health care professionals focused on nutrition support and education, as well as nutrition education programs targeted and delivered to older adults *(16)*.

In summary, numerous national health policy reports and professional organizations' statements in the last two decades have emphasized the importance of promoting health and preventing disease and the significance of maintaining nutritional well-being as a strategy towards achieving this end. As well, the older population is consistently identified as a cohort at particular risk for nutritional problems that requires a range of integrated services spanning both health and social service realms. These reports have also stressed the need for integrated nutrition services, particularly screening, education, assessment and intervention throughout the continuum of care as well as increased access to meal assistance programs. Many of these reports recognized that several strategies are required to address these needs, including increasing education and awareness of nutritional problems in older adults among health care professionals and caregivers, recognizing the critical role of nutrition professionals in providing nutrition services and coordinating care, and improving coverage of nutrition services by third-party payment systems. In spite of the growing recognition of the importance of nutrition services in the health and medical care of the older population, major disparities and limitations exist in the provision and availability of nutrition services for elders. The next section presents the current mechanisms for the delivery of nutrition services throughout the continuum of care.

5. CURRENT MECHANISMS FOR THE DELIVERY OF NUTRITION SERVICES TO OLDER AMERICANS

The provision of nutrition services to the older population is currently complicated by a wide range of funding streams. No single agency of coverage provides the full range of services needed. In addition, many coverage limitations exist throughout the continuum of care, based on clinical or financial eligibility requirements. Nutrition services currently fall between medical and social service systems and few mechanisms exist for coordinating care across these systems. The principal mechanism for the provision of nutrition services to older Americans within the traditional health care system is through the third-party payment system, particularly the Medicare and Medicaid programs. These programs set guidelines for the reimbursement of medical and health-related services for beneficiaries in acute care settings, ambulatory settings, post-acute, long-term care, and community and home health programs. The availability of nutrition services in some institutional settings may also be regulated by specific requirements of the Joint Commission on Accreditation of Healthcare Organizations (JCAHO) if the institution seeks JCAHO accreditation. Outside the traditional health care system, additional federal programs exist to provide nutrition services and food assistance to elders, in particular the Elder Nutrition Program and the Food Stamp Program. The following section discusses the major mechanisms within each program for the provision of nutrition services across the continuum of care.

5.1. The Medicare Program

Within the traditional health care system, Medicare is the major provider of health care coverage for older Americans. This public health insurance program currently provides health insurance for over 95% of Americans aged 65 or older (78). In 1998, approx 33.8 million older individuals were enrolled in Medicare and total program disbursement for this population reached $118.2 billion (79). Since the program's inception in 1965, under Title XVIII of the Social Security Act, Medicare's primary focus has been to defray costs associated with hospital and physician services. Traditionally, Medicare has excluded coverage of preventive services. Medical nutrition therapy services have not been covered specifically or even considered under Medicare as a distinct method of therapeutic intervention. Throughout the continuum of care, Medicare historically has not provided separate payment for nutrition services; yet nutrition services may be provided in various health care settings and included as a component of a facility's provided health services (80). In acute care settings, professional nutrition services, including parenteral nutrition support, are covered by Medicare as part of a bundled payment for all services rendered per patient. The reimbursement rate for all patient services is a fixed cost based upon the specific diagnostic related group (DRG) designation. This reimbursement framework provides an incentive for hospitals to limit services and lengths of hospitalizations, potentially limiting utilization of nutrition services.

Under Medicare's conditions of participation, in order to receive Medicare reimbursement, hospitals must employ a qualified dietitian on a full-time, part-time or consultant basis. The dietitian acts as a liaison with medical staff and provides guidance on dietetic policies impacting patient treatment. General requirements of the qualified dietitian also include supervising all aspects of nutritional care, such as assessing nutritional status and adequacy of nutritional regimen; planning, in writing, therapeutic diets when prescribed by the practitioner responsible for the patient's care; and providing patient and family dietary instruction, and counseling. The dietitian must also document periodic monitoring of the patient's nutritional status, adequacy of the nutritional regimen, and patient response to prescribed therapeutic diets in the patient's medical record. Medicare regulations require that patients' nutritional needs must be met in accordance with the Recommended Dietary Allowances (RDAs) or Dietary Reference Intakes (DRIs) of the Food and Nutrition Board of the National Academy of Science, and National Research Council. Dietary therapy must also adhere to orders of the practitioner responsible for the patients' care. Menus must be approved by the dietitian and a current therapeutic diet manual (approved by the dietitian) must be available to all medical, nursing, and food service personnel *(81,82)*. Beyond these Medicare requirements, additional standards for the provision of expanded nutrition services provided by dietitians are required for hospitals electing to participate in JCAHO accreditation procedures *(83)*.

As in hospital settings, skilled nursing facilities (SNFs) and nursing homes are reimbursed by Medicare through a prospective payment system and nutrition services are included within a bundled per diem rate. Federal mandates for the employment of qualified dietitians are similar to hospital conditions for participation, and nutrition assessment, monitoring and treatment of identified problems is required through a mandatory comprehensive assessment instrument. Medicare also specifies requirements for food services in SNFs and nursing homes related to menu planning, nutritional adequacy, the provision of therapeutic diets, frequency of meals, and sanitary conditions *(81,84)*.

Home health-care service agencies must have nutrition expertise available as a provision of Medicare certification. These services are paid by Medicare as part of associated administrative costs. However, separate in-home visits by dietitians are excluded from Medicare reimbursement *(84)*. Under the prosthetic device benefit, limited coverage for outpatient and home enteral and parenteral nutrition support does exist. Medicare allows reimbursement for nutrition support only for beneficiaries who are unable to meet nutritional requirements via an oral diet for greater than 90 d. In hospice settings, dietary counseling is provided when required, although nutrition professionals are not required providers and are not mandated to be full time employees *(85)*. Payment for dietary counseling is included in the per diem rate.

In ambulatory settings, nutrition services may be covered if deemed "medically necessary" and provided "incident" to a physician's services. Therefore, registered dietitians practicing in collaboration with physicians may be reimbursed for initial and follow up patient treatment contingent on a physician's referral. In hospitals' outpatient department, the provider of these nutrition services meeting the specified criteria must by an employee of the hospital. In a private physician practice, such services must be rendered by an employee of the physician. Traditionally, independently practicing registered dietitians providing nutrition services have not been eligible for Medicare reimbursement *(38)*.

With the passage of the Balanced Budget Act of 1997, several noteworthy changes in the Medicare program arose which pertain to the expanded provision of preventive services including nutrition services. Some of these changes include the creation of the Medicare + Choice program, the development of an outpatient diabetes self-management training benefit, and congressional calls for investigations of expanded coverage for more preventive services. The Institute of Medicine's investigation, noted previously *(8)*, arose from this mandate. In response to this report, Medicare benefits will be extended to cover Medical Nutrition Therapy (MNT) for beneficiaries with diabetes and renal disease.

The Medicare + Choice program was created to expand coverage options for all Medicare beneficiaries. Medicare + Choice allows beneficiaries to elect to enroll in either a Medicare managed care health plan, such as a health maintenance organization (HMO), or a private fee-for-service plan offered through private insurance companies who contract with Medicare. This choice replaces the original federally administered Medicare plan. In addition to traditional Medicare benefits, these plans may offer more preventive services, including nutrition services such as MNT at their discretion *(86)*. Therefore, benefit packages vary across plans and by state. In 2001, approx 5.6 million Medicare beneficiaries were enrolled in Medicare HMOs *(87)*. Despite the potential advantages of these coverage options, the Medicare + Choice market is incomplete or unstable and may leave older persons with limited or no opportunities to participate in this program. For example, there may be no service providers or only very limited providers opting for Medicare + Choice participation in certain geographic locations. As well, providers may have dropped their participation in Medicare + Choice in other areas *(88)*.

A major stride in Medicare coverage expansion is the recent inclusion of an outpatient diabetes self-management training program for patients diagnosed with either insulin dependent or non-insulin dependent diabetes. The benefit was included in the Balanced Budget Act of 1997 and was scheduled to become effective in February 2001. The expanded benefit includes an initial hour long individual training or assessment session, 9 h of group training within a continuous 12-mo period, and up to 2 h of annual follow-up training. Training sessions must be provided by a team comprised of at least a diabetic educator and a registered dietitian, except for in rural areas where shortages of health care professionals exist. Training will assist patients in managing their condition by focusing on 15 content areas. A brief overview of the subject areas include: information on the pathophysiology of diabetes; the relationship between nutrition, exercise, medications and blood glucose levels; strategies for behavior modification; and preventing, detecting, and treating acute and chronic diabetic complications. This benefit is for newly diagnosed patients, those with altered treatment regimens, patients at high risk for diabetic complications as evidenced by poor glycemic control, and for patients experiencing specified diabetic complications. In order to receive this benefit, training must be ordered by the beneficiary's physician or a qualified non-physician practitioner *(89)*.

Another monumental advance in Medicare coverage for preventive services is currently underway. Ambulatory coverage is being implemented for MNT for beneficiaries with diabetes or chronic renal insufficiency and for post renal transplant patients provided by registered dietitians or qualified nutritionists. The proposed rule was published in the Federal Register, August 2, 2001, by the Centers for Medicare and Medicaid Services, Medicare program: Revisions to Payment Policies Under the Physician Fee Schedule for Calendar Year 2002. Current provisions of the new MNT benefit state that this benefit will be limited to beneficiaries who have not yet received the diabetes outpatient self-management training, beneficiaries not receiving Medicare subsidized maintenance dialysis, and beneficiaries who meet other yet to be determined eligibility criteria. For beneficiaries with diabetes, care under this benefit must be coordinated with the diabetes outpatient self-management training benefit. Services defined as MNT under this provision are: "...nutritional diagnostic, therapy, and counseling services provided by a registered dietitian or nutrition professional for the purpose of managing disease" *(90)*. In order to receive this benefit, beneficiaries must be referred to the registered dietitian or qualified nutrition professional by their "treating physician." The regulation will allow independently employed registered dietitians and qualified nutrition professionals to be directly reimbursed for these services by Medicare. This new benefit became effective January 1, 2002 *(90)*.

5.2. The Medicaid Program

Beyond Medicare, which is available to all older Americans, some elders may be "dually eligible" and qualify for Medicaid as well. The Medicaid program is a medical assistance program established under Title XIX of the Social Security Act of 1965. It is an entitlement program funded jointly by federal and state governments to provide medical assistance to individuals or families with low incomes and limited resources *(91)*. In 1998, 4.7 million people aged 65 or older were Medicaid recipients, accounting for 13.6% of all program participants *(78)* and representing 28.5% of total Medicaid payments *(92)*. State participation in Medicaid is voluntary.

The federal government provides broad national guidelines under which each state establishes its own eligibility standards, determines the type, amount, duration and scope of services, sets the rate of payment for services, and administers its own program. Therefore, each Medicaid program varies to a large extent from state to state. State Medicaid programs are required by the federal guidelines to provide certain services to the categorically needy in order to receive federal matching funds. Federal matching funds are also available to states for the provision of certain optional services. There are no federal guidelines regarding the provision of nutrition services through Medicaid *(91)*, however, most state Medicaid plans provide some level of nutrition services as a state option *(86)*. Similar conditions of participation apply to Medicaid funded health care settings as described in Medicare guidelines and likewise, nutrition services may be covered if furnished "incidental" to medical care. Recently, in an effort to reduce costs, many Medicaid recipients were being shifted into HMOs *(91)*, which may provide nutrition service benefits.

5.3. The Elder Nutrition Program

Outside the traditional health care system, other fundamental federally-funded programs exist to deliver nutrition services and enhance food security for elders. The most extensive program, providing coordinated community and home-based health and social services for older Americans is the Elder Nutrition Program (ENP). ENP was created in 1972 as an amendment to the Older Americans Act of 1965 (OAA). Under Title IIIc of the OAA, ENP provides grants to state units on aging and their associated Area Agencies on Aging. The program also distributes funding under Title VI to Native American Tribal Organizations *(93)* *(see* Fig. 1). Collectively, these grants help to maintain a broad national network of nutrition programs providing congregate and home delivered meals in addition to other health-related supportive social services to older Americans. Nutrition programs must serve at least one meal per day, 5 or more days per week. Meals must provide at least one-third of the RDAs. Elder Nutrition Programs are also required to provide nutrition screening for meal program participants. Use of NSI screening tools is encouraged although agencies may use other screening tools provided the tools maintains the ability to identify individuals at high nutritional risk *(94)*. In addition, the ENPs may provide nutrition assessment, education, and counseling to clients.

The ENP emphasizes the opportunity for older Americans to form social networks at congregate meal sites in addition to receiving important nutrition services. All older Americans (aged 60 yr and older) and their spouses (of any age) are eligible for ENP benefits and client donations are strictly voluntary. The ENP attempts to target those individuals with the greatest social and economic need, in particular low income minori-

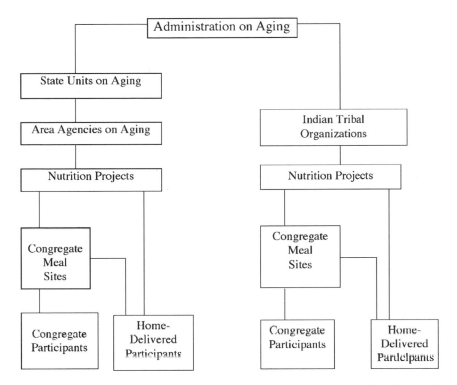

Fig. 1. Administrative framework of the elderly nutrition program in the United States.

ties, by strategically placing services in vicinities with the greatest number of needy persons. The OAA 2000 Amendments extended targeting of programs to rural elders as well *(94)*.

A comprehensive, congressionally mandated evaluation of ENP *(48)* demonstrated the success of the program in reaching targeted members of the older population. The national evaluation also demonstrated that clients' mean daily intakes approached or exceeded the RDAs for persons aged 50 yr and older for virtually all nutrients. Intakes were consistently higher among program participants for almost all essential nutrients examined, compared with matched nonparticipating elders. The social aspect of the program was also shown to be successful in that ENP clients experienced a 17% increase in monthly social contacts compared to nonparticipating matched elders *(48)*.

An array of additional valuable services are also provided under Title III to meet clients' needs, including personal care, homemaker, and chore assistance, adult day care/ adult day health services, case management, transportation including assisted transportation, legal assistance, information, and assistance regarding available community services, and outreach to older Americans or their caregivers to encourage the use of existing services and benefits. These services are often provided by the same local organization that administers the ENP, facilitating linkage for ENP recipients to other home- and community-based services.

In 2000, total funding for ENP reached over $500 million, accounting for over 50% of the Administration on Aging's budget. Fifty-six grant awards were disbursed to states and related jurisdictions under Title III. These grants included $373 million for congregate nutrition services and $146 million for home-delivered nutrition services *(95)*. In that same year, 225 tribal organizations and 2 Native Hawaiian organizations were awarded Title VI grants amounting to $16 million *(96)*. Most current participation rates indicate that 6.5 million people received at least one type of service provided under Title III as described above. Of those served, 36% lived in poverty, nearly 20% were minorities, 60% both lived in poverty and were minorities, and nearly 34% lived in rural areas. In 1998, approx 130 million and 114 million home delivered meals and congregate meals were served, respectively *(97)*. Home delivered meals accounted for 53% of the total meals served in 1998, representing an 11% increase as a percentage of total meals served by ENP since 1990. Conversely, during this period the number of congregate meals served fell by about 20% *(98)*. With earlier hospital discharges and more elders needing home based services, the demand for home delivered meals is expected to continue to rise *(48)*.

Despite the demonstrated success and effectiveness of ENP, many older Americans who are eligible for the program do not participate for a variety of reasons. Some personal factors for nonparticipation include the reluctance to accept food assistance or simply being unaware of such programs. In addition, structural constraints such as funding limitations within the program hinder others from participating. Funding limitations combined with an increased need for home-delivered meals have resulted in long waiting lists for this service, and to a smaller degree, for congregate meals *(48)*. In an attempt to meet this growing unmet need, funds are being shifted from congregate meal programs to home-delivered meal services in some organizations. However, even with this transfer of funds, the demand for home-delivered meal services continues to rise. Some program directors report that the reallocation of funds from congregate meal programs has negatively impacted this service in some locations *(98)*.

The US Department of Agriculture (USDA) provides an additional funding source to supplement the Title IIIc and Title VI grants through the Nutrition Services Incentives Program (NSIP). States and Tribes elect to receive this supplement in the form of either cash, commodities, or a combination of the two. The allocation formula for support provided by NSIP (formerly known as the Nutrition Program for the Elderly) was changed from a reimbursement model to a performance incentive model by the Older Americans Act Amendments of 2000. Allocations are now a function of the number of meals served in the previous year by a state agency on aging or tribal organization compared to the national total *(94)*. Other sources of funding for national nutrition programs are derived from state, tribal, local, and other federal funds as well as client contributions *(93)*.

5.4. The Food Stamp Program

Another federally funded program exists to combat hunger and assist individuals in meeting nutritional needs. Those who meet specific income eligibility criteria may be eligible for income supplements in the form of food stamps. The USDA Food Stamp Program is currently the largest federally funded food assistance program *(98)*. The program is administered by the Food and Nutrition Service of the USDA and is operated through state agencies. Coupons or electronic benefits are provided to low income households that can be used as a means to purchase food. By 2002, all states must switch to electronic benefit systems *(98)*.

In 2000, over 1.7 million Food Stamp Program participants were older persons (aged 60 yr or older) who accounted for 10% of all program participants. The average monthly food stamp benefit for older individuals was $59 (99). Unlike the general population who must meet both gross and net income limits to qualify for Food Stamps, elders are only required to meet the net income limit. Elders also have a higher limit on allowable assets. Individuals who are incapable of accessing the Food Stamp Program office or food store may designate a personal representative to apply for and use their Food Stamp benefits. Despite these special provisions in place for older persons, the USDA estimates that 65% of older individuals eligible for the Food Stamp Program do not receive benefits. Some of the major reasons cited for elder nonparticipation in a General Accounting Office (GAO) telephone survey of state food stamp directors included the perceived burden of the application process in comparison to the potential benefits and feelings of embarrassment because of the stigma associated with being a Food Stamp recipient (98).

5.5. Summary

Because of the numerous and diverse funding streams supporting nutrition services and the inconsistent coverage for nutritional care and treatment within the traditional health care system, current delivery mechanisms for the provision of nutrition services are complex and often uncoordinated. These structural barriers and gaps in services and reimbursement place elders at increased risk for malnutrition and nutrition-related conditions. The implementation of the expanded MNT benefits and nutrition training for certain Medicare beneficiaries will not only provide many older Americans with necessary, beneficial, and potentially cost-saving treatments, but may also serve to increase awareness within the medical community of the importance of nutrition therapies and services for improving patient outcomes. Moreover, the expanded benefits provide a direct mechanism for increased elder contact with qualified nutrition professionals. Through these referred visits, nutrition professionals can play an instrumental role in improving the coordination of care within the health care system and social service programs described, by increasing awareness of available programs and helping elders gain access to appropriate services.

5.6. Conclusions, Recommendations, and Future Challenges

The rapid growth of the older population will have serious implications for our health care system. While the older population in general appears to be healthier and less functionally impaired than in the past, certain segments of this population such as the oldest old, women, and minorities are expected to grow the most rapidly and are more likely to be poor, in poorer health, more disabled, and require more medical and social services. To be effective, mechanisms to maintain health and prevent or delay costly institutionalization require recognition that elders need a range of social and medical services and that these services must be coordinated throughout the continuum of care.

Nutritional problems are widely prevalent in the older population and range from conditions of undernutrition to overnutrition. Nearly 90% of the older population has a nutrition-related chronic condition in which nutritional intervention may be of benefit. Research demonstrates nutritional status impacts health outcomes, length of hospital stays, readmission rates, discharge disposition, morbidity, and mortality. Despite recent attention and increased concern over nutritional status and its role in health maintenance for the older population, significant inconsistencies exist in the provision of nutrition services throughout the continuum of care. These inconsistencies create gaps in services and barriers to existing services, placing an already at-risk population at greater risk for nutritional problems.

Many experts have recommended strategies to improve existing frameworks, including implementation of nutrition screening, education, and appropriate interventions as well as expanded Medicare coverage for necessary nutrition services. The recent inclusion of Medicare coverage for medical nutrition therapy among beneficiaries with diabetes and renal disease attenuates one of the greatest barriers to nutrition care, but only for a select group of individuals. Although this expansion is encouraging and demonstrates progress (expert panel recommendations are being heeded), many elders who may benefit from nutritional interventions and therapies will remain uncovered by the Medicare program.

These circumstances present the near-term challenges for nutritionists and other health care professionals. Mechanisms are slowly emerging to coordinate the provision of a continuum of nutrition services for the older population. As research continues to develop in this important area, the factors which contribute to nutritional risk in diverse older populations will become more evident. The efficacy of dietary interventions and medical nutrition therapies will also be documented. This evidence will surely facilitate movement towards the improved provision and delivery of nutrition services to vulnerable elders.

REFERENCES

1. Federal Interagency Forum on Aging-Related Statistics. Older Americans 2000: Key Indicators of Well-Being. Federal Interagency Forum on Aging-Related Statistics, US Government Printing Office, Washington, DC, 2000.
2. National Center for Health Statistics. National Vital Statistics Report, vol 48, no. 18, Table 12. http://www.cdc.gov/nchs/fastats/pdf/48_18t12.pdf, 2001, accessed June 19, 2001.
3. Liao Y, McGee DL, Cao G, Cooper RS. Recent Changes in the Health Status of the Older U.S. Population: Findings from the 1984–1994 Supplement on Aging. J Am Geriatr Soc. 2001;49:443–449.
4. US Census Bureau. USA Statistics in Brief. Health. http://www.census.gov/statab/www/part3.html, 2001, accessed July 26, 2001.
5. Administration on Aging. A Profile of Older Americans 2000. http://www.aoa.gov/aoa/stats/profile/, 2001, accessed June 19, 2001.
6. Haupt BJ. An Overview of Home Health and Hospice Care Patients: 1996 National Home and Hospice Survey. National Center for Health Statistics. Advance Data No.297. http://www.cdc.gov/nchs/data/ad/ad297.pdf, 1998, accessed June 21, 2001.
7. Gabrel C, Jones A. The National Nursing Home Survey 1997: summary. National Center for Health Statistics. Vital Health Stat 13 (147), 2000.
8. Institute of Medicine, Committee on Nutrition Services for Medicare Beneficiaries. The Role of Nutrition in Maintaining Health in the Nation's Elderly: Evaluating coverage of nutrition services for the Medicare population. National Academy Press, Washington, DC, 2000.
9. US Department of Health and Human Services. Healthy People 2010. 2nd ed. With Understanding and Improving health and Objectives for Improving Health. 2 vols. US Government Printing Office, Washington DC, 2000.
10. Dawson-Hughes B, Harris SS, Krall EA, Dallal GE. Effect of calcium and vitamin D supplementation on bone density in men and women 65 yr of age or older. N Eng Med 1997;337:670–676.
11. Gallagher-Allred CR, Voss AC, Finn SC, McCamish MA. Malnutrition and clinical outcomes: the case for medical nutrition therapy. J Am Diet Assoc 1996;96:361.
12. Gallagher-Allred CR, Voss AC, Koop K. The effect of medical nutrition therapy on malnutrition and clinical outcomes. Nutrition 1999;6:512–514.
13. Sikand G, Kashyap ML, Wong ND, Hsu JC. Dietitian intervention improves lipid values and saves medication costs in men with combined hyperlipidemia and a history of niacin noncompliance. J Am Diet Assoc 2000;100:218–224.

14. Whelton PK, Appel LJ, Espeland MA, Applegate WB, Ettinger WH Jr, Kostis JB, et al. Sodium reduction and weight loss in the treatment of hypertension in older persons. A randomized controlled trial of nonpharmacologic interventions in the elderly (TONE). JAMA 1998;279:839–846.

15. Centers for Disease Control and Prevention, US Department of Health and Human Services. Chronic diseases and their risk factors: The nation's leading causes of death. 1999. http://www.cdc.gov/nccdphp/statbook/pdf/cdrf1999.pdf, 1999, accessed June 21, 2001.

16. American Dietetic Association. Position of the American dietetic Association: Nutrition, aging and the continuum of care. J Am Diet Assoc 2000;100:580–595.

17. Erlinger TP, Pollack H, Appel LJ. Nutrition related cardiovascular risk factors in older people: results from the Third National Health and Nutrition Examination Survey. J Am Geriat Soc 2000;48:1486–1489.

18. Kramarow E, Lenztner H, Rooks R, Weeks J, Saydah S. Health and Aging Chartbook. Health, United States. National Center for Health Statistics, Hyattsville, MD, 1999.

19. US Census Bureau. Statistical Abstract of the United States 2000. Vital Statistics section, no. 129. Deaths by Age and Leading Cause: 1997. http://www.census.gov/prod/2001pubs/statab/sec02.pdf, 2001, accessed July 26, 2001.

20. Williams DR, Collins C. US socioeconomic and racial differences in health: patterns and explanations. Ann Rev Sociol 1995;21:349–386.

21. Mirowski J, Hu PN. Physical impairment and the diminishing effects of income. Social Forces 1996;74:1073–1096.

22. Nutrition Screening Initiative. Report of nutrition screening 1: Toward a common view. Greer, Margolis, Mitchell, Grunwald, Washington, DC, 1991.

23. Geronimus AT, Bound J, Waidmann TA, Colen CG, Steffick D. Inequality in life expectancy, functional status, and active life expectancy across selected black and white populations in the United States. Demography 2001;38:227–251.

24. Buchowski MS, Sun M. Nutrition in minority elders: current problems and future directives. J Health Care poor Underserved 1996;7:184–209.

25. House JS, Lepkowski JM, Kinney AM, Mero RP, Kessler RC, Herzog AR. The social stratification of aging and health. J Health Soc Behav 1994;35:213–234.

26. Klein GL, Kita K, Fish J, Sinkus B, Jensen GL. Nutrition and health for older persons in rural America: A managed care model. J Am Diet Assoc 1997;97:885–888.

27. Jensen GL. Nutritional problems of free living elderly, the rural elderly: Living the good life? Nutr Rev 1996;54:S17–S21.

28. Hewitt M. Defining "rural" areas: impact on health care policy and research. In: Sociocultural and Service Issues in Working with Rural Clients. Jones, S. (ed.) Rockefeller College, Albany, 1993, pp. 9–32.

29. Geronimus AT, Bound J, Waidmann TA. Poverty, time and place: variation in excess mortality across selected US populations,1980–1990. J Epidemiol Community Health 1999;53:325–334.

30. Bernstein AB, Hing E, Burt CW, Hall MJ. Trend data on medical encounters: tracking a moving target. Health Aff 2001;20:58–72

31. Dwyer JT. Screening older Americans' nutritional health: Current practices and future responsibilities. Nutrition Screening Initiative. Washington, DC, 1991.

32. US Department of Health and Human Services, Public Health Service. The Surgeon General's Report on nutrition and health: summary and recommendations. US Government Printing Office; DHHS (PHS) Publication no. 88–50211, Washington, DC, 1988.

33. Vailas LI, Nitzke SA, Becker M, Gast J. Risk indicators for nutrition are associated inversely with quality of life for participants in meal programs for older adults. J Am Diet Assoc 1998;98:548–553.

34. Nutrition Screening Initiative. Incorporating Nutrition Screening and Interventions into Medical Practice: A Monograph for Physicians. Greer, Margolis, Mitchell, Grunwald, Washington, DC, 1994.

35. Posner BM, Jette A, Smigelski C, Miller D, Mitchell P. Nutritional risk in New England elders. J Gerontol Med Sci 1994;49:M123–M132.

36. US Department of Health and Human Services, Public Health Service. Healthy People 2000 Full Report, With Commentary US Government Printing Office DHHS (PHS) Publication no. 91–50212, Washington, DC, 1991.

37. Bales C. What does it mean to be "at nutritional risk"? Seeking clarity on behalf or the elderly. Am J Clin Nut 2001;74:155–156.

38. Millen BE, Levine E. A continuum of nutrition services for older Americans. In: Chernoff R (ed.). Geriatric Nutrition: The Health Professional's Handbook. 2nd ed. Aspen Publishers, Gaithersburg, MD, 1999. pp. 435–467.

39. Jensen GL, Friedmann JM, Coleman CD, Smiciklas-Wright H. Screening for hospitalization and nutritional risks among community-dwelling older persons. Am J Clin Nutr 2001;74:201–205.
40. Horwath CC. Dietary intake studies in elderly people. World Rev Nutr Diet 1989;59:1–70.
41. Lee JS, Frongillo EA. Understanding needs is important for assessing the impact of food assistance program participation on nutritional and health status in U.S. elderly persons. J Nutr 2000;131:765–773.
42. Alaimo K, McDowell MA, Briefel RR, et al. Dietary intake of vitamins, minerals, and fiber of persons ages 2 months and over in the United States: Third National Health and Nutrition Examination Survey, Phase I, 1988–91. US Department of Health and Human Services. National Center for Health Statistics. Advance Data 1999;258:1–28.
43. McDowell MA, Briefel RR, Alaimo K, et al. Energy and micronutrient intake of persons ages 2 months and over in the United States: Third National Health and Nutrition Examination Survey, Phase I, 1988–91. USDHHS. NCHS. Advance Adata 1994;255:1–24.
44. Cid-Ruzafa J, Caulfield LE, Barron Y, West SK. Nutrient intakes and adequacy among an older population on the eastern shore of Maryland: the Salisbury Eye Evaluation. J Am Diet Assoc 1999;99: 564–571.
45. Marshall JA, Lopez TK, Shetterly SM et al. Indicators of nutritional risk in a rural elderly Hispanic and non-Hispanic population: San Luis Valley Health and Aging Study. J Am Diet Assoc 1999;99:315–322.
46. Jensen GL, Kita K, Fish J, Heydt D, Frey C. Nutrition risk screening characteristics of rural older persons: relation to functional limitations and health care charges. Am J Clin Nutr 1997;66:819–828.
47. Millen BE, Silliman RA, Cantey-Kiser J, Copenhafer DL, Ewart CV, Ritchie CS, et al. Nutritional risk in an urban homebound older population: The nutrition and healthy aging project. J Nutr Health Aging 2001;5:269–277.
48. Ponza M, Ohls JC, Millen BE. Serving Elders at Risk: The older Americans act nutrition programs, national evaluation of the elderly nutrition program, 1993–1995. Mathematica Policy Research, Inc., Princeton, NJ, 1996.
49. Kuczmarski RJ, Flegal KM, Cambell SM, et al. Increasing prevalence of overweight among US adults. JAMA 1994;272:205–211.
50. National Center for Health Statistics. Health, United States, 2000 With Adolescent Health Chartbook. Hyattsville, MD, 2000.
51. Jensen GL, Rogers J. Obesity in older persons. J Am Diet Assoc 1998;98:1308–1311.
52. Heiat A, Vaccarino V, Krumholz HM. An evidence-based assessment of Federal guidelines for overweight and obesity as they apply to elderly persons. Arch Intern Med 2001;161:1194–1203.
53. Langlois JA, Harris T, Looker AC, Madans J. Weight change between age 50 years and old age is associated with risk of hip fracture in white women aged 67 years and older. Arch Intern Med 1996; 156:989–994.
54. Mussolino ME, Looker AC, Madans JH, Langlois JA, Orwoll ES. Risk factors for hip fracture in white men: The NHANES I epidemiologic follow-up study. J Bone Miner Res 1998;13:918–924.
55. French SA, Folsom AR, Jeffery RW, Williamson DF. Prospective study of intentionality of weight loss and mortality in older women: The Iowa Women's Health Study. Am J Epidemiol 1999;149:504–514.
56. Constans T, Bacq Y, Brechot JF, Guilmot JL, Choutet P, Lamisse F. Protein-energy malnutrition in elderly medical patients. J Am Geriat Soc 1992;40:263–268.
57. Sullivan DH, Walls RC, Bopp MM. Protein-energy undernutrition and the risk of mortality within one year of hospital discharge: a follow-up study. J Am Geriat Soc 1995;43:507–512.
58. Sullivan DH, Walls RC. The risk of life-threatening complications in a select population of geriatric patients: the impact of nutritional status. J Am Coll Nut 1995;14:29–36.
59. Corti M-C, Guralnik JM, Salive ME, Sorkin JD. Serum albumin level and physical disability as predictors of mortality in older persons. JAMA 1994;272:1036–1042.
60. Salive ME, Cornoni-Huntley J, Phillips C, Guralinik JM, Cohen HJ, Ostfeld AM, Wallace RB. Serum albumin in older persons: Relationship with age and health status. J Clin Epidemiol 1992;45:213–221.
61. Ritchie CS, Burgio KL, Locher JL, Corwell A, Thomas D, Hardin M, Redden D. Nutritional status of urban homebound adults. Am J Clin Nutr 1997;66:815–818.
62. Agarwal N, Acevedo F, Leighton LS, Cayten CG, Pitchumoni CS. Predictive ability of various nutritional variables for mortality in elderly people. Am J Clin Nutr 1988;48:1173–1178.
63. D'Erasmo E, Pisani D, Ragno A, Romagnoli S, Spagna G, Acca M. Serum albumin level at admission: mortality and clinical outcome in geriatric patients. Am J Med Sci 1997;314:17–20.
64. Friedmann JM, Jensen GL, Smiciklas-Wright H, McCamish MA. Predicting early nonelective hospital readmission in nutritionally compromised older adults. Am J Clin Nutr 1997;65:1714–20.

65. Marinella MA, Markert RJ. Admission serum albumin level and length of hospitalization in elderly patients. South Med J 1998;91:851–854.

66. Volkert D, Kruse W, Oster P, Schlierf G. Malnutrition in geriatric patients. Ann Nutr Metab 1992; 36:97–112.

67. Reuben DB, Ix JH, Greendale GA, Seeman TE. The predictive value of combined hypoalbuminemia and hypocholesterolemia in high functioning community-dwelling older persons: Macarthur studies of successful aging. J Am Geriat Soc 1999;47:402–406.

68. Sahyoun NR, Jacques PF, Dallal G, Russell RM. Use of albumin as a predictor of mortality in community dwelling and institutionalized elderly populations. J Clin Epidemiol 1996;49:981–988.

69. Chima CS, Barco K, Dewitt MLA, Maeda M, Teran JC, Mullen KD. Relationship of nutritional status to length of stay, hospital costs, and discharge status of patients hospitalized in the medicine service. J Am Diet Assoc 1997;97:975–978.

70. Covinsky KE, Martin GE, Beyth RJ et al. The relationship between clinical assessments of nutrition status and adverse outcomes in older hospitalized medical patients. J Am Geriat Soc 1999;47:532–538.

71. US.Department of Health, Education, and Welfare, Public Health Service. Healthy People: The surgeon general's report on health promotion and disease prevention. US Government Printing Office; DHEW (PHS) Publication no. 79–55071, Washington, DC, 1979.

72. Surgeon General's Workshop on Healthy Promotion and Aging. US Government Printing Office; Publication no. 1988-201-875/83669, Washington, DC, 1988.

73. Nutrition Screening Initiative. Nutrition Interventions Manual for Professionals Caring for Older Americans. Greer, Margolis, Mitchell, Grunwald, Washington, DC, 1992.

74. Nutrition Screening Initiative. Nutrition screening manual for professionals caring for older Americans. 73 Nutrition Screening Initiative, Washington, DC. Nutrition Interventions Manual for Professionals Caring for Older Americans. Greer, Margolis, Mitchell, Grunwald, Washington, DC, 1991.

75. White JV, ed. The Role of Nutrition in Chronic Disease Care. Nutrition Screening Initiative, Washington, DC, 1997.

76. Wellman N. Nutrition Care Alerts Promote Health and Function. Geriatric Times July/August vol I, Issue 2, 2000, http://www.medinfosource.com/gt/g000826.html.

77. Institute of Medicine, Division of Health Promotion and Disease Prevention. The second fifty years: promoting health and preventing disability. National Academy Press, Washington, DC, 1992.

78. Health Care Financing Administration. HCFA Statistics: Populations http://www.hcfa.gov/stats/hstats99/blusta99.htm, 2001, accessed August 10, 2001.

79. US Census Bureau. Statistical Abstract of the United States 2000. Health and Nutrition section, no. 164. Medicare Enrollees 1980–1998 and no. 165. Medicare Disbursements by Type of Beneficiary 1980–1999. http://www.census.gov/prod/2001pubs/statab/sec03.pdf, 2001, accessed August 14, 2001.

80. Health Care Financing Administration. HCFA Legislative Summary - Title 1: Medicare Beneficiary Improvements: Section 105. http://www.hcfa.gov/regs/sum-title1.htm, 2001, accessed August 7, 2001.

81. Code of Federal Regulations. Health Care Financing Administration. 42CFR482-484. U.S. Government Printing Office via GPO Access; http://www.access.gpo.gov/nara/cfr/index.html, 2001, accessed August 2, 2001.

82. Health Care Financing Administration. State Operations Manual. Appendices, Appendix A: Interpretive Guidelines-Hospitals. 482.28 Condition of Participation and Interpretive Guidelines: Food and dietetic services. A61–A68. http://www.hcfa.gov/pubforms/07_som/somap_a_061_to_061.htm, 2001, accessed July 14, 2001.

83. Escott-Stump S, Krauss B, Pavlinac J, Robinson G. Joint Commission on Accreditation of Healthcare Organizations: Friend, not foe. J Am Diet Assoc 2000;100:839.

84. American Dietetic Association. The Medicare Program and Nutrition Services. www.eatright.org/medicare.html, 2001, accessed 2001 various dates July–August.

85. Health Care Financing Administration. State Operations Manual. Appendix M - Survey Procedures and Interpretive Guidelines for Hospices. 418.88(b) Standard and Guidelines: Dietary Counseling. Tag Number L-201, M-39. http://www.hcfa.gov/pubforms/07_som/somap_m.htm, 2001, accessed July 14, 2001.

86. Mathieu M. Changing managed-care model offers opportunities for nutrition coverage. J Am Diet Assoc 2000;100:415.

87. Health Care Financing Administration Press Office. Medicare News: HMO Plan Expands To Include More Medicare Beneficiaries In Hampshire County, Mass. http://www.hcfa.gov/news/pr2001/pr010326.htm, 2001, accessed August 7, 2001.

88. Gold M. Medicare+Choice: An Interim Report Card. Health Affairs (Millwood). 2001;20:120–138.
89. Federal Register. Health Care Financing Administration, Rules, Medicare: Outpatient diabetes self-management training services; expanded coverage, vol. 65, no. 251:83129-83154. US Government Printing Office via GPO Access http://www.access.gpo.gov/su_docs/index.html, 2000, accessed July 14, 2001.
90. Federal Register. Centers for Medicare and Medicaid Services. Medicare program: Revisions to Payment Policies Under the Physician Fee Schedule for Calendar Year 2002, proposed rule. vol. 66, no. 149:40371-40420. US Government Printing Office via GPO Access http://www.access.gpo.gov/su_docs/index.html, 2001, accessed August 10, 2001.
91. American Dietetic Association. The Medicaid Program and Nutrition Services. www.eatright.org/medicaid.html, 2001, accessed July 14, 2001.
92. Health Care Financing Administration. HCFA Statistics: Expenditures. Table 34 http://www.hcfa.gov/stats/hstats99/blus2y99.html, 2001, accessed August 10, 2001.
93. Administration on Aging. The Elderly Nutrition Program. http://www.aoa.gov/factsheets/enp.html, 2001, accessed Aug. 6, 2001.
94. Administration on Aging. Resources and Information about the Older Americans Act Amendments of 2000. http://www.aoa.gov/Oaa/status/default.htm, 2001, accessed August 6, 2001.
95. Catalog of Federal Domestic Assistance June 2001 Update. Special Programs for the Aging: Title III, Part C: Nutrition Services 93.045 http://aspe.os.dhhs.gov/cfda/p93045.htm, 2001, accessed August 9, 2001.
96. Catalog of Federal Domestic Assistance June 2001 Update. Special Programs for the Aging: Title VI, Part A, Indian Programs_Grants to Indian Tribes and Part B, Grants to Native Hawaiians 93.047 http://aspe.os.dhhs.gov/cfda/P93047.htm#i33, 2001, accessed August 9, 2001.
97. Administration on Aging. National Aging Program Information System. State Program Reports: http://www.aoa.gov/napis/98spr/default.htm, 1998, accessed August 9, 2001.
98. US General Accounting Office. Report to Congressional Requesters. Food Assistance. Options for improving nutrition for older Americans. GAO/RCED00-238. http://www.gao.gov/new.items/rc00238.pdf, 2000, accessed August 9, 2001.
99. US Department of Agriculture, Food and Nutrition Service. Office of Analysis, Nutrition and Evaluation. Characteristics of food stamp households: fiscal year 2000 (advance report), 2001, http://www.fns.usda.gov/oane/MENU/Published/FSP/Participation.htm#2000AdvChar, accessed August 9, 2001.

3

The Progression from Physiological Aging to Disease

The Impact of Nutrition

Roger B. McDonald and Rodney C. Ruhe

1. INTRODUCTION

Biologic aging is a complex and multifactoral phenomenon that is not well understood. Deficiencies in our understanding of the aging process are particularly evident with regard to the interface between normal deteriorative changes observed in all individuals (e.g., gray hair, loss of muscle mass, etc.) and clear, definable disease (e.g., cancer, Alzheimer's disease, etc.). For example, what factors contribute to the progression of the age-related dysregulation of glucose homeostasis into type II diabetes, and why does this disease occurs in only 8% of the older population, even though all individuals over the age of 80 yr show loss in insulin regulation?

Adding to the complexity of the age-disease interface is the impact of nutrition. Current data indicate unequivocally that changes in nutritional patterns can significantly influence the risk of disease in a population (e.g., the direct relationship between saturated fat and the incidence of heart disease). However, aging is not a disease, but a normal physiological process that can occur without definable pathology. For example, numerous investigations have demonstrated that rats and nonhuman primates live significantly longer and have less pathology when restricted in calories than do animals fed *ad libitum* *(1)* That is, nutritional alterations resulted in reduced pathology, but the animals still aged and died. Also, vitamin E supplementation in experimental animals resulted in extended median life span without an increase in maximal life span *(2)*. This finding is generally interpreted to mean that vitamin E impacts disease (increased median life span), but not aging (no change in maximal life span). Together, the results of these investigations demonstrate that nutrition can alter rates of aging and the development of disease.

In this review, we focus on the interaction between the normal process of aging and the development of disease, and whether or not nutrition can modify this interaction. However, it is not possible to discuss all areas of aging or to provide an in-depth review on the topics covered. For that, we will refer the reader to more thorough reviews. The purpose of this brief review is to discuss issues that we believe have the greatest clinical

From: *Handbook of Clinical Nutrition and Aging*
Edited by: C. W. Bales and C. S. Ritchie © Humana Press Inc., Totowa, NJ

relevance. To this end, we have limited our discussion to type 2 diabetes, gastrointestinal disorders, and the anorexia of aging.

2. AGING, GLUCOSE METABOLISM, AND TYPE 2 DIABETES

2.1. Glucose Metabolism in Aging

It has long been recognized that changes in glucose metabolism as a result of aging may lead to the development of a variety of health problems, particularly cardiovascular disease and type 2 diabetes. However, the relationship among aging, glucose metabolism, and disease is complex and not well understood. For example, the once strong correlation between aging and the development of type 2 diabetes has been undermined by recent observations that the greatest increase in incidence of this disease is occurring in younger populations *(3)*. An important concept that has emerged from recent epidemiological and experimental studies is that cardiovascular disease and type 2 diabetes are not caused by aging *per se*, nor are they inevitable consequences of aging. Rather, changes in glucose metabolism, which may occur as a function of age, render the body more vulnerable to the development of these diseases.

In the healthy individual, blood glucose concentration is well-regulated and maintained within a relatively narrow range (80–100 mg/100 mL in the postabsorptive state). An increase in blood glucose concentration, as occurs after the ingestion of carbohydrates, elicits rapid and precise secretion of insulin from the β-cells within the islets of Langerhans. Insulin acts to decrease hepatic glucose output and to accelerate the uptake of glucose into the peripheral tissues, therefore lowering blood glucose concentration. The secretion of insulin operates under a feedback control mechanism, i.e., plasma insulin concentration is determined by the rate of insulin secretion, which, in turn, is determined by blood glucose concentration. Any alterations in this finely-regulated system may lead to a disruption in glucose homeostasis and the subsequent development of hyperglycemia, hypoglycemia, and insulinemia.

2.2. Diseases of Altered Glucose Regulation

Chronic and acute changes in glucose homeostasis are associated with several pathologies, the most severe and prevalent of which are cardiovascular disease and type 2 diabetes. Cardiovascular disease (CVD), which includes macrovascular disease (coronary heart disease, cerebrovascular disease, and peripheral vascular disease) and microvascular complications (neuropathy, renal disease, and retinopathy), is directly related to the progression and severity of type 2 diabetes. The leading cause of mortality in people with type 2 diabetes is CVD, and it is well documented that all forms of CVD, including coronary heart disease, stroke, and peripheral vascular disease, are much more common in persons with type 2 diabetes than in nondiabetic individuals *(4)*. Numerous studies have provided strong evidence that the causal link between type 2 diabetes and CVD is hyperglycemia, the chronic or acute increase in fasting or postprandial blood glucose concentration above those levels that are considered normal. Even mild increases in fasting and postprandial blood glucose concentration are known to contribute to macrovascular injury and atherosclerotic changes *(5)*. A meta-analysis of 20 different studies of 95, 783 individuals followed for 12 yr led to the conclusion that an increase in fasting or postprandial blood glucose concentration above normal levels is a risk factor for cardiovascular events even within a range below the diabetic threshold of blood glucose concentration (<126 mg/dL), and that glucose is likely to be a continuous cardiovascular risk factor, similar to total cholesterol and blood pressure (6). A close relationship has been established between hyperglycemia and microvascular damage, and the progression of diabetic retinopathy, nephropathy, and polyneuropathy (7).

Hyperglycemia, a hallmark of type 2 diabetes, is the direct consequence of disrupted glucose homeostasis. In persons with type 2 diabetes, there occurs an inefficient uptake of glucose from the blood by peripheral tissues, a condition known as glucose intolerance. Glucose intolerance is caused, in part, by insulin resistance, an attenuation in the biological response to normal concentrations of insulin. In addition, type 2 diabetes is often associated with a diminution in the sensitivity of the pancreatic β-cells to glucose stimulation, with a subsequent decrease in insulin secretion. In time, the combination of increased insulin resistance and diminished insulin secretion in response to a glucose challenge will result in hyperglycemia. High concentrations of glucose in the blood and tissues can promote the production of free radicals, which can cause general damage to proteins through cross-linking, fragmentation, and lipid oxidation. Free radicals may also mediate some of the changes associated with the development of atherosclerosis, e.g., activation of coagulation, vasoconstriction, increased expression of adhesion molecules, and oxidative modification of low density lipoproteins (8). Another adverse effect of hyperglycemia is the nonenzymatic glycosylation of proteins. As a function of time and glucose concentration, protein amino groups react with glucose to eventually form advanced glycosylation endproducts (AGEs). AGEs can accumulate over time and induce excess crosslinking of collagen and other extracellular matrix proteins. Macrovascular and microvascular complications are the most common and significant consequences of glycosylation. The AGE-induced crosslinking of proteins in the vascular wall has been implicated in pathological changes associated with atherosclerosis, such as the accumulation of low density lipoprotein (LDL) particles (9). The glycosylation of vascular proteins may contribute to the thickening, loss of elasticity, and increased permeability of blood vessel walls associated with diabetic microvascular complications.

2.3. Causes of Type 2 Diabetes

If glucose intolerance and insulin resistance result in hyperglycemia, which may in turn, cause the vascular damage related to CVD and type 2 diabetes, then what factors contribute to the development of glucose intolerance and insulin resistance? Until recently, the aging process was considered the primary factor associated with the appearance of glucose intolerance and insulin resistance. This supposition was supported by several studies that examined insulin action in healthy, non-obese young and older individuals with clinically normal oral glucose tolerance (10–12). In general, the results of these studies demonstrated that older people were insulin resistant despite having normal glucose tolerance and physical activity. Epidemiological studies have long indicated that the prevalence of both type 2 diabetes and glucose intolerance increases with age. For example, a study in 1976 showed that the average annual incidence of type 2 diabetes per 100,000 persons triples between the ages of 50 and 70 when compared with a less than 25% increase between the ages of 30 and 50 yr (13). It is estimated that between 25% and 30% of the US population aged 65 and older has type 2 diabetes or impaired glucose tolerance (14).

However, more recent studies provide compelling evidence that aging *per se* has very little, if any, effect on glucose intolerance and insulin resistance *(15–17)*. For example, numerous studies have demonstrated that glucose-stimulated insulin secretion is well maintained in the aging human and that endogenous factors, such as changes in insulin receptor number and affinity, do not play a significant role in the development of type 2 diabetes *(18)*. The loss of skeletal muscle, a major site of glucose utilization, occurs commonly with advancing age, but this does not contribute to the development of glucose intolerance *(18)*. Although it is true that some aspects of glucose homeostasis may deteriorate with age, it must be emphasized that aging is not always associated with glucose intolerance, as seen in the fact that the vast majority of elderly persons in the United States do not suffer from impaired glucose tolerance. It should also be noted that the incidence of type 2 diabetes has increased in all age groups over the past 10 yr, with the greatest increase occurring among persons 30–50 yr of age *(19)*. More specifically, the incidence of type 2 diabetes among people aged 30–39 yr increased approx 70% during the past decade, whereas the incidence among persons over the age of 65 remained stable *(19)*. The dramatic increase in the rate of type 2 diabetes among younger populations is evidence that this disease is not simply the result of aging, but rather, the consequence of modifiable environmental factors. The most significant factors contributing to the development of type 2 diabetes are obesity and physical inactivity.

Decreased physical activity is becoming more common in the United States and throughout the world because of the decrease in demand for physical labor, an increase in sedentary occupations, and less emphasis on physical education, particularly in the younger age groups. Almost one-third of the adult population in the United States does not participate in exercise or other physical activity *(19)*. Physical inactivity increases the risk of obesity and results in decreased insulin sensitivity and diminished glucose tolerance *(20)*, each of which is associated with the development of type 2 diabetes. Lack of physical activity is a potentially reversible factor contributing to glucose intolerance.

Obesity is perhaps the most important factor contributing to the development of glucose intolerance in all age groups. The prevalence of obesity in the US population as a whole is approx 20% *(21)*. During the past decade, the percentage of Americans defined as obese (30 lbs over ideal weight) has increased by approx 33%. It is not a coincidence that these figures mirror the 33% rise in type 2 diabetes over the same 10-yr period *(3)*. The association between obesity and the incidence of type 2 diabetes is very strong. In contrast to the findings of earlier studies, the vast majority of recent studies in humans and rodents have demonstrated a positive relationship between obesity and insulin resistance. A likely reason for the disparate findings between earlier and more recent studies is the emergence of information in the past 15 yr that insulin resistance in aging is largely attributable to abdominal obesity rather than to total degree of adiposity *(22)*. Several cohort studies indicate that weight gain during adulthood, the degree and type of obesity (abdominal fat vs total fat), and the duration of obesity are all strong and independent risk factors for the development of type 2 diabetes *(23)*. The results of numerous studies highlight the importance of weight loss to control or prevent glucose intolerance and diabetes. It is estimated that 65% to 75% of cases of type 2 diabetes in Caucasians could be avoided if individuals in this subgroup did not exceed their ideal weight *(24)*. For individuals who are already overweight, even modest weight loss is associated with significantly reduced diabetes risk *(25)*. Skeletal muscle responds to exercise training by increasing glucose transporter concentration, resulting in more effective insulin action and improved glucose tolerance *(26)*. In combination with weight control, exercise is an effective means of preventing and treating glucose intolerance and type 2 diabetes in persons who already suffer from, or are at risk for, developing these conditions, regardless of age.

Over the past decade, the results of experimental studies and data from epidemiologic investigations have indicated that the development of glucose intolerance and type 2 diabetes is time-dependent, not age-dependent. That is, glucose intolerance, accompanied by hyperglycemia and subsequent damage to the cardiovascular system, can be initiated at any age, can progress during any given period within the life span, and can be halted and even reversed at any time during the life span. For most individuals, the appearance, progression, and severity of glucose intolerance and type 2 diabetes is determined by the presence and degree of exogenous factors, particularly obesity and a sedentary lifestyle, and by the duration of these factors, independent of chronological age. Because these exogenous factors are modifiable, the development and deleterious effects of type 2 diabetes are largely preventable.

3. AGING AND THE GASTROINTESTINAL TRACT

The gastrointestinal tract is a unique system that from mouth to anus is actually outside the internal milieu of the body. The primary role of the gastrointestinal system is to modify food (digestion and absorption) for metabolic use by other physiological systems and, through its highly developed immune system, to protect the body from food-borne contaminants. Thus, any age-related changes to this system can lead to an increase in risk for disease. However, although physical and morphological changes are common in advanced age, the gastrointestinal system appears to function well during aging in the absence of a primary disease. The elderly population does show a greater incidence of acute disorders, such as constipation, gastric reflux, and mild gastritis. Undoubtedly, these disorders are distressing problems, but can be treated effectively with diet and over-the-counter drugs, and they do not significantly increase the risk of other health problems. A comprehensive review of such age-related changes to the gastrointestinal tract are beyond the scope of this chapter. The reader is referred to Chapter 26 in this text and to an excellent discussion by Holt *(27)*.

3.1. Macronutrient Absorption

Given the many clinical conditions associated with nutrient malabsorption in the elderly, the perception that there is a general decrease in intestinal absorption with age comes as no surprise. Investigations evaluating the absorption rates of carbohydrate in both human and laboratory animals have consistently shown a small, but significant, decline with age *(28–30)*. The small differences in absorption rates of carbohydrates between the ages have prompted most researchers to conclude that these alterations are unlikely to be of physiological importance. Findings similar to that of carbohydrate absorption have been reported for lipid *(31)*, whereas the data on the rate of protein absorption with age are insufficient to make definitive conclusions.

3.2. Micronutrient Absorption

The data for age-related changes in intestinal absorption of several micronutrients appear to be unequivocal. Several investigations have shown a significant decrease in absorption of various micronutrients in elderly populations *(27,32)*. For example, calcium absorption declines in both men and women and appears to be related to alterations in vitamin D metabolism *(33–35)*. The prevalence of cobalamin (B_{12}) malabsorption may be as high as 15% of the elderly population *(36,37)*. Decreased absorption of riboflavin, niacin, and vitamin D have also been reported *(32)*. Although there is considerable evidence to suggest a diminution of micronutrient absorption in the older population, it remains to be determined if this decrease reflects "normal" age-related changes in intestinal physiology or is a result of intestinal diseases/disorders.

Much of the experimental work evaluating the cellular and physiological mechanisms that underlie the age-related decrease in micronutrient absorption has been unable to demonstrate a clear and unequivocal disruption in function. Using the inverted gut sac technique, Ferraris et al. *(38)* reports a significant decline in glucose absorption rates when expressed per millimeter of tissue in 24- vs 6-mo-old mice. However, these investigators find that cellular density per millimeter of jejunum was significantly increased in the older rats, suggesting that total absorption would not be different. The fact that total absorption of micronutrients does not change with age in mice has been supported *(39,40)*. Investigations in humans designed to determine the physiological/biochemical basis of altered micronutrient absorption have been hampered by inappropriate subject population (i.e., patients in long-term care facility or other clinical populations) and the lack of precise methodology. Thus, a normal biological mechanism that underlies any age-related malabsorption remains to be clearly demonstrated.

3.2.1. COBALAMIN MALABSORPTION

An excellent example of the influence of disease on age-related physiological change is the report of low serum B_{12} concentration in the elderly vs younger populations *(41)*. Low serum B_{12} concentration can be indicative of cobalamin deficiency associated with megaloblastic anemia or neurological complications. However, investigations performed in a healthy aged population have shown that supplementation with B_{12} does not increase serum levels even though the serum levels were below the normal range for younger individuals *(42)*. Other investigators have found that the decline in mean serum B_{12} concentrations in older vs younger populations reflects only a strong influence of small subgroups of elderly individuals, with the majority of the population having normal B_{12} concentrations *(41)*. These findings have led most investigators to conclude that subnormal serum B_{12} concentration in the elderly population is not solely the result of aging.

It is more likely that the low serum B_{12} concentrations seen in the elderly are because of malabsorption resulting from intestinal disorders. Specifically, it appears that chronic infection by the *Helicobacter pylori* bacterium may be responsible for the higher incidence of B_{12} malabsorption in the elderly population *(27,43)*. Investigations have shown that *H. pylori* infection significantly reduces the secretion of an intrinsic factor resulting in hypochlorhydria and the risk of atrophic gastritis. Atrophic gastritis is recognized as the leading risk factor associated with B_{12} malabsorption in the elderly. The *H. pylori*-associated hypochorhydria prevents the stomach from reaching a pH low enough for the food-bound cobalamin to be released in free form, a necessary condition for proper intestinal absorption *(41)* *(see* Table 1). When antibiotic therapy is given to patients with low serum B_{12} concentrations and atrophic gastritis, the serum level of this vitamin rises.

Table 1
Food-Cobalamin Malabsorption[a] and Presence of *H. pylori* Bacteria

	Percent of subjects with H. pylori	
	All subjects	*Low serum cobalamin only*
Severe Malabsorption (*n* = 27)	78%	78%
Mild Malabsorption (*n* = 27)	45%	41%
Normal Absorption (*n* = 44)	42%	41%

[a] Determined by egg yolk-cobalamin absorption test. Data adapted from Carmel et al. *(75)*.

Table 2
Mean Daily Kilocalorie (kcal)[a] Intake by Age Group—Third National Health
and Nutrition Examination Survey, Phase 1, 1988–1991

		Daily kcal intake	
Age group (yr)	*Sample size*	*No.*	*(SE[b])*
20–29	1682	2484	(±44.4)
30–39	1526	2372	(±43.4)
40–49	1228	2146	(±41.5)
50–59	929	1967	(±30.7)
60–69	1106	1822	(±39.0)
70–79	851	1624	(±25.3)
≥80	609	1484	(±27.4)

[a] Kilocalories derived from reported consumption of foods and beverages.
[b] Standard error. Data adapted from NHANES III *(44)*.

These findings provide strong evidence that bacterial infection of the stomach may be the key to malabsorption and low serum levels of B_{12}.

Nonetheless, the question remains, why does *H. pylori* infection with subsequent B_{12} malabsorption occur primarily in the elderly population? As with many questions dealing with aging, the answer is not clear and the current data are insufficient to determine a precise cause. Regardless, it is prudent for clinicians suspecting nutrient malabsorption to test for intestinal disorders rather than to accept the premise that absorption declines as a function of age.

4. ENERGY BALANCE AND THE AGE-RELATED DECREASE IN FOOD INTAKE

4.1. Prevalence of Decreased Food Intake with Age

Several investigations, including cross-sectional and longitudinal studies, have suggested a progressive decline in food intake at advanced ages *(44–46)* (*see* Table 2). The decline in energy intake is commensurate with a reduction in energy expenditure during middle age, resulting in a rise of percent adiposity through the fifth and sixth decades of life *(47)*. The increase in percent adiposity with age appears to slow and even decrease after the age of 70 such that energy balance often becomes negative and losses in lean body mass and body fat occur *(48,49)*. Dietary intake studies involving elderly subjects frequently report inadequate caloric intake *(50–52)*, and unintentional weight loss has been described in up to 35% of aged community-dwellers *(53)* and 70% of nursing home residents *(54)*. This decrease in caloric intake appears to develop without definitive cause in otherwise healthy elderly persons *(55)*.

4.2. Energy Balance Homeostasis and Aging

Several investigations provide evidence that age-related alterations in the homeostatic mechanisms of energy balance influence the development of diminished food intake. For example, Roberts *(56)* reports that older men (mean age 68 yr) do not adjust their energy intake to the same degree in response to under- or overfeeding as do younger subjects (23 yr). Other investigators have found that elderly men (60–84 yr) compensated less precisely for changes in caloric intake than do younger men (18–35 yr) *(57)*. The older subjects in this study reported less hunger and greater fullness when compared to the younger group. Similarly, desire to eat after a test meal is diminished more in aged (70–84 yr) vs younger (23–50 yr) men and women *(58)*.

Although the age-related decrease in food intake appears to be a "normal" biological manifestation of the aging process, it often results in undernutrition and secondary problems, such as sarcopenia *(59)*, impaired immunity *(60)*, and physical frailty *(61)*, all of which can substantially impact the quality of life. Moreover, it is not inconceivable that some of the symptoms and/or diseases seen at the time of clinical screening are the direct result of undiagnosed age-related anorexia. The problem of undiagnosed age-related anorexia persists despite continued research in clinical and laboratory settings because declining food intake is often subtle and not recognized until confounding illnesses have developed.

4.3. Psychological and Pathological Determinates of Anorexia of Aging

The evidence of a disruption in a physiological mechanism underlying age-related anorexia is substantial. Nonetheless, psychosocial states are known to influence energy regulation and their effect on age-related anorexia are addressed in detail elsewhere *(47,62,63)*. Briefly, investigations evaluating possible psychological mechanisms effecting age-related anorexia have found that depression is the leading cause of weight loss *(64)*. This finding is significant when considering that the rates of depression are significantly greater in the elderly than the rates observed in younger age groups, due primarily to the greater likelihood of life-altering events (i.e., death of spouse, loneliness, social isolation, and so on). Most investigations have found that when the depression is treated by antidepressant drug therapy and/or conventional psychological counseling, the refusal to eat is eliminated. The key to successful treatment of depression-related anorexia of aging is early detection and treatment.

The initial descriptive accounts of possible biological mechanisms that may underlie age-related anorexia tended to focus on physical and pathological conditions that result in a decrease in food intake. For example, patients with Alzheimer's disease will often forget to eat and/or eat less during mealtime as a result of a heightened degree of distraction. Athlin et al. *(65)* reported that patients with Parkinson's disease have altered taste and smell perception, have difficulty with the motor skills necessary for eating, and may

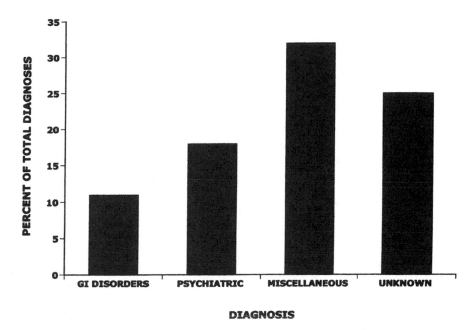

Fig. 1. Weight loss associated with a specific diagnosis in an outpatient population. (Adapted with permission from Wallace and Schwartz [66].)

take drugs that decrease hunger. Other descriptive investigations attribute an age-related decrease in food intake to underlying disease (e.g., cancer and stroke), drug interactions, indirect self-destructive behavior, and immobility.

4.4. Possible Biological Mechanisms of Age-Related Anorexia

Psychosocial and pathological causes of age-related anorexia account for less then 25% of the cases reported (66) (see Fig. 1). At least 35% of diagnosed cases of age-related anorexia or excessive body-weight loss are idiopathic. This finding supports the suggestion that the development of age-related anorexia has, at least in part, a biological basis that is independent of a primary disease. The identification of the mechanism underlying the age-related decrease in hunger is confounded by the fact that control of food intake involves an extensive array of effectors and proposed mechanisms that are not completely understood. Because of the interaction of biology and behavior in the control of food intake, the majority of investigations evaluating the biological mechanism of age-related anorexia have focused on a possible disruption in neural regulation.

Various investigators have noted that older subjects feel satiated sooner during meals as compared to younger individuals. These findings have led some to suggest that regulatory signals from the gut may stimulate the satiety center of the brain, in turn, decreasing long-term food intake. Although the precise signal involved is undetermined, cholecystokinin (CCK), a well-characterized short-term satiating hormone arising from the gut and acting on the vagus nerve, may have a role. At least one animal study has found an increase in satiety in older vs younger rats following intraperitoneal injection of CCK-8 (68). However, we are unaware of investigations directly evaluating the effect of CCK on the vagus nerve, and no studies on the role of CCK in human age-related anorexia have been published. Morely et al. *(69)* suggest that early satiation may reflect diminished concentration of nitric oxide (NO). Nitric oxide may delay gastric emptying and, in turn, may increase CCK release and satiation. These investigators found a decrease in mRNA for gastric NO synthase in aging rats and suggested that the diminution of NO leads to gastric relaxation and feelings of satiation. The effect of NO on the age-related increase in meal satiation is unknown.

The importance of the hypothalamus in the control of food intake has been identified in earlier experiments *(67)*, and current experiments have continued to elucidate the role of this neural center in the development of age-related anorexia. Neural peptide Y (NPY), a hypothalamic neural transmitter, stimulates food intake and is a long-term modulator of energy balance. Several investigations have shown decreased concentrations of hypothalamic NPY in aging vs younger rats *(70–72)*. Our laboratory has conducted several investigations that suggest a role for NPY in the mechanism that underlies diminished food intake of senescent rats. We found that senescent rats displaying rapid spontaneous weight loss (our model of age-related anorexia) have significantly smaller meals of shorter duration than do age-matched rats that are maintaining weight *(73)*. Moreover, meal frequency did not differ between presenescent (weight stable) and senescent rats, clearly demonstrating altered feeding behavior as one cause of age-related anorexia. The consumption of shorter, smaller meals despite progressively declining body weight (which averaged 5% at the end of the experiment) implies dysfunction in both short- and long-term regulation of energy balance.

Given the importance of NPY to the control of food intake, we then tested the hypothesis that the dysfunction in the regulation of energy balance seen in our model for age-related anorexia reflected altered response to this neural transmitter. We found that the senescent (rapid weight loss) rats ate 75% less food following an intrahypothalamic injection of NPY than during their weight-stable (presenescent) period *(74)* (*see* Fig. 2). This investigation supports our general hypothesis that age-related anorexia has a biological component independent of psychological behavior.

Although our data provide compelling evidence that NPY has a substantial role in the development of age-related anorexia, many questions remain. Because the expression of NPY is regulated, in part, by leptin, what is the interaction between this hormone and NPY during age-related anorexia? Most importantly, what effect, if any, does NPY have on food intake in the aged and how can this knowledge be transferred to an effective preventative/curative agent for age-related anorexia?

5. SUMMARY

The deficiencies in our understanding of the process of biological aging are particularly evident with regard to the interface between normal deteriorative changes observed in all individuals and clear, definable disease. The interaction between normal aging and disease is further complicated by the effects of nutrition. Recent studies confirm that whereas 25–30% of the US population aged 65 yr and older has type 2 diabetes or impaired glucose tolerance, aging *per se* has little effect on glucose tolerance. This fact is underscored by the observation that the most rapid increase in the rate of type 2 diabetes is not in the elderly but in adults aged 30–50 yr. It is more likely that the dramatic increase in the incidence of type 2 diabetes is a result of a higher prevalence of obesity (up by approx 33% in the past decade), resulting from changing dietary habits and lack of

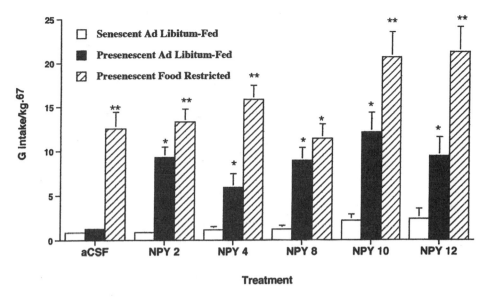

Fig. 2. Food intake at the first meal post-intracerebroventricular injection of neuropeptide Y (NPY) in old (24–30 mo; $n = 11$) rats. aCSF, artificial cerebrospinal fluid; NPY2–NPY12 is doses in μg of NPY. (With permission from Blanton et al. *[74]*.)

physical activity. In the case of gastrointestinal function, a biological mechanism for age-related nutrient malabsorption has not been determined. However, micronutrient malabsorption, particularly of cobalamin, may result from intestinal disorders such as chronic infection with *H. pylori*, an infection prevalent in the elderly population. A decline in food intake is also prevalent in the elderly. Although there are psychosocial and pathological causes of reduced food intake with aging, the "anorexia of aging" may also have a biological basis that is independent of any primary disease.

6. RECOMMENDATIONS FOR CLINICIANS

1. Aging is not a disease and should not be viewed as such. The process of aging comprises numerous physiological and psychological changes that may be beneficial (wisdom) or troublesome (presbyopia), but rarely are these changes life-threatening.
2. Aging *per se* does not cause disease, but the incidence of various diseases often increases as a function of age. Most forms of cardiovascular disease and cancer are more prevalent in older vs younger populations, however, it is important that clinicians look for an underlying cause of disease in older individuals, as is done with any other patient, and not view disease in the elderly as an inevitable consequence of aging.
3. Although genetics is known to be a critical component of the aging process, modifiable environmental factors also play an important role in determining the length and quality of an individual's life. Most of these factors, including obesity, smoking, physical inactivity, and diet, are subject to clinical intervention.

7. ACKNOWLEDGMENTS

This work was supported by National Institutes of Health Grant AG06665 and a gift from the California Age Research Institute.

REFERENCES

1. Weindruch R. Animal models. In: Masoro EJ (ed.) Handbook of Physiology: Aging. Oxford University Press, New York, 1995, pp. 37–52.
2. Holloszy J. Longevity of exercising male rats: effect of an antioxidant supplemented diet. Mech Ageing Dev 1998;100:211–219.
3. King H, Aubert RE, Herman WH. Global burden of diabetes 1995–2025. Prevalence, numerical estimates and projections. Diabetes Care 1998;21:1414–1431.
4. Hsueh WA, Law RE. Cardiovascular risk continuum: implications of insulin resistance and diabetes. Am J Med 1998;105:4S–14S.
5. Kawamori R. Asymptomatic hyperglycaemia and early atherosclerotic changes. Diabetes Res Clin Pract 1998;40 (Suppl):S35–S42.
6. Coutinho M, Gerstein HC, Wang Y, Yusuf S. The relationship between glucose and incident cardiovascular events: a metaregression analysis of published data from 20 studies of 95,783 individuals followed for 12.4 years. Diabetes Care 1999;22:233–240.
7. Fedele D, Giugliano D. Peripheral diabetic neuropathy. Current recommendations and future prospects for its prevention and management. Drugs 1997;54:414–421.
8. Watts GF, Playford DA. Dyslipoproteinaemia and hyperoxidative stress in the pathogenesis of endothelial dysfunction in non-insulin dependent diabetes mellitus: an hypothesis. Atherosclerosis 1998;141:17–30.
9. Diwadkar VA, Anderson JW, Bridges SR, Gowri MS, Oelgten PR. Postprandial low-density lipoproteins in type 2 diabetes are oxidized more extensively than fasting diabetes and control samples. Proc Soc Exper Biol Med 1999;222:178–184.
10. Fink RI, Wallace P, Olefsky JM. Effects of aging on glucose-mediated glucose disposal and glucose transport. J Clin Invest 1986;77:2034–2041.
11. Reaven GM, Chen N, Hollenbeck C, Chen Y-D. Effect of age on glucose tolerance and glucose uptake in healthy individuals. J Am Geriat Soc 1989;37:735–740.
12. Rowe JW, Minaker KL, Pallotta JA, Flier JS. Characterization of the insulin resistance of aging. J Clin Invest 1983;71:1581–1587.
13. Palumbo PJ, Elveback LR, Chu CP, Connolly DC, Kurland LT. Diabetes mellitus: incidence, prevalence, survivorship, and causes of death in Rochester, Minnesota. Diabetes 1976;25:566–573.
14. Kreisberg RA. Aging, glucose metabolism, and diabetes: current concepts. Geriatrics 1987;42:67–76.
15. Boden G, Chen X, DeSantis RA, Kendrick Z. Effects of age and body fat on insulin resistance in healthy men. Diabetes Care 1993;16:728–733.
16. Ferrannini E, Vichi S, Beck-Nielsen H. Insulin action and age. European Group for the Study of Insulin Resistance (EGIR). Diabetes 1996;45:947–953.
17. Paolisso G, Gambardella A, Ammendola S. Glucose tolerance and insulin action in healthy centenarians. Am J Physiol 1996;270:E890–E894.
18. Ruhe RC, McDonald RB. Carbohydrate metabolism and aging. In: Watson RR, ed. Handbook of Nutrition in the Aged. CRC Press, Boca Raton, 2000, pp. 205–237.
19. Mokdad AH, Ford ES, Bowman BA, et al. Diabetes trends in the US: 1990–1998. Diabetes Care 2000;23:1278–1283.
20. Heath GW, Gavin JR, Hinderliter JM, Hagberg JM, Bloomfield SA, Holloszy JO. Effects of exercise and lack of exercise on glucose tolerance and insulin sensitivity. J Appl Physiol 1983;55:512–517.
21. Flegal KM, Carroll MD, Kuczmarski RJ, Johnson CL. Overweight and obesity in the United States: prevalence and trends, 1960–1994. Int J Obes 1998;22:39–47.
22. Kohrt WM, Kirwan JP, Staten MA. Insulin resistance in aging is related to abdominal obesity. Diabetes 1993;42:273–281.
23. Wannamethee SG, Shaper AG. Weight change and duration of overweight and obesity in the incidence of type 2 diabetes. Diabetes Care 1999;22:1266–1272.
24. Seidell JC. Time trends in obesity: an epidemiological perspective. Horm Metab Res 1998;21:155–158.
25. Resnick HE, Valsania P, Halter JB, Lin X. Relation of weight gain and weight loss on subsequent diabetes risk in overweight adults. J Epidemiol Community Health 2000;54:596–602.
26. Cox JH, Cortright RN, Dohm GL, Houmard JA. Effect of aging on response to exercise training in humans: skeletal muscle GLUT4 and insulin sensitivity. J Appl Physiol 1999;86:2019–2025.

27. Holt PR. The gastrointestinal tract. In: Masoro EJ (ed.) Handbook of Physiology: Aging. Oxford University Press, New York, 1995, pp. 505–554.

28. Feibush JM, Holt PR. Impaired absorptive capacity for carbohydrate in the aged. Dig Dis Sci 1982;27:1095–1100.

29. Dubick WG, Armbrecht HJ. Changes in intestinal glucose transport over the lifespan of the rat. Mech Ageing Dev 1987;39:91–102.

30. Kendall MJ. The influence of age on the xylose absorption test. Gut 1970;11:498–501.

31. Hollander D, Dadufalza VD. Intestinal exsorption of oleic acid: influence of aging, bile, pH and ethanol. J Nutr 1983;113:511–518.

32. Russell RM. The aging process as a modifier of metabolism. Am J Clin Nutr 2000;72:529S–32S.

33. Nordin BE, Need AG, Steurer T, Morris HA, Chatterton BE, Horowitz M. Nutrition, osteoporosis, and aging. Ann NY Acad Sci 1998;854:336–351.

34. Agnusdei D, Civitelli R, Camporeale A, et al. Age-related decline of bone mass and intestinal calcium absorption in normal males. Calcif Tissue Int 1998;63:197–201.

35. Wood RJ, Fleet JC, Cashman K, Bruns ME, Deluca HF. Intestinal calcium absorption in the aged rat: evidence of intestinal resistance to 1,25(OH)2 vitamin D. Endocrinology 1998;139:3843–3848.

36. Lindenbaum J, Rosenberg IH, Wilson PW, Stabler SP, Allen RH. Prevalence of cobalamin deficiency in the Framingham elderly population. Am J Clin Nutr 1994;60:2–11.

37. Pennypacker LC, Allen RH, Kelly JP, et al. High prevalence of cobalamin deficiency in elderly outpatients. J Am Geriat Soc 1992;40:1197–1204.

38. Ferraris RP, Hsiao J, Hernandez R, Hirayama B. Site density of mouse intestinal glucose transporters declines with age. Am J Physiol 1993;264.G285–G293.

39. Toillet L, Tacnet F, Ripoche P, Corman B. Effect of aging on zinc and histidine transport across rat intestinal brush-border membranes. Mech Ageing Dev 1995;79:151–167.

40. Ferraris RP, Vinnakota RR. The time course of adaptation of intestinal nutrient uptake in mice is independent of age. J Nutr 1995;25:2175–2182.

41. Carmel R. Cobalamin, the stomach, and aging. Am J Clin Nutr 1997;66:750–759.

42. Hughes D, Elwood PC, Shinton NK. Clinical trial of the effect of vitamin B12 in elderly sujects with low serum B12 levels. Br Med J 1970;2:458–460.

43. Stabler P, Lindernbaum J, Allen R. Vitamin B12 deficiency in the elderly: current dilemmas. J Clin Nutr 1997:741–749.

44. Daily dietary fat and total food energy intakes. Third National Health and Nutrition Examination Survey, phase III 1988–1991, Morbid Mortal Weekly Rep 1994;43:116–125.

45. Hallfrisch J, Muller D, Drinkwater D. Continuing trends in men: the Baltimore Longitudinal Study of Aging (1961–1987). J Gerontol 1990;45:M186–M191.

46. Koehler KM. The New Mexico Aging Process Study. Nutr Rev 1994; 8 (Suppl):S34–S37.

47. Morley JE. Anorexia of aging: physiologic and pathologic. Am J Clin Nutr 1997;66:760–773.

48. Chumlea WC, Garry PJ, Hunt WC, Rhyne RL. Distributions of serial changes in stature and weight in a healthy elderly population. Hum Bio 1988;60:917–925.

49. Steen B, Isaksson B, Svanborg A. Body composition at 70 and 75 years of age: a longitudinal population study. J Clin Exper Gerontol 1979;1:185–192.

50. McGandy RB, Russell RM, Hartz SC, et al. Nutritional status survey of healthy noninstitutionalized elderly: Energy and nutrient intakes from three-day diet records and nutrient supplements. Nutr Res 1986;6:785.

51. Mowe M, Bohmer T, Kindt E. Reduced nutritional status in an elderly population (> 70 y) is probable before disease and possibly contributes to the development of disease. Am J Clin Nutr 1994;59:317–324.

52. O'Hanlon P, Kohrs MB. Dietary studies of older Americans. Am J Clin Nutr 1978;31:1257.

53. Launer LJ, Harris T, Rumpel C, Madans J. Body mass index, weight change, and risk of mobility disability in middle-aged and older women. The epidemiologic follow-up study of NHANES I. JAMA 1994;271:1093–1098.

54. Silver AJ, Morley JE, Strome SS, Jones D, Vickers L. Nutritional status in an academic nursing home. J Am Geriat Soc 1988;36:487.

55. McCue JD. The naturalness of dying. JAMA 1995;273:1039–1043.

56. Roberts S. Effects of Aging on Energy Requirements and the Control of Food Intake in Men. J Gerontol Series A 1995;50A:101–106.

57. Rolls B, Dimeo K, Shide D. Age-related impairments in the regulation of food intake. Am J Clin Nutr 1995;62:923–931.
58. Clarkston WK, Pantano MM, Morley JE, Horowitz M, Littlefield JM, Burton FR. Evidence for the anorexia of aging: gastrointestinal transit and hunger in healthy elderly vs. young adults. Am J Physiol 1997; 272.
59. Evans WJ, Campbell WW. Sarcopenia and age-related changes in body composition and functional capacity. J Nutr 1993;123:465–846.
60. Thompson JS, Robbins J, Cooper JK. Nutritional and immune function in the geriatric population. Clin Geriat Med 1987;3:309.
61. Folstein MF, Folstein SE, McHugh PR. Mini-mental state. J Psych Res 1975;12:189–198.
62. Egbert AM. The dwindles: failure to thrive in older patients. Nutr Rev 1996;54:S25–S30.
63. Marcus E-L, Berry EM. Refusal to eat in the elderly. Nutr Rev 1998;56:163–171.
64. Morley JE, Morley P. Psychological and social factors in the pathogenesis of weight loss. Ann Rev Gerontol Geriat 1995;15:83–109.
65. Athlin E, Norberg A, Axelsson K, Möller A, Nordström G. Aberrant eating behavior in elderly parkinsonian patients with and without dementia: analysis of video-recorded meals. Res Nurs Health 1989;12:41–51.
66. Wallace JI, Schwartz RS. Involuntary weight loss in elderly outpatients: recognition, etiologies, and treatment. Clin Geriat Med 1997;13:717–735.
67. Anand BK, Brobeck JR. Hypothalamic control of food intake in rats and cats. Yale J Biol Med 1951;24:123–140.
68. Miyasaka K, Kanai S, Ohta M, Funakoshi A. Aging impairs release of central and peripheral cholecystokinin (CCK) in male but not in female rats. J Gerontol 1997;52A:M14–M18.
69. Morley JE, Kumar VB, Mattammal MB, Farr S, Morley PM, Flood JF. Inhibition of feeding by a nitric oxide synthase inhibitor: effects of aging. Euro J Pharmacol 1996;311:15–19.
70. Cha C, Young I, Lee E. Age-related changes of VIP,NPY and somatostatin-immunoreactive neurons in the cerebral cortex of aged rats. Brain Res 1997;753:235–244.
71. Kowalski C, Micheau J, Corder R, Gaillard R, Conte-Devolx B. Age-related changes in cortico-releasing factor, somatostatin, neuropeptide Y, methionine enkephalin and B-endorphin in specific rat brain areas. Brain Res 1992;582:38–46.
72. Lemierre S, Rouch C, Nicolaidis S, Orosco M. Combined effect of obesity and aging on feeding-induced monoamine release in the rostromedial hypothalamus of the Zucker rat. Int J Obes 1998;22:993–999.
73. Blanton CA, Geitzen DW, Griffey SM, Horwitz BA, McDonald RB, Murtagh-Mark C. Meal patterns associated with the age-related decline in food intake in the Fischer 344 rat. Am J Physiol: Regulatory, Integrative, and Comparitive Physiololgy. 1999;275:R1494–R1502.
74. Blanton CA, Horwitz BA, Blevins JE, Hamilton JS, Hernandez EJ, McDonald RB. Reduced feeding response to neuropeptide Y in senescent Fischer 344 rats. Am J Physiol: Regulatory, Integrative, Comparitive Physiology 2001;280:R1052–R1060.
75. Carmel R, Perez-Perez GI, Blaser MJ. Helicobacter pylori infection and food-cobalamin malabsorption. Dig Dis Sci 1994;39:309–314.

4

The Status of Nutrition in Older Adults

A European Perspective

Lisette C. P. G. M. de Groot
and Wija A. van Staveren

1. INTRODUCTION

In the European Community the major causes of mortality at old age are diseases in which lifestyle plays an important role *(1)*. Internationally, cardiovascular disease is the leading cause of death in people over the age of 65, with deaths from cancer ranking a close second. At the age of 65, men and women in developed countries have a life expectancy of 15–20 yr. The evidence suggests that improvements in nutrition, along with changes in other lifestyle factors, may make these years healthier, more active, and allow elders to be less dependent on others *(2,3)*. Nutrition, physical activity, and the use of medicine are among the major modifiable lifestyle factors of concern. These factors are affected by societal and cultural influences that have contributed to pronounced diversity in food patterns and, consequently, in health patterns among elderly Europeans *(4,5)*. Approximately 10 yr ago, it was acknowledged that in order to obtain information on how to age in good health, this diversity should receive research attention, and this should be accomplished before Europe reaches a situation with much less variability in food intake. Therefore, in 1988, a major longitudinal European multicenter study, Survey on Nutrition and the Elderly, a Concerted Action (SENECA), was initiated to study cross-cultural differences in nutritional issues and lifestyle factors affecting health and performance of elderly people in Europe. Seneca was also the name of a philosopher, who stated in one of his letters to Lucilius: "Do not compare the incomparable." Using strictly standardized methodologies both over time and across Europe, this statement was put to the test in the SENECA surveys in 1988/89 (baseline), in 1993/94 (follow-up), and in SENECA's FINALE in 1999.

2. PURPOSE AND METHODS OF THE STUDY

The purpose of SENECA was to examine the relationships of health and survival in relation to the variable dietary and lifestyle patterns of elderly people in Europe. The study was carried out in several stages. All protocols in this multistage study were highly

From: *Handbook of Clinical Nutrition and Aging*
Edited by: C. W. Bales and C. S. Ritchie © Humana Press Inc., Totowa, NJ

Table 1
Towns and Parent Countries of the SENECA Study

Site, country	Abbreviation	Latitude in degrees north
Elverum, Norway	E/N	61
Roskilde, Denmark*	R/DK	56
Marki, Poland	M/PL	52
Monor, Hungary	M/H	47
Culemborg, The Netherlands*	C/NL	52
Hamme, Belgium*	H/B	51
Haguenau, France*	H/F	49
Chateau Renault		
Amboise, France	Ca/F	48
Romans, France*	R/F	45
Bellinzona, Switzerland	Be/CH	46
Yverdon, Switzerland*	Y/CH	47
Burgdorf, Switzerland	Bu/CH	47
Bentazos, Spain*	B/E	43
Fara Sabina-Magliano		
Sabina-Poggio Mirteto, Italy	FMP/I	42
Padua, Italy*	P/I	46
Vila Franca de Xira, Portugal*	V/P	39
Coimbra, Portugal	C/P	40
Anogia-Archanges, Greece	AA/GR	35
Markopoulou, Greece	M/GR	30

*Towns included in stage 2 follow-up and FINALE of SENECA.

standardized because of the cross-cultural nature of this study. To insure that the data collection was consistent across participating sites and countries, a common core protocol prescribed the methodology for the study and laid out a common manual of operations. In addition, blood sampling materials were supplied from a central source, and blood analyses were conducted in central laboratories.

2.1. Stage 1

The first SENECA (1988–1989), consisted of an initial baseline survey of 2586 subjects randomly selected from 18 towns across 12 European countries (*see* Table 1).

The sample population was stratified by sex and limited to persons born between the years 1913 and 1918. Criteria for exclusion included those persons living in a psychogeriatric nursing home, persons not fluent in the language of their current country of residence, and persons not able to answer the questions independently. The participation rate for stage one was about 51%. All subjects were asked to complete questionnaires, providing a range of information, e.g., sociodemographic information, dietary food habits, lifestyle, and overall health.

Subjects completed a modified dietary history, designed to capture the subjects' food and nutrient intake, along with the subjects' anthropometry. A blood sample was analyzed for serum concentrations of vitamins, A, D, E, B_6, B_{12}, folic acid, and carotenes, serum lipids, and blood levels of albumin, hemoglobin, and hematocrit. All diet data were analyzed and compared to the Mediterranean diet score developed by Trichopoulou *(6)*

Table 2
Number of Participants Per SENECA Center at Baseline,
BMI (kg/m^2) and Percentage Deceased at FINALE

	Men				Women			
	Total				Total			
	N	BMI	SD	Deceased	N	BMI	SD	Deceased
H/B	126	25.2	3.3	56	105	28.3	4.1	29
R/DK	101	25.5	3.2	54	101	5.2	4.7	36
H/F	109	27.1	3.6	54	110	27.6	5.7	23
R/F	142	26.5	3.5	54	137	25.4	4.6	23
P/I	97	26.1	3.5	48	93	24.9	4.2	22
C/NL	114	26.1	3.0	59	124	27.6	4.2	32
V/P	111	27.0	3.6	46	111	27.5	4.5	33
B/E	88	27.7	3.6	49	119	28.6	4.4	28
Y/CH	123	26.8	3.9	48	126	26.3	4.2	25
Bu/CH	30	27.4	4.0	47	30	27.7	5.1	23
Be/CH	30	26.9	4.6	47	30	27.6	3.7	38
M/PL	19	27.4	5.7	67	23	30.5	7.9	36
Total	1090			52	1109			28

See Table 1 for abbreviations.

to assess quality. The diet data was scaled to a median value of 10.5 MJ (2500 kcal) for men and 8.4 MJ (2000 kcal) for women. Items in the subjects' intake that closely resembled those items in the Mediterranean diet were coded "one," and all other items were coded, "zero."

2.2. Follow-Up Survey

A follow-up survey of 1170 subjects living in 9 of the selected 18 towns (Table 1), ranging in age from 74 to 79 was conducted in 1993. The follow-up survey consisted of the same measures collected in stage one, but also included a physical performance test of Reuben and Sin *(7)*, the Geriatric Depression Scale *(8)*, the Mini-Mental State Examination described by Folstein et al. *(9)*, and some additional biochemical measures in certain testing areas.

2.3. FINALE

In 1999, a final longitudinal assessment of the subjects in the nine towns selected for stage two was conducted. Survival rates and causes of death for the subjects were recorded. No data on food consumption was collected during this stage, and not all testing centers obtained blood samples.

3. HIGHLIGHTS OF THE STUDY

Table 2 summarizes the number and distribution of SENECA participants and also shows the percentage decline in numbers of surviving subjects at the final assessment in 1999. Results from the comparative cross-sectional phase of the study showed that, in general, the variability from site to site was great for many of the parameters studied *(4)*.

Although participation was somewhat selective (the most healthy and active subjects were more willing to continue their involvement), 4-yr changes in diet, indicators of nutritional status and health were all in an unfavorable direction *(5)*, with numbers of living subjects at each site at the 10-yr finale, ranging from 33% to 64% for men and 62% to 78% for women.

3.1. Anthropometry

A geographical gradient was found for height, with the tallest subjects (both male and female) residing in the northern European towns. In all centers, women were smaller than men, weighed less, had thicker triceps skinfold, and a lower waist-hip ratio. Mean body mass index (BMI) varied at baseline for the 12 towns from 25.2 to 27.7 kg/m^2 for men and 24.9 to 30.5 kg/m^2 *(see* Table 2) for women. The prevalence of BMI values exceeding 30 kg/m^2 was high, ranging from 8% to 43% in men and 4% to 56% in women. These results indicated an increased risk for disabilities. In contrast, BMI values below 20 kg/m^2 were also found in a significant number of subjects in several towns. Low BMIs reflect low lean body mass reserves and possible malnutrition; subnormal BMI may also be a sign of an ongoing and as yet undiagnosed disease. Although small-to-modest average changes in height, body weight, and circumferences emerged over SENECA's 10-yr follow-up period, a significant proportion of subjects had considerable gains or losses of body weight. In particular, a weight loss of >3 kg over the 10 yr period emerged as predictive for mortality *(10)*.

3.2. Malnutrition

A number of risk factors for malnutrition or weight loss are included in Morley's mnemonic MEALS on WHEELS *(11)*, in Robbins's 9 D's *(12)*, as well in the list of 11 dwindles of failure to thrive by Egbert *(13)* *(see* Fig. 1). Several of these factors were highly prevalent among SENECA's follow-up participants, e.g., dementia 9% and depression 20% *(14)*. Correspondingly, according to the Mini-Nutritional Assessment, a tool for the application of nutritional screening *(15)*, 44% of the study population was at risk for malnutrition *(16)*. Despite the limited value of this risk-appraisal questionnaire for identifying malnutrition in the apparently healthy elderly *(16)*, it emphasizes the importance of timely signaling of impending poor nutritional status. These previously mentioned findings indicate that some "healthy" elderly people are on the edge of a negative energy balance. Not only do they have increased energy requirements relative to the recommendations, but they also exhibit a profound loss of ability to control energy intake *(17)*. Their taste sensitivity may also decline substantially with age *(18)*. An understanding of all physical, social, and psychological conditions that may lead to failure to thrive is needed for the early detection and prevention of malnutrition.

3.3. Obesity

Although the SENECA results did reveal problems with undernutrition, our data also raised concern about the prevalence of obesity, which is growing among older persons. In SENECA, a reduction of 1.5–2 cm in height over an age span of 10 yr was observed *(10)*.

As a result of such a decrease in height with age, the BMI will be overestimated. The utility of the BMI index is further affected in the elderly by changes in body composition with aging. Relative obesity (BMI > 30) was highly prevalent among men and women,

Dwindles and D's

delirium	disease	dentition
drinking alc.	dementia	diarrhoea
desertion	drugs	dysfunction
destitution	dysphagia	
despair	dysgeusia	
	depression	

Fig. 1. Based on the D's and Dwindles: a mnemonic for the precipitants of geriatric failure to thrive. Adapted from Egbert 1996 *(13)* and Robbins 1989 *(12)*.

Table 3
Mean Serum Total Cholesterol (in mmol/L) in SENECA Participants

Site*	Latitude degrees North	N	Cholesterol Men (Mean)	N	Women (Mean)
R/DK	56	64	5.7	53	6.7
C/NL	52	46	5.5	59	6.4
H/B	51	64	6.0	60	6.2
H/F	49	49	5.6	46	6.0
Y/CH	47	59	5.8	64	6.3
R/F	45	65	5.6	54	6.4
B/E	43	31	5.5	41	6.2
V/P	39	68	5.3	70	6.0

*For abbrevations, *see* Table 1. Not all sites participated in the follow-up study.

approx 20%, however, an increase of intra-abdominal body fat based on changes in waist circumference in the SENECA might be more indicative for increased risk. Unfortunately, there is no clear criteria for what constitutes excessive body fat in old age *(5,19,20)*. More longitudinal observations of obese older subjects and well-controlled intervention studies inducing weight loss in overweight or obese elders are needed before we can understand the best way to achieve intentional weight loss in the overweight elderly.

3.4. Serum Albumin, Hemoglobin, Hematocrit, and Lipids

The baseline serum albumin, hemoglobin and hematocrit levels and also the longitudinal changes observed in 1993/94 indicated a relative good overall health of the SENECA population. However, these parameters are known to be better indicators of disease status than indicators of the nutritional or health status *(21)* *(see* Chapter 5).

The trends of serum lipid levels, especially those of LDL cholesterol, indicate that on average the participants from the Southern centers had slightly lower lipid levels than those in Northern centers *(see* Table 3). In addition, total cholesterol concentrations decreased substantially, 12% in men and 10% in women during the first 4 yr of the study. In contrast, concentrations of high-density lipoprotein (HDL) cholesterol and triglycerides over the same time period remained quite stable (5). Despite selective mortality, a number of cohort studies in the elderly support the notion that serum cholesterol and lipoprotein abnormalities predict cardiovascular disease in older adults. The more favorable survival rates in the southern European centers as compared to the northern centers are in agreement with this line of thinking (22).

3.5. Serum Vitamin D and Vitamin B_{12}

Additional nutritional concerns have emerged concerning the adequacy of the circulating levels of vitamins D and vitamin B_{12}. Regardless of geographical location, elderly Europeans were at substantial risk of having an inadequate vitamin D status in the winter. Unexpectedly, lower median 25 hydroxyvitamin D [25(OH)D], serum concentrations were observed in elderly southern Europeans than were found in elderly northern Europeans. These low 25(OH)D concentrations could generally be explained by reduced sunlight exposure and indicators of physical health status (23). This tendency of reduced sun exposure, accompanied by the age-associated decline in the capacity to synthesize provitamin D_3 in skin and hydroxylate vitamin D_3 in kidneys may lead to a reduced "endogenous" vitamin D supply. Additionally, as Western diets generally provide only 25–50% of the current recommended vitamin D intake, supplementation at old age would appear to be advisable in the population represented in SENECA, especially in the winter.

Because atrophic gastritis is suspected to be common in older people, the presence of this disorder was studied in relation to cobalamin deficiency in the Dutch SENECA cohort. Mild cobalamin deficiency (prevalence of 23.8%) was common in this cohort of the elderly. Unfortunately, this could be explained in only 28% of the study population by inadequate cobalamin intake (median intake: 5 µg/d) or severe atrophic gastritis, which was present in 13% of the follow-up participants. In another 20% of participants, the low cobalamin levels had no clear explanation (24). These findings have raised many questions that need further investigation: addressing vitamin B_{12} metabolism in the elderly; bioavailability of vitamin B_{12} from various food sources; and the clinical significance of various markers of low of vitamin B_{12} status (25,26).

3.6. Evaluation of Micronutrient Intakes

Population-based nutritional surveys—including SENECA—have shown a gradual decline in total energy intake at old age (27,28). This decline in total food intake inevitably jeopardizes the adequacy of micronutrient intake. To ensure an adequate micronutrient supply for elderly people, a minimum daily energy intake level of 1500 kcal/d has been suggested (29). Although in the SENECA study, the prevalence of inadequate micronutrient intake decreased gradually as energy intake increased, no single criterion cut-off value for energy intake could be identified. Overall, 24% of the men and 47% of the women had inadequate intakes of one or more micronutrients, according to the lowest European Recommendations (30). However, in the SENECA participants with energy intakes above the reference value of 1500 kcal/d, 19% of men and 26% of women had an inadequate nutrient intake (31).

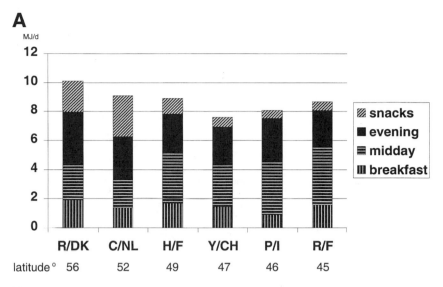

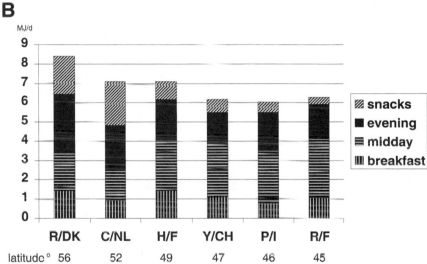

Fig. 2. Energy intake at different meals as percentage of total energy intake, MJ/d, SENECA follow-up study in 1993 in six study centers for men (**A**) and women (**B**). Adapted from de Groot et al. *(32)*.

3.7. Meal Patterns, the Selection of Food Groups, and Dietary Quality

The identification of meal patterns and the selection of food groups is essential for improving diet and nutritional status. Energy intake at different meals in six study centers during the follow-up study is given in Fig. 2 for men (A) and women (B), respectively. A significant negative relation was observed between energy intake at midday and geographical latitude of the study town. For other main meals, no such relationship emerged. In general, the number of meals, including snacks or between meals, were higher in the northern centers than in the south *(32)*.

A

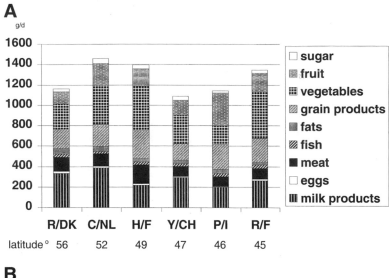

B

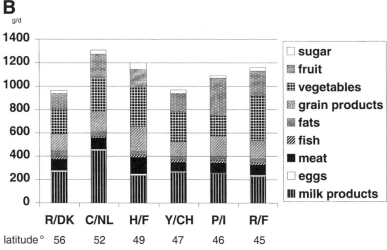

Fig. 3. Mean food group intake in men (**A**) and women (**B**), SENECA 1993. Adapted from de Groot et al. *(32).*

Dietary quality was evaluated in relation to the Greek variant of the traditional Mediterranean diet in several SENECA cohorts. Important characteristics of such a Mediterranean diet are *(32)*: a high contribution of olive oil, providing a high ratio of monounsaturated to saturated fatty acids even with a high total fat intake; a relatively high intake of omega-3 fatty acids, believed to play a role in the improvement of blood lipid parameters, blood clotting, arthritis, and depression; and a high intake of plant foods, good sources of several nutrients, such as folate and vitamin B_6, which are at risk of deficiency in older adults.

In Fig. 3A, B, food group intake data are ranked based on latitude. No clear north vs south pattern could be distinguished. However, in the northern towns (R/DK and C/NL), the elderly tended to eat more hard fats, luxury bread (e.g., croissants or Danish pastry)

Table 4
Hazard Ratios (HR)1 of Single Food Items and Totals of the Original and Adapted
Mediterranean Diet Score, for Male and Female Participants of the SENECA Population

	Men (N = 631) HR (95% CI)	Women (N = 650) HR (95% CI)
Monounsaturated: saturated fat ratio	0.87 (0.67–1.15)	0.88 (0.61–1.25)
Grains	0.80 (0.63–1.02)	1.00 (0.73–1.38)
Fruits and products	0.97 (0.76–1.22)	1.08 (0.78–1.49)
Vegetables	1.10 (0.88–1.39)	0.99 (0.72–1.36)
Legumes/nuts/seeds	0.97 (0.76–1.22)	1.07 (0.78–1.46)
Alcoholic beverages	1.17 (0.93–1.47)	1.18 (0.86–1.62)
Meat and poultry	0.74 (0.58–0.94)	1.35 (0.98–1.86)
Milk and milk products	0.92 (0.73–1.15)	1.12 (0.83–1.53)
oMDS	0.94 (0.74–1.19)	1.09 (0.78–1.54)
Fruits and products and vegetables	1.04 (0.83–1.31)	0.89 (0.65–1.22)
Alcoholic beverages	1.17 (0.93–1.47)	0.91 (0.63–1.30)
Meat and poultry	0.74 (0.58–0.94)	1.17 0.84–1.64)
Milk and milk products	1.01 (0.81–1.27)	0.68 (0.50–0.93)
aMDS	0.74 (0.55–1.00)	0.79 (0.55–1.13)

oMDS: cut-off values ≤ 3, > 3;aMDS: cut-off values ≤ 4, >> 4.

*HR adjusted for age at baseline, physical activity, smoking, region, and albumin. oMDS, original
Mediterranean Diet Score; aMDS, adapted Mediterranean Diet Score.

and sugar products than the participants in R/F and P/I. In the more southern towns,
subjects consumed more vegetable oils and fruits. H/F and Y/Ch had intermediate
intakes (32).

In our analyses, we adapted the original Mediterranean score as described by Haveman-
Nies et al. (33), so that the cutoff values for milk and meat are in more agreement with
dietary guidelines. With data from SENECA's FINALE, we looked into the predictive
value for survival of the original and adapted Mediterranean Diet Score (oMDS and
aMDS, respectively). Table 4 shows the data for both the total scores and the specific food
items comprising that score. As is shown in Table 4, the MDS coincided with improved
survival time in men and women, although the values did not reach significance in
women. The individual food items did not provide a clear predictive value. In women, the
adaptations to alcohol, meat, and milk in the model resulted in more favorable scores for
the three items (34).

In the southern centers, the mean MDS was better than the mean score observed in the
northern centers. Table 5 shows the mean scores of these centers and the predictive value
of both scores for survival. The oMDS did not seem to coincide with a beneficial effect
on survival. However, after adjustment for men and women in northern and southern
Europe, the hazard ratio's pointed for all groups in the same direction: a favorable score
is related to a better survival time (34).

Table 5
SENECA Mediterranean Diet Score (MDS) as Predictor of Survival Time: Rate Ratio Estimates
(Confidence Intervals) Derived From Cox's Models[*]

	Men				Women			
	N	Mean	HR	Score	N	Mean	HR	Score
North	391				392			
oMDS		3.4	0.91	(0.69–1.21)		3.5	0.95	(0.64–1.40)
aMDS		2.9	0.78	(0.50–1.20)		3.5	0.68	(0.40–1.16)
South	241				258			
oMDS		4.8	1.06	(0.63–1.77)		4.8	1.85	(0.74–4.65)
aMDS		4.3	0.73	(0.48–1.10)		4.5	0.90	(0.54–1.51)

[*] Models adjusted for age, smoking, physical activity, and albumin. oMDS, original Mediterranean Diet Score; aMDS, adapted Mediterranean Diet Score.

4. SUMMARY AND CONCLUSION

The purpose of the SENECA study was to study cross-cultural differences in nutritional issues and lifestyle factors affecting health and performance of the elderly in Europe. The study population in SENECA tended to represent the more healthy and better educated elderly in the towns studied. Large variability between, but also within, centers was observed in diet, lifestyle, health, and performance. In this chapter, we have focused on the food habits and food consumption data. Dietary quality was in general, better in the southern centers as opposed to the northern centers. The overall conclusion is that, in our elderly population, diet still matters for the optimal maintenance of health. Further analyses may reveal other lifestyle factors related to health and survival and may help to develop future intervention programs in this age group to maintain their quality of life. At least, these programs may partly answer the important questions raised approx 2000 yr ago by the philosopher SENECA: "You want to live? Do you know how to?"

REFERENCES

1. de Groot CPGM, van Staveren WA. SENECA's accomplishments and challenges. Nutr 2000;16:541–543.
2. World Health Organisation, Nutritional Guidelines for Healthy Aging, in press.
3. World Health Organisation, World Atlas of Aging. WHO Tech Ser 98.1, 1998.
4. de Groot CPGM, van Staveren WA, Hautvast JGAJ (eds.). EURONUT-SENECA. Nutrition and the elderly in Europe. Eur J Clin Nutr 1991;45(Suppl. 3):1–196.
5. de Groot CPGM, van Staveren WA, Dirren H, Hautvast JGAJ. SENECA, Nutrition and the elderly in Europe. Follow-up study and longitudinal analysis. Eur J Clin Nutr 1996;50(Suppl. 2):1–127.
6. Trichopoulou A, Kouris-Blaza A, Vassilakou T, Gnardellis C, Polychronopoulos E, Venizelos M, et al. Diet and survival of elderly Greeks: a link to the past. Am J Clin Nutr 1995;61(Suppl.):1346S–1350S.
7. Reuben DB, Sin AL. An objective measure of the physical function of elderly outpatients. JAGS 1990;38:1105–1112.
8. Sheikh JI, Yesavage JA. Geriatric depression scale (GDS). Recent evidence and development of a shorter version. Clin Geron 1986;5:165–173.
9. Folstein MF, Folstein SE, McHugh PR. "Mini-mental state". A practical method for grading the cognitive state of patients for the clinican. J Psychiatr Res 1975;12:189–198.

10. de Groot CPGM, Enzi G, Matthys C, Moreiras O, Roszkowski W, Schroll M. Ten-year changes in anthropometric characteristics of elderly Europeans. J Nutr Health Aging 2002;6:4–8.
11. Morley JE. Anorexia of ageing: physiologic and pathologic. Am J Clin Nutr 1997;66:760–773.
12. Robbins LJ. Evaluation of weight loss in the elderly. Geriatrics 1989;44:31–37.
13. Egbert AM. The dwindles: failure to thrive in older patients. Nutr Rev 1996;54:S25–S30.
14. Haller J, Weggemans RM, Ferry M, Guigoz Y. SENECA. Nutrition and the elderly in Europe. Mental health: minimental state examination and geriatric depression score of elderly Europeans in the SENECA study of 1993. Eur J Clin Nutr 1996;50(Suppl. 2):S112–S116.
15. Guigoz Y, Vellas B, Garry PJ. Assessing the nutritional status of the elderly: the Mini Nutritional Assessment as part of the geriatric evaluation. Nutr Rev 1996;54:S59–S65.
16. de Groot CPGM, Beck AM, Schroll M, van Staveren WA. Evaluating the DETERMINE Your Nutritional Health Checklist and the Mini Nutritional Assessment as tools to identify nutritional problems in elderly Europeans. Eur J Clin Nutr 1998;52:877–883.
17. Roberts SB, Fuss P, Heymann MB, et al. Control of food intake in older men. JAMA 1994;272:1601–1606.
18. de Graaf C, Polet P, van Staveren WA. Sensory perception and pleasantness of food flavors in elderly subjects. J Gerontol 1994;49:P93–P99.
19. Stevens J, Cai J, Pamuk ER, Williamson DF, Thun M, Wood JL. The effect of age on the association between body-mass index and mortality. N Eng J Med 1998;338:1–7.
20. Visser M, Langlois J, Guralnik JM, Cauley JA, Kronmal RA, Robbins J, et al. High body fatness but not low fat-free mass, predicts disability in older men and women: the Cardiovascular Health Study. Am J Clin Nutr 1998;68:584–590.
21. Whicher J, Spence C. When is serum albumin worth measuring? Ann Clin Biochem 1987;24:572–580.
22. Harris TB, Launer LJ, Madan J, Feldman JJ. Cohort study of the effect of being overweight and change in weight on risk of coronary heart disease in old age. BMJ 1997;314:1791–1794.
23. van der Wielen RPJ, Löwik MRH, van den Berg H, de Groot CPGM, Haller J, Moreiras O, van Staveren WA. Serum vitamin D concentrations among elderly people in Europe. Lancet 1995;346:207–210.
24. van Asselt DZB, de Groot CPGM van Staveren WA et al. Role of cobalamin intake and atrophic gastritis in mild cobalamin deficiency in older Dutch subjects. Am J Clin Nutr 1998;68:328–34.
25. Russell RM. Mild cobalamin deficiency in older Dutch subjects. Am J Clin Nutr 1998;68:222–223.
26. Dickinson CJ. Does folic acid harm people with vitamin B12 deficiency? Q J Med 1995;88:357–364.
27. Hallfrisch J, Muller D, Drinkwater T, Tobin J, Andres R. Continuing diet trends in men: The Baltimore Longitudinal Study of Aging (1961–1987). J Gerontol 1990;45:M186–M191.
28. Sjogren A, Osterberg T, Steen B. Intake of energy, nutrients and food items in a ten year cohort comparison and in a six year longitudinal perspective: A population study of 70- and 76- year old Swedish people. Age Ageing 1994;23:108–112.
29. Lowenstein F. Nutritional status of the elderly in the United States of America, 1971–1974. J Am Coll Nutr 1982;1:165–177.
30. Trichopoulou A, Vassilakou T. Recommended dietary intakes in Europe. Eur J Clin Nutr 1990; 44(Suppl 2):51–100.
31. de Groot CPGM, van den Broek T, van Staveren WA. Energy intake and micronutrient intake in elderly Europeans: seeking the minimum requirement in the SENECA study. Age Ageing 1999;28:469–474.
32. de Groot CPGM, Schlettwein-Gsell D, Schroll-Bjornsbo K, van Staveren WA. Meal patterns and food selection of elderly people from six European towns. Food Quality and Preference 1998;9:479–486.
33. Haveman-Nies A, Tucker KL, de Groot CPGM, Wilson PWF, van Staveren WA. Evaluation of dietary quality in relationship to nutritional and lifestyle factors in elderly people of the US Frammingham Heart Study and the European SENECA study. Eur J Clin Nutr 2001;55:870–880.
34. van Staveren WA, de Groot CPGM, Haveman-Nies A. The SENECA-study: potentials and problems in relating diet to survival over ten yr time. Public Health Nutr 2002;5:901–905.

II   Fundamentals of Geriatric Nutrition

5

Nutritional Assessment and Support in Chronic Disease Management

Margaret-Mary G. Wilson and John E. Morley

1. INTRODUCTION

Chronic disease, as defined by the National Center for Chronic Disease Prevention and Health Promotion refers to prolonged illnesses that rarely undergo spontaneous resolution or complete cure. More than 90 million Americans live with chronic disease. Such illnesses constitute the single largest cost to the US health care system, accounting for 60% of the US total health care costs (1). The increase in the prevalence of chronic disease over the past few decades is probably the result of the positive effect of lifestyle modifications and emerging therapeutic modalities on longevity. Therefore, the trade-off for increasing length of life in the older adult is inevitably an increase in the burden of chronic disease. Consequently, within the geriatric arena, treatment regimens focusing on secondary prevention prevail.

Research has shown that the primary causes of chronic morbidity and mortality in older adults are all influenced by diet (2). Nevertheless, existing evidence indicates that persons with chronic disease often receive inadequate nutritional management (3). Emerging data continues to spur a change in the traditional therapeutic approach to the management of chronic disease. Current therapeutic trends favor broadening manage ment goals to include related pathological and psychosocial domains of disease impact. This holistic approach has encouraged the development of highly efficient system level strategies and the delivery of well-integrated and coordinated multidisciplinary treatment plans (4). Nutritional evaluation and intervention is a critical and integral component of these management strategies.

2. PATHOPHYSIOLOGICAL CONSIDERATIONS

Weight loss is common in older adults with chronic disease (5,6). However, the effect of chronic diseases on body weight regulation in older adults has not been clearly elucidated. Previous studies using indirect calorimetry demonstrated an increase in resting energy expenditure in several chronic diseases. However, a review of recent studies using the doubly labeled water technique challenges the widely held notion that increased total energy expenditure is the pathophysiological mechanism underlying weight loss in

From: *Handbook of Clinical Nutrition and Aging*
Edited by: C. W. Bales and C. S. Ritchie © Humana Press Inc., Totowa, NJ

chronic diseases, such as dementia, Parkinson's disease, and cardiac failure. Paradoxically, in these studies, persons with Alzheimer's disease and significant unexplained weight loss demonstrated lower total daily energy expenditure. Similar findings have been obtained in those with Parkinson's disease and chronic heart failure (7–9). This observation may be explained by a disproportionate reduction in physical activity expenditure. The magnitude of the reduction in physical activity energy expenditure has been shown to exceed the increase in resting energy expenditure, resulting in a net reduction in total daily energy expenditure. These findings lend credence to the enduring intuitive concept that weight loss related to chronic disease, regardless of etiology, results primarily from reduced energy intake. One exception to this may be chronic obstructive pulmonary disease (COPD). In severe cases, the energy expended during breathing may result in a net increase in daily physical activity expenditure and consequent weight loss. However, reduced appetite and premature satiety associated with hypoxia may reduce food intake and precipitate weight loss in such cases. Therefore, nutritional intervention in persons with chronic disease should be considered a parallel intervention and addressed as a separate management issue. The traditional watch-and-wait approach, whereby it is expected that specific treatment of the underlying illness must have a positive therapeutic effect on nutritional status, is no longer justified based on objective data. Factors involved in the pathophysiology of weight loss in various chronic diseases are outlined in Table 1.

3. NUTRITIONAL ASSESSMENT

Evaluation of nutritional status is a critical, though often overlooked, component of comprehensive geriatric evaluation. Efficient evaluation strategies must acknowledge the dynamic interplay between psychosocial factors, physical function, and health status in determining nutritional status.

3.1. History

Initial history taking should seek to identify risk factors other than medical illness that pose a threat to the nutritional well-being of the older adult (see Table 2). The inevitable social transition that occurs with aging may have a deleterious effect on the nutritional status of the older adult. Regardless of economic circumstances, the aging adult will be challenged by compromised mobility of varying degrees. The inevitable thinning of the intimate support system and social network, resulting from bereavement and relocation, pose additional obstacles. Ongoing changes within the community may elicit a sense of insecurity within a previously safe environment. Additionally, the emergence of more sophisticated technology in a climate of aggressive consumerism may abruptly compromise purchasing and bargaining skills. Coexisting poverty introduces the added burden of multiple competing expenses, notably compromising the older adults ability to fulfill recommended dietary needs. Poorer older adults are also more likely to live in neighborhoods with higher rates of crime, threatening their safety even further and posing another obstacle to grocery shopping. Diseases and age-related pathophysiological changes occurring in this social milieu operate as synergistic factors that threaten optimal nutrition. Thus, nutritional surveillance is critical in chronically ill patients, as the inevitable interaction between protracted morbidity, functional status, and socioeconomic factors exponentially increases the risk of nutritional compromise.

Table 1
Pathophysiology of Weight Loss in Chronic Diseases

	Anorexia	Early satiation	Malabsorption	Increased metabolism	Cytokine mediated	Impaired physical function
Parkinson's disease	√			√		√
COPD	√	√		√		√
Rheumatoid arthritis	√				√	√
Heart failure	√		√		√	√
Depression	√	√				
Chronic pancreatitis	√		√			
Gluten enteropathy			√			
Gallstones		√				
Cancer	√	√			√	
Hyperthyroidism	√*		√	√		
Hypoadrenalism	√		√			
Hypercalcemia	√					
Pheochromocytoma	√			√		

*Apathetic variant.

Table 2
Meals on Wheels Acronym: Common Causes of Undernutrition in Older Adults

Medications
Emotional (depression, psychoses)
Anorexia (tardive)
Late-life paranoia
Swallowing disorders

Oral factors (tooth loss, periodontal infections, gingivitis)
No money (poverty)

Wandering (dementia)
Hyperthyroidism
Enteral problems (malabsorption syndromes)
Eating problems (ill-fitting dentures)
Low nutrient diets (low salt/low cholesterol/antidiabetic diets)
Shopping and food preparation problems

The cornerstone of nutritional intervention in younger adults frequently revolves around the prescription of therapeutic diets that are specifically tailored to the underlying disease. In chronically ill older adults, the pathological classification of chronic disease is less important than the potentially negative impact of chronic illness on functional status. Evaluation of each patient to assess the degree of dependence on caregivers for basic and instrumental activities of daily living is a critical component of history taking (12,13). Relevant psychosocial domains, specifically mood and cognitive function, warrant focused evaluation. Available evidence implicates depression as the most common cause of weight loss in community-dwelling and institutionalized older adults (14).

Similarly, dementia is a well-recognized cause of weight loss in older adults *(15)*. Current guidelines from the National Institute of Neurological and Communicative Disorders and Strokes Task Force on Alzheimer's disease includes weight loss as a clinical feature consistent with Alzheimer's disease *(16)*. However, it should be recognized that early in the disease, there may be weight gain. Persons with chronic pain syndrome are also at particular risk of compromised nutritional status. This may result from either the anorectic effect of persistent pain or anorexigenic analgesic regimens. Therefore, direct inquiry should be made regarding the presence and severity of pain. The adequacy of pain relief and the effect of pain relieving medications on food intake should also be closely monitored.

Meticulous attention should be paid to medication history (*see* Table 3). Prescription, nonprescription, and recreational drug use should be reviewed. Special efforts should be directed toward identifying inappropriate polypharmacy and adverse effects of medication. Specific questions should be asked regarding the inappropriate use of opiates and sedatives. All patients should be screened with the CAGE questionnaire to identify persons at risk for alcohol dependence *(17)*. The CAGE questionnaire is a simple, validated screening tool comprising four questions as follows:

1. Do you feel you should cut down the amount of alcohol that you drink?
2. Do you get annoyed when you are asked about your alcohol drinking habits?
3. Do you feel guilty about the amount of alcohol that you drink?
4. Do you need a drink first thing in the morning (an eye-opener)?

A positive response to two or more questions indicates a high risk of alcohol problem drinking.

Nicotine use should also be addressed as a component of nutrition risk assessment. Environmental and aesthetic factors exert a notable influence on eating habits. Therefore, all patients should be interviewed regarding their dining habits, food preferences, cooking skills, and dining environment.

3.2. Nutritional Screening

The prevalence of factors that threaten nutritional status mandate the incorporation of nutritional screening as an integral component of effective geriatric health maintenance. This strategy is not only effective in optimizing functional status, but also enhances the cost-effectiveness of therapeutic intervention *(18,19)*. Several screening tools have been developed for use in a variety of clinical settings. SCALES is a well validated, highly sensitive screening tool (*see* Table 4). This tool possesses the advantages of speed and ease of administration that notably enhances the practical utility in a wide range of clinical settings *(20)*. The mini-nutritional assessment (MNA) tool is a validated tool with a positive predictive value for detecting undernutrition of 97%. The sensitivity and specificity of this tool have been shown to be 96% and 98%, respectively. The MNA incorporates several domains, including functional status, lifestyle, diet, self-perception of health, and anthropometric indices *(21)*. The DETERMINE tool is another readily available screening instrument that targets community-dwelling older adults. DETERMINE is designed as a self-administered tool, consequently serving the added purpose of enhancing community awareness of nutritional risk factors *(19)*. This tool is yet to be validated.

Table 3
Medication-Related Symptoms That May Affect Nutritional Status

Symptom	Examples
Nausea/vomiting	Antibiotics
	NSAIDS*
	Opiates
	Digoxin
	Theophylline
	Cytotoxic drugs
Anorexia	Theophylline
	Fluoxetine
	Digoxin
Hypogeusia	Metronidazole
	Calcium channel blockers
	Angiotensin-converting enzyme inhitibors
	L-dopa
	Iron supplements
	Metformin
Dysphagia	Potassium supplements
	NSAIDS*
	Iron supplements
	Alendronate
	Prednisone
	Anticholinergia medications
Early satiety	Anticholinergic agents
	Sympathomimetic agents
Reduced feeding ability	Sedatives
	Opiates
	Psychotropic agents
Diarrhea	Laxatives
	Antibiotics
	Sertraline
	Theophylline
Hypermetabolism	Thyroxine
	Natural supplements: thyroid extracts, ephedra

* NSAIDs, nonsteroidal anti-inflammatory agents.

Table 4
SCALES Protocol for Evaluating Risk of Undernutrition in the Elderly

	1 Point	2 Points
Sadness*	10–14	15
Cholesterol	160 mg/dL	–
Albumin	3.5–4 g/dL	<3.5 g/dL
Loss of weight	1 kg in 1 mo	3 kg in 6 mo
Eating problems	Needs feeding assistance	–
Shopping and cooking	Needs assistance	–

* Measured using the Yesavage Geriatric Depression Scale. Score > 2 indicates increased risk of undernutrition.

Inherent in the threat of chronic disease is nutritional compromise. Thus, in evaluating the chronically ill older adult, screening is essentially superfluous, as the presumption of nutritional risk is critical to effective interdisciplinary management. This approach renders the sensitivity and predictive value of the chosen screening tool as relatively unimportant. In the setting of chronic illness, nutritional screening assessment tools are best directed toward risk stratification as opposed to diagnostic exclusion.

4. EVALUATION

4.1. Anthropometry

Traditionally, anthropometric methods have formed the cornerstone of physical examination of undernourished persons. However, associated pathophysiological changes that accompany chronic disease may confound the role of body weight as a prime index of nutritional status. Notably, such changes include sarcopenia (loss of skeletal muscle mass, quality, and strength), pathological fluid shifts, and obesity, which may either complicate disease or constitute the disease process. Therefore, examination of the chronically ill patient for features of protein, energy, or micronutrient deficiency is critical, as these are valuable subtle markers of coexisting undernutrition (*see* Table 5).

Body weight must be evaluated in the context of the underlying illness. In the absence of significant confounding factors, an abnormally low body weight is empirically defined as <80% of the recommended body weight using age-adjusted norms *(22,23)*. However, the accurate interpretation of weight mandates serial monitoring of weight measurements over time. Clinically significant weight loss is considered a decrease in weight exceeding 2% of baseline body weight in 1 mo, 5% in 3 mo, or 10% in 6 mo *(24)*. Additionally, regardless of the temporal profile and baseline body weight, unintentional weight loss in excess of 10 lbs should arouse strong suspicion of associated nutritional compromise.

Body mass index (BMI) is mathematically derived from the weight-to-height ratio and has been shown to correlate better with body fat than absolute body weight. The BMI is calculated as body weight (kg) divided by the square of the height in meters. Accepted normal values for BMI are between 22 and 27 *(25)*. The accuracy of this index is confounded by the age-related loss of disc height that complicates vertebral osteoporosis. Additionally, measurements of height may be inaccurate and difficult in persons with severely limited mobility or limb loss. In such persons, formulas using surrogate parameters of height, such as arm span and knee-floor height, may enhance the accuracy of this anthropometric index *(26–28)*.

Indices based on skin-fold thickness (SFT) and mid-arm circumference (MAC) have been advocated as adjunct parameters to assess nutritional status. Available evidence indicates a significant correlation between SFT, MAC, and total body fat in older adults *(29)*. However, the utility of these unidimensional indices in detecting serial changes in body fat is limited because of their inability to accurately evaluate differential changes in fat and muscle mass. Furthermore, the accuracy of MAC is based on the theoretical model of uniform circumferential fat distribution around the arm *(30)*. The latter model does not hold true for older adults because of age related skin changes and alterations in fat distribution. In the aging process, there is increased compressibility of the skin and, consequently, altered soft tissue contours from atrophy of the subcutaneous adipocytes, resulting from redistribution of fat centrally. There is also a reduction in the elasticity of

Table 5
Clinical Features of Common Micronutrient Deficiencies

Micronutrient	Clinical features
Vitamin A	Xerosis, night blindness, keratomalacia Bitot's spots, gingivitis, hypogeusia
Thiamine (vitamin B)	Delirium, muscle weakness, cardiac failure, edema, hypesthesia, hyporeflexia
Riboflavin (vitamin B_2)	Cheilosis, angular stomatitis, gingivitis, glossitis
Pyridoxine (vitamin B_6)	Glossitis, delirium, sensory peripheral neuropathy
Vitamin B_{12}	Macrocytic anemia, sensory ataxia, dementia, peripheral neuropathy, optic neuritis
Niacin	Photosensitive dermatitis, delirium, glossitis, diarrhea
Iron	Microcytic anemia, dysphagia (Plummer-Vinson syndrome), glossitis, koilonychia
Folic acid	Macrocytic anemia, stomatitis, glossitis
Vitamin C	Follicular hyperkeratoses, gingival hypertrophy petechiae, ecchymoses
Vitamin D	Osteomalacia, proximal myopathy
Vitamin K	Impaired clotting function

the skin from age-related changes in collagen content *(31)*. Measurement of the mid-arm muscle area has been proposed as a more accurate index. This is a two-dimensional mathematical index derived from the MAC and SFT. Evidence indicates that this index may be a more accurate index of somatic mass and may be more sensitive to weight changes *(30)*.

Awareness of the clinical implications of sarcopenia have prompted further definition of the components of weight loss in the older adult. Sarcopenia describes age-related loss of muscle mass and is technically defined as lean body mass more than two standard deviations below the young normal mean. Epidemiological data indicates that sarcopenia may be associated with impaired functional status. Further research is needed to examine the disease outcomes of the sarcopenic elderly. Nevertheless, available data is sufficient to justify efforts to determine the predominant compartment responsible for weight loss in undernourished older adults *(32)*. Bioelectric impedance (BEI) is a valuable tool in this regard. BEI is based on the theory that the resistance to electrical current flowing through an object is proportional to the object's volume and length. Because electrical current applied to the human body is transmitted mainly through fat free mass (FFM), BEI measurement allows for the specific evaluation of FFM *(33,34)*.

Direct imaging techniques, such as computerized tomographic (CT) scanning and magnetic resonance imaging (MRI), can also be employed in the evaluation of body mass composition. CT scanning enables visualization and quantification of subcutaneous and intracavitary fat. MRI has the added advantage of allowing visualization and quantification of both adipose and muscle tissue in different body compartments *(35–37)*.

Direct photon absorptiometry (DPA) measurements are based on the difference in tissue attenuation of photons transmitted at two different energy levels. This technique permits measurement of different tissue compartments. DPA is most frequently used for bone-density measurement, however, fat mass and fat-free mass can also be measured using this technique *(38)*. A major drawback to the use of these techniques in the evaluation of body mass is the lack of validation of these tools for clinical use.

Research into the diagnosis and stratification of nutritional status has been notably enhanced by the advent of more sophisticated technology. Regardless, available clinical data comparing the correlation between body weight, BMI, and nutritional status, with the degree of correlation obtained using more sophisticated anthropometric tools, fails to demonstrate any significant difference. Therefore, for practical clinical purposes, the most cost-effective parameter of proven clinical utility in monitoring nutritional status is body weight measurement *(39)*.

4.2. Laboratory Evaluation

Laboratory evaluation of nutritional status provides objective data that guide nutritional risk stratification and the definition of optimal nutritional therapeutic strategies. A major drawback to the use of laboratory parameters is the effect of multiple confounding factors on the specificity of these indices in assessing nutritional status. These factors are even more prevalent in the setting of chronic illness *(see* Table 6). A well-designed nutritional surveillance program should not be dependent on laboratory data. Thus, the hallmark of effective screening is the recognition of threats to nutritional status long before abnormal biochemical indices are sought.

4.2.1. Serum Albumin

Traditionally, hypoalbuminemia has been considered indicative of protein-energy undernutrition. The nutritional significance of this index has been unjustifiably strengthened by evidence linking low albumin levels to increased morbidity and mortality *(40,41)*. Current evidence does not support the use of serum albumin as an objective marker of nutritional status because the causality between undernutrition and low serum albumin has yet to be substantiated. Furthermore, there is a paucity of data documenting an improvement in outcomes following serum albumin repletion *(42)*.

The specificity of hypoalbuminemia as a predictive index of undernutrition is even further compromised in the setting of protracted or chronic illness in older adults. Available studies suggest that there is an age-related decline in serum albumin levels at a rate of 0.8 g/L for every decade following the seventh decade of life *(43)*. Additional factors contributing to hypoalbuminemia in the setting of chronic illness include overexpression of cytokines, such as TNF-α, IL-2, and IL-6, that inhibit albumin gene expression *(44)*. Hypoalbuminemia may be further exacerbated in such cases by cytokine-induced increases in vascular permeability, thereby further depleting serum albumin levels *(45)*. Disease states that directly affect gastrointestinal, hepatic, or renal function may further compromise the predictive value of hypoalbuminemia as an index of undernutrition. Acute fulminant liver disease or chronic liver disease, in the form of hepatitis or liver cirrhosis, may reduce hepatic albumin synthesis. Tubulo-interstitial nephritis and glomerular disease manifesting with proteinuria may result in significant visceral protein depletion. Similarly, gastrointestinal diseases that manifest with protracted vomiting, chronic diarrhea, or malabsorption syndromes may result in hypoalbuminemia.

Table 6
Factors Confounding Laboratory Evaluation of Nutritional Status

Parameter	Confounding factors
Albumin	Cytokines, nephrotic syndrome, liver cirrhosis, malabsorption syndrome, acidosis, paraproteinemias, posture
Prealbumin	Liver cirrhosis, renal failure, steroids, inflammation, stress, iron deficiency
Isulin growth factor-1	Renal failure, hepatic failure, autoimmune diseases, inflammation, stress
C-reactive protein	Catabolic states, trauma, infection, sepsis
Transferrin	Iron deficiency, acute hepatitis, antibiotics, estrogen supplements, liver cirrhosis, nephrotic syndrome, malignancies
Cholesterol	Stress, cytokines

Artefactual factors may limit accurate interpretation of albumin levels. Changes in intravascular osmotic pressure and altered tissue fluid flux may alter serum albumin concentration despite the presence of unchanged visceral protein stores. Data also indicates that moving from the recumbent to the upright position may result in an increase in serum albumin concentration (42,46). The pathophysiological mechanism responsible for the latter observation is unknown.

Overall, the long half-life of serum albumin (18–21 d) and the susceptibility of this protein to multiple confounding factors renders serum albumin measurement highly unreliable as either a diagnostic or prognostic index (47).

4.2.2. PREALBUMIN

The relatively short half-life of prealbumin (2 d) contributes to the popularity of this index (48). Low prealbumin levels are associated with increased morbidity and prolonged hospital stay among frail older adults. However, comparative data does not identify any correlation with increased mortality (49). The lack of association of low prealbumin levels with increased mortality may be attributed to the sensitivity of this index to alterations in nutritional status, allowing prompt intervention. Admittedly, data is lacking regarding the beneficial effects of repleting prealbumin levels. However, there is evidence to indicate that a failure to adequately replete prealbumin stores in the presence of optimal protein intake may suggest an increase in mortality. Generally, an increase of prealbumin levels in excess of 10 mg/dL indicates adequate repletion (50,51).

As with albumin, prealbumin levels are subject to multiple confounding factors. A gender differential in prealbumin levels has been noted, with females having lower levels than men. However, this differential disappears in the tenth decade of life (43). In contrast to the trend that occurs with serum albumin levels, renal failure results in elevated serum prealbumin levels. This is attributed to delayed renal clearance of prealbumin. Chronic liver disease, acute inflammatory processes, stress, and anemia may lower prealbumin levels (52–54) although the underlying pathophysiological mechanism is unclear. It is plausible that cytokine expression and impaired prealbumin production, as in the case of albumin, will eventually be implicated.

4.2.3. INSULIN GROWTH FACTOR

Insulin growth factor (IGF-1) is a single-chain peptide produced by the liver under the stimulation of growth hormone. The effects of growth hormone on the tissues are mediated by IGF-1 *(55)*. IGF-1 levels have been shown to fall very rapidly during periods of starvation. Nutritional repletion produces an equally prompt return to normal levels. This characteristic, which is attributed to a short half-life of 2–4 h and a relatively small body reservoir, renders IGF-1 one of the most sensitive indices of alterations in nutritional status. Low IGF-1 levels in hospitalized older adults are associated with an increase in morbidity and, specifically, the occurrence of life-threatening complications. Data has shown that normalizing IGF-1 levels in undernourished chronically ill adults decreases the risk of dying from the underlying illness *(56–58)*. Regardless of the proven sensitivity and predictive value of this index, the cost of this investigation precludes routine clinical use.

4.2.4. C-REACTIVE PROTEIN

Attempts have been made to use C-reactive protein (CRP) as a marker of nutritional status. CRP is an acute-phase reactant that exhibits a very rapid response to inflammatory processes. However, as with all acute-phase reactants, CRP levels are primarily indicative of ongoing catabolic processes *(59)*. Therefore, in the chronically ill patient, CRP levels are, at best, an inaccurate and indirect reflection of the nutritional response to disease. Some workers advocate the use of the Prognostic and Inflammatory Nutritional Index (PINI) to enhance the correlation between CRP measurements and nutritional status *(60)*. The PINI is mathematically derived according to the following formula:

$$PINI = \frac{\alpha\text{-1 acid glycoprotein (mg/L)} \times CRP \text{ (mg/L)}}{albumin \text{ (g/L)} \times prealbumin \text{ (mg/L)}}$$

However, the fact that serum CRP, albumin, and prealbumin levels are all influenced by ongoing inflammatory processes may notably increase the margin of error when the PINI is used as an index of undernutrition.

4.2.5. TRANSFERRIN

Evidence-based data justifying the use of transferrin as an objective index of nutritional status is lacking. Recent studies indicate that transferrin values correlate very poorly with nutritional status *(61)*. Additional data indicates that adequate nutritional repletion frequently fails to result in corresponding normalization of transferrin levels *(62)*. Finally, transferrin levels are of limited value in predicting outcomes in chronically ill older adults *(61)*. The limited role of this index is further compromised by the myriad factors that reduce transferrin levels. Therefore, objective review of the available evidence precludes objective utilization of transferrin values in the evaluation of undernutrition.

4.2.6. CHOLESTEROL

Serum cholesterol values less than 160 mg/dL are considered indicative of low lipoprotein levels and, therefore, reflective of visceral protein depletion. However, serum cholesterol shares the limitations of other biochemical parameters, in that the causal link between hypocholesterolemia and undernutrition is indirect. Available data shows a significant increase in mortality in nursing home and hospitalized older adults with low serum cholesterol levels. In contrast, there is also evidence that reveals a higher risk of death in older adults with hypercholesterolemia *(63–66)*. Therefore, in caring for the older adult, dissociating the clinical benefits of treating persistently high cholesterol levels from the increased morbidity and mortality associated with low cholesterol levels, is a complex task based mainly on intuition and clinical consensus. The lack of an analytical objective approach to interpreting cholesterol levels in relation to nutritional status severely curtails the utility of this index as a nutritional parameter.

4.3. Immunological Indices

Undernutrition is associated with absolute lymphopenia and a decrease in the CD4/CD8 ratio *(67)*. The degree of absolute lymphopenia reflects the extent of nutritional compromise. A total lymphocyte count (TLC) less than $800/mm^3$ is indicative of severe undernutrition and an exponential increase in mortality *(68,69)*. Likewise, alterations in the nutritional status are closely reflected in the degree of activation of the cytokine system. Thus, IL-1, IL-2 soluble receptor, complement levels, and other quantitative parameters of immune function, such as leucocyte terminal deoxynucleotidyl transferase and monocyte function, have been used as research tools to evaluate nutritional status. Similarly, qualitative aspects of immune function, such as chemotaxis and opsonization, have been explored in this regard *(70)*. From a practical standpoint, the expense of these tests cannot be clinically justified, as knowledge of the immunological profile outside the arena of immune-based disease, is unlikely to alter the nutritional management plan.

5. NUTRITIONAL SUPPORT

Effective nutritional support is dependent on the development and execution of a clinically appropriate nutritional therapeutic strategy *(see also* Chapters 11 and 26). Unjustifiably, nutritional intervention is often confined to a single domain in the overall organizational management scheme. The latter strategy has propagated the unfounded hypothesis that disease outcomes are dependent on the additive results of different domains of management. Based on this concept, each therapeutic domain is considered responsible for a variably determined fraction of the overall outcome. Available data renders the latter concept very unlikely, as nutritional intervention is an important independent predictor of outcomes *(19,40)*. Thus, regardless of the success within other domains of management, effective nutritional management must be instituted as a parallel intervention in all chronically ill adults.

5.1. Nutritional Requirements

Successful intervention mandates careful estimation of the patient's nutritional needs. The method of estimation varies with the clinical setting. Indirect calorimetry using a bedside metabolic cart that measures oxygen consumption and carbon dioxide production is an accurate means of measuring resting energy expenditure *(71)*. This method is most frequently employed in critically ill older adults. In most other cases, the Harris-Benedict equation provides an adequate estimate of the basal energy expenditure *(72)*. Physical activity and coexistent metabolic stressors are also relevant to deciding the optimal energy intake. Empirical correction factors are used in the setting of acute illness to compensate for the catabolic effect of coexistent stress *(71)*. A drawback to the use of these correction factors in chronically ill patients is the paucity of objective data regarding stress-related energy expenditure in chronically ill patients. For practical clinical purposes, initiation of nutritional supplementation in the older adult should be based on a presumed daily requirements of at least 40 kcal/kg *(73)*. Subsequent measurement of CRP values and cytokine profiles to evaluate the degree of ongoing active inflammation may prove useful in the evaluation of patients that fail to respond to ongoing nutritional supplementation.

An alternative method of estimating the daily energy requirements involves the use of the calculated protein requirement. Under basal metabolic conditions, the healthy older adult usually requires 0.8–1 g/kg body weight. However, under identical conditions, the protein requirement of the chronically ill older patient is approx 1.2 g/kg body weight. The daily energy requirements may be estimated using the calculated protein requirement as a reference parameter. A daily balanced diet constructed to provide the protein requirements should fulfill total dietary energy needs *(74)*.

5.2. Enteral Nutritional Support

Clinical evidence supports enteral feeding over parenteral nutrition. The only absolute contraindication to enteral feeding is mechanical intestinal obstruction. Relative contraindications should be considered in the clinical context of the individual patient (*see* Table 7). The option of enteral tube feeding should be considered when a patient is unable to orally ingest sufficient energy to sustain or achieve ideal body weight. Health professionals involved in the decision to start enteral tube feeding should be cognizant of the fact that available data indicates that this will not alter the rate of survival *(75,76)*. Patient expectations and benefits of tube feeding must be carefully weighed against the risks and complications of this procedure. The availability of trained personnel is an additional important consideration. Patient and family preferences must be carefully considered and ethical, spiritual, or legal counseling sought where relevant. Emerging data has rendered the decision to initiate feeding extremely complicated. Studies of patients with dementia indicate that nutritional status often fails to improve with tube feeding *(77)*. Additionally, the insertion of enteral tubes in patients with pharyngeal dysphagia does not reduce the risk of aspiration *(78)*.

Surgical and endoscopic enteral tube placement have a complication rate ranging from 32% to 70% *(79)*. This data challenges both the efficacy and safety of enteral tube placement (*see* Table 8). Health professionals should ensure that decisions regarding enteral tube feeding are ultimately made by the patient or surrogate decision maker. Such decisions should be preceded by a careful and individualized review of objective information relating to prognosis and expected outcomes.

Chronically ill older adults who are candidates for enteral tube placement are unlikely to require alternative enteral access for less than 4–6 wk. Tube enterostomy should be the initial intervention in these patients. In cases where patient or family are undecided regarding long-term enteral tube feeding, nasogastric tube placement may be considered as initial intervention. Similarly, the clinical suspicion of gastric dysmotility may mandate a period of nasogastric tube feeding to enable evaluation of gastric residuals and tolerance of feeds. However, the routine use of nasogastric tubes in most long-term patients should be discouraged because of the significant associated morbidity. Complications of nasogastric tube placement include aspiration pneumonitis, airway obstruction and pneumothorax. Nasogastric tubes also require frequent replacement because of

Table 7
Contraindications to Enteral Tube Feeding

Absolute contradindication	Relative contraindications
Mechanical intestinal obstruction	Acute pancreatitis
	Pancreatic fistula
	Enterocutaneous fistula
	Severe gastrointestinal bleeding
	Massive small bowel resection

Table 8
Complications of Enteral Tube Feeding

Mechanical	Pulmonary
Obstruction	Aspiration pneumonitis
Dislodgement	Pneumonia
Leakage	
Site infection	
Gastrointestinal	*Metabolic*
Nausea/vomiting	Dehydration
Gastric fullness/discomfort	Electrolyte imbalance
Abdominal distension	Hyperglycemia
Diarrhea	Azotemia/prerenal failure
Constipation	
Anorexia	*Psychological*
	Anxiety
	Depression
	Body image dysphoria
	Agitation

accidental dislodgement or clogging, notably increasing the cost associated with this procedure. The negative aesthetic qualities and the discomfort associated with nasogastric tube placement and positioning are added disadvantages.

The site of enteral tube placement has significant impact on surgical technique and efficiency with regard to nutrient and medication delivery (*see* Table 9). Clinical indications for jejunal tube placement include severe gastric atony, mechanical gastric outlet obstructions, proximal intestinal fistulas, severe pancreatitis and severe gastroesophageal reflux disease. The choice between gastrostomy and jejunostomy tube placement, when in question, may be facilitated by clinical observation during nasogastric tube feeding.

5.3. Parenteral Nutritional Support

Early morbidity associated with parenteral nutrition is often associated with the creation of vascular access. Parenteral nutrition may be delivered through central or peripheral veins. The mode of access determines composition of the infused solutions. Delivery through peripheral veins mandates a reduction in osmolality when compared with solu-

Table 9
Enteral Ostomy Tubes: Advantages and Disadvantages

Mechanical factors	Gastrostomy	Jejunostomy
Insertion method	Endoscopic/surgical	Surgical only
Laparotomy technique	Small (modified)	Full
Tube replacement	Simple	Complicated
Infusion method	Intermittent bolus or continuous	Continuous only
Tube bore size	Large (ideal for medication administration)	Small (interferes with medication administration)
Clogging	Infrequent	Frequent

tions infused through larger, central veins. Consequently, a higher volume of free water is required to maintain adequate energy delivery when peripheral parenteral nutrition (PPN) is utilized. Additionally, the provision of adequate fat is precluded by the requirement for lower osmolality. This renders PPN inadequate to sustain long-term energy requirements. Therefore, PPN is best reserved for patients in whom parenteral feeding is not expected to exceed 10–14 d. Long-term parenteral nutrition is also more time- and cost-effective when delivered through larger central veins rather than peripheral veins. The latter are more susceptible to dislodgement and mechanical disruption of flow. Metabolic considerations are critical to reducing the morbidity associated with parenteral nutrition. Therefore, patients on parenteral nutrition must be closely supervised and monitored by an experienced nutritionist. Close daily monitoring of the patient's metabolic and electrolyte status is essential as the electrolyte composition of the infused solution is based on serum electrolyte values. Overwhelming evidence implicates intestinal mucosal atrophy as a source of morbidity following prolonged periods of total bowel rest. The presence of glutamine within the gut lumen, is critical to maintaining mucosal integrity. Studies indicate that intestinal mucosal atrophy increases bacterial translocation and consequently increases the risk of endotoxemia (80,81). The immunosuppressive effects of age and coexistent chronic disease increase the risk of sepsis and multiorgan dysfunction in such cases. Therefore, regardless of the underlying pathology, exclusive parenteral nutrition should be discouraged. In most cases, simultaneous enteral stimulation can be maintained by slow continuous enteral infusion of dextrose-containing solutions.

5.4. Choice of Nutritional Formulation

Logic and intuition dictate that first-line intervention in patients able to eat should consist of natural foods. Fortifying meals during the cooking process provides the option of providing energy-dense natural foods as a means of nutritional supplementation. Innovative strategies include the incorporation of increased amounts of butter, oils, mayonnaise, sugar, milk, and syrups in standard recipes. The addition of pureed meats, cheese or cream to soups and casseroles are other methods by which the nutrient density of meals may be enhanced. The advantage of naturally enhancing the energy density of foods facilitates the preservation of natural tastes and odors, which contribute significantly to the pleasurable qualities of meals. This facilitates the process of positive allisthesia. Positive allisthesia refers to the positive feedback effect that the pleasurable qualities of food have on further food intake during a meal. Available evidence indicates that pleasant sensory information obtained from gustatory, olfactory, and visual receptors serve to encourage continued meal consumption and are the major factors that influence food intake during the initial 15–20 min of a meal *(82)*. Additional advantages of using nutrient-dense natural foods include the familiarity and cultural adaptability of the food items. The preservation of the visual aesthetic qualities of meals may also enhance consumption. Fortified foods also allow for manipulation of the prescribed diet to suit individual patient food preferences and allows for flavor enhancement. Emerging data highlights the importance of flavor-enhanced foods as a means of enhancing energy intake. Studies have shown that flavor enhancement among nursing home residents may encourage food intake and weight gain in nursing home residents. Nevertheless, flavor enhancement should be used with caution, as in older persons with relatively unimpaired chemosensory function, there may be a paradoxical decrease in food intake *(83,84)*.

5.5. Commercially Formulated Nutritional Supplements

The use of commercially formulated nutritional liquid supplements is inevitable in persons with enteral tubes. However, in persons able to eat, oral commercial supplements should only be used as a second line intervention when natural foods fail to fulfill energy requirements. Unfortunately, intensive advertising within the current climate of consumerism and fast foods encourages the use of commercially formulated oral supplements as first line intervention in undernourished patients. Health professionals must be aware that several disadvantages may be associated with the indiscriminate prescription of commercial supplements. The inevitable monotony of formulated commercial supplements, with regard to flavor, palatability, and visual presentation, may discourage long-term consumption. The liberal use of oral commercial supplements also discourages the creative utility of cheaper means of dietary supplementation. Additionally, the resultant extra financial burden arising from supplement purchase may further limit access to adequate nutrition in persons with limited income.

In certain situations, commercial supplements are an appropriate choice. Particularly finicky eaters may have a range of food preferences that precludes the delivery of adequate energy. Commercial supplements should be encouraged if preferred by such patients. Patients with chronic neurological diseases, such as dementia, Parkinson's disease, familial essential tremor, and hemiballismus may be unable to eat large enough meals to compensate for the significant increase in energy expenditure. In such cases, small volume nutrient dense formulated supplements may be valuable adjuncts to meals. Functionally impaired adults that live alone may experience great difficulty with cooking and meal preparation. The availability of balanced formulated supplements may ease the burden of meal preparation in such adults and provide a greater sense of security within the home environment. Caregivers may also appreciate the availability of this option for periods when the burden of care giving is perceived as excessive.

Appropriate consideration must be given to product selection when prescribing commercially formulated supplements for either oral or enteral tube feeding. Because of the relative paucity of data relating to vehicle efficiency, the choice between solid and liquid supplements is generally made empirically or based on patient preference or swallowing ability. Additional considerations involved in supplement decision-making include cost-effectiveness and nutritional benefit. Nutritional supplements are generally classified as either balanced or modified. Balanced supplements contain polymeric forms of proteins, carbohydrates, and lipids constituted in proportions similar to those contained in a balanced meal. Modified supplements have either been enriched or deprived of particular nutrients as dictated by the underlying disease process (*see* Table 10). Modified supplements may be significantly more expensive than balanced supplements. Despite the fact that such supplements are marketed as disease specific, there is little objective evidence in support of the efficacy of such diets *(71)*. Evidence-based data indicates that older adults with chronic disease that may be considered candidates for commercial supplements should be started on a balanced supplement, regardless of the underlying disease pathology. Modified supplements should be reserved for patients unable to tolerate balanced formulations.

Traditionally, oral nutritional supplements are offered in most settings during the meal. However, available data has shown that the administration of liquid supplements at least 60 min before meals in older patients results in higher energy intake compared with simultaneous administration of supplements with meals *(85)*. Based on this evidence, oral liquid nutritional supplements should be administered between meals in older adults, as this strategy may be more effective in increasing energy consumption.

5.6. Orexigenic Agents

The use of orexigenic agents is increasing in popularity. However, the use of these agents in older patients should be restricted to those that have failed to respond to management of identified underlying risk factors. Orexigenic agents may also be a useful adjunct in end of life care. The choice of effective agents is limited (*see* Table 11). Several proposed agents have fallen out of favor because of the absence of sufficient evidence to support their clinical efficacy. The indiscriminate use of antidepressants as orexigenic agents, in the absence of a simultaneous thorough screen for depression should be avoided. Early recognition of depression and prompt institution of appropriate pharmacological and nonpharmacological treatment are pivotal factors in reducing the associated morbidity and mortality. One-third of depressed older adults manifest with weight loss *(86)*. Effective antidepressant therapy should result in weight gain within this subset of patients. The choice of antidepressant therapy may also influence body weight. Selective serotonin inhibitors can cause significant weight loss at the onset of therapy. Evidence in younger adults suggests that this is a transient phenomenon with baseline body weight being restored as treatment progresses *(87)*. However, age-related changes in energy regulation and adaption to chronic disease may delay or prevent return to baseline body weight.

Mirtazapine has proved useful in the management of depressed patients exhibiting weight loss. Mirtazapine is a well-tolerated and effective antidepressant. This agent inhibits presynaptic α_2 adrenergic receptors and postsynaptic 5-HT2 and 5HT3 receptors. Paradoxically, common side effects of mirtazapine, namely increased appetite and weight gain, serve as a clinical advantage and have encouraged its use as an orexigenic agent in older depressed persons exhibiting weight loss *(88,89)*. Recent evidence indicates that megesterol acetate may enhance weight gain in nursing home residents *(90,91)*. However, associated serious side effects, such as thromboembolic disease and adrenal suppression, mandate cautious use.

Dronabinol (delta-9-tetrahydrocannabinol), the active ingredient of Cannabis sativa, is approved for use by the Food and Drug Administration (FDA) as an orexigenic agent

Table 10
Disease-Specific Nutritional Supplements

	Amino acid content	Lipid content
Hepatic	Increased ratio of branched chain to aromatic amino acids	Unchanged
Renal	Esssential amino acids only	Unchanged
Respiratory	Unchanged	Increased ratio of long-chain triglycerides; increased lipid: carbohydrate ratio
Critically ill	Increased branched-chain amino acids	Medium-chain triglycerides
Gastrointestinal	Short-chain peptides Increased glutamine	Medium-chain triglycerides
Immune system	Increased arginine	Unchanged

Table 11
Orexigenic Agents

Corticosteroids	Dronabinol (delta 9 tetrahydrocannabinol)
Cyproheptadine	Oxoglutarate
Loxiglumide (cholecystokinin antagonist)	Anabolic agents (testosterone, anadrol)
Megesterol acetate	Oxandrin
Mirtazapine	Growth hormone

in patients with Acquired Immune Deficiency Syndrome (AIDS) and as an antiemetic in chemotherapy-induced nausea and vomiting. Dronabinol is also an effective anti-emetic in cancer-associated anorexia (92,93). Additional evidence indicates that Dronabinol induces weight gain in persons with dementia. Research is yet to determine whether weight gain in such patients is because of an orexigenic effect or a reduction in agitation, behavioral abnormalities and consequently physical energy expenditure (94). Further studies are required to determine the precise role of Dronabinol as an orexigenic agent in chronically ill older persons.

6. INTERDISCIPLINARY TEAM MANAGEMENT

Design of an effective nutritional intervention team mandates multidisciplinary effort. Intensive efforts should be directed toward enhancing the aesthetic qualities of their physical dining environment. Persons suffering from chronic illness are very often, unintentionally, subjected by caregivers to a regimented environment. This may be entirely at odds with the individual's personal preferences. Specific inquiry should be made by the interdisciplinary team regarding the person's preferred dining environment, meal times, and dining company.

Persons with chronic disabilities that compromise upper extremity function may benefit from the use of adaptive devices. Sensory impairment has a major effect on the pleasurable qualities of meals. Efforts should be made to develop compensatory strategies to preserve qualities that enhance energy intake. Thus, persons who are visually impaired should be given a detailed description of the individual food items presented during the meal to enable them to exercise choice and preference as the meal is ingested.

Health professionals directly involved in assisting older adults with feeding should be made aware that their role far exceeds that of physical assistance with the mechanical process of eating. Dining assistance must be approached as a dynamic continuing education process between caregiver and patient. Effective interaction between the dyad is critical to a positive outcome. Educational programs that emphasize the integration of feeding programs into ongoing rehabilitative care should be incorporated into the overall management plan.

7. PALLIATIVE CARE

Paradoxically, emerging evidence indicates that nutritional supplementation in the setting of incurable chronic disease may increase the burden of illness. Data analysis suggests that the morbidity associated with enteral tube feeding in such cases may outweigh any nutritional benefit *(75,76)*. Within the realm of end-of-life care, the issue of nutritional support is more likely to be complicated by bioethical and legal considerations. Decisions issued by the Supreme Court indicate clearly that nutritional support is a form of medical therapy *(95)*. Additionally, there are legitimate bioethical arguments in support of decisions to withhold enteral tube feeding as a component of end-of-life care, if this is in line with the patient's wishes *(96,97)*. Health professionals should resist the urge to make decisions regarding nutritional intervention in terminally ill patients based on sentiment or personal values. An ideal nutritional intervention plan in such cases mandates extensive informed discussion and involvement of the patient or surrogate decision makers. Health professionals should attempt to elicit the patient's expectations and subsequently define realistic goals of care. Effective communication in this regard usually protects against the violation of the patient's beliefs and values systems.

Age-specific mortality rates have declined over the past three decades. Analysis of this trend indicates that this observation may be attributed to decreasing mortality from chronic disease. The inevitable outcome of reducing mortality in older persons is an increase in the number of chronically ill older patients. This sociological phenomenon has been described by sociologists as the "failure of success" *(98)*. This erroneous sense of failure is further propagated by the perceived increase in the caregiving burden associated with increased longevity of the chronically ill and frail older adult. Fortunately, advancing technology and medical research continue to improve nutritional support strategies available for the chronically ill. Health professionals involved in nutritional care must continue to develop effective interdisciplinary, well-integrated plans that may be adapted to any clinical setting. An effective evidence-based approach to nutritional surveillance and management of chronically ill patients in long-term care facilities has been developed by the Council of Nutrition *(see* Figs. 1 and 2) *(99)*.

Finally, educational programs targeting allied health professionals, legislative officials, consumer organizations, and the lay public are critical to ensuring optimal nutritional health in chronically ill older adults. Interdisciplinary nutritional surveillance integrated with a coordinated and comprehensive management plan is a pivotal strategy in ensuring efficient nutritional care. Ultimately, execution and compliance with such nutritional strategies may eventually succeed in eroding, or at least tarnishing, the cynical Unchangedimage of the "illusion of failure" *(98)*.

Clinical Guide to Prevent and Manage Malnutrition in Long-Term Care

FOR PHYSICIANS, PHARMACISTS, AND DIETICIANS (EVALUATE, DOCUMENT AND TREAT)

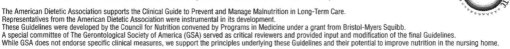

The American Dietetic Association supports the Clinical Guide to Prevent and Manage Malnutrition in Long-Term Care.
Representatives from the American Dietetic Association were instrumental in its development.
These Guidelines were developed by the Council for Nutrition convened by Programs in Medicine under a grant from Bristol-Myers Squibb.
A special committee of The Gerontological Society of America (GSA) served as critical reviewers and provided input and modification of the final Guidelines.
While GSA does not endorse specific clinical measures, we support the principles underlying these Guidelines and their potential to improve nutrition in the nursing home.

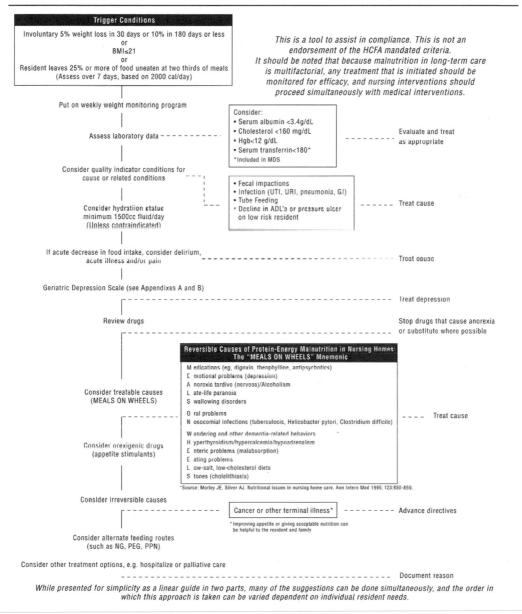

Fig. 1. Clinical guide to prevent and manage malnutrition in long-term care for physicians, pharmacists, and dietitians.

Clinical Guide to Prevent and Manage Malnutrition in Long-Term Care

FOR NURSING STAFF AND DIETARY STAFF AND DIETICIANS

The American Dietetic Association supports the Clinical Guide to Prevent and Manage Malnutrition in Long-Term Care.
Representatives from the American Dietetic Association were instrumental in its development.
These Guidelines were developed by the Council for Nutrition convened by Programs in Medicine under a grant from Bristol-Myers Squibb.
A special committee of The Gerontological Society of America (GSA) served as critical reviewers and provided input and modification of the final Guidelines.
While GSA does not endorse specific clinical measures, we support the principles underlying these Guidelines and their potential to improve nutrition in the nursing home.

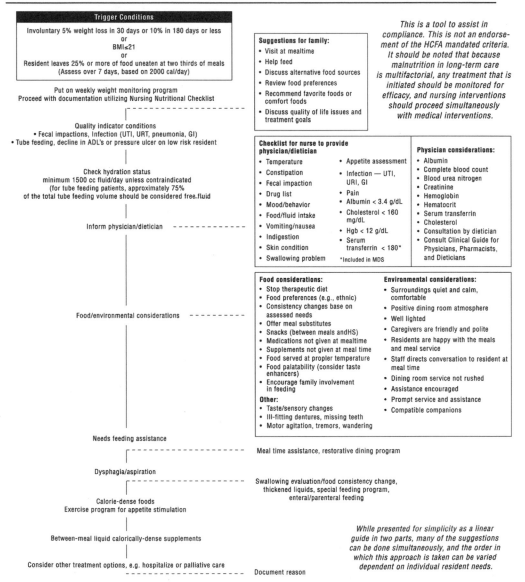

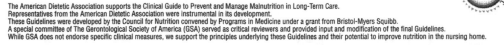

Fig. 2. Clinical guide to prevent and manage malnutrition in long-term care for nursing staff, dietary staff, and dietitians.

8. RECOMMENDATIONS FOR CLINICIANS

1. Nutritional assessment includes history taking, nutritional screening (with a focus on risk stratification), and a nutritional evaluation, including anthropometry and laboratory evaluation. However, a well-designed nutritional surveillance program should recognize threats to nutritional status before full-blown malnutrition is detected using biochemical indices.

2. Surveillance of risk factors can lead to early intervention. Some of the most important causes of weight loss in the elderly include depression, dementia, and chronic pain syndrome.

3. Nutritional intervention in persons with chronic disease should occur parallel with other aspects of medical management. A "wait-and-watch" approach while treatment of the underlying condition is attempted is not a justified approach.

4. In patients who are able to eat, the first line of intervention should consist of natural foods, which can also be fortified during the cooking/preparation process. This approach optimizes the acceptance and enjoyment of meals and promotes positive feedback on future food intake (positive allisthesia).

5. The use of commercial supplements carries the potential disadvantages of monotony and high costs, although in situations where circumstances prevent the consumption of adequate amounts of natural foods, these products can be useful. In most cases "balanced" supplements are the best choice; the use of more expensive "modified" supplements should be reserved for patients unable to tolerate balanced formulations.

6. The use of orexigenic agents should be restricted to patients for whom other approaches to reduce risk factors and enhance food intake have failed. An ideal pharmacologic choice is not available; agents currently showing the most promise include Mirtazapine and Dronabinol.

7. Clinical evidence favoring enteral feeding over parenteral nutrition continues to mount. The option of enteral tube feeding should be considered when a patient is unable to orally ingest sufficient energy to sustain or achieve ideal body weight. However, expectations of benefits must be weighed against known potential risks and complications. For example, it should be noted that the extension of survival is not a likely outcome.

8. Although enteral feeding is ideal, in certain situations when adequate nutrition cannot be achieved by this route, parenteral nutrition offers a useful alternative. However, parenteral nutrition should not be the exclusive form of feeding because of the risk of mucosal atrophy and associated morbidities. In most cases, simultaneous enteral stimulation can be maintained by slow continuous enteral infusion of dextrose-containing solutions.

9. When palliation is the objective, nutritional supplementation may increase, rather than decrease, the burden of illness. Decisions about nutrition support in end-of-life care should include extensive informed discussion and involvement of the patient or surrogate decision makers.

REFERENCES

1. About chronic disease: definition, overall burden, and cost-effectiveness of prevention. US Centers for Disease Control and Prevention, National Center for Chronic Disease Prevention and Health Promotion. www.cdc.gov/nccdphp/about.htm, accessed June 9, 2001.
2. Shikany JM, White GL. Dietary guidelines for chronic disease prevention. South Med J 2000;93:1138–1151.

3. National Committee for Quality Assurance. NCQA's state of managed care quality report–1998. National Committee for Quality Assurance, Washington, DC, 1998. www.ncqa.org/pages/communications/state%20of%20managed%20care/report98.htm, accessed June 14, 2001.

4. Wagner EH. Chronic disease management: what will it take to improve care for chronic illness? Eff Clin Prac 1998;1:2–4.

5. Wilson MG, Vaswani S, Liu D, Morley JE, Miller DK. Prevalence and causes of undernutrition in medical outpatients. Am J Med 1998;104:56–63.

6. Wallace JI, Schwartz RS, LaCroix AZ, et al. Involuntary weight loss in older outpatients: incidence and clinical significance. J Am Geriatr Soc 1995;43:329–337.

7. Poehlman ET, Scheffers J, Gottlieb SS, et al. Increased resting metabolic rate in patients with congestive cardiac failure. Ann Intern Med 1994;121:860–862.

8. Wolfe-Klein GP, Silverstone FA, Lansey SC, et al. Energy requirements in Alzheimer's disease patients. Nutrition 1995;11:264–268.

9. Levi SL, Cox M, Lugon, M, et al. Increased energy expenditure in Parkinson's disease. BMJ 1990;301:1256–1257.

10. Toth MJ, Fishman PS, Poehlman ET. Free living daily energy expenditure in patients with Parkinson's disease. Neurology 1997;48:88–91.

11. Toth MJ, Gottlieb SS, Goran MI, et al. Daily energy expenditure in free-living heart failure patients. Am J Physiol 1997;272:E469–E475.

12. Katz SD, Downs TD, Cash HR, Grotz RC. Progress in the development of the index of ADL. Gerontologist 1970;10:20–30.

13. Lawton MP, Brody EM. Assessment of older people: self-maintaining and instrumental activities of daily living. Gerontologist 1969;9:179–186.

14. Wilson MMG, Vaswani S, Liu D, Morley JE, Miller DK. Prevalence and causes of undernutrition in medical outpatients. Am J Med 1998;104:56–63.

15. Poehlman ET, Dvorak RV. Energy expenditure, energy intake, and weight loss in Alzheimer's disease. Am J Clin Nutr 2000;71(Suppl):650S–655S.

16. McKhann G, Drachman D, Folstein M, Katzman R, Price D, Stadlam EL. Clinical diagnosis of Alzheimer's disease: report of the NINCDS-ADRDA Work group under the auspices of the Department of Health and Human Services Task Force on Alzheimer's Disease. Neurology 1984;34:939–944.

17. Mayfield D, Mcleod G, Hall P. The CAGE questionnaire: validation of a new alcoholism screening instrument. Am J Psych 1974;131:1121–1123.

18. American Dietetic Association Council on Practice Quality Management Committee. ADA Definition for nutrition screening and nutritional assessment. J Am Diet Assoc 1994;94:838–839.

19. Position of the American Dietetic Association: Nutrition, aging and continuum of care. J Am Diet Assoc 2000;100:580–595.

20. Morley JE. Nutritional assessment is a key component of geriatric assessment. Facts Res Gerontol 1994;2:5.

21. Guigoz Y, vellas B. The Mini-nutritional assessment for grading the nutritional state of elderly patients, presentation of the MNA, history and validation. Facts, Res and Intervention Geriatr Newsletter: Nutrition 1997;6:2.

22. Master AM, Lasser RP, Beckman G. Tables of average weight and height of Americans aged 65–94 years. JAMA 1960;172:658–662.

23. Andres R, Elahi D, Tobin JD, Muller DC, Brant L. Impact of age on weight goals. Ann Intern Med 1985;103:1030–1033.

24. Zawada ET. Malnutrition in the elderly. Postgraduate Medicine 1996;100:207–222.

25. Committee for Diet and Health, Food and Nutrition Board. National Research Council Diet and Health. Diet and Health: implications for reducing chronic disease risk. National Academy, Washington, DC, 1989.

26. Kwok T, Whitelaw MN. The use of arm span in the nutritional assessment of the elderly. J Am Geriatr Soc 1991;39:492–496.

27. Chumlea WC, Roche AF, Mukherjee D. Nutritional assessment of the elderly through anthropometry. Ross Laboratories, Columbus, OH, 1987.

28. Rabe B, Thamarin A, Gross R et al. Body mass index of the elderly derived from height and arm span. Asia Pac J Clin Nutr 1996;5:79.

29. Jensen TG, Dudrick SG, Johnson DA. A comparison of triceps, skinfold upper arm circumference measurements taken in standard and supine positions. JPEN 1981;5:519–521.

30. Heymsfield SB, McManus C, Smith J, et al. Anthropometric measurement of muscle mass: revised equations for calculating bone-free arm muscle area. Am J Clin Nutr 1982;36:680–690.
31. Sullivan DH, Patch GA, Baden AI, et al. An approach to assessing the reliability of anthropometrics in elderly patients. J Am Geriatr Soc 1989;37:607–613.
32. Evans WJ. What is sarcopenia? J Gerontol 1995;50A:5–8.
33. Segal KR, Van Loan M, Fitzgerald PI, et al. Lean body mass estimation by bioelectrical impedance analysis: a four site cross-validation study. Am J Clin Nutr 1988;47:7–14.
34. Hoffer EC, Meador CK, Simpson DC. Correlation of whole body impedance with total body water volume. J Appl Physiol 1969;27:531–534.
35. Sobol W, Rossner S, Hinson B, et al. Evaluation of a new magnetic resonance imaging method for quantifying adipose tissue areas. Int J Obes 1991;15:589–599.
36. Fowler PA, Fuller MF, Glasbey CA, et al. Validation of the in vivo measurement of adipose tissue by magnetic resonance imaging of lean and obese pigs. Am J Clin Nutr 1992;56:7–13.
37. Rossner S, Bo WJ, Hiltbrandt E, et al. Adipose tissue determinations in cadavers -a comparison between cross-sectional planimetry and computerized tomography. Int J Obes 1990;14:893–902.
38. Heymsfield SB, Wang J, Heshka S, et al. Dual-photon absorptiometry: comparison of bone mineral and soft tissue measurements in vivo with established methods. Am J Clin Nutr 1989;49:1283–1289.
39. Blaum CS, O'Neill EF, Clements KM, et al. The validity of the Minimum data set for assessing nutritional status in nursing home residents. Am J Clin Nutr 1997;66:787–794.
40. Knaus WA, Wagner DP, Draper ER, et al. The APACHE III prognostic system risk prediction of hospital mortality for critically ill hospitalized adults. Chest 1991;100:1619–1636.
41. Gillum RF, Makuc DM. Serum albumin, coronary artery disease and death. Am Heart J 1992;123: 507–513.
42. Omran ML, Morley JE. Assessment of protein-energy malnutrition in older persons: Laboratory evaluation. Nutrition 2000,16.131–140.
43. Tietz N, Shuey D, Wekstein R. Laboratory values in fit aging individuals-sexagenarians through centenarians. Clin Chem 1992;38:1167–1185.
44. Doweiko JP, Nompleggi DJ. The role of albumin in human physiology and pathophysiology, part III: albumin and disease states. JPEN 1991;15:476–483.
45. Ballmer-Weber BK, Drummer R, Kung E, et al. Interleukin-2 induced increase of vascular permeability without decrease of the intravascular albumin pool. Br J Cancer 1995;71:78–82.
46. Courtney ME, Greene HL, Folk CC, et al. Rapidly declining serum albumin values in newly hospitalized patients: prevalence, severity and contributory factors. JPEN 1982;6:143–145.
47. Rothschild MA, Oratz M, Schreiber SS. Albumin synthesis. N Engl J Med 1972;286:748–757.
48. Robbins J, Cheng SY, Gershengorn MC, et al. Thyroxine transport proteins of plasma: molecular properties and biosynthesis. Rec Prog Horm Res 1978;34:477–519.
49. Ferguson RP, O'Connor P, Crabtree B, et al. Serum albumin and prealbumin as predictors of clinical outcomes of hospitalized elderly nursing home residents. J Am Geriatr Soc 1993;41:545–549.
50. Bourry J, Milano G, Caldani C, et al. Assessment of nutritional proteins during the parenteral nutrition of cancer patients. Ann Clin Lab Sci 1982;12:158–162.
51. Katz MD, Lor E, McGhan WF. Comparison of serum prealbumin ans transferrin for nutritional assessment of TPN patients: a preliminary study. Nutr Supp Serv 1986;6:22.
52. Carpentier YA, Barthel J, Bruyns J. Plasma protein concentrations in nutritional assessment. Proc Nutr Soc 1982;4:405–417.
53. Delpeuch F, Cornu A, Chevalier P. The effect of iron deficiency anemia on two nutritional indices of nutritional status, prealbumin and transferrin. Br J Nutr 1980;43:375–379.
54. Rask L, Anundi H, Bohme J, et al. Structural and functional studies of vitamin A binding proteins. Ann NY Acad Sci 1981;359:79–90.
55. Hall K, Tally M. The somatomedin-insulin-like growth factors. J Intern Med 1989;225:47–54.
56. Jacob V, Le Carpentier JE, Salzano S, et al. IGF-1, a marker of undernutrition in hemodialysis patients. Am J Clin Nutr 1990;52:39–44.
57. Unterman TJ, Vazquez RM, Slas AJ, et al. Nutrition and somatomedin. XIII. Usefulness of somatomedin-C in nutritional assessment. Am J Med 1985;78:228–234.
58. Sullivan DH, Carte WJ. Insulin-like growth factor I as an indicator of protein-energy undernutrition among metabolically stable hospitalized elderly. J Am Coll Nutr 1994;13:184–191.
59. Deodhar SD. C-reactive protein: the best laboratory indicator available for monitoring disease activity. Cleveland Clin J Med 1989;56:126–130.

60. Ingenbleek Y, Carpentier YA. A prognostic inflammatory and nutritional index scoring critically ill patients. Intern J Vit Nutr Res 1985;55:91–95.
61. Roza AM, Tuitt D, Shizgal HM, et al. Transferrin—a poor measure of nutriitonal status. JPEN 1984; 8:523–528.
62. Gergieff MK, Amrnath UM, Murphy EL, et al. Serum transferrin levels in the longitudinal assessment of protein-energy status in preterm infants. J Pediatr Gastroenterol Nutr 1989;8:234–239.
63. Rudman D, Mattson DE, Nagraj HS, et al. Prognostic significance of serum cholesterol in nursing home men. JPEN 1988;12:155–158.
64. Noel MA, Smith TK, Ettinger WH. Characterisitcs and outcomes of hospitalized older patients who develop hypocholesterolemia. J Am Geriatr Soc 1991;39:455–461.
65. Forette B, Tortrat D, Wolmark Y. Cholesterol as a risk factor for mortality in elderly women. Lancet 1999;1:868–870.
66. Kaiser FE. Cholesterol and the older adult. South Med J 1993;86:2511–2514.
67. Kaiser FE, Morley JE. Idiopathic CD4+ T lymphopenia in older persons. J Am Geriatr Soc 1994;42:1291.
68. Blackburn GL, Bistrian BR, Maini BS, et al. Nutritional and metabolic assessment of the hospitalized patient. JPEN 1977;1:11–22.
69. Seltzer MH, Bastidas JA, Cooper DM, et al. Instant nutrittional assessment. JPEN 1979;3:157–159.
70. Rosenthal AJ, Sanders KM, McMurtry CT, et al. Is malnutrition over diagnosed in older hospitalized patients? Association between the soluble interleukin-2 receptor and markers of malnutrition. J Gerontol A Biol Sci Med Sci 1998;53:M81.
71. Rolandelli RH, Ullrich JR. Nutritional support in the frail elderly surgical patient. Surg Clin North Am 1994;74:79–92.
72. Harris J, Benedict F. A biometric study of basal metabolism in man. Publication #279. Carnegia Institution, Washington, DC, 1919.
73. Lipkin EW. In: Enteral/parenteral alimentation. Hazzard WR, Bierman EL, Blass JP, et al. (eds.) McGraw-Hill, New York, NY, 1994, pp. 333–342.
74. Gersovitz M, Motil K, Munro HN, et al. Human protein requirements: Assessment of the current recommended dietary allowance for dietary protein in elderly men and women. Am J Clin Nutr 1982;35:6–14.
75. Mitchell S, Kiely DK, Lipsitz LA. Does artificial enteral nutrition prolong the survival of institutionalized elders with chewing and swallowing problems. J Gerontol 1998;53A:M207–M213.
76. Glick MR. Rethinking the role of tube feeding in patients with advanced dementia. N Engl J Med 2000;342:206–210.
77. Mitchell SL, Kiely DK, Lipsitz LA. The risk factors and impact on survival of feeding tube placement in nursing home residents with severe cognitive impairment. Arch Int Med 1997;157:327–332.
78. Finucane TE, Christmas C, Travis K. Tube feeding in patients with advanced dementia: A review of the evidence. JAMA 1999;282:1365–1370.
79. Peterson TI, Kruse A. Complications of percutaneous endoscopic gastrostomy. Eur J Surg 1997;163: 351–356.
80. Papaconstantinou HT, Chung DH, Zhang W, et al. Prevention of mucosal atrophy: role of glutamine and caspases in apoptosis in intestinal epithelial cells. J Gatrointestinal Surg 2000;4:416–423.
81. Wiepkema PR. Positive feedbacks at work during feeding. Behavior 1971;39:266–273.
82. Mathey MAM, Siebelink E, de Graaf C, Van Staveren WA. Flavor enhancement of food improves dietary intake and nutritional status of nursing home elderly. J Gerontol 2001;56A:M200–M205.
83. Schiffman SS, Warwick ZS. Use of flavor-amplified foods to improve nutritional status in elderly persons. In: Nutrition and the Chemical Senses in Aging: Recent Advances and Current Research Needs. Murphy C, Cain WS, Hegsted DM (eds.). Acad Sci, New York, NY, 1989, pp. 267–276.
84. Wilson MG, Purushothaman R, Morley JE. Effect of liquid dietary supplements on energy intake in the elderly. Am J Clin Nutr 2002;75:944–947.
85. Wilson MMG, Vaswani S, Liu D, Morley JE, Miller DK. Prevalence and causes of undernutrition in medical outpatients. Am J Med 1998;104:56–63.
86. Gram LF. Fluoxetine. N Engl J Med 1994:331;1354–1360.
87. Puzantian T. Mirtazapine, an antidepressant. Am J Health Syst Pharm 1998;55:44–49.
88. Kasper S, Praschak-Rieder N, Tauscher J, Wolf R. A risk-benefit assessment of mirtazapine in the treatment of depression. Drug Saf 1997;17:251–264.
89. Jakobs MK. Megesterol Acetate: a medical nutrition therapy tool to effect positive weight outcomes in the elderly. J Am Diet Assoc 1997;89:A119.

90. MacIntosh C, Morley JE, Cahpman I. The anorexia of aging. Nutrition 2000;16:983–995.

91. Voth EA, Schwartz RH. Medicinal applications of delta-9-tetrahydrocannabinol and marijuana. Ann Intern Med 1997;126:791–798.

92. Nelson K, Walsh D, Deeter P, Sheehan F. A phase II study of delta-9-tetrahydrocannabinol for appetite stimulation in cancer-associated anorexia. J Palliative Care 1994;10:14–18.

93. Volicer L, Stelly M, Morris J, McLaughlin J, Volicer BJ. Effects of Dronabinol on anorexia and disturbed behavior in patients with Alzheimers disease. Int J Geriat Psychiatry 1997;12:913–919.

94. Weir RF, Gostin L. Decisions to abate life-sustaining treatment for nonautonomous patients: ethical standards and legal liability for physicians after Cruzan. JAMA 1990;264:1846–1853.

95. Steinbrook R, Lo B. Artificial feeding-solid ground, not a slippery slope. N Engl J Med 1988;318: 286–290.

96. Lynn J, Childless J. Must patients always be given food and water? In: By No Extraordinary Means. Lynn J, (ed.), Indiana University Press, Bloomington, IN, 1986, pp. 47–60.

97. Waidmann T, Bound J, Schoenbaum M. The illusion of failure: Trends in self-reported health of the US elderly. Milbank Quarterly 1995;73:253–286.

98. Manton KG, Corder LS, Stallard E. Estimates of change in chronic disability and institutional incidence and prevalence rates in the US elderly population from 1982, 1984 and 1989. National Long Term Care Survey. J Gerontol 48:S153–S166.

99. Council for Nutrition: Clinical Strategies in Long Term Care: Clinical Guide to Prevent and Manage Malnutrition in Long-Term Care. Programs in Medicine, Philadelphia, PA, 2000.

6

Common Nutrient Deficiencies in Older Adults

Christopher J. Bates

1. INTRODUCTION

Older adults are at risk for nutrient deficiencies for a wide variety of reasons. They range from poverty, to impairment of appetite and senses of taste and smell, poorly fitting dentures, underlying illness, and the effects of medication or impaired physiology. The latter encompasses maldigestion and malabsorption, impaired retention of nutrients, therefore possibly increased nutrient requirements. Because of the complexity of the social, biochemical, and physiological processes that are involved, it has proved to be a difficult and complex task to obtain reliable evidence about the nature and relative importance of these deficiencies. Not everyone in a particular age group encounters similar problems associated with the aging process. One of the characteristics of aging is that the observed range of indices and intakes is broadened, so the most healthy of the elderly remain comparable with younger adults into extreme old age, whereas their less healthy counterparts may deteriorate sooner and diverge more quickly from the norms seen in young healthy adults.

The purpose of the present chapter is to list some of the ways in which nutrient deficiency states can be recognized and assessed (most of which are generally similar to those used for younger people). Second, the reasons why some older people are especially vulnerable are outlined. Third, it will provide some direct evidence as to the prevalence of biochemical deficiencies from recent surveys of people living in Britain.

2. ASSESSMENT OF DEFICIENCY

Nutrient deficiencies can be recognized or assessed in a number of different ways. Several different types of assessments are required to build a complete picture of the problem, and each provides a different and complementary window. Estimation of long-term food and nutrient intake requires considerable cooperation from the individual, and is subject to unavoidable inaccuracies, but is the most direct way to recognize the origin of a diet-related problem. Biochemical indices of nutrient status, measured in body fluids such as blood or urine, or in surface tissues for some trace elements, such as hair or fingernails, are more objective and potentially more accurate than intake estimates. However,

From: *Handbook of Clinical Nutrition and Aging*
Edited by: C. W. Bales and C. S. Ritchie © Humana Press Inc., Totowa, NJ

their interpretation in relation to nutrient intakes, adequacy of body-stores, and other physiological processes, needs careful individual assessment. Functional indices of status, which may be either biochemical or physiological, can help answer whether variations in nutrient supply have an effect on essential biochemical pathways, homeostasis, and bodily function. Clinical signs of deficiency usually arise only after severe and prolonged dietary and biochemical deficiency, and they only occur below the extreme lower end of the spectrum of nutritional adequacy and homeostatic control. In many cases, the clinical signs of deficiency are insufficiently specific to provide an unequivocal diagnosis on their own, but the resolution of a clinical abnormality following supplementation with one or more nutrients often can provide strong evidence for the nutritional origin of a clinical lesion.

2.1. Dietary Intake Assessment

Estimations of nutrient intake by individuals are dependent on the provision of a reliable food intake record by the individual, followed by its conversion to nutrient intake by means of tables providing the nutrient contents of foods. Food tables can only provide the average content of each nutrient derived from a number of food samples and analyses, usually performed by many different laboratories using different assay procedures. Some nutrients, notably certain vitamins, can vary considerably according to the genetic variety of the food item, its ripeness, storage duration, and conditions. The mineral content of plant foods often varies with the mineral content of the soil in which the plants are grown. Therefore, any nutrient intake calculation will inevitably suffer from some measurement error or uncertainty, which is an inherent problem in the assumptions arising from the use of food table nutrient values. However, in practice, these errors are usually smaller than those arising from other inevitable inaccuracies that occur during the collection of food intake estimates.

Food intake records may be obtained in a variety of ways, which vary in their reliability and in the level of demand imposed on the subject and the investigator. One of the simplest records is a 24-h recall of the previous day's diet, which may be either structured (i.e., prompted) or unstructured and may make use of portion size estimates (e.g., small, medium, or large) or household measures (e.g., cups and tablespoonfuls) as an approximate measure of quantity. Second, a written descriptive food intake record may be kept for periods, such as 3 or 7 d. A third approach, which is more time-consuming, but more accurate, usually covering a longer period, is a 3, 4, or 7-d weighed intake diary, in which the subject is provided with a device for the direct weighing of all the food they consume. There is a distinct possibility that subjects may change (i.e., simplify) their eating habits because of the extra effort required for the recording and because of their conscious focus on their dietary behavior. For instance, the subjects may avoid having second helpings or may consciously avoid foods perceived as "unhealthy." This means that a weighed intake estimate may underestimate or bias the records in relation to a subject's "usual" intakes. A fourth recording method is the "food frequency questionnaire," in which the subject is asked how many times in a defined period (i.e., during the last month or per week during the last year) they have eaten specified foods from a list. This assumes good memory, truthfulness, and effective communication with the investigator. It can be useful in establishing general food patterns and preferences, but is less useful for quantitative measurements.

None of the dietary assessment methods are foolproof and entirely reliable, and all need to be carefully assessed and validated for the particular purpose of the study or survey in question. The effects of random inaccuracies can be reduced by increasing the number of replications, either per individual or by increasing the number of individuals included, but the effects of bias are more difficult to resolve. It is important to ensure, by careful design, that any inevitable bias will not invalidate the conclusions of the study, and that confirmatory evidence is included wherever possible.

2.2. Biochemical and Functional Status Indicators

The procedures used for status index measurements of body fluids, such as blood and urine, and in tissues, such as hair and fingernails, are not age-specific in their operation. Therefore, they can be applied equally to all age groups of subjects, although it may for some purposes be necessary to define age- and gender-specific normal ranges.

As laboratory assay techniques are progressively refined and more powerful, it is becoming possible to measure wider range of status analytes in biological samples, as well as to measure them precisely and accurately. However, the following caveats must be noted. The interpretation of status measurements is frequently not straightforward, as the concentrations of nutrients in samples (e.g., such as blood serum or plasma, blood cells, urine, etc., or functional status indices) can be influenced by many different confounding biological factors, along with the relevant nutrient intakes. In addition, the status indices may reflect either short-term (hours) or long-term (days, weeks, months) nutrient intake patterns. Any comparisons made between population groups for diagnostic purposes must be done in a strictly controlled way and with knowledge of the most important confounding factors.

The use of external quality assessment schemes and quality-control materials of appropriate biological origin can harmonize methods between laboratories and between studies. Also, it is very important to be aware of the influence of factors, such as the acute-phase reaction (induced by infection and/or inflammation), and the possible influence of drugs used for medication on the index values.

Table 1 lists the procedures that are now most frequently used for vitamin status assessment, and Table 2 lists those that are used for mineral status assessment. As indicated in these tables, the investigator may choose a straightforward concentration assay, in which the actual concentration of the micronutrient or of a specific carrier protein is measured in a body fluid, such as serum, plasma, or urine. Alternatively, he or she may opt for a specific tissue compartment, such as the circulating red cells (erythrocytes), the buffy coat (total white cell) layer, or a specific white cell fraction. Finally, an indirect "functional" assay may be chosen. The term "functional assay" most commonly implies the measurement of an analyte, an enzyme, or a physiological function, which is modulated with some degree of specificity by the nutrient in question. For convenience, this is expanded to include analytes (e.g., transferrin receptors) that are induced by a relative deficiency of a nutrient (in this case, iron), but which are not simple binding proteins for that nutrient. There could be many categories of indirect or functional status assays, based on different aspects of the range of possible biochemical or physiological responses to variations in nutrient supplies. The question is, how useful are they in determining the adequacy of a nutrient supply to the essential tissues? Do they effectively reflect homeostasis or the risk of long-term tissue damage and eventual disease risk given the additional

Table 1
Vitamin Status Assessment Procedures

Vitamin	Concentration assay	Functional assay	Usual sample choice
Vitamin A (retinol) None available	HPLC separation with optical density detection	Dark adaptation; conjunctival impression cytology	Plasma (for the HPLC assay)
Carotenoids (some are vit. A precursors)	HPLC separation with optical density detection	None available	Plasma, combined with HPLC vitamin A assay
Vitamin E (mainly α and γ tocopherols)	HPLC separation with optical density detection	Erythrocyte lysis after peroxide stress[a]	Plasma, combined with HPLC vitamin A assay
Vitamin D	25-hydroxy vitamin D by HPLC or radioimmunoassay	Parathyroid hormone (PTH) levels	Plasma
Vitamin K	Plasma phylloquinone by HPLC with fluorescence assay	PIVKA[b]; undercarboxylated osteocalcin	Plasma
Vitamin C	HPLC or fluorescence or dye-reduction assay	None available	Plasma
B₁ (thiamine)	Fluorescence assay, with or without HPLC, in urine or red cells	Transketolase activation in vitro by thiamine pyrophosphate	Red cell lysate for transketolase assay
B₂ (riboflavin)	Fluorescence assay, with or without HPLC, in urine, plasma or red cells	Glutathione reductase activation by flavin adenine dinucleotide	Red cell lysate for glutathione reductase assay
B₆ (pyridoxine)	Fluorescence or enzyme activation assays for plasma pyridoxal phosphate (PLP)	Red cell aspartate aminotransferase activation by PLP	Red cell and plasma assays are both widely used
Folate	Microbiological or competitive protein binding assays	Homocysteine in plasma	Serum or whole blood for folate concentration assay
Vitamin B₁₂	Competitive binding (intrinsic factor) assay	Methylmalonic acid in plasma	Serum or plasma

[a]Developed for studies on premature infants; now only rarely used.
[b]Protein induced by vitamin K absence or antagonism. *See* refs. *5* and *15*.

106

Table 2
Mineral and Trace Element Assessment Procedures

Mineral/trace element	Concentration assays	Functional assays	Interpretation and comments
Iron	Serum ferritin by immunoassay; plasma iron concentrations and transferrin % saturation by colorimetric assay	Transferrin (TF) receptors by immunoassay in plasma; free protoporphyrin by fluorescence in blood	Ferritin is the most sensitive for body stores but TF receptors are less affected by the acute phase reaction
Zinc	Plasma zinc by colorimetric or atomic absorption assays or by ICPMS	No widely-accepted functional assay available	Deficiency is best recognized by its physiological effects. Difficult to study
Copper	Can be measured by colorimetric, atomic absorption or ICPMS assays. Not very useful	Red cell superoxide dismutase or serum diamine oxidase	Difficult to study; biochemical indicators still at research stage
Selenium	Plasma or red cell selenium by fluorescence assay or ICPMS	Glutathione peroxidase activity in plasma or red cells	Several newer assays being developed
Iodine	Urinary iodide by colorimetric assay	Goiter; plasma thyroid hormones; hormone binding proteins	Concept of "iodine deficiency diseases" (IDD)
Fluorine	Urinary fluoride by ion-specific electrode	None available	Narrow range of intake for optimum tooth protection
Sodium, potassium, calcium, magnesium	Assays in urine or plasma by atomic emission or absorption spectroscopy, etc.	None available	Used mainly to monitor intakes (urine Na,K), or hormone status

likelihood of insults from toxins, infective agents, and physical stresses? Clearly, the concept of "optimal nutrition" in relation to "optimal tissue protection" is a complex one, which has not been adequately defined, but the continuous development of a range of alternative functional indices and probes is gradually broadening the arsenal of procedures for this purpose.

The basic approach to designing useful status measurements is similar for all age groups. However, the "normal ranges" for both nutrient concentration and functional assays may also be age-specific, and the choice of the most informative assays may sometimes also be age-specific, in view of the special characteristics of the vulnerability of the elderly. For instance, it has recently been argued that tissue vitamin B_{12} status in older people is not always adequately reflected in their serum vitamin B_{12} levels, which is the traditional assay for vitamin B_{12} status. Instead, it has been suggested that plasma methylmalonic acid measurements are needed in order to complement the vitamin B_{12} concentration assay, because an important functional deficiency may still be present even when serum vitamin B_{12} levels lie within the normal range *(1,2)*. To illustrate this with another example, many older people have chronic inflammatory conditions, which can complicate the interpretation of traditional status indices (such as serum ferritin for iron status) *(3)*. In such a situation, another index describing iron status (e.g., the recently developed soluble plasma transferrin receptor concentration), which is less affected by the acute phase reaction and, hence, by inflammation, may prove more reliable and useful.

2.2.1. Vitamin Indices

Table 1 summarizes the principal biochemical assessment procedures that are available for the measurement of vitamin status.

For the fat-soluble vitamins (Table 1), vitamins A, E, and the carotenoid pigments may be measured together in a single high-pressure liquid chromatography (HPLC) run, starting with a lipid (usually hexane) extract of serum or plasma. The appropriate choice of stationary phase, mobile phase, and selected (multiple) wavelengths for optical density detection can ensure reliable quantitation even from small plasma samples of 50 μL or less. A photodiode array (PDA) detector can provide the range of simultaneous optical density recording channels at different wavelengths that are needed for this type of assay. The US National Institute of Science and Technology (NIST) runs a useful round-robin comparison scheme for interlaboratory harmonization. For retinol, accepted cut-off points are: <0.35 μM = deficient; <0.7 μM = low. There are generally no accepted defined normal ranges for the serum (or plasma) carotenoids, but the risk of functional vitamin A deficiency increases when both retinol and the provitamin A carotenoids (α- and β-carotenes and cryptoxanthins) fall to low concentrations. There are a number of alternative and older assay procedures available, especially for vitamin A, which depend on its native fluorescence or chemical conversion to a colored derivative, but most of these either require much larger amounts of sample, or are less accurate.

For vitamin E (the major component in most plasma samples being α-tocopherol), severe deficiency is associated with values less than 1.1 μmol/g lipid or <2.2 μmol/mol cholesterol.

The preferred index for vitamin D status is the concentration of 25-hydroxy vitamin D [25(OH)D] in serum or plasma. This can be measured either by HPLC separation followed by optical density or by radioimmunoassay, the latter being based on an antibody to a vitamin D derivative and is available in the form of a commercial assay kit *(4)*. There is an external quality assurance scheme available in the United Kingdom *(5)*. The most commonly accepted cut-off point below which biochemical deficiency is considered to occur is set at 25 nM, although some researchers have recently argued, on the basis of completeness of normalization of parathyroid hormone levels, that a higher cut-off for 25(OH)D should be used. The 25-(OH)D concentration varies with both the supply of vitamin D from the action of sunlight on the skin and the supply from the diet. However, the concentration of 1,25-dihydroxy vitamin D (calcitriol), the hormonal form of the vitamin, is homeostatically regulated and is much less affected by the vitamin D supply. Therefore, the hormonal form is less informative in nutritional terms, although it is of interest at the functional, homeostatic level of control, especially for the regulation of calcium supplies and bone metabolism.

Interest in vitamin K status has received a new stimulus in recent years from the discovery that several key vitamin K-dependent protein carboxylation reactions and, hence, γ-carboxyglutamate (GLA)-containing proteins not involved in the blood-clotting cascade, are functionally important for calcium homeostasis. Thus, they are potentially important with respect to several degenerative diseases that affect older people, including bone and cardiovascular diseases *(6)*. Traditionally, vitamin K status has been assessed by indirect (functional) blood clotting assays. Recently, however, the direct measurement of vitamin K in plasma has become possible, and a promising new and sensitive functional index of vitamin K status is the degree of undercarboxylation of circulating osteocalcin *(6)*. However, normal ranges have not yet been defined.

Of the water-soluble vitamins, vitamin C is usually measured in serum or plasma. The buffy coat vitamin C assay used to be favored a few decades ago, because under certain circumstances, it reflects tissue vitamin C levels more accurately, but it is difficult to perform, and its advantages have been questioned. The measurement of vitamin C can be achieved in many ways *(5)*. HPLC separation is specifically called for, if an isomer of the vitamin (erythorbic or D isoascorbic acid), which has a very low biological potency, is present in human diets as a result of the use of manufactured foods containing this substance as a preservative. Plasma vitamin C levels below 11 μM represent serious biochemical deficiency.

Tissue status of the three B vitamins, thiamine (B$_1$), riboflavin (B$_2$) and pyridoxine (B$_6$), can be assayed by measuring the three red cell enzymes (transketolase, glutathione reductase, and aspartate aminotransferase). Their enzymic activities are dependent on the B-vitamin-derived coenzymes, thiamine pyrophosphate (=cocarboxylase), flavin adenine dinucleotide, and pyridoxal phosphate, respectively. Enzyme activity is measured in a reaction rate analyzer, both with and without the appropriate coenzyme, which enables the extent of cofactor "activation," expressed as an "activation coefficient," to be calculated. The greater the activation coefficient, the more vitamin-depleted the enzyme in vivo and the more deficient the subject. For the transketolase activation coefficient, severe biochemical thiamine deficiency is usually associated with values above 1.25 (activity ratio); for the glutathione reductase activation cofficient the cut-off value varies with different versions of the assay, being typically in the range 1.2 to 1.4. For the aspartate aminotransferase activation coefficient, the cut-off is higher, usually around 1.8 to 2.2. This type of assay is now preferred over the older urine B vitamin concentration assays that were widely used 50 yr ago. Although the direct measurement of the B vitamin concentrations in plasma or red cell extracts may have some advantages, only a few laboratories possess the necessary analytical expertise and facilities, and the normal ranges are not well defined. For vitamin B_6 status assessment, however, several laboratories prefer to measure plasma pyridoxal phosphate (or total B_6 concentrations). Whichever B_6 index is selected, there are potential confounding factors that complicate the interpretation of the results (7,8). Plasma pyridoxal phosphate concentrations are usually found to be lower in frail elderly people than in younger adults (7), but the explanation and functional interpretation of this observation has not yet been fully resolved.

Folate status is usually measured by serum or plasma folate concentration assays or by red cell folate concentrations (derived from whole blood folate measurements), the latter being considered the better index of long-term status. For analytical convenience, the older microbiological assay (growth of the test microorganism, *Lactobacillus casei*, in a folate-deficient growth medium with added sample extract) has now been largely replaced by commercial kit assays based on milk folate-binding proteins, using radioassay or fluorescence endpoints. There is some disagreement over whether these are reliable and interchangeable, and folate assays are among the most difficult to harmonize between different laboratories (9). There are several external quality assurance methods (5). Severe biochemical deficiency is associated with serum or plasma folate levels below 7 nM or red cell levels below 250 nM. Functional tests for folate adequacy include the response of plasma homocysteine to folate supplementation and the occurrence of multilobed nuclei in circulating polymorphonuclear leucocytes, which may respond to folate supplements.

Vitamin B_{12} status is usually measured in serum or plasma by assays based on the specific vitamin B_{12} recognition and binding properties of intrinsic factor. Intrinsic factor is the binding protein that is secreted into the stomach to enable vitamin B_{12} to be absorbed efficiently in the upper ileum. There are several commercial kits that are based on this interaction. The agreement between these appears to be somewhat better than for the folate assay kits. Microbiological assays were also in common use for vitamin B_{12} analysis until a few years ago. Serum or plasma levels below 75 or 100 pM are considered to indicate severe biochemical deficiency and 150 pM is often taken as the limit of mild deficiency. The most specific functional indicator of tissue vitamin B_{12} deficiency is a raised serum or plasma concentration of methylmalonic acid. This sensitive functional test can reveal tissue deficiency states even in some subjects who have serum B_{12} levels within the normal range (1,2).

The other B vitamins (niacin, biotin, and pantothenic acid) are infrequently included in micronutrient status investigations in Western countries, because most diets are adequately supplied with them. It is rare to find evidence of deficiency, except in cases of uncommon genetic disorders, bizarre diets, or the deliberate use of vitamin antagonists.

2.2.2. Mineral Indices

Table 2 summarizes the principal biochemical assessment procedures that are available for the measurement of mineral micronutrient status.

Of the mineral micronutrients, deficiency of iron is perceived as a public health problem of worldwide significance, although it is becoming clear that optimum biochemical status does not always correspond with optimum clinical protection. Iron status assays are most commonly included in nutritional investigations, partly because iron-deficiency anemia is a relatively common condition, and partly because iron status, unlike that of most other minerals, can be measured in several complementary ways. The main characteristics of iron-deficiency anemia are low-blood hemoglobin concentration, low hematocrit, and low-mean cell volumes (MCV), i.e., a microcytic anemia. However, this is not unequivocal evidence for iron deficiency, because conditions (such as lead poisoning) can produce a similar picture by interfering with the incorporation of iron into hemoglobin. More direct assays for iron deficiency are based on serum or plasma assays. The percentage saturation of transferrin (known as "total iron binding capacity") is a good measure of circulating iron availability; serum ferritin is a measure of tissue iron stores, and the recently introduced serum soluble transferrin receptor assay provides a third index of iron adequacy at the level of feedback control. Only the latter index partially avoids a common scourge of many micronutrient status assays based on serum or plasma: the acute phase reaction. If acute phase-initiated inflammation or infection is present (as it is in many older people with chronic illnesses), then serum ferritin levels increase markedly and serum iron levels decrease, regardless of the true magnitude of the body iron stores. For this and for other reasons related to the extent of iron depletion, the soluble transferrin receptor assay is considered a valuable new addition to the available options for the measurement of iron status.

In the British National Diet and Nutrition Survey (NDNS) of people aged 65 yr and over (see Section 4.), an analysis of iron status indices (10) revealed more values in the low or deficient range in the group aged 75 yr and over than in the group aged 65–74 yr. However, a recent study of iron status of people aged 67–96 yr, who were participating in the Framingham Heart Study in the United States, found that abnormally high iron stores may be a greater cause for health-related concern than iron deficiency in this age group. Only 3% of the Framingham study group had depleted iron stores, whereas approx 13% had elevated stores (11,12).

Blood assays for zinc and copper are less well developed and less satisfactory than those available for iron, mainly because the concentrations of these elements in blood fractions are difficult to interpret. They have been traditionally measured in blood plasma, either by flame atomic absorption spectrometry or by colorimetric assays, e.g., on a clinical chemistry analyzer. Recently, developments in inductively coupled plasma mass spectrometry (ICPMS) have enabled such elements to be measured more efficiently in multielement mode. Plasma zinc concentrations give some information about zinc status, but plasma levels do not correlate well with zinc concentrations in other tissue compartments (3), and plasma zinc is also a negative acute-phase reactant. The best evidence for suboptimal zinc status is a positive functional or health response to zinc supplements. In the elderly, this evidence might be derived from improved indices of immune function (13), although the proposal remains controversial. Copper status may be reflected by changes in activity of zinc-copper superoxide dismutase in red cells, and a recent study has suggested that the diamine oxidase activity of serum can also provide useful information about copper status (14). However, total plasma copper is a positive acute-phase reactant, like ferritin, thus its interpretation is not straightforward.

Magnesium has received relatively little attention in nutrition surveys and clinical investigations, partly because there is no robust and generally accepted way of estimating the prevalence of a marginal or functional deficiency of this essential nutrient. Estimates of the concentration in plasma can be made by atomic absorption spectroscopy or by

ICPMS, but their interpretation is controversial. Although links to acute vascular function have been studied, investigations of the implications of long-term magnesium status in healthy people are lacking.

Assays of selenium in plasma and blood and of glutathione peroxidase activity as a functional index of selenium status, are beginning to yield useful information about selenium status in human populations. Selenium can be measured by conversion to a fluorescent product, and recent advances in ICPMS have enabled it to be measured with minimal interference from artefacts arising from the carrier inert gas used. Although plasma selenium is a negative acute-phase reactant, it is also highly responsive to population variations in selenium intakes and can reveal evidence of selenium overload, as well as of deficiency, whereas glutathione peroxidase activity reaches a plateau at high selenium intakes. Several other potential selenium indices are now being actively investigated.

Iodine status is usually assessed from urinary iodine levels, measured by a colorimetric assay based on its catalytic action on the reduction of ceric salts with arsenious acid. The urine concentration is a direct reflection of recent dietary intake. Blood assays of thyroid hormones may be useful as confirmatory indicators, because a lack of iodine produces an increase in thyroid-stimulating hormone and can alter the ratio of thyroxine to tri-iodothyronine.

2.3. Clinical Signs of Specific Nutrient Deficiencies

Paradoxically, although clinical deficiency signs and symptoms are the ultimate predicted result of severe and prolonged nutrient deficiencies, they are generally less useful as indices of status in population studies than the biochemical index values. This is partly because they tend to be nonspecific, in the sense that several types of nutrient deficiency or non-nutritional insult (infection, trauma, side effects of medication, and so on) can produce the same pathological end result. This is especially true of older people, for whom the most characteristic and common pathological states are frequently multifactorial. For a number of micronutrients, the clinical-pathological picture seen in older people is quite different from that seen in children with the same deficiencies or even in young adults; therefore, the clinical examination needs to be age-oriented and carefully interpreted. In addition, the pathological effects of deficiency are often slow to resolve after removal of the primary causative factor, especially if this is nutritional, and this may complicate the diagnostic procedure. Nevertheless, a clinical examination and/or record of recent illnesses is an important part of the investigation of a suspected nutritional inadequacy.

Signs and symptoms of vitamin A deficiency are rare in Western countries, especially among older people. It is a characteristic of the normal physiological developmental process that vitamin A stores build up gradually in the liver throughout life, being lowest in the fetus and highest in older adults. In countries where vitamin A deficiency is widely prevalent, toddlers and young children are especially vulnerable, exhibiting signs like xerophthalmia and keratomalacia, and an increased risk of severe life-threatening infections. However, even in these vulnerable communities, older people appear to be spared.

Vitamin E deficiency in humans is a controversial topic. Overt clinical deficiency of the type and severity that has been demonstrated in experimental animals is virtually unknown in humans, except in individuals with genetic defects that severely impair vitamin E stores, such as abetalipoproteinemia. On the other hand, vitamin E is one of a small group of micronutrients whose antioxidant, free radical chain-breaking properties make them ideally suited for quenching prooxidant free radicals and, thus, preventing or reversing their potential damaging effects. There is current research interest in the proposition that vitamin E may protect against certain pathological events in older people, even though straightforward vitamin E deficiency states are virtually unknown. However, the evidence is conflicting and incomplete, and most authorities currently advise against large increases in vitamin E intake or the excessive use of supplements, because the balance of health advantage versus possible (subtle) disadvantage remains controversial.

For the remaining two fat-soluble vitamins, vitamin D and vitamin K, there is considerable evidence that older people living in Western countries are frequently functionally deficient, to the extent that such deficiency may have important clinical consequences. Although the causes of the current epidemic of osteoporosis in older people living in northern Europe and North America are likely to be complex and only partly nutritional in origin, there is good evidence that inadequate vitamin D status is a significant candidate. Exposure to sunlight and dietary vitamin D intakes is frequently low (16). Although classical osteomalacia, attributable directly to simple vitamin D deficiency, is not especially common (see Section 3), the more complex condition of osteoporosis (see Chapter 29) with a component of vitamin D deficiency appears to be widespread, prompting the setting of a reference nutrient intake (RNI) of 10 μg/d of vitamin D for adults aged 65+ yr in the United Kingdom (17) and an adequate intake (AI) of 10 μg/d for adults aged 51–70 yr and 15 μg/d for adults aged 70+ yr in the United States (18).

The clinical consequences of poor vitamin K status are more controversial and less well-established. However, recent research has pointed toward the possibility of important clinical outcomes for bone and artery health, resulting from undercarboxylation of two proteins whose key functional Gla-residues are vitamin K-dependent, namely osteocalcin and matrix Gla-protein (6). Unlike the consequences of undercarboxylation of the proteins of the blood-clotting cascade, which have been known for much longer, these newly discovered functions of vitamin K are especially relevant to older people. Indeed, there is now a potential conflict between the use of warfarin (a vitamin K antimetabolite) as a means of reducing the hazards of excessive intravascular blood clotting and the maintenance of the essential extra-hepatic functions of vitamin K.

Turning to the water-soluble vitamins, the perceived problems for older people appear to be the greatest for vitamins C and B_{12}. For vitamin C deficiency, similar to vitamin A deficiency in children, it is likely to be a major weakening of the body's defenses against infections, which leads to severe morbidity and mortality. Whereas classical vitamin C deficiency signs characteristic of scurvy are rare in Western society, vitamin C status in older people appears to be a powerful predictor of mortality from a wide variety of degenerative diseases (19). From this study, the authors have concluded that it is most likely that vitamin C is acting as a marker for the protective action of fruit and vegetables, as it is an important component.

Vitamin B_{12} is important for older people because of the increase in the prevalence of those gastrointestinal malfunction states that interfere with vitamin B_{12} absorption with age. Human diets vary in their content of vitamin B_{12}, even in Western countries (vegetarian diets are much poorer in B_{12} than meat-containing ones). Nevertheless, it is the efficiency of absorption that dominates B_{12} status in humans. In older people, not only does the prevalence of pernicious anemia and related gastrointestinal malfunction increase, but atrophic gastritis and partial or complete gastrectomy can also affect B_{12} absorption, i.e., by interfering with the release of protein-bound vitamin B_{12} from the food matrix. The clinical consequences of severe vitamin B_{12} deficiency are megaloblastic anemia and (if undetected for a prolonged period), combined subacute degeneration of the spinal cord, resulting in neurological abnormalities that can become permanent and irreversible if untreated. Because of this risk of irreversible damage, the need to detect and treat vitamin B_{12} deficiency at an early stage of its development is widely recognized. With increasing longevity in Western populations, effective monitoring of vitamin B_{12} status of older people is an important preventive measure.

Among the other B vitamins, both folate and riboflavin may be critical for older people. The strong relation between folate and homocysteine status, with potential implications for health status, is discussed in Chapter 15. Riboflavin status of older people was of considerable concern in the United Kingdom during the 1960s, when evidence of clinical mouth symptoms (angular stomatitis and cheilosis) was thought to be widespread among older people. However, the specificity and interpretation of this evidence was later questioned, and two government surveys in the1960s and 1970s *(20,21)* concluded that clinical evidence of riboflavin deficiency was lacking, although biochemical deficiency was widespread. More recently, interest in riboflavin status has reemerged in the context of its key interaction with folate economy as an essential cofactor for a critical enzyme controlling folate metabolism; methylene tetrahydrofolate reductase, for which there are common genetic polymorphisms with probable functional significance.

Clinical thiamine deficiency in the United Kingdom and other Western countries is rare, and where it does occur it is most frequently associated with alcoholism, as exemplified by the Wernicke-Korsakoff syndrome. Vitamin B_6 deficiency, although common at the biochemical level in older people, is rarely seen at the clinical level. Clinical deficiency of the other B vitamins is extremely rare in Western society except in people with specific genetic defects, bizarre diets, or if exposed to vitamin antagonists.

Clinical signs of iron deficiency in older people are connected mainly with anemia, which has a range of functional side effects, in addition to the general appearance of a characteristic pallor. Poor iron status is also thought to affect immune function, although the evidence in man is not entirely conclusive, and it may affect the appearance of fingernails, causing growth distortion (koilonychia).

The severe, genetically determined zinc deficiency state of acrodermatitis enteropathica, with characteristic skin lesions, has been described in children but not in older people, and the effects of poor zinc status in older people is likely to be manifested in more subtle ways, such as changes in immune function. The same is true of the other essential trace metals such as copper, manganese, or chromium, requiring biochemical tests as they are difficult to detect by clinical examination.

One nutritionally essential element for which clinical deficiency is particularly widespread in the developing world is iodine. Clinical signs of goiter are both a sensitive, and reasonably specific indicator of insufficiency. In older people, goiters are often difficult to reverse by iodine supplements, although their biochemical thyroid function usually responds quite readily. In some parts of the world, goiters may be the result of a combined deficiency of both iodine and selenium. Clinical selenium deficiency in the absence of accompanying iodine deficiency has been described in some parts of China, but this deficiency is now less common, following the introduction of selenium-containing fertilizers.

3. REASONS FOR INCREASED VULNERABILITY OF OLDER PEOPLE TO MALNUTRITION, WITH PARTICULAR REFERENCE TO BONE HEALTH

Several vitamins, notably vitamins D and K, and several mineral and trace elements play an essential and specific role in bone, and for many of these nutrients, older people are potentially vulnerable to deficiency states for both dietary and other physiological reasons. The following sections highlight some of the evidence for, and characteristics of, this problem, beginning with vitamin D. Chapter 29, which discusses osteoporosis, also addresses aspects of this subject.

In the British NDNS of people aged 65 yr and over *(22)*, vitamin D status as measured by plasma 25(OH)vitamin D levels was lowest during the winter months and highest during the late summer months in free-living elderly people. In people living in long-stay institutions (e.g., nursing homes), however, vitamin D status was equally low throughout the whole year, and the summer increase was not observed. In the latter group, approx 40% had 25(OH)D levels below 25 nM (a commonly accepted cut-off for biochemical deficiency), whereas in the free-living group, only 8% overall had such low-index values. In both groups of elderly people, the mean dietary intake of vitamin D was only 3.4 µg/d and the median was less than 3 µg/d, compared with a reference nutrient intake of 10 µg/d for people aged 65 yr and over *(17)*. The majority of respondents in the survey were Caucasian, however, it is known from other UK studies that minority ethnic groups, especially those from the Indian subcontinent, have even poorer vitamin D status and a correspondingly greater risk of overt clinical deficiency. There is evidence that light-catalyzed vitamin D synthesis on the skin of older people is reduced when compared to younger people, because of a reduced concentration in the vitamin D precursor, 7-dehydrocholesterol in their skin *(23–25)*. In addition, elderly people with osteoporosis exhibit impaired conversion of 25(OH)D to the hormonally active effector, 1,25(OH)$_2$D, when stimulated by parathyroid hormone *(26)*.

Provision of a 10-µg daily vitamin D supplement to elderly American subjects during the winter months prevented a seasonal loss of bone mineral *(27)*. A vitamin D intake of 20 µg/d was more effective than approx 5 µg/d in preventing bone mineral loss at the femoral neck *(28)*. Thus, the combination of old age, infrequent exposure to sunlight (especially likely for people living in nursing homes), and low dietary intake of vitamin D, especially during the winter months may result in bone mineral loss. Because older people find it difficult to achieve an appropriate intake of vitamin D from unfortified food, it is likely desirable to increase their vitamin D intakes by fortification or supplementation during the winter months. However, it should be noted that the safety margin between adequacy and overdosage is not very wide for vitamin D. For this reason, a fixed daily supplement may be safer than the fortification of food, because the latter may result in a wide spectrum of intakes consequent on idiosyncratic food choices.

The involvement of vitamin K in a range of metabolic processes that are critical for good health and normal tissue homeostasis in older people has become a major research topic in recent years *(6)*. For instance, it has recently been shown that men aged 65+ yr had a significantly greater percentage of undercarboxylation of their circulating osteocalcin than men aged 18–30 yr *(29)*. In both age groups and both sexes, vitamin K (phylloquinone) supplements reduced the extent of osteocalcin undercarboxylation. The authors of this study note that in other studies, a high serum level of undercarboxylated osteocalcin has been associated with increased skeletal turnover, low bone mineral density, and increased risk of osteoporotic fracture. The use of vitamin K antagonists has also been related to low bone mineral density and an increased risk of fracture. However, the role and importance of vitamin K insufficiency in skeletal health remains unclear.

Several groups have also shown that calcium supplements can increase bone mineral density in older people. Dawson-Hughes reported that a 500-mg daily calcium supplement increased bone density in people with food calcium intakes less than 400 mg/d *(30)*. Subsequent studies suggested that women with higher basal calcium intakes can also benefit from calcium supplements *(31–33)*. Some of these effects are produced by intakes that would be difficult to achieve from food alone, and it remains unclear whether they represent true "deficiency" or a pharmacological effect of high intakes.

Vitamin C is the fourth micronutrient that plays a significant role in bone metabolism. Inadequate vitamin C status is often observed in older people. Several studies have reported a cross-sectional relationship between greater vitamin C intake from food or the use of vitamin C supplements and higher bone mineral density *(34–36)*. However, no evidence from any intervention studies is currently available. It is clear from the British NDNS survey that circulating vitamin C levels are generally lower in older adults and is not entirely accounted for in terms of low dietary intakes. Low vitamin C status is one of the best markers for risk of mortality in older people *(19)*, although there is little evidence that a reduction in mortality can be achieved by increasing vitamin C intakes. Inflammatory processes and an altered economy of transition metal ions, such as iron and copper, may increase the rate of turnover of vitamin C. However, the causes of low vitamin C status in the elderly are not fully understood.

Vulnerability to nutrient deficiencies that affect bone status is, of course, only the tip of the iceberg with respect to the range of nutritional vulnerabilities that are faced by older people. Other examples include vitamins E and B_6 e.g., in relation to immune function *(37,38)*. Low vitamin B_6 intakes and poor vitamin B_6 status indices have been documented in a considerable number of studies of elder populations *(39–50)*. The functional significance of this is uncertain, not least because different vitamin B_6 status indices give different pictures, and it is possible that the blood picture is not representative of the critical tissues and their supply of B_6 cofactors *(51)*. Clearly, further studies are needed to clarify the interpretation of status index measurements in older people and to define their dietary micronutrient requirements and how these differ from those of younger, more healthy, adults.

4. AN APPRAISAL OF THE EVIDENCE THAT OLDER PEOPLE MIGHT DIFFER FROM YOUNGER ADULTS, WITH RESPECT TO NUTRIENT INTAKES AND NUTRIENT STATUS INDICES

A report by the Department of Health published in 1992 summarized the knowledge of the nutritional vulnerability of elderly people in Britain *(52)*.

In this report, it was concluded that protein intakes are generally adequate, except possibly for some severely malnourished older people who might, for instance, be recovering from a bone fracture or other illness. For thiamin, there is no simple relationship between intake and status. For riboflavin, a considerable proportion of older people have poor biochemical status, but nondietary factors, as well as riboflavin intake, may also affect status *(53)*. For vitamin B_{12}, there is evidence of poor status in hospitalized elderly people, but less evidence of any decline in status with age in healthy elderly people. With the exception of some vegans and very strict vegetarians, vitamin B_{12} deficiency is not usually caused by dietary deficiency. Vitamin B_{12} deficiency is much more likely to be the result of impaired absorption, which could have several possible causes. Biochemical folate deficiency may be present, but little evidence of clinical deficiency exists. The same is true for vitamin C, although one study *(54)* found clinical benefit from a 1-g daily supplement of vitamin C in older people living in an institution. Both vitamin C and vitamin E are thought to have wide potential implications for the reduction of degenerative disease risk through the reduction of tissue damage by oxidative-free radicals, although the extent and significance of such protective effects remains to be defined.

Of the mineral elements considered in the 1992 report, the functional significance of magnesium and its requirement is poorly understood. It is likely that cardiac arrhythmias are exacerbated by magnesium deficiency, especially when other electrolyte imbalances are present. The assessment of iron status is not easy because traditional measures, such as blood hemoglobin, mean cell volume, and serum ferritin all have shortcomings. In older people, there is a greater risk of iron malabsorption than in younger adults, attributable to conditions like hiatal hernia, peptic ulcer, diverticular disease, hemorrhoids, or cancer. Older men are more likely than younger men to have poor iron status indices, but the reverse is true among women. Zinc status is especially at risk for older people living in institutions; however, cellular immunity can be impaired by inappropriately high zinc intakes as well as by low intakes. A similar concern was expressed about the use of selenium supplements, suggesting that these "should be avoided because high intakes are toxic." Since the 1992 report was written, concern about generally low selenium intakes in the United Kingdom has increased, and more selenium-containing over-the counter (OTC) multinutrient supplements are now available in the United Kingdom. Hospitalized elderly people tend to have low leucocyte copper levels, but the potential health significance of this is not known.

Nutrients significant for bone health are of major public health and research importance in the United Kingdom, because of the increasing prevalence of bone disease, particularly osteoporotic fractures, in the population. The reference nutrient intake for calcium in people aged 65 yr and over stands at 700 mg/d for both sexes, and there is some limited evidence that intakes below 500 mg/d are associated with lower cortical (but not trabecular) bone mass. Around 30 yr ago, there was histological evidence of high prevalence of osteomalacia in older Britons living in the Northern half of the British Isles (12%–47% prevalence, estimated from several studies), although this high prevalence was not seen in London and Cardiff (the Southern half of the country). In recent years, this high prevalence of overt clinical deficiency in northern Britain has likely declined. Nevertheless, there remains a high prevalence of low biochemical index values, notably of 25(OH) vitamin D, especially during the late winter months. Daily dietary intakes of vitamin D remain far below the UK RNI of 10 µg/d for people aged 65 yr and over. A typical daily intake is approx 3–4 μg. Naturally rich sources of vitamin D include fatty fish, eggs, meat (especially liver), and fortified foods including margarine (with compulsory fortification in the United Kingdom) and breakfast cereals (with voluntary, permissive fortification). The 1992 report notes that for those at high risk of vitamin D deficiency, a 6-mo or annual depot injection of vitamin D can be given. Raised fluoride intakes (approx 4–6 ppm in drinking water) have been claimed to be associated with increased bone mass and/or decreased fracture incidence in older people, but this is controversial and has not been detected at the lower levels of fluoride used for water fluoridation in the United Kingdom.

During the past 15 yr, a rolling series of diet and nutrition surveys of different age groups have provided information about nutrient intakes and selected status indices for the most nutritionally critical nutrients in mainland Britain. With the completion and publication of the Report of the NDNS of people aged 65 yr and over *(22)* in 1998, it became possible to compare nutrient intakes and biochemical status indices between younger and older British adults. Although the surveys of the different age groups in Britain have not all been carried out by the same organizations or by the same methods, and intersurvey harmonization may not be perfect, some useful intergroup comparisons can be derived, which are consistent with studies of other populations.

Table 3 shows that for daily food energy and for micronutrient intake estimates, there is a greater median intake of nutrients by men than by women at all ages. For micronutrients other than retinol (vitamin A) and vitamin D, there is evidence of a decline in intakes with increasing age, in parallel with a decline in energy intake, which corresponds with the well-established declines in energy expenditure and lean body mass with increasing age. However, the nutrient density of the diets remain essentially unchanged with increasing age, so that although total daily nutrient intakes go down, the quality of the diet apparently does not.

In Table 4, a comparison of blood status indices is made between surveys and, hence, between age groups. (The reason for including the 15–18-yr age group is that the assay methodology was generally the same, and the analytical laboratory was the same as the survey of older adults.) For some of the status indices, there was a clear gender difference, which was likely hormonally driven. For plasma cholesterol and two of the fat-soluble vitamins (retinol and α-tocopherol), the median concentrations increased during early adulthood, peak, then declined to a modest extent in old age. A greater decline in old age was seen for 25(OH)D, confirming the prediction that older people are especially vulnerable to poor vitamin D status in Northern climes. This is probably because of their tendency to avoid sunlight exposure and also because of reduced rates of vitamin D production for a given level of sunlight exposure.

For the water-soluble vitamins, vitamin C and folate, there was a steady decline in blood levels from young adulthood to old age. This was especially steep for vitamin C. Vitamin B_{12} status also declined in older people. Vitamin B_6 status as measured by plasma pyridoxal phosphate concentrations was found to be considerably lower in the elderly survey participants than in the younger ones *(7,8)*.

The indices of mineral status yielded a less consistent picture than that seen for the indices of vitamin status. Iron status was poorer in young menstruating women than in young or older men and older women; however, there was also a modest decline in some of the iron indices with increasing age in the oldest groups. There was also a moderate

Table 3
Median Energy and Nutrient Intakes by Adults Participating in Two Major British Diet and Nutrition Surveys During the Period 1986–1995

Age	Males				Females			
	35–64 yr[a]	65–74 yr[b]	75–84 yr[b]	85+ yr[b]	35–64 yr[a]	65–74 yr[b]	75–84 yr[b]	85+ yr[b]
N	619	271	265	96	668	256	217	170
Estimated daily intake of:								
Food energy (MJ)	10.13	8.15	7.73	6.96	7.03	6.01	5.80	5.58
Retinol (µg)	665	795	787	780	541	653	632	642
Vitamin D (µg)	3.32	3.61	3.28	2.78	2.45	2.67	2.68	2.09
Vitamin E (mg)	9.1	8.4	7.5	5.8	9.1	6.4	5.9	5.2
Vitamin C (mg)	59.6	62.6	51.4	46.0	59.4	56.8	45.9	42.2
Folate (µg)	300	276	237	232	213	211	188	172
Total iron (mg)	13.5	10.6	10.7	9.7	10.3	8.7	8.1	7.6
Calcium (mg)	951	848	807	717	735	683	641	619
Magnesium (mg)	314	255	226	218	229	195	177	173
Zinc (mg)	11.1	8.8	8.1	7.9	8.6	7.1	6.9	6.5
Sodium (mg)	3365	2722	2673	2475	2307	2002	2004	1852

[a]The data for the 35–64 yr age group is amalgamated from two age groups from the Adults' Survey (55), whose fieldwork was in 1986–1987.
[b]The data for the three older groups were from the free-living sample of the National Diet and Nutrition Survey: People aged 65 Years and Over (22). The fieldwork was in 1994–1995.

The Adult Survey diet record was kept for 7 d by each participant. That of the 65+ year survey was kept for 4 d for each participant. The recording procedures in the two surveys were similar, but were administered by different organizations.

119

Table 4

Median Nutritional Status Indices for Young People and Adults Participating in Three Major British Surveys During the Period 1986–1997

Age	Males					Females				
	15–18 yr[a]	35–64 yr[b]	65–74 yr[c]	75–84 yr[c]	85+ yr[c]	15–18 yr[a]	35–64 yr[b]	65–74 yr[c]	75–84 yr[c]	85+ yr[c]
N	164	520	216	207	72	169	547	194	165	115
Status index										
Plasma cholesterol (mmol/L)	3.85	6.15	5.70	5.40	4.80	4.05	6.20	6.09	6.29	5.83
HDL cholesterol (μmol/L)	1.09	1.10	1.09	1.10	1.06	1.18	1.40	1.29	1.35	1.33
Plasma retinol (μmol/L)	1.49	2.25	2.15	2.14	2.04	1.46	1.90	2.05	2.07	2.11
α-Tocopherol (μmol/L)	18.7	27.7	35.8	33.4	30.0	18.2	27.7	39.1	37.7	35.8
25(OH)vitamin D (nmol/L)	46.1	nm	59.6	48.1	43.4	50.8	nm	52.4	46.9	36.3
Plasma vitamin C (μmol/L)	51.6	nm	41.4	36.1	29.9	56.9	nm	55.2	47.3	35.4
Serum folate (nmol/L)	17.0	nm	12.8	11.6	12.1	15.2	nm	14.7	13.4	12.2
Red cell folate (nmol/L)	515	nm	437	400	477	474	nm	436	429	406
Serum vitamin B_{12} (pmol/L)	265	273	210	203	195	251	302	230	213	197
Serum pyridoxal phosphate (nmol/L)	58.5	nm	36.4	33.3	29.3	49.3	nm	36.9	33.3	29.3
Blood hemoglobin (g/dL)	13.2	14.7	14.7	14.4	13.4	13.2	13.3	13.7	13.4	13.1
Iron % saturation	23.8	nm	27.3	26.7	25.1	18.9	nm	24.8	22.4	23.4
Serum ferritin (μg/L)	44	95	93	95	67	23	43	61	52	51
Plasma zinc (μmol/L)	14.6	nm	14.5	14.1	12.7	14.5	nm	14.2	13.8	13.3

[a]The 15–18 yr group is from the National Diet and Nutrition Survey: Young People Aged 4 to 18 Years (56), whose fieldwork was performed in 1997.

[b, c]See footnotes a and b, respectively in Table 3.

[d]Numbers of samples shown for hemoglobin. For the other analytes, they were slightly less, because of limitations of blood volumes available for some of the samples. nm = not measured. The assay methods used were not necessarily the same between the three surveys, and for the adults' survey, they were performed in a different laboratory from that used for the other two surveys. However, for the cholesterol indices, the three fat-soluble vitamins (A, D, and E), vitamin C, iron % saturation, and zinc, essentially the same assays were used in both the young people's and the 65+ yr surveys.

decline in plasma zinc levels with increasing age. However, some of the indices are affected by chronic inflammation and by the acute-phase reaction, so one has to exercise caution in concluding that there is a decline in body stores from a decline in plasma levels.

In conclusion, recent British surveys have indicated that older people have poor status for vitamins D, C, B_{12}, and B_6, with more modest declines for other blood vitamins. Mineral indices are generally less vulnerable.

5. SUMMARY AND RECOMMENDATIONS FOR FURTHER RESEARCH

Clearly, people age at different rates depending on their genetic constitution and their exposure to those insults that may enhance the rate of aging or to those protective factors that may retard it. Diet is a source of enhancers and retardants of the aging process. Older people who are physiologically young for their years generally have nutritional characteristics (food choices, nutrient intakes, and status indices) that are very similar to those of younger adults. In contrast, those who are frail and ill often have poorer appetites, reduced nutrient intakes, impaired status indices, and a high risk of clinical deficiency or of suboptimum functional status.

With respect to the macronutrients, the available status indices are only crude indicators; thus, weight loss or a very low body mass index will signal that "something is likely to be wrong," but cannot indicate exactly what the problem is. Even measures such as plasma albumin, are relatively crude indices of status (see Chapter 5). Lipid indices, such as plasma cholesterol, can provide some degree of risk assessment, but only in conjunction with other indicators. A reduction in cholesterol may be desirable for an older person who is at high risk of vascular disease, but is undesirable in another who is underweight, frail, and generally malnourished (see Chapter 5).

The micronutrient indices and their associated intakes are potentially more specific sources of information about particular physiological risks and types of malnutrition. In countries like the United Kingdom, which are far from the equator, the effects of reduction in load-bearing exercise, together with increasing longevity, have resulted in an epidemic of age-related bone disease. Therefore, there is a growing interest in those micronutrients (e.g., calcium, vitamins D, K, and C, phosphorus, and zinc) whose modulation may reduce the rate of bone loss and associated fracture risk. A recent Committee on Medical Aspects of Food Policy (COMA) report on Nutrition and Bone Health in the United Kingdom (16) has highlighted the need for new research on adaptive responses to different diets studies on nutrient-gene interactions and the importance of environmental influences in early life. The results and mechanisms of seasonally low vitamin D status on osteoporosis risk also need to be investigated. Groups at risk of low vitamin D status should be studied, particularly for the best practical way of providing vitamin D supplements in the community and in the institutional setting.

A considerable body of research has underpinned the concept of the health benefit of a relatively high level of fruit and vegetable inclusion in the diet. It is unclear whether this benefit is attributable to the so-called "antioxidant," free radical-scavenging nutrients, vitamin C, vitamin E, bioflavonoids, and trace element components of radical-scavenging enzymes, or to other components, such as the nonstarch polysaccharide ("fiber") components. The B vitamins; especially folate and vitamin B_{12}, have recently been propelled into prominence in the context of homocysteine-lowering, reduction of endothelial damage, and reduction of the associated risks of vascular disease. The potential roles of folate and vitamin B_{12}, and possibly other micronutrients, in reducing the risk of dementia and of cognitive decline in older people represents another very active area of research. The functional significance of low plasma pyridoxal phosphate levels in older people also needs to be further explored.

The "graying" or blunted responsiveness of the immune system and especially cell-mediated immunity in older people is undoubtedly a major research challenge *(37)*, both in terms of its cause and its possible alleviation, eg by judicious micronutrient supplementation. Of the many functional markers of immune robustness, we need to select those that are most useful and meaningful in terms both of their importance in protecting the body against attack or malfunction and their measurable responsiveness to nutritional modulation.

The 20th century has witnessed major advances in the dissection of the discrete mechanisms of physiological chemistry and nutrition and of the characteristic functions of single nutrients. During the 21st century, the synthesis, control, and interlocking of these mechanisms and, in particular, the long-term effects of dietary choices and other lifestyle factors in determining longevity and health in old age, are likely to take center stage.

6. RECOMMENDATIONS FOR CLINICIANS

1. Two complementary nutritional assessment techniques are the estimation of dietary intakes of macronutrients (e.g., energy and protein) and micronutrients (vitamins and minerals) and the measurement of biochemical and functional indices of micronutrients. Clinical signs and symptoms of deficiency may also be useful, but can be nonspecific and confounded by age-related changes.
2. Dietary assessment techniques include the 24-h recall, the written food record, the weighed intake diary, and the food frequency questionnaire.
3. Biochemical assays may directly measure the concentration of a nutrient or sometimes the carrier that specifically transports it in a body fluid, such as serum, plasma, or urine, or else its concentration in a specific tissue compartment (e.g., red blood cells). Functional assays measure enzymes, metabolites, or physiological functions that are specifically modulated by the nutrient in question.
4. Many biochemical and functional measures may be affected independently by the aging process. Ideally, age-adjusted norms should be used for evaluation, but well-validated age-related norms are not always available in practice.
5. Clinical deficiency of vitamin B_{12} is a relatively common problem for older people because of the age-related increase in prevalence of impaired vitamin B_{12} absorption. Clinical evidence of deficiency of vitamins D and C is observed in some older people, and there is increasing concern about the adequacy of their vitamin K and vitamin B_6 status. Folate is also potentially important, partly in relation to homocysteine and vascular disease risk.
6. Iron deficiency anemia and suboptimum zinc status are perhaps the most frequently described mineral insufficiencies in older people, and calcium and selenium intakes may be suboptimal. In certain developing countries, poor iodine status may also be an issue.

REFERENCES

1. Lindenbaum J, Rosenberg IH, Wilson PWF, Stabler SP, Allen RH. Prevalence of cobalamin deficiency in the Framingham elderly population. Am J Clin Nutr 1994;60:2–11.

 2. Stabler SP, Allen RH, Fried LP, et al. Racial differences in prevalence of cobalamin and folate deficiencies in disabled elderly women. Am J Clin Nutr 1999;70:911–919.
 3. Wood RJ, Suter PM, Russell RM. Mineral requirements of elderly people. Am J Clin Nutr 1995;62:493–505.
 4. Hollis BW, Kamerud JQ, Selvaag SR, Lorenz JD, Napoli JL. Determination of vitamin D status by radioimmuno assay with a ^{125}I-labelled tracer. Clin Chem 1993;39:529–533.
 5. Bates CJ. Vitamin Analysis. Ann Clin Biochem 1997;34:599–626.
 6. Shearer MJ. Role of vitamin K and Gla proteins in the pathphysiology of osteoporosis and vascular calcification. Curr Opin Clin Nutr Metab Care 2000;3:433–438.
 7. Bates CJ, Pentieva KD, Prentice A, Mansoor MA, Finch S. Plasma pyridoxal phosphate and pyridoxic acid in a representative sample of British men and women aged 65 years and over and their relationship to plasma homocysteine. Br J Nutr 1999;81:191–201.
 8. Bates CJ, Pentieva KD, Prentice A. An appraisal of vitamin B_6 status indices and associated confounders, in young people aged 4–18 years and in people aged 65 years and over, in two national British surveys. Publ Hlth Nutr 1999;2:529–535.
 9. Gunter EW, Bowman BA, Caudell SP, Twite DB, Adams MJ. Results of an international round robin for serum and red cell folate. Clin Chem 1996;42:1689–1694.
10. Doyle W, Crawley H, Robert H, Bates CJ. Iron deficiency in older people: Interactions between food and nutrient intakes with biochemical measures of iron: further analysis of the National Diet and Nutrition Survey of people aged 65 years and older. Eur J Clin Nutr 1999;53:552–559.
11. Beard J. Iron status of free-living elderly individuals. Am J Clin Nutr 2001;73:503–504.
12. Fleming DJ, Jacques PF, Tucker KL, et al. Iron status of the free-living, elderly Framingham Heart Study cohort: an iron-replete population with a high prevalence of elevated iron stores. Am J Clin Nutr 2001;73:638 646.
13. Boukaiba N, Flamant C, Acher S, et al. A physiological amount of zinc supplementation: effects on nutritional, lipid, and thymic status of an elderly population. Am J Clin Nutr 1993;57:566–572.
14. Kehoe CA, Turley E, Bonham MP, et al. Response of putative indices of copper status to copper supplementation in human subjects. Br J Nutr 2000;84:151–156.
15. Bates CJ. Vitamins: fat and water soluble, analysis of. In: Encyclopedia of Analytical Chemistry: Instrumentation and Applications. Meyers RA (ed.) John Wiley & Sons Ltd, Chichester, 2000, pp. 7390–7425.
16. Department of Health. Nutrition and Bone Health with particular reference to calcium and vitamin D. Report on Health and Social Subjects, no. 49. The Stationery Office, London, England, 1998.
17. Department of Health. Dietary reference values for food energy and nutrients for the United Kingdom. Report on Health and Social Subjects no. 41. HMSO, London, England, 1991.
18. Standing Committee on the Scientific Evaluation of Dietary Reference Intakes, Food and Nutrition Board, Institute of Medicine. Dietary Reference Intakes for Calcium, Phosphorus, Magnesium, Vitamin D and Fluoride. National Academy Press, Washington DC, 1997.
19. Khaw K-T, Bingham S, Welch A, et al. Relation between plasma ascorbic acid and mortality in men and women in EPIC–Norfolk prospective study: a prospective population study. Lancet 2001;357:657–663.
20. Department of Health and Social Security. Report on Health and Social Subjects, no. 3. A Nutrition Survey of the Elderly. Report by the Panel on the Nutrition of the Elderly. HMSO, London, England, 1972.
21. Department of Health and Social Security. Report on Health and Social Subjects no.16. Nutrition and Health in Old Age. The cross-sectional analysis of the findings of a survey made in 1972/3 of elderly people who had been studied in 1967/8. Report by the Committee on Medical Aspects of Food Policy. HMSO, London, England, 1979.
22. Finch S, Doyle W, Lowe C, et al. National Diet and Nutrition Survey: People Aged 65 Years or Over, vol. 1. Report of the Diet and Nutrition Survey. The Stationery Office, London, England, 1998.
23. MacLaughlin JA, Holick MF. Aging decreases the capacity of human skin to produce vitamin D. J Clin Invest 1985;76:1536–1538.
24. Webb AR, Kline L, Holick MF. Influence of season and latitude on the cutaneous synthesis of vitamin D_3. Exposure to winter sunlight in Boston and Edmonton will not promote vitamin D_3 synthesis in human skin. J Clin Endocrinol Metab 1988;76:1536–1538.
25. Webb AR, Pilbeam C, Hanafin N, Holick MF. An evaluation of the relative contributions of exposure to sunlight and of diet to the circulating concentrations of 25–hydroxyvitamin D in an elderly nursing home population in Boston. Am J Clin Nutr 1990;51:1075–1080.

26. Slovik D, Adams JS, Neer RM, Holick MF, Potts JT Jr. Deficient production of 1,25–dihydroxyvitamin D in elderly osteoporotic patients. N Engl J Med 1981;305:372–374.

27. Dawson-Hughes B, Dallal GE, Krall EA, Harris S, Sokoll D, Falconer G. Effect of vitamin D supplementation on wintertime overall bone loss in healthy postmenopausal women. Ann Intern Med 1991; 115:505–512.

28. Dawson-Hughes B, Harris SS, Krall EA, Dallal GE, Falconer G, Green CL. Rates of bone loss in postmenopausal women randomly assigned to one of two dosages of vitamin D. Am J Clin Nutr 1995;61: 1140–1145.

29. Binkley NC, Krueger DC, Engelke JA, Foley AL, Suttie JW. Vitamin K supplementation reduces serum concentrations of under-γ-carboxylated osteocalcin in healthy young and elderly adults. Am J Clin Nutr 2000;72:1523–1528.

30. Dawson-Hughes B, Dallal G, Krall EA, Sadowski L, Sahyoun D, Tannenbaum S. A controlled trial of the effect of calcium supplementation on bone density in postmenopausal women. N Engl J Med 1990; 323:878–883.

31. Heaney RP, Recker RR, Saville PD. Menopausal changes in calcium balance performance. J Am Coll Nutr 1995;14:1–5.

32. Neives JW, Komar L, Cosman F, Lindsay R. Calcium potentiates the effect of estrogen and calcitonin on bone mass: Review and analysis. Am J Clin Nutr 1998;67:18–24.

33. Reid IJ, Ames RW, Evans MV, Gamble GD, Sharpe SJ. Effect of calcium supplementation on bone loss in postmenopausal women. N Engl J Med 1993;1993:460–464.

34. Hall S, Greendale GA. The relation of dietary vitamin C intake to bone mineral density: Results from the PEPI study. Calc Tiss Res 1998;63:183–189.

35. Morton DJ, Barratt-Connor EL, Schneider DL. Vitamin C supplement use and bone mineral density in postmenopausal women. J Bone Min Res 2001;16:135–140.

36. New SA, Bolton-Smith C, Grubb DA, Reid DM. Nutritional influences on bone mineral density: A cross-sectional study in premenopausal women. Am J Clin Nutr 1997;65:1831–1839.

37. Chandra RK. Graying of the immune system. Can nutrient supplements improve immunity in the elderly? J Am Med Assoc 1997;277:1398–1399.

38. Meydani SN, Meydani M, Blumberg JB, et al. Vitamin E supplementation and in vivo immune response in healthy elderly subjects: a randomized controlled trial. J Am Med Assoc 1997;277:1380–1386.

39. Bailey AL, Maisey S, Southon S, Wright AJA, Finglas PM, Fulcher RA. Relationships between micronutrient intake and biochemical indicators of nutrient adequacy in a 'free-living' elderly UK population. Br J Nutr 1997;1997:225–242.

40. Ferroli CE, Trumbo PR. Bioavailability of vitamin B-6 in young and older men. Am J Clin Nutr 1994;60:68–71.

41. Kant AK, Moser-Veillon PB, Reynolds RD. Effect of age on changes in plasma, erythrocyte, and urinary B-6 vitamers after an oral vitamin B-6 load. Am J Clin Nutr 1988;48:1284–1290.

42. Löwik MHR, van den Berg H, Westenbrink S, Wedel M, Schrijver J, Ockhuizen T. Dose-response relationships regarding vitamin B-6 in elderly people: a nationwide nutritional survey (Dutch Nutritional Surveillance System). Am J Clin Nutr 1989;50:391–399.

43. Lowik MRH, Schrijver J, van den Berg H, Hulshof KFAM, Wedel M, Ockhuizen T. Effect of dietary fiber on the vitamin B6 status among vegetarian and non-vegetarian elderly (Dutch Nutrition Surveillance System). J Am Coll Nutr 1990;9:241–249.

44. Lowik MRH, van den Berg H, Kistemaker C, Brants HAM, Brussard JH. Interrelationships between riboflavin and vitamin B_6 among elderly people (Dutch Nutrition Surveillance System). Int J Vit Nutr Res 1994;64:198–203.

45. Manore MM, Vaughan LA, Carroll SS, Leklem JE. Plasma pyridoxal 5' phosphate concentration and dietary vitamin B_6 intake in free-living, low-income elderly people. Am J Clin Nutr 1989;50:339–345.

46. Pannemans DLE, van den Berg H, Westerterp KR. The influence of protein intake on vitamin B_6 metabolism differs in young and elderly humans. J Nutr 1994;124:1207–1214.

47. Ribaya-Mercado JD, Russell RM, Sahyoun N, Morrow FD, Gershoff SN. Vitamin B_6 requirements of elderly men and women. J Nutr 1991;121:1062–1074.

48. Riggs KM, Spiro AI, Tucker KL, Rush D. Relations of vitamin B_{12}, vitamin B_6, folate and homocysteine to cognitive performance in the Normative Aging Study. Am J Clin Nutr 1996;63:306–314.

49. Rose CS, Gyorgy P, Butler M, et al. Age differences in vitamin B_6 status of 617 men. Am J Clin Nutr 1976;29:847–853.

50. Russell RM, Suter PM. Vitamin requirements of elderly people: an update. Am J Clin Nutr 1993;58:4–14.
51. Driskell JA. Vitamin B_6 requirements in humans. Nutr Res 1994;14:293–324.
52. Department of Health. Report on Health and Social Subjects, no. 43. The Nutrition of Elderly People. Report of the Working Group on the Nutrition of Elderly People of the Committee on Medical Aspects of Food Policy. HMSO, London, England, 1992.
53. Rutishauser IHE, Bates CJ, Paul AA, Black AE, Mandal AR, Patnaik BK. Long term vitamin status and dietary intake of healthy elderly subjects. Riboflavin. Br J Nutr 1979;42:33–42.
54. Schorah CJ. Inappropriate vitamin C reserves. In: The Importance of Vitamins to Human Health. Taylor T (ed.). MTP, Lancaster, 1979, pp. 61–72.
55. Gregory J, Foster K, Tyler H, Wiseman M. The Dietary and Nutritional Survey of British Adults. HMSO, London, 1990.
56. Gregory J, Lowe S, Bates C, et al. National Diet and Nutrition Survey: Young People Aged 4 to 18 Years. Volume 1: Report of the diet and nutrition survey. The Stationery Office, London, England, 2000, p. 796.

7

Dietary Supplements for Health Maintenance and Risk Factor Reduction[*]

Rebecca B. Costello, Maureen Leser, and Paul M. Coates

1. INTRODUCTION

In the last 20 years, there has been increased recognition of the direct relationship between diet and health *(1,2)*. Gerontologists and nutritionists are now more interested in the level of a nutrient that it takes to prevent and/or manage a chronic disease state, rather than the level of a nutrient needed to prevent a deficiency disease state. In terms of nutritional needs, the elderly population is one of the most diverse and heterogeneous of any age group. Determining the nutritional needs of older adults is challenging because their physiology, medical conditions, lifestyles, and social situations are different from those of younger people.

Health-promoting food components found directly in food, added to functional foods, and/or available in dietary supplements may offer older adults treatment options not formerly available. For example, antioxidant intake from food or supplements may offer protection against oxidative destruction of tissues, which can lead to chronic disease and possibly even aging itself *(3)*. Dietary supplements may help manage or lessen the impact of age-associated diseases, disorders, and conditions. These include cardiovascular disease, diabetes mellitus, osteoporosis and hip fractures, joint disorders, atrophic gastritis, benign prostatic hyperplasia, infectious diseases, vision disorders, Alzheimer's disease, and other degenerative diseases of the nervous system. There is increasing information that B vitamins, such as folic acid, vitamin B_6 and B_{12}, play a role in preventing blood vessel diseases and maintaining normal neurologic function *(4–9)*. The need for vitamin D and calcium in the prevention of osteoporosis because of bone mineral loss is well established *(10–12)*.

Evidence is emerging from well-designed randomized clinical trials to suggest that some herbal supplements may have beneficial effects. Herbs are sold in many forms,

---

[*] The findings and views reported in this chapter represent those of the contributing authors and not necessarily those of the National Institutes of Health and are not intended to constitute an "authoritative statement" under the Food and Drug Administration rules and regulations.

From: *Handbook of Clinical Nutrition and Aging*
Edited by: C. W. Bales and C. S. Ritchie © Humana Press Inc., Totowa, NJ

including fresh, dried, liquid, or solid extracts, and as tablets, capsules, powders, and tea bags. However, with many herbal preparations, it is not fully understood how they work, nor is the active component always known. Although approx 30% of all drugs used today are derived from plants *(13,14)*, very few of the herbal supplements on the market have been vigorously tested in clinical studies for efficacy and toxicity. Products used by the elderly to address aging concerns include a number of herbal supplements, such as evening primrose oil, *Ginkgo biloba*, ginseng, kava, saw palmetto, St. John's wort, valerian, and black cohosh. A number of specialty supplements, such as glucosamine and chondroitin, coenzyme Q10, dehydroepiandrosterone (DHEA), melatonin, omega-3 fatty acids, and soy proteins, are also popular with the elderly *(15)*. Among the herbal products that have data from clinical trials showing promise for common ailments in the elderly are St. John's wort, valerian, *Ginkgo biloba*, horse chestnut seed extract, saw palmetto, and yohimbe *(16)*.

In many cases, the lack of scientific evidence makes it extremely difficult to quantify the true risks and benefits of supplements. Also, the risk of interactions between supplements and other medications may be higher among the elderly because they take more prescription medicines on average than do younger adults. This review focuses on the rationale and evidence base for the use of dietary supplements for health maintenance and risk factor reduction. Need assessment tips and resource references are also provided through the use of tables and figures.

1.1. Overview of Dietary Supplement Use

Total sales of dietary supplements in 2001 were estimated to be $17.7 billion in the United States. Between the years 1990 and 1997, the prevalence of high-dose vitamin and herbal use increased by 130% and 380%, respectively *(17)*. However, the enthusiasm for and use of herbal products has fallen off in the last few years. According to consumer usage model estimates, 4.5% of US adults (10 million people) are committed or "heavy" users of supplements, and 35% (75 million people) are "regular" users *(17)*. Supplement use has been shown to increase with age and gender (use is higher among women than among men), is consistent with more healthy lifestyles and healthy weight status, and is correlated with higher family income and level of education. Findings from the Third National Health and Nutrition Examination Survey, 1988–1994 (NHANES III) suggest that 40% of Americans use dietary supplements *(18)*. Approximately 56% of middle age and older adults consume at least one supplement on a regular basis. Use of supplements among the elderly was highest (55%) in women 80 yr and above when compared to 42.3% in men of the same age group *(18)*. As noted previously, herbal medicine has experienced a rapid growth in popularity with 8% of older aged individuals (65 and above) consuming herbal products in the past year *(19)*.

Information on the use of dietary supplements from regional surveys and disease-oriented studies in older-aged individuals provides information that is similar to the nationwide surveys. The Beaver Dam Eye Study is a study of 2152 middle- and older-aged adults in a primarily Caucasian community in southcentral Wisconsin designed to evaluate the effects of nutritional factors on aging. Dietary supplement use was documented by in-person interviews and questionnaires between 1988–1990. Thirty-three percent of women aged 65–74 yr were found to consume a multinutrient supplement (defined as a broad-spectrum multivitamin product), 14% consumed a vitamin C supplement, and 31% consumed a vitamin E supplement. Multinutrient intakes for men aged

65–74 were slightly lower than the women at 27% with comparable vitamin C and E supplemental intakes *(20)*.

Nutrient and non-nutrient dietary supplement use is highly prevalent among women at risk for breast cancer recurrence. Newman and colleagues evaluated supplement intakes in 435 women (mean age 53 yr) living in the western United States who entered into a dietary intervention study to prevent recurrence of breast cancer. They found that 80.9% of the participants had a past history of dietary supplement use. Vitamin E was the most commonly reported supplement (49%), followed by vitamin C (47%), multivitamin and mineral supplements (46%), and herbal products (21%) *(21)*.

1.2. Regulation of Dietary Supplements

The Dietary Supplement Health and Education Act (DSHEA) *(22)* laid the foundation for the current regulatory framework for dietary supplements. This law amended the Federal Food, Drug, and Cosmetic Act of 1938 "to establish standards with respect to dietary supplements." Dietary supplements have been defined by DSHEA to include a product (other than tobacco) intended to supplement the diet that bears or contains one or more of the following dietary ingredients: vitamins, minerals, herbs, or other botanicals, amino acids, dietary substances to supplement the diet by increasing the total dietary intake, or concentrates, metabolites, constituents, extracts, or any combination of the ingredients described previously. Under DSHEA, the US Food and Drug Administration (FDA) regulates safety, manufacturing, and product information, such as claims in product labels, package inserts, and accompanying literature. The FDA cannot require testing of dietary supplements prior to marketing (except for new dietary ingredients); however, although manufacturers are prohibited from selling dangerous products, DSHEA gives the FDA permission to remove a product from the marketplace only when the FDA proves that the product is dangerous to the health of Americans. If in the labeling or marketing of a dietary supplement product, a claim is made that the product can diagnose, treat, cure, or prevent disease (e.g., cures cancer), the product is said to be an unapproved new drug and is thus being sold illegally.

The Federal Trade Commission regulates the advertising of dietary supplements, including claims in print and broadcast advertising, infomercials, catalogs, the Internet, and similar direct marketing materials. Advertisements for any products, including dietary supplements, must be truthful, nonmisleading, and claims must be substantiated.

1.3. Recommended Dietary Intakes for the Elderly

Nutrients and other dietary components are essential for normal growth and development, prevention of specific nutrient deficiencies, and prevention of chronic degenerative diseases. Since 1941, the Recommended Dietary Allowances (RDAs) have served as a tool for assessing the adequacy or inadequacy of observed nutrient intakes for individuals and groups, as well as developing recommendations for food intake in the United States *(23)*. The RDAs have been updated on a periodic basis. However, when it came time to update in 1989, the Food and Nutrition Board of the Institute of Medicine, National Academy of Sciences, decided to replace them with a comprehensive set of Dietary Reference Intakes (DRIs) that have broader and more useful applications *(23–25)*. DRIs are recommended nutrient intakes that promote functional endpoints associated with good health and limit adverse health effects associated with deficient

Table 1
Dietary Reference Intakes

Estimated average requirement (EAR) is the nutrient intake value that is estimated to meet the requirement for a specific criterion of adequacy for half of the healthy individuals within a specific age, sex, life stage, and physiologic state.

Recommended dietary allowance (RDA) is the dietary intake level that is sufficient to meet the nutrient requirements of nearly all (97–98%) healthy individuals within a specific age, sex, life stage, and physiologic state.

When insufficient data is available for setting a RDA, observed or experimentally determined approximations or estimates of nutrient intakes by a group (or groups) of healthy people that are assumed to have adequate intake are used to establish an *adequate intake* (AI).

Tolerable upper intake level (UL) is the highest usual daily nutrient intake level that is likely to pose no risk of adverse health effects for almost everyone in the general population. As intake increases above the UL, the risk of adverse effects increases.

From ref. *143*.

or excess intakes. DRIs are used to assess the adequacy of nutrient intake for individuals and groups, set national nutrition policies, and plan nutrition programs for populations. Four sets of values were defined to address the full scope of the DRIs as described in Table 1 *(24,25)*.

New findings indicate that nutrient requirements change along with physiologic function during the aging process. The committee expanded the age groups targeted by the DRIs to establish recommendations for adults aged 19–30, 31–50, 51–70, and >70 yr in addition to infants and children. DRIs are based on normal needs of healthy representatives of each life stage and gender group. The American Dietetic Association (ADA) takes the position that the best way to meet the DRIs is to wisely choose a wide variety of foods. Additional vitamins and minerals from fortified foods and/or supplements can help some people meet their nutritional needs as specified by science-based nutrition standards, such as the DRIs *(26)*. When making a decision to recommend fortified foods and/or dietary supplements, particularly when doses exceed the RDA, dietary and physiologic circumstances that may depart from the norm should be considered.

The 2000 Dietary Guidelines for Americans states that different foods contain different nutrients and other healthful substances *(27)*. No single food can supply all the nutrients in the amounts needed. Science-based recommendations, such as the Dietary Guidelines for Americans and the Food Guide Pyramid, provide guidance for a healthy diet. The Jean Mayer USDA Human Nutrition Research Center on Aging at Tufts University has developed a modified food pyramid for adults over 70 yr (www.hnrc.tufts.edu). In addition to suggesting numbers of servings of each food group consistent with the USDA pyramid, it includes guidelines for water equivalents and advises adults in this age group to consult with their health care provider about the use of calcium, vitamin D, and vitamin B_{12} supplements (*see* Fig. 1).

There is evidence that some individuals have difficulty following these dietary recommendations and that dietary supplementation may even be beneficial for those consuming fortified foods. Foote and colleagues evaluated the dietary intakes of 1740 healthy, free-living US adults from 51 to 85 yr of age and found that more than 60% had low intakes of vitamin D, vitamin E, folate, and calcium *(28)*. Fewer than half consumed the daily servings of dairy, grain, and fruits and vegetables recommended in the USDA Food

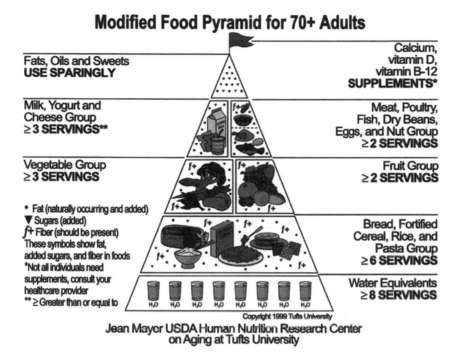

Fig. 1. Food pyramid for 70+ adults. Reprinted with permission, Tufts University, 1999.

Guide Pyramid. An 8-wk, double-blind, placebo-controlled clinical trial among 80 adults ranging in age from 50 to 87 yr indicated that a multivitamin supplement providing 100% of the daily value was able to decrease the prevalence of suboptimal levels of several vitamins and improve micronutrient status beyond what was achieved through a diet rich in fortified foods (29). This evidence suggests that older adults may not be heeding current dietary messages and may benefit from multivitamin supplements; however, elders *must be* cautioned against indiscriminate use of supplements. A recent survey found no association between the choice of dietary supplement and specific dietary deficiencies among 130 community-dwelling adults aged 70 yr in two rural North Carolina counties. This further highlights the importance of nutritional counseling and guidance for this population (30). Targeting nutrition messages through age-adjusted tools, such as the modified Food Pyramid, for adults over 70 yr may be especially helpful.

2. DIETARY SUPPLEMENTS IN THE MANAGEMENT OF CARDIOVASCULAR DISEASES

Among the dietary supplements utilized in the prevention and treatment for cardiovascular disease are B vitamins, antioxidants, plant sterols, omega-3 fatty acids, soy and garlic. Most extensively studied are the B vitamins for lowering elevated blood homocysteine levels, antioxidants for preventing atherosclerotic heart disease, plant sterols, garlic, and soy for lowering elevated blood cholesterol, along with omega-3 fatty acids for decreasing cardiac arrhythmias and sudden death. A number of these supplements are described below and in Tables 2–4.

Table 2
Individual Vitamin and Mineral Dietary Supplements Commonly Used by the Elderly

Supplement	Reported uses	Potential interactions	Adverse effects/concerns/comments
Calcium (Ca)	• Preventing and treating osteoporosis • Reducing the risk of colorectal cancer • Reduce the risk of hpertension	• Estrogen ↑ calcium absorption • Mineral oil, stimulant laxatives and dilantin ↓ calcium absorption • Loop and thiazide diuretics, Mg and Al salts ↑ urinary excretion of calcium • Calcium supplements ↓ absorption of levothyroxine, and tetracycline • Bisphosphonates bind calcium; used to treat hypercalcemia of malignancy • Concomitant calcium supplementation improves absorption of vitamin D • Concomitant administration ↑ vitamin D absorption • Loop and thiazide diuretics as well as Mg and Al salts ↑ urinary excretion of calcium. • Mineral oil and stimulant laxatives ↓ calcium absorption • Corticosteroids deplete calicum. • Estrogen ↑ calcium absorption	• Safe when used orally and appropriately in amounts not exceeding the UL of 2.5 g/d • Can cause GI irritation, belching, and flatulence • Calcium should not be given at the same time with other minerals supplements —known to decrease absorption of iron, and zinc • Calcium absorption ↓ as dose ↑ above 500 mg; if >500 mg/d is needed, divide the dose
Chromium (Cr)	• Improves glycemic control in type 2 diabetes • Lowers blood cholesterol • Promotes weight loss	• Vitamin C may ↑ absorption • Chromium may mitigate corticosteroid-induced ↑ in blood sugar • In combination with nicotinic acid, may produce a synergestic effect in improving control of blood glucose	• Doses 50–200 µg/d are likely safe • Doses >200 µg/d may lead to cognitive, perceptual and motor dysfunction. • Chromium may exacerabate renal insufficiency • Trivalent chromium (III) is available in several orms: Cr chloride, Cr nicotinate, Cr picolinate, and high-chromium yeast • At higher amounts, can lead to cognitive, perceptual, and motor dysfunction

132

	Reduce risk of...	Interactions	Safety
Chromium (Cr) *(continued)*			• Hexavalent Cr (VI) is toxic and should not be used as a dietary supplement
Folic acid	• Reduce risk of CVD (CHD, stroke, and peripheral vascular disease) • Reduce risk of cancer (particularly for breast and colorectal) • Reduce risk of alzheimer's disease and cognitive impairment	• NSAIDs may interfere with folate metabolism • Dilantin may inhibit intestinal absorption • Methotrexate may ↓ folate stores	• Safe when used orally and appropriately. • Large doses of folic acid can mask B_{12} deficiency; do not exceed UL of 1000 µg/d • There is significant interaction between methotrexate and folate metabolism; MD consult indicated on appropriate dose of folic acid when taking methotrexate
Magnesium (Mg)	• Reduce risk of osteoporosis CVD, and hypertension	• Magnesium ↓ absorption of digoxin • Long-term use of lasix and thiazide diuretics may ↑ urinary excretion of magnesium • Can ↓ efficacy of chlorpromazine, penicillamine, oral anticoagulants, and some antibiotics	• Safe when used orally and appropriately; not to exceed the UL of 350 mg/d from supplements unless prescribed for repletion by a MD • Most forms of oral magnesium supplements can cause diarrhea, dose-dependent • Individuals with impaired kidney function are at higher risk for adverse effects
Selenium (Se)	• Reduce risk of cancer • Enhance immune function	• Selenium ↑ cytotoxic effects of cisplatin in presence of EDTA • Insufficient reliable information regarding possible interactions with herbs and other dietary supplements	• Likely safe when taken orally in amounts not exceeding the UL of 400 µg daily • Can cause acute toxicity at higher doses: nausea, vomiting, fatigue, irritability, and nail changes • Selenium supplements are available in several inorganic (sodium selenite and sodium selenate) and organic (selenomethionine and selenium yeast) forms—all have different absorption efficiency. Selenomethionine is the form being utilized in ongoing cancer clinical trials.

continued

Table 2 (Continued)
Individual Vitamin and Mineral Dietary Supplements Commonly Used by the Elderly

Supplement	Reported uses	Potential interactions	Adverse effects/concerns/comments
Zinc (Zn)	• Improve performance and strength • Enhance immune function • Reduce the risk of macular degeneration	• Concomitant use may ↓ copper absorption • Coffee may ↓ zinc absorption • Captopril and thiazide diuretics ↑ urinary zinc excretion • Zinc ↑ cytotoxic effects of cisplatin in presence of EDTA • Zinc ↓ absorption and levels of tetracycline • Zinc ↓ absorption and serum levels of fluoroquinolones	• Likely safe when taken orally in amounts not exceeding the UL of 40 mg/d; however, use should be limited to the RDA of 15 mg/d (men) or 12 mg/d (women) unless otherwise prescribed • Chronic intakes of 25 mg can ↓ the bioavailability of copper • Side effects: intakes of 150–450 mg have been associated with altered iron function, reduced immune function, reduced levels of HDL; at very high intakes (2000 mg/d) GI irritation, nausea, and vomiting • Contraindicated in individuals with known hypersensitivity to zinc compounds
Vitamin B6 (Six forms; pyridoxal 5' phosphate [PLP] is active coenzyme form)	• Reduce the risk of CVD (CHD, stroke, and peripheral vascular disease) • Enhance immune function • Enhance mental function	• Antituberculosis medications and penicillamine may ↑ B6 requirement • B6 may antagonize therapeutic effect of L-dopa (anti-Parkinsonian drug)	• Safe when used orally in amounts not exceeding the UL of 100 mg/d • B6 ↑ risk for sensory neuropathy at intakes > 1000 mg/d • High doses have been found to ↓ the efficacy of anticonvulsants such as phenobarbitol and dilantin. With L-dopa, avoid supplemental vitamins that contain >5 mg pyridoxine in a daily dose
Vitamin B12 methyl-cobalamin and 5-deo-xyadenosyl cobalamin	• Reduce the risk of CVD • Reduce the risk of depression and Alzheimer's disease • Replacement therapy	• B12 absorption ↓ by proton pump inhibitors (omeprazole and lansoprazole) and H2-receptor antagonists (tagamet, pepcid, zantac), cholestyramine, chloramphenicol, neomycin, and colchicine and metformin (glucophage)	• Safe when used orally • Methylcobalamin and 5-deoxyadenosyl cobalamin are the forms of B12 used in the body. Cyanocobalamin is the form used in most supplements and is readily converted to 5-deoxyadenosyl and methylcobalamin

Vitamin B12 (continued)

- B12 replacement therapy can be administrered orally or parenterally. Tablets have a low bioavailability—use crystalline form of B12
- Avoid large doses of folic acid (>1000 μg) to prevent masking of an undiagnosed B12 deficiency

---

Vitamin C
ascorbic
acid

- Reduce the risk of CVD (CHD and stroke), glaucoma, and cataracts
- Reduce the risk of glaucoma and cataracts

- Aspirin, barbiturates, estrogen and OCs, nicotine and tetracyclines ↑ the elimination of vitamin C
- Vitamin C ↑ Fe absorption (esp of heme iron)
- Large doses of vitamin C may attenuate effects of oral anticoagulants

- Safe when used orally in amounts not exceeding the UL of 2000 mg/d
- Side effects of doses > UL: GI discomfort, headache, flushing, insomnia, precipitation of urate, oxalate, or cysteine renal stones
- Increased rate of carotid wall thickening has been documented in clinical study in patients with CVD consuming large doses of vitamin C
- Suggest avoiding gram-size doses during cancer treatments because of possible pro-oxidant effects
- Take vitamin C 2 h before or 4 h after aluminum antacid

Vitamin D
(cholecal-
ciferol)

- Building bone mass and preventing bone loss
- Reduce the risk of post-menopausal osteoporosis
- Reduce the risk of cancer
- Enhance immune function

- Caution when administering with cardiac glycoside containing herbs as well as corticosteroids, digoxin, thiazide diuretics, phenytoin, phenobarbital and mineral oil
- Some drugs may deplete levels: bile acid sequestrants, carbamazepine, phenytoin & fosphenytoin, phenobarbital, mineral oil and stimulant laxatives

- Safe when used orally in amounts not exceeding the UL of 50 μg/d
- Conversion factor: 1 μg vitamin D = 40 IU. Excess vitamin D can promote hypercalcemia, leading to cardiac arrhythmias
- Use with caution in patients with renal impairment, monitor serum calcium and phosphorus levels

continued

135

Table 2 (Continued)
Individual Vitamin and Mineral Dietary Supplements Commonly Used by the Elderly

Supplement	Reported uses	Potential interactions	Adverse effects/concerns/comments
Vitamin E (family of 8 fat-soluble antioxidants, α-tocopherol most active form)	• Reduce the risk of CVD (CHD, stroke), cancer and cataracts. • Enhance immune function.	• May ↑ effect of anticoagulants/ antiplatelet drugs and herbal medicines with anticoagulant and antiplatelet potential • Vitamin E may impair the hematologic reponse to iron therapy in patients with iron deficiency anemia. Avoid large doses of vitamin E during treatment of iron deficiency • May ↑ effectiveness of cancer chemotherapy and may prevent tolerance to nitrates • The weight loss agent, Orlistat (Xenical) is reported to block the absorption of vitamin E by up to 60%	• Relatively nontoxic. Safe when used orally in amounts not exceeding the UL of 1000 mg/d. Doses higher than 1200 mg/d may result in headache, fatigue, nausea, diarrhea, cramping, weakness, blurred vision, and gonadal dysfunction • Conversion factor: 1 mg =1.26 IU; RDA of 15 mg = 22 IU (natural form) or 33 IU (synthetic form) • Possible risk of bleeding for those on anticoagulants or with vitamin K deficiency • Possible ↑ risk of hemorrhage in high risk groups • Monitor INR in patients taking warfarin and vitamin E > 800 IU daily

CHD, coronary heart disease; CVD, cardiovascular disease; INR, international normalized ratio; NSAIDs; nonsteroidal anti-inflammatory drugs; UL, upper tolerable limit. Adapted from refs. *50,143,215–217.*

Table 3
Herbal Supplements Commonly Used by the Elderly

Supplement	Reported uses	Compounds of interest	Potential interactions	Adverse effects/concerns/comments
Aloe vera—gel (*A. barbadensis*)	• Orally: relief from gastroduodenal ulcers and asthma • Can also be used topically for burns and wound healing, inflammation, and arthritis	• Magnesium lactate, polysaccharide glucomannan, and bradykininase		• Aloe gel products sold for internal consumption can be contaminated with anthraquinones present in aloe juice or latex that may act as cathartic laxatives • Monitor blood glucose in individuals on diabetic medications • Few side effects reported with topical use
Aloe, dried juice from leaf, latex (*A. vera, A. fevox*)	• Relief from constipation, used as a laxative or cathartic	• Anthraquinone glycosides derived from dried leaf juice and latex constituents	• May ↓ absorption of other drugs • Long term use of digoxin or cardiac glycosides containing herbs, anti-arrhythmics, diuretics, and corticosteroids may ↑ loss of potassium	• Approved in Germany for treatment of constipation—limit use to 2 wk • There is no evidence that aloe is effective in treating cancer • Aloe injections (T-UP, concentrated aloe) are illegal in the United States • Side effects: abdominal pain, nausea, vomiting, diarrhea and electrolyte (potassium losses) imbalance at higher doses • Contraindicated in individual with intestinal obstruction, Crohn's disease, ulcerative colitis, appendicitis, and kidney disorders

continued

137

Table 3 (Continued)
Herbal Supplements Commonly Used by the Elderly

Supplement	Reported uses	Compounds of interest	Potential interactions	Adverse effects/concerns/comments
Astragalus (*Astragalus membranaceus*)	• Enhance immune function • Relief of cold and respiratory infections • Antioxidant • Treatment for cancer • Reduce toxic effects of chemotherapy • Protect against heart disease	• Astralagus root contains varied constituents such as cycloartane triterpene saponins, flavonoids, polysaccharides, trace minerals, amino acids, and coumarins	• Theoretical concern that astralagus can minimize the immunosuppressive effects of cyclosporine and corticosteroids based on T-cell-stimulating activity	• Astragalus is most commonly used in combination with other herbs • There is no scientific evidence that astragalus can prevent or cure cancer in humans or ↓ toxic effects of chemotherapy • Generally considered safe • Side effects: abdominal bloating, loose stools, hypotension, and dehydration • Avoid in individuals with autoimmune diseases
Black Cohosh (*Cimicifuga racemosa*)	• Reduce postmenopausal symptoms: dysmenorrhea, nervous tension, hot flashes	• Triterpene glycosides, organic acids and esters, flavonoids	• May ↑ effects of anti-hypertensives • Insufficient information regarding interactions with other herbs and supplements	• Black cohosh is the primary ingredient in an over-the-counter product called Remifemin. Has been used extensively in Germany. Possibly effective for symptoms of menopause. Treatment for 4 wk is usually required before significant improvement in symptoms is noted • Has been used orally and safely in studies lasting up to 6 mo; long-term data lacking • Side effects: mild GI discomfort, headaches, nausea, dizziness, bradycardia and weight gain • Not recommended for use in individuals with hormone-sensitive cancers (breast, uterine, ovarian) and in individuals with endometriosis and uterine fibroids as safety data is lacking

138

Herb	Uses	Active Constituents	Drug Interactions	Comments
Cat's Claw (*Uncaria tomentosa*)	• Enhance immune function • Treatment for cancer • Antihypertensive • Relief from diverticulitis, peptic ulcers, colitis	• Root and bark contain numerous quinovic acid glycosides and Alkaloid constituents, such as pentacyclic oxindole alkaloid. Active constituents can vary greatly depending on time of harvest	• Avoid use with anti-hypertensives and anticoagulants	• Cat's claw is a popular herb in the United States; however, very little scientific information available regarding safety and efficacy exists • No serious side effects have been reported • There is concern with use in individuals with autoimmune disease, multiple sclerosis, and tuberculosis • Has been used in individuals that are HIV(+) on zidovudine (AZT)
Chasteberry (*Vitex agnus-castus*)	• Reduce symptoms of menopause	• Primarily rotundifuran, labdane diterpenes, aucubin, agnuside, casticin, and vitexilactone.	• Possible interactions with dopamine antagonists and dopamine-receptor blocking agents.	• Possibly safe when used orally and appropriately; however, abnormal frequency of menstrual bleeding has been reported • Possibly effective for menopausal symptoms
Echinacea (*E. angustifolia, E. pallida, E. purpurea*)	• Prevent and reduce symptoms of cold and flu	• No single active component isolated; contains alkylamides, phenoic glycosides, polysaccharides	• Avoid use with immunosupressant therapies	• *E. pallida* is approved in Germany for treatment of the common cold • Relatively safe with short-term use; limit use to no longer than 8 wk • Echinacea has been reported to cause allergic reactions
Essiac	• Enhance immune system • Reduce tumor size of cancers	• Essiac is a combination of several herbs; burdock root, the inner bark of slippery elm, and Turkish rhubarb that is pre-pared as a tea	• Turkish rhubard acts as a stimulant laxative and long-term use could cause electrolyte (potassium) losses and could potentiate action of cardiac glycosides or anti-arrhythmic drugs	• There is no scientific evidence to support use for the treatment of cancer • Side effects: may produce a laxative-like effect, nausea, headache, vomiting, and increased urination

continued

139

Table 3 (*Continued*)
Herbal Supplements Commonly Used by the Elderly

Supplement	Reported uses	Compounds of interest	Potential interactions	Adverse effects/concerns/comments
Fenugreek (*Trigonella foenum-graecum*)	• Control of blood glucose levels • Reduce the risk of CVD • Lowering blood cholesterol levels	• Seed components and constituents	• May ↓ blood sugar levels • High mucilage content of fenugreek may ↓ or delay absorption of oral drugs • There have been reports of enhanced anticoagulant drug activity. Therefore, do not take fenugreek at the same time as other drugs, separate administration by an hour or two • Fenugreek may interfere with hormone therapies and MAO inhibitors • Fenugreek may alter blood glucose control	• Fenugreek has GRAS status in the United States, therefore likely safe when seed—preparations are used in amounts commonly found in foods • Side effects include diarrhea and flatulence • Monitor insulin levels in diabetics
Garlic (*Allium sativum*)	• Lowering blood cholesterol • Lowering blood pressure • As an antimicrobial for mild respiratory and digestive tract infections • Reduce the risk of cancer	• Allylic sulfur compounds such as allicin, thiosulfinates, polysulfides, ajoene, and saponins	• Isolated reports of interaction with anti-coagulants and anti-platelet drugs • Concomitant use with EPA/fish oils may ↑ antithrombotic effects • Additive effects on cholesterol lowering are seen when taken with lipid-lowering agents	• Somewhat effective for lowering blood cholesterol short term • Insufficient evidence to support a specific role in cancer prevention • Has been used in clinical studies up to 4 yr without reports of toxicity. • Might ↓ blood sugar levels and interfere with control • Can irritate GI tract (more likely with fresh garlic), use with caution in individuals with infections or inflammatory GI conditions

Garlic (*continued*)			• Massive doses can cause hemolytic anemia (more likely with fresh garlic) • Monitor individuals on anti-coagulant and antiplatelet drugs
Gingko biloba Ginkgo leaf (extract)	• Flavonoid glycosides and diterpene lactones (ginkgolides and bilobalides), flavonoids	• Aids in circulation to improve cognitive function • Relief of pain from intermittent claudication • Decrease the risk of dementias associated with Alzheimer's disease	• May have an additive effect with other blood-thinning agents such as herbs and/or drugs with anticoagulant or antiplatelet potential • May also affect bio-availability of other drugs • Likely safe when used orally and appropriately • Contraindicated in individuals with epilepsy or who are prone to seizures • Avoid in individuals with diabetes. • Five cases of cerebral hemorrhage have been reported in those taking prescription anticoagulants with ginkgo products • Avoid in individuals who are hypersensitive to poison ivy, cashews or mangoes (may vary among supplement products)
Ginseng root, Asian (*Panax ginseng*)	• Ginsenosides are the main active components derived from the root and leaves	• Acts as an adaptogen to enhance energy levels, relieve stress and eases symptoms of anxiety • Enhance immune function • Delays or reduces the effects of aging • Improve control of blood sugar	• There have been reports of potential interaction with warfarin • There have been reports of interaction with MAO inhibitors, stimulants and phenelzine sulfate (an antidepressant) • May enhance the effect of hypo-glycemics • Ginseng has been used for medicinal purposes for over 2000 yr • Generally considered safe when used orally and appropriately. Safety of long term (>3 mo) use unknown • May have benefits enhancing cognitive function

continued

Table 3 (*Continued*)
Herbal Supplements Commonly Used by the Elderly

Supplement	Reported uses	Compounds of interest	Potential interactions	Adverse effects/concerns/comments
Ginseng root, Asian (*continued*)				• Most common side effect is insomnia • Not recomended for individuals with HTN • Monitor individuals on warfarin • Discontinue use 7 d before surgery
Ginseng, eleuthero (formerly called Siberian ginseng) (*Eleutherococcus senticosus*)	• Restorative tonic for the enhancement of mental and physical capacities • Enhance immune function	• Eleutherosides are the main active compounds derived from the root. Also includes saponins, β-sitosterol glycosides, coumarin derivatives	• Can increase excretion of thiamin, riboflavin and vitamin C • Reports have suggested to avoid use with alcohol, drugs with sedative properties, anticoagulants and antiplatelet drugs • May interact with spicy foods and bitter substances	• Likely safe when used appropriately and shortterm. Siberian Ginseng is often misidentified or adulterated • Side effects: infrequent but may include insomnia, drowsiness, change in heart rhythm, anxiety, muscle spasms • Monitor blood glucose levels in diabetics • Can possibly exacerbate blood pressure
Gymnema or Gurmar (*Gymnema sylvestre*)	• Control of blood glucose levels	• Gymnema leaf contains gymnemic acid	• Enhances the action of insulin and can have an additive hypoglycemic effect when given in combination with glyburide or tolbutamide	• Safety data is lacking • May affect taste sensation of sweetness and bitterness • Monitor blood glucose in diabetes

142

Horse chestnut seed extracts (*Aesculus hippocastanum*)	Reduce swelling and discomfort due to chronic venous insufficiency, varicose veins, and phlebitis	Aescin, a triterpene saponin and aesculin, a glycoside which is also a hydroxycoumarin	• May ↑ effects of anticoagulants and antiplatelet drugs • Possibly induces hypoglycemic effects. • Do not administer with drugs known to cause nephrotoxicity	• Most widely prescribed oral antiedema venous remedy in Germany • Treatment for 1–3 mo may be required before full therapeutic effects are apparent • Side effects uncommon, but GI irritation and toxic nephropathy may occur • Contraindicated in individuals with infectious or inflammatory GI conditions • Monitor individuals on warfarin • Monitor blood glucose levels in diabetics
Hoxsey herbal treatment	Treatment of cancer	Internal preparation consists of a combination of numerous herbs. External preparation used as a paste or salve contains antimony trisulfide, zinc chloride and blood root		• One of the oldest alternative cancer treatments in the United States • There is no scientific evidence that this preparation is effective in treating cancer and the sale of Hoxsey is currently illegal in the United States • Contains chapparal which has been reported to be hepatotoxic
Kava (*Piper methysticum*)	Short-term reduction of stress and anxiety	Kavalactones and pyrones from the rhizome and roots	• May potentiate effects of alcohol, barbiturates, and antianxiety agents such as valium • Should not be taken with antidepressants or antipsychotics	• FDA Consumer Advisory posted March 25, 2002 for cases of reported severe liver injury caused by kava extracts • Aqueous infusions of kava have traditionally been used as a ceremonial beverage in the Pacific Islands

continued

Table 3 (*Continued***)**
Herbal Supplements Commonly Used by the Elderly

Supplement	Reported uses	Compounds of interest	Potential interactions	Adverse effects/concerns/comments
Kava (*continued*)			• Has been shown to ↓ the efficacy of L-dopa	• At high doses, may reduce motor reflexes and judgment when driving or operating heavy machinery • Side effects appear to increase with large doses and long-term use and can result in temporary skin problems, allergic reactions and GI discomfort. Serious adverse effects of hepatitis, cirrhosis, and liver failure have been reported from Germany and Switzerland • Should not be taken for more than 3 mo without medical advice • Avoid use in individuals with liver or gall bladder problems • Discontinue use at least 24 h prior to surgery • Avoid use with alcohol and hepatotoxic drugs
Milk Thistle (*Silybum marianum*)	• As an anti-oxidant to prevent damage to cells • Reduce risk of liver damage from drugs and alcohol	• Silymarin, a milk thistle fruit and seed extract. • Complex consists of four flavanolignans	• May ↑ effectiveness of aspirin in patients with cirrhosis • May worsen blood sugar control • Can ↓ toxicity of hepatotoxic drugs	• Safety data lacking, but possibly safe when purified extract is used appropriately • Can cause allergic reactions in individuals sensitive to ragweed, chrysanthemus, marigolds, daisies, and other herbs

PC-SPES	• Enhance immune function • Prevent or delay the recurrence of prostate cancer	• Preparation consists of a combination of 8 herbs, including saw palmetto	• FDA Advisory and Recall of products adulterated with prescription drugs posted February 8, 2002 • Concern exists for inappropriate self-treatment for cancers • Can cause laxative effects • Side effects: estrogenic effects such as breast enlargement and nipple tenderness • May ↓ testosterone levels • ↑ risk for blood clots
Red clover (*Trifolium repens*)	• Reducing menopausal symptoms • Help maintain bone density in the lower spine	• Isoflavones (form-ononetin, biochanin A, daidzein, genistein) • Coumarins	• Enhances effects of anticoagulants and digoxin • Labeling of products may be confusing as the same amount of isoflavones can be stated several ways and can differ significantly depending on how the isoflavones are calculated (with or without related sugar constituents) • Presently, contraindicated in women with a history of estrogen receptor-positive cancers • Long-term data is lacking
Saw palmetto (*Serenoa repens*)	• Relief from urinary symptomatology associated with BPH • Also used as a mild diuretic	• Extracts containing fatty acids and β sito-sterol	• No drug interactions have been reported • Evidence for benefit for enlarged prostate • Long-term effects (> 48 wk) and safety are unknown. Treatment for 1–2 mo is usually necessary to achieve significant improvement

continued

145

Table 3 (*Continued*)
Herbal Supplements Commonly Used by the Elderly

Supplement	Reported uses	Compounds of interest	Potential interactions	Adverse effects/concerns/comments
Saw Palmetto (*continued*)				• Side effects are not common but may include mild GI side effects (nauseas, vomiting, constipation, diarrhea) and dizziness • May alter prostate-specific antigen test results
Soy and related phytoestrogen constituents and soy protein	• Prevention of CVD • Lowering blood cholesterol levels • Reduce postmenopausal symptoms • Reduce the risk of osteoporosis	• Isoflavone glycosides, saponins, and soy protein	• In theory may competitively inhibit ERT; ↑ TSH levels and ↑ breast cancer risk	• In October 1999, the FDA authorized a health claim concerning the relationship between a daily diet, low in saturated fat and cholesterol, that contains 25 g of soy protein, and the reduction in risk of heart disease • Mild GI side effects: bloating and flatulence • Possible allergic reactions • Phytic acid in soy protein isolate can decrease absorption of non-heme iron from foods • Isolated soy isoflavones may not be safe for women with estrogen receptor-positive breast cancer or for pregnant or lactating women • For those with low iodine levels, may block production of thyroid hormones and ↑ TSH levels

146

Herb	Uses	Active constituents	Drug interactions	Safety/comments
St. John's Wort (*Hypericum perforatum*)	• Reduce symptoms associated with depression (fatigue, loss of appetite, insomnia) • Reduce anxiety and mood disturbances associated with menopause	• Hypericin, pseudohypericinin, hyperforin, and flavonoids	• May ↑ effects of digoxin • May ↑ photosensitivity with other such drugs • Avoid use with protease inhibitors (Indinavir) or nonnucleoside reverse transcriptase inhibitors • ↓ efficacy of cyclosporin	• Likely safe when used orally and appropriately • Therapeutic effects may take 2–4 wk to achieve • Long-term safety not known • Most common side effect is insomnia. Photosensitivity at high doses • Contraindicated for treatment of bipolar disorder or schizophrenia • Discontinue use at least 5 d before surgery
Valerian (root, tea, extract) (*Valerian officinalis*)	• Sleep aid, sedative • Also used for mood disorders and restlessness	• Bornyl acetate and valerenic acids Valepotriates may be toxic, if present	• Although valerian has not been reported to interact with any drugs or to influence laboratory tests, this has not been rigorously studied	• In Germany, approved as a sleep aid and mild sedative • Approved in United States as food additive • Generally safe when used orally and appropriately for short-term periods (<1 mo) • Minor side effects: headache, excitability, dizziness, and GI distress, possibly insomnia • Long-term use or excessive use is not recommended owing to potential side effects, which include headaches, blurred vision, heart palpitations, excitability, hypersensitivity reactions, insomnia and nausea and upset stomach

continued

Table 3 (*Continued*)
Herbal Supplements Commonly Used by the Elderly

Supplement	Reported uses	Compounds of interest	Potential interactions	Adverse effects/concerns/comments
Valerian (*continued*)				• Liver toxicity is also a concern with long-term use • May need to taper dose several weeks before surgery
Yohimbe (*Pausinystalia yohimbe*)	• All forms of erectile dysfunction	• Yohimbine and related indole alkaloids	• Taken by itself can cause HTN, avoid use with antihypertensives • Lower doses may have favorable effect in orthostatic hypotension induced by tricyclic antidepressants	• Yohimbine-HCl is available as an FDA-approved drug for the treatment of organic impotence. Other forms, such as yohimbe bark extracts and yohimbine (drug form) sold in health food stores may contain varying amounts of yohimbine as well as other ingredients • Yohimbe bark is on the German Commission E's list of unapproved herbs • Side effects include: HTN, anxiety, headache, GI symptoms • Large doses can cause severe hypotension, cardiac arrhythmias, psychotic reactions, skin eruptions, and death • Should not be used by the elderly or in individuals with HTN, heart, kidney, or liver disease

BPH, benign prostatic hypertrophy. CVD, cardiovascular disease; ERT, estrogen replacement therapy: GRAS, generally recognized as safe; HTN, hypertension; MAO, monoamine oxidase; TSH, thyroid-stimulating hormone. Adapted from refs. *187,198,215,218–224.*

Table 4
Other Dietary Supplements Used by the Elderly

Supplement	Reported uses	Potential interactions	Adverse effects/concerns/comments
Alpha lipoic acid	• Lower blood glucose levels • As an antioxidant to decrease oxidative stress • Treat and prevent peripheral nephropathy	• Possibly additive effects with herbs or drugs that ↓ blood glucose levels	• Functions as a coenzyme involved in carbohydrate metabolism. It is both water and lipid soluble • Approved in Germany for the treatment of diabetic neuropathy. Oral and IV administration forms • Oral alpha lipoic acid has been used safely in clinical trials lasting 4 mo to 2 yr • Side effects: rash • Adverse effects more common with IV therapy • Monitor blood glucose levels in diabetics • Take on an empty stomach
Coenzyme Q10 (ubiquinone)	• Slow aging • Increase energy • Improve cardiac performance • As an antioxidant to decrease blood pressure • Enhance immune function • Decrease oxidative stress	• HMG-CoA reductase inhibitors (statins) and some oral hypoglycemic agents can reduce serum CoQ10 levels • CoQ10 can reduce the anticoagulation effects of warfarin	• The Japanese government has approved CoQ10 for treatment of congestive heart failure • Preparations should be consumed with meals and may need to be taken in divided doses • Side effects include gastritis, loss of appetite, nausea, and diarrhea • Monitor in patients taking warfarin
DHEA Dehydroepiandrosterone	• Slows aging • Improves memory • Boosts energy • Protects against heart disease • Prevents growth and recurrence of some cancers • Eases symptoms of depression • Protects against diseases as diabetes, Parkinson's and Alzheimer's	• Triazolam ↑ plasma concentrations • Potentially can ↑ levels of drugs metabolized through the cytochrome P450 3A (CYP3A) enzyme system	• Side effects: increased facial hair, oily skin, mood swings, altered hormone profiles, liver abnormalities, menstrual cycle irregularities, ↑ risk of heart disease, diabetes, stroke, prostate cancer in man, and breast and endometrial cancer in women • ↓ levels of HDL cholesterol • Can ↑ insulin resistance or sensitivity • Can exacerbate liver dysfunction • Can exacerbate mental illness • DHEA is banned by the National Basketball Association

continued

149

Table 4 (*Continued*)
Other Dietary Supplements Used by the Elderly

Supplement	Reported uses	Potential interactions	Adverse effects/concerns/comments
Glucosamine (HCL) or sulfate	• Reverses osteoarthritis • Protects joints and tendons from injury and decreases inflammation	• Antidiabetic drugs may ↑ blood glucose levels and thus theoretically alter insulin sensitivity as reduced insulin secretion has been seen in animal studies • Contraindicated with anticoagulants	• Available in several formulations: glucosamine sulfate, glucosamine HCl, and N-acetylglucosamine • Side effects: mild GI discomfort • Potential allergic reactions in people allergic to shellfish. Avoid products containing excessive amounts of manganese (>11 mg/d) as one could exceed the UL • Long-term safety remains to be determined
Hydrazine sulphate	• Reduces cachexia and symptoms associated with cancer	• Do not take with tranquilizers, barbiturates, alcohol or foods high in tyramine	• Hydrazine sulphate is a chemical commonly used in industrial processes. It is not approved for use in cancer patients in the United States and was removed from the market in the 1970s; however, may be available in supervised clinical trials. NCI/NIH clinical trials have not demonstrated benefit. • Available by prescription in Canada and is widely used in Europe and Russia • Side effects uncommon but include: mild-to-moderate levels of nausea, vomiting, itching, dizziness, poor motor coordination, and/or tingling or numbness in hands and feet
Melatonin N-acetyl-5-methoxytryptamine)	• Reduces symptoms of jet lag • Aids in sleep disorders • Aids in shift-work disorders • Slows aging • May inhibit growth of breast cancer cells	• Theoretically, concomitant use with herbs that have sedative properties might enhance therapeutic and adverse effects • Effective for treating benzodiazepine withdrawal • Can reverse the negative effects of some β-blockers on nocturnal sleep	• Melatonin is a hormone produced by the pineal gland in the brain. It is manufactured synthetically and used as a supplement • The optimal oral dose has not been established • Classified as an orphan drug by FDA for use in circadian rhythm sleep disorders in blind children and adults with minimal light or no light perception • Studies have been mixed and inconclusive regarding

Melatonin (*continued*)		• Theoretically, concomitant use with alcohol, benzodiazepines and other sedative drugs might cause additive sedation • Avoid use with immunosuppressive drugs • Verapamil can increase melatonin excretion	the use of melatonin to improve the quality of life or increase survival time in individuals with cancer • Has been used safely from 7 d up to 2 mo, long-term safety is not known • Side effects include headaches, transient depressive symptoms, dtime fatigue, and drowsiness, dizziness, abdominal cramps, and irritability • Avoid driving or operating machinery for 4–5 h after taking melatonin • Avoid in individuals with immune-system disorders, autoimmune diseases, immune-system cancers • Avoid in individuals with severe mental illness or those taking steroids
Omega-3-fatty acids or fish oils	• Lower blood cholesterol and triglycerides • Relieve pain of rheumatoid arthritis • Relieve symptoms of depression • Relieve symptoms of allergies, asthma, and skin disorders • Reduce the risk of breast, prostate, and colon cancers	• Long-term use may ↑ risk of vitamin E deficiency • Avoid drugs and herbs with anticoagulant/antiplatelet potential, antihypertensive drugs, cyclosporin, and etretinate	• Fish oils have GRAS status in the United States • Safe when used orally and appropriately • Clinical trials have shown that fish oils significantly ↓ triglyceride levels by 20–50%, and is effective in reducing acute cardiac events • Studies in animals have found that fish oils suppress cancer formation and metastasis; however, there is no direct evidence for such in humans • May cause belching, halitosis, GI upset (1–3 g/d) or clinical bleeding (>3 g/d). • Worsening glycemia may occur at >3 g/d
SAMe (S-adenosyl-L-methionine)	• Relieve symptoms of osteoarthritis • Relieve symptoms of depression	• Concurrent use with anticepressants may cause additive serotonergic effects and serotonin syndrome-like effects	• SAMe is a naturally occurring substance in the body; not found in foods • Can be administered orally, IV, or IM

continued

Table 4 (*Continued*)
Other Dietary Supplements Used by the Elderly

Supplement	Reported uses	Potential interactions	Adverse effects/concerns/comments
SAMe (*continued*)	• Support liver health • Slow the aging process • Improve intellectual performance	• Protects against hepatic dysfunction caused by acetaminophen, alcohol, estrogens, MAO inhibitors, phenobarbital, phenytoin and steroids	• Controlled trials have shown SAMe to be superior to placebo and comparable to NSAIDs for ↓ symptoms associated with osteoarthritis in studies lasting several wk to 2 yr. SAMe also found effective for short-term treatment of major depression • Side effects more common at higher doses and include flatulence, vomiting, diarrhea, headache, and nausea • Significant symptom relief may require up to 30 d of treatment • Not recommended for use in individuals with bipolar disorders
Shark cartilage	• Inhibit development of some tumors (inhibits angiogenesis)	• Can cause hypercalcemia, do not use with supplemental calcium	• There is no scientific evidence that shark cartilage is an effective treatment for cancer • Laboratory and animal data is limited • Clinical trials are currently underway • Side effects: nontoxic, but may cause nausea, vomiting, dyspepsia, constipation, hyperglycemia, hypercalcemia, fatigue, fever, and dizziness

GRAS, generally recognized as safe; HMG-CoA, hydroxymethylglutaryl-coenzyme A reductase; MAO, monoamine oxidase. Adapted from refs. *215* and *218*.

2.1. B Vitamins

Evidence is accumulating that an elevated blood level of homocysteine, an amino acid normally found in blood, is an independent risk factor for cardiovascular and cerebrovascular disease. It has been estimated that lowering homocysteine by 5 µmol/L may reduce the risk of cardiovascular death by 10% (31). Folate (naturally as occurring in foods) and folic acid (the synthetic form occurring in supplements and fortified foods), along with vitamins B_6 and B_{12}, play a crucial role in modulating blood levels of homocysteine. Since the folic acid fortification program took effect in January 1998, dietary intake of folate equivalents has increased. Jacques et al. demonstrated that folic acid fortification resulted in a decreased prevalence of low levels of folate and high levels of homocysteine in the blood of middle-aged and older adults (32). A recent meta-analysis showed that treatment with 0.5–5.0 mg/d of folic acid lowered serum homocysteine by 15–40% within approx 6 wk. Additionally, a further 7% reduction in homocysteine levels was documented with the addition of vitamin B_{12} (mean 0.5 mg/d). Vitamin B_6, however, did not contribute to any additional lowering of homocysteine levels (33). McKay et al. found that a multivitamin/mineral formulated at 100% of the daily value for folate taken for 8 wk, in addition to a folic acid-fortified diet decreased homocysteine concentrations by 9.6% in 80 healthy men and women aged 50–87. Homocysteine concentrations were unaffected in the placebo group (34). In another study, 65 free-living subjects aged 36–71 with homocysteine concentrations greater than or equal to 9 µmol/L participated in a randomized controlled trial to compare the effects of folic acid supplementation, consumption of folic acid-fortified breakfast cereals, and increased consumption of folate-rich foods on plasma homocysteine levels. Daily consumption of folic acid-fortified breakfast cereals and the use of folic acid supplements was shown to be the most effective strategy for reducing homocysteine concentrations (35). This study suggests that folic acid supplementation can further reduce homocysteine levels in healthy middle-aged and older adults who consume a folic acid-fortified diet.

A 6-mo treatment regimen with a combination of folic acid (1 mg), vitamin B_{12} (400 µg) and vitamin B_6 as pyrioxidine (10 mg) in patients with coronary artery disease was found to significantly decrease blood homocysteine levels, the rate of vessel restenosis, and the need for revascularization after coronary angioplasty (36). Although research clearly indicates that B vitamins will help lower homocysteine levels, it is premature to recommend folic acid supplementation for the prevention of heart disease until results of ongoing randomized controlled clinical trials positively link increased folic acid intake with decreased homocysteine levels and decreased risk of cardiovascular disease (37). Clinical intervention trials are ongoing to determine whether supplementation with folic acid, vitamin B_{12}, or vitamin B_6 can lower the risk of developing coronary heart disease, recurrent stroke, and reduction of arteriosclerosis in renal transplant recipients. The optimum dose of folic acid has not yet been determined, but a daily dose as low as 400 µg/d as part of a multivitamin/multimineral supplement, in addition to a folate-rich diet, may be significantly relevant for older adults because blood homocysteine levels tend to increase with age.

2.2. Antioxidants

Preliminary research has led to a widely held belief that antioxidants, such as vitamins E and C, and β-carotene, may help prevent or delay coronary heart disease (38).

However, results from subsequent studies have been conflicting, in part because of differences in the dosage and formulation of supplements used and underlying disease pathology of the study population. Antioxidant therapies may be useful in preventing both the initiation of atherosclerotic disease and its complications by retarding low-density lipoprotein (LDL) oxidation, inhibiting the proliferation of smooth muscle cells, platelet adhesion and aggregation, expression and function of adhesion molecules, and attenuating the synthesis of leukotrienes *(39)*. Some population surveys *(40)* and observational studies have associated lower rates of heart disease with higher intake of antioxidants. A study of approx 90,000 nurses suggested that the incidence of heart disease was 30–40% lower among nurses with the highest intake of vitamin E from diet and supplements *(41)*. A randomized controlled trial that provided 400–800 IU of vitamin E to patients with coronary heart disease (Cambridge Heart Antioxidant Study or CHAOS) found a significant reduction in nonfatal myocardial infarctions, however, this was coupled with a nonsignificant increase in cardiovascular death and all-cause mortality in the group receiving vitamin E *(42)*. In addition, two large intervention trials have failed to show any significant effects of vitamin E on coronary heart disease. The Heart Outcomes Prevention Evaluation (HOPE) Study followed almost 9500 Canadian men and women for 4.5 yr who were at high risk for heart attack or stroke *(43)*. In this intervention study, subjects who received 265 mg (400 IU) of vitamin E daily had the same rates of cardiovascular events and hospitalizations for heart failure or chest pain as did those who received placebo. The GISSI (Gruppo Italiano per lo Studio della Sopravvivenza nell'Infarto Miocardico) prevention trial is a secondary prevention trial that enrolled 11,324 Italian patients who had survived a recent myocardial infarction. The GISSI trial investigators utilized 300 IU of vitamin E concurrent with a Mediterranean-type diet for 3.5 yr and also failed to show benefit from vitamin E supplementation in the reduction of death, nonfatal myocardial infarction, and stroke *(44)*. Supplementation with a combination of vitamin E and C has been shown to reduce the rate of disease progression in men, but not women *(45)*. Most recently, no effect of vitamin E was seen among high-risk patients enrolled in the Collaborative Group of the Primary Prevention Project *(46)*.

Some researchers have raised concern over the antiplatelet effect of vitamin E and its potential for increasing bleeding time and possible hemorrhagic stroke *(47)*. Researchers at the Human Nutrition Research Center on Aging at Tufts University demonstrated the safety of supplementation with 60, 200, or 800 IU of a synthetic vitamin E supplement (all-rac-α-tocopherol) per day for 4 mo in adults over 65 yr of age. Supplementation did not affect levels of plasma total proteins, lipid levels, liver or kidney function, thyroid hormones, indices of red and white blood cell counts, or bleeding time *(48)*. When patients receiving chronic warfarin therapy were given either 800 or 1200 IU of vitamin E or a placebo for 1 mo in a double-blind clinical trial, no significant alterations in prothrombin time or in the international normalized ratio (INR) were seen *(49)*. Long-term safety, however, has not been as closely studied.

The Institute of Medicine feels that it is still premature to recommend vitamin E supplementation for older adults, as recently published randomized clinical trials raise questions about the benefit of vitamin E supplements for preventing or controlling cardiovascular disease *(50)*. The American Heart Association (AHA) *(51)* also supports this position. However, the suggested association between vitamin E and heart health has enough scientific potential that physicians may feel it is beneficial for some individuals with cardiovascular disease. Recommending safe intakes under such circumstances is within their scope of clinical practice and may be prudent *(52)*, particularly in light of the fact that the amounts of vitamin E that exerted beneficial effects in epidemiological and intervention studies are not achievable by dietary means.

A number of large-scale prospective cohort studies have examined the relationship between vitamin C intake and cardiovascular disease. The results from those studies have been even less consistent than those for vitamin E, and the majority of the studies do not support a relationship between vitamin C intake and cardiovascular disease protection. However, more recently, clinical intervention studies with daily doses of 500 mg of vitamin C or acute doses of 1–3 g have shown significant improvement in endothelial function and vasodilation. Endothelial dysfunction with impaired biological activity of nitric oxide is emerging as a significant risk factor for angina pectoris, myocardial infarction, and stroke *(53)*.

2.3. Magnesium

Epidemiologic studies have suggested that individuals or groups ingesting hard water that contains magnesium, consuming a diet higher in magnesium, or using magnesium supplements, have decreased morbidity from cardiovascular disease *(55)*. Similarly, epidemiologic evidence suggests that magnesium may play an important role in regulating blood pressure *(54–58)*. However, intervention studies with magnesium therapy in hypertensive patients have led to conflicting results. In the Atherosclerosis Risk In Communities Study (ARIC), a cross-sectional study, magnesium intake was found to be inversely associated with carotid artery thickness in women, but not in men. A recent study in 50 men and women with stable coronary artery disease found that 6 mo of oral magnesium supplementation improved arterial dilation in response to brachial artery pressure testing *(59)*. Additionally, another study of patients with coronary artery disease found that 3 mo of oral magnesium supplementation inhibited platelet-dependent thrombosis; these effects were independent of aspirin therapy *(60)*. Magnesium depletion is associated with cardiac complications, including electrocardiographic changes, arrhythmias, and increased sensitivity to cardiac glycosides *(61)*. In patients with heart failure, a population at high risk for magnesium deficiency, oral magnesium replacement results in a decrease in the frequency of ventricular arrhythmias *(62,63)*. Average dietary intakes in the United States are estimated to be below the RDA, thus increasing the risk of nominal magnesium deficiency in those consuming typical American dietary patterns. Therefore, in at-risk populations, such as the elderly with chronic diseases, supplementation may be a reasonable means of precluding such deficiency. Health care professionals should note that individuals with impaired renal function are at a greater risk of magnesium toxicity from the use of dietary supplements and intakes should not exceed the RDA. Also, older adults who are dependent on magnesium-based laxatives may be at risk for toxicity. Given the common use of diuretics, some of which may increase urinary loss of magnesium, high incidence of marginal or inadequate dietary magnesium intake, use of magnesium-based laxatives, and incidence of renal insufficiency in older populations, a medical doctor may be the best person to evaluate all of the factors potentially promoting magnesium deficiency or toxicity and determine a need for magnesium supplementation.

2.4. Omega-3 Fatty Acids

Omega-3 and omega-6 fatty acids, along with their metabolites, are vital to human health. In addition dietary omega-3 fatty acids (α-linolenic acid [ALA], eicosapentaenoic acid [EPA], and docosahexaenoic acid [DHA]) act to prevent heart disease through a variety of actions, as suggested by results obtained in several secondary prevention trials.

Four prospective controlled intervention trials with either oily fish *(64)* or omega-3 fatty acid capsules *(44,65,66)* have provided direct evidence for a cardioprotective effect. The GISSI-Prevenzione study is the largest of the controlled trials to prospectively test the ability of omega-3 fatty acid supplements to alter coronary heart disease risk in 11,324 patients surviving a recent myocardial infarction. Patients were randomly assigned to receive either omega-3 fatty acids (1 g/d), vitamin E (300 mg daily), both, or neither for 3.5 yr *(44)*. In this trial, total mortality was reduced by 20% and sudden death by 45% in patients consuming omega-3 fatty acids. It appears that this reduction in mortality is through decreased incidences in sudden death *(44)*.

Salmon, trout, tuna, lake whitefish, bluefish, swordfish, herring, anchovies, mackerel, and sardines are the predominate sources of DHA and EPA omega-3 fatty acids. At this time, the AHA encourages consumption of at least 2 servings of fatty fish per week to confer cardioprotective effects *(51)*. Farm raised fish contain less omega-3 fatty acids unless they were fed other fish or algae. Alternatively, a fish oil supplement that would result in an omega-3 fatty acid intake of approx 900 mg/d could be taken. This amount has been shown to be beneficial in lowering coronary heart disease mortality rates in patients with coronary artery disease. In consultation with their physician, these individuals could consider supplementation for coronary heart disease risk reduction. In addition to fatty cold-water fish (e.g., salmon and mackerel), data supports the inclusion of vegetable oils. Canola oil, flax seed (ground) and flax oil, and some nuts (e.g., almonds and walnuts) are good dietary sources of ALA omega-3 fatty acids. Soybean oil is often listed as a good source of omega-3 fatty acids, but the overwhelming amount of omega-6 fats present (ratio of omega-6 to omega-3 fatty acids is 33:1) limits the conversion of ALA to EPA and DHA, making soy oil a poor source of omega-3. Flax oil pills provide another option for increasing omega-3 fatty acids. For those individuals concerned about the consumption of fish with high levels of environmental contaminants, the best approach would be to consume a wide variety of species to minimize the exposure. However, for middle-age and older adults, the health benefits derived from the consumption of fish far outweighs the risk of toxicity from fish that may possess toxic levels of contaminants.

Increases in LDL cholesterol with omega-3 supplementation have been a concern, but are modest (usually <5%), more than offset by marked reductions (30–40%) in atherogenic triglyceride levels *(67)*. Similarly, in high-risk individuals, supplements could also be a component of the medical management of hypertriglyceridemia. Recommended intake is 2–4 g/d of EPA and DHA in capsule form *(68)*.

2.5. Plant Sterols

Plant sterols or phytosterols have been known to have a cholesterol-lowering effect since the 1950s *(69–71)*. The esterification of plant stanols renders them soluble in dietary fat, which has been shown to be an effective vehicle for delivering plant stanols and sterols to the site of cholesterol absorption in the small intestine. In food preparations, such as spreads that provide 3.4 to 5.1 g/d of plant stanol esters, these substances have been shown to significantly reduce serum total and LDL cholesterol levels without affecting high-density lipoprotein (HDL) cholesterol or triglycerides. Both unsaturated (sterol ester) and saturated (stanol ester) forms of plant sterols have been used in a number of clinical studies, demonstrating that consumption of these fats is beneficial in lowering blood cholesterol in both normolipidemic and dyslipidemic individuals, including those treated with lipid-lowering agents *(69–75)*. Both the AHA and the National Education Cholesterol Project Adult Treatment Panel III (NCEP ATP III) *(76)* report recommends the use of plant stanols for individuals who need to lower total and LDL cholesterol. Concern has been raised about the potential for plant sterol-containing foods to decrease antioxidant levels, such as β-carotene or α-tocopherol. Results of long-term studies are needed before health professionals and groups can unequivocally recommend plant stanols for the prevention of cardiovascular disease *(51)*.

2.6. Soy

Epidemiologic studies have suggested that populations consuming large amounts of soy protein in place of animal protein appear to have less cardiovascular disease. The active components in soy are the soy protein, the phytoestrogen component that includes isoflavones, and alcohol-extractable components. Favorable effects of soy phytoestrogens on blood lipid profiles, vascular reactivity, thrombosis, and cellular proliferation have been reported *(77)*. The mechanism underlying the cholesterol lowering effect of soy remains to be elucidated, but is most likely multifactorial *(78)*. Daily consumption of soy protein with its associated phytoestrogens can improve lipid profiles in hypercholesterolemic individuals. Although the clinical response to soy relates to the initial blood cholesterol level, even in subjects with normal lipid levels, a soy diet has resulted in lowering plasma lipids. Newer research suggests that soy supplementation may increase the levels of HDL cholesterol, regardless of whether or not an individual is hypercholesterolemic. Anderson and colleagues *(79)* conducted a meta-analysis of 38 clinical trials of soy protein consumption in humans that demonstrated an improvement in total cholesterol by 9% and LDL cholesterol by 13%, as well as a decrease in triglyceride levels of 10%. Results from double-blind placebo-controlled trials of mildly hypercholesterolemic subjects following the NCEP Step I diet suggested that consuming 20–50 g soy protein daily can significantly reduce LDL cholesterol *(80,81)*. However, most recently, dietary soy has been shown to have both beneficial and potentially adverse cardiovascular effects in a randomized controlled trial. In a group of normotensive men and postmenopausal women, supplementation with soy improved blood pressure and lipids, but also decreased endothelial function (an indicator of vascular function and health) in men and increased lipoprotein (a) [Lp(a)] concentrations, a risk factor for cardiovascular, in both groups *(82)*.

Since 1999, the FDA has allowed labels on foods that contain > 6.25 g of soy protein per serving, one-fourth of the daily intake (25 g) shown to significantly lower cholesterol level, to claim reduced risk of heart disease. The AHA encourages a greater intake of soy proteins containing isoflavones, along with other heart-healthy diet modifications for high-risk populations with elevated total and LDL cholesterol. However, they point out that some commercial soy protein concentrates may be processed via techniques that remove isoflavones and other potentially active compounds *(51)*. The optimal doses, forms, and duration of treatment of isoflavones, and the interaction of various soy components on cardiovascular disease risk factors remain to be clarified.

2.7. *Garlic (*Allium sativum*)*

The lipid-lowering effects of garlic have been demonstrated in animal experiments and in randomized clinical trials. Evidence from numerous studies points to the fact that garlic may normalize plasma lipids, enhance fibrinolytic activity, inhibit platelet aggregation, and reduce blood pressure and blood glucose concentrations. However, the use of different formulations or preparations of garlic and different study designs has led to contradictory results in clinical studies. A systematic review of the literature and a review of 36 randomized trials conducted by the Agency for Healthcare Research and Quality *(83)* noted only modest short-term effects of garlic supplementation on lipid and antithrombotic factors. In the treatment of high blood pressure, the majority of the studies, which were small in scale and of short duration, used various doses of garlic, providing approx 3–6 mg of allicin per day. These studies found that garlic did not reduce blood pressure when compared to placebo. Another meta-analysis conducted by Stevinson and colleagues *(84)* that included 13 randomized placebo-controlled trials demonstrated a modest, but significant, difference in the reduction of total cholesterol level in hypercholesterolemic subjects given garlic when compared with placebo. However, the six diet-controlled trials of high-methodologic quality showed a nonsignificant difference between the garlic and the placebo groups. Therefore, the authors of this review concluded that the use of garlic for hypercholesterolemia was of questionable value. Garlic has been reported to increase the risk of bleeding, likely because of its antiplatelet action, but this has not been well established *(85)*.

3. DIETARY SUPPLEMENTS IN THE MANAGEMENT OF CANCER

Most dietary supplements used by cancer patients are derived from native plants and foods from around the world. Extracts from green tea, garlic, soybeans, rosemary, and crucifers that contain folic acid, minerals (including calcium and selenium), and antioxidants (e.g., vitamins E and C) are common in the cancer patient's regimen. Current evidence suggests a protective effect against almost all major cancers primarily from vegetable consumption, with less of an effect for fruit consumption *(86)*. However, a recent meta-analysis of eight prospective studies in over 350,000 women suggests this may not the case for breast cancer *(87)*. A number of these dietary supplements used for cancer are described below and in Tables 2–4.

3.1. *Antioxidants*

Antioxidants, such as vitamins E and C, selenium, and the carotenoids, help protect against the damaging effects of free radicals, which may contribute to the development of cancer *(50)*. However, most antioxidants can behave as prooxidants under certain conditions, which complicates the search for optimal doses of antioxidant supplements.

3.1.1. Vitamin E

Human trials and surveys that have tried to associate vitamin E with the incidence of major cancers have been generally inconclusive. Large randomized trials indicate that the relationship between specific micronutrient intakes and cancer risk is complex. Some evidence associates higher intake of vitamin E with a decreased incidence of breast cancer, lung, prostate, and colon cancer. The weight of evidence does not support a strong association, with the exception of prostate cancer. The most significant finding was from the follow-up phase of the Alpha-Tocopherol Beta-Carotene (ATBC) study, which randomly assigned 29,133 50–69-yr-old male smokers to 50 mg α-tocopherol, 20 mg β-carotene, both, or a placebo for 5–8 yr. This study demonstrated a 32% decrease in the incidence and a 41% decrease in mortality from prostate cancer among subjects who received α-tocopherol supplements (88). Two other studies support an association between vitamin E and decreased prostate cancer risk (89,90). An examination of the effect of dietary factors, including vitamin E, on incidence of postmenopausal breast cancer in over 18,000 women from New York, however, did not associate a greater vitamin E intake with a reduced risk of developing breast cancer (91). A study of women in Iowa provided evidence that an increased dietary intake of vitamin E may decrease the risk of colon cancer, especially in women under 65 yr of age (92). On the other hand, vitamin E intake was not associated with risk of colon cancer in almost 2000 adults with cancer, when compared to controls without cancer (93). Despite the intriguing results from the ATBC study, the overall evidence is inconclusive and precludes researchers from recommending vitamin E supplements for the prevention or treatment of cancer.

3.1.2. CAROTENOIDS

Surveys suggest an association between diets rich in carotenoids and a lower risk of many types of cancer (94–96). The best evidence is for lung, colon, breast, and prostate cancers. In particular, there is evidence that increased consumption of green and yellow vegetables or food sources of β-carotene and/or vitamin A may decrease the risk of lung cancer (97). Only β carotene has been studied as a supplement in randomized trials with consistently negative results. A number of studies, examining a protective role for β-carotene in cancer prevention, have yielded unexpected results. In the ATBC study, previously described, vitamin E was found to be beneficial for reducing the incidence of prostate cancer, but a daily dose of β-carotene increased the incidence of lung cancer in the group of smokers (98,99). The Carotene and Retinol Efficacy Trial (CARET), a lung cancer chemoprevention trial that randomized subjects to receive either supplements of β-carotene and vitamin A or placebo was stopped when subjects in the intervention group had a 46% higher risk of dying from lung cancer (100). Results of studies of β-carotene supplementation do not appear to decrease colorectal cancer risk, and the results for prostate cancer have been mixed. The epidemiological evidence linking carotenoids to breast cancer remains inconclusive. As the evidence of benefit is lacking, the Institute of Medicine concluded that β-carotene supplements are not advisable for the general population, although they also state that this advice "does not pertain to the possible use of supplemental β-carotene as a provitamin A source for the prevention of vitamin A deficiency in populations with inadequate vitamin A nutriture" (50). Preliminary results from observational studies of other carotenoids, including lycopene, are promising for lowering the risk of lung and prostate cancer; however, there have been no clinical trials of lycopene supplementation for prostate cancer.

3.1.3. VITAMIN C

Epidemiological evidence that vitamin C reduces the risk of cancers of the oral cavity, esophagus, and stomach is fairly robust (101). Vitamin C is thought to inhibit the intragastric formation of carcinogenic nitrosamines. Infection with H. pylori has been shown to deplete ascorbic acid content of gastric juice. Higher serum ascorbic acid has been associated with a decreased risk of the progression of precancerous lesions to gastric cancer in a population with a high prevalence of *H. pylori* infection. In a recent multicenter case-control study evaluating the nutrient intake and risk of developing four types of esophageal and gastric cancer, both dietary and supplemental vitamin C were significantly and inversely associated with the risk of noncardiac gastric adenocarinoma *(102)*. Significant protective effects were also seen for dietary folate and vitamin B_6, but not for vitamin B_{12}. Further studies are needed to confirm these exciting findings before supplementation with vitamin C can be recommended for the reduction of risk for gastric cancers.

3.2. Calcium

Currently, there is a lack of scientific agreement regarding the association between the intake of dairy products, calcium, and decreased the risk of colorectal cancer. In colonic mucosa, decreased levels of calcium can have a direct effect on stimulating cell proliferation in cells undergoing neoplastic transformation that can lead to colorectal adenomas, the precursors of colorectal cancer. Another possible mechanism for the protective effects of calcium may be related to interference with the metabolism of bile acids and ionized fatty acids. A meta-analysis in 1996 and a review in 1998 found inconclusive epidemiological evidence about the effect of calcium intake on colon cancer *(103,104)*. In one study in patients with a history of polypectomy for adenomatous polyps, increasing daily calcium up to 1200 mg/d via low-fat dairy products not only reduced the proliferation of colonic epithelial cells, but also caused the cells to return to their normal differentiation patterns *(105)*. Baron and colleagues demonstrated a moderate association between calcium supplementation, 3 g (1200 mg of elemental calcium) daily, and a 20% decreased risk of the recurrence of colorectal adenomas over a 4-yr period *(106)*. On the other hand, a study recently published in patients with colorectal cancer found that calcium and vitamin supplementation did not decrease markers of cell kinetics of colon epithelium, suggesting a lack of clinical efficacy in preventing new adenomas *(107)*. Wu and colleagues recently examined dietary intake information, medical history, and lifestyle factors from the Nurses' Health Study (87,998 women) and the Health Professionals Follow-up Study (47,344 men) to examine the association between calcium intake from foods and supplements and colon cancer risk. The investigators found an inverse association between distal colon cancer and higher total calcium intakes (>1250 mg/d compared to 500 mg/d). Those subjects who consumed 700–800 mg of calcium per day had a 40–50% lower risk of developing cancer *(108)*. Presently, it is not clear whether increasing calcium intake will ultimately translate into reduced cancer risk.

3.3. Selenium

Selenium is an important constituent of antioxidant enzymes that protect cells against the effects of free radicals. Researchers have long been interested in selenium's potential to delay the onset of carcinogenesis. Some studies indicate that mortality from cancer, including lung, colorectal, and prostate cancers, is lower among people with higher blood levels or intake of selenium *(109–115)*. The effect of selenium supplementation on the recurrence of basal and squamous cell skin cancers was studied in seven dermatology clinics in the United States from 1983 through the early 1990s. Supplementation with 200 µg selenium daily did not affect recurrence of skin cancer, but significantly reduced total mortality and resulted in a two-thirds reduction of mortality as a result of lung and colorectal cancer (116).

The largest-ever prostate cancer prevention trial sponsored by the National Cancer Institute at the National Institutes of Health will enroll 32,000 healthy men to test the efficacy of vitamin E (400 mg) and selenium (200 µg) in men 55 yr or older. The Selenium and Vitamin E Cancer Prevention Trial (SELECT) will determine if these two dietary supplements can protect against prostate cancer. The trial, initiated in July 2001, will take up to 12 yr to achieve the final results (117).

3.4. Folic Acid

Folic acid is being investigated for a role in cancer development and progression because of its natural involvement in the synthesis and repair of DNA. Researchers have demonstrated that a deficiency of folate can result in misincorporation of uracil into DNA that may result in chromosome breaks. Such breaks may contribute to the increased risk of cancer and cognitive defects associated with folate deficiency in humans (118). Several studies have linked diets low in folate (119,120) and low blood folate levels (121) with increased risk of breast, pancreatic, and colon cancer. Findings from a study of over 121,000 nurses suggested that long-term folic acid supplementation (for 15 yr) was associated with a decreased risk of colon cancer in women aged 55–69 yr of age (119). Another prospective study found reductions in colon cancer associated with higher dietary folate in men, but not in women (122). Among women consuming alcohol regularly when compared to nondrinkers, higher folate intake was associated with decreased breast cancer risk (123–125). Researchers are continuing to investigate whether enhanced folate intake from foods or folic acid supplements may reduce the risk of cancer. Until results from such clinical trials are available, folic acid supplements should not be recommended to reduce the risk of cancer.

3.5. Herbal Supplements

Approximately 35% of older patients diagnosed with cancer have reported using complementary therapies, most frequently, herbal therapy (126). Some of the most frequently used supplements by patients with cancer include astralagus, saw palmetto, cat's claw, aloe vera, mistletoe, milk thistle, Hoxsey, Essiac, and PC-SPES. There is little to no clinical evidence for the efficacy of these supplements, and several are noted to have the potential for serious side effects, as described in Table 3. PC-SPES, an herbal medicine, is a formula consisting of a combination of eight herbs that shows some promise as a treatment for prostate cancer. PC-SPES has been shown to reduce serum testosterone concentrations and the level of prostate-specific antigen (PSA) in a small group of study subjects (127). Additional clinical trials are pending further evaluation of the safety and efficacy of PC-SPES for the treatment of prostate cancer.

3.6. Other Dietary Supplements

A number of other unconventional cancer treatments have been promoted, but are as yet unproven for cancer. It is imperative that cancer patients discuss the use of dietary supplements with their physicians before attempting to include such therapies with prescribed medications.

4. DIETARY SUPPLEMENTS IN THE MANAGEMENT OF DIABETES

In adult patients with diabetes, the risk of cardiovascular disease is 3–5-fold greater than in the general population. Prevention and treatment of long-term micro- and macrovascular complications remain critical problems in the management of type 2 diabetes mellitus. A number of studies have suggested that patients with diabetes appear to have decreased antioxidant defense capability, measured as lower levels of specific antioxidants, such as vitamin C or vitamin E, or reduced activities of antioxidant enzymes. A number of supplements, such as magnesium, chromium, α-lipoic acid, vitamin E, omega-3 fatty acids, ginkgo biloba, gurmar, and fenugreek, have been used for the treatment of diabetes, but few have strong scientific evidence to support their effectiveness. It is interesting to note that the prescription drug, metformin, originated from the herb, *Galega officinalis* (goat's rue or French lilac) extract. French lilac extract was used in medieval times to treat diabetes. Metformin is the only hypoglycemic drug with its roots from a botanical source *(13,14)*. Several of these supplements will be discussed, and others are included in Tables 2–4.

4.1. Magnesium

Magnesium deficiency may play a role in insulin resistance and carbohydrate intolerance. Elevated blood glucose levels increase the loss of magnesium in the urine, which in turn lowers blood levels of magnesium; low magnesium levels, in turn, can impair glucose tolerance. Correcting magnesium depletion in the elderly has been found to improve glucose handling by improving insulin response and action *(128)*. Low blood levels of magnesium have also been associated with some of the long-term complications of diabetes such as neuropathy. In 1999, the American Diabetes Association (ADA) issued a position statement that concluded by saying, adequate dietary magnesium intake can generally be achieved by a nutritionally balanced meal plan. The available data suggest that routine evaluation of serum magnesium levels is recommended only in patients at high risk for magnesium deficiency. Levels of magnesium should be repleted only if hypomagnesemia can be demonstrated *(129)*.

4.2. Chromium

Several studies have suggested that chromium supplementation might be beneficial in individuals with glucose intolerance, diabetes mellitus, gestational diabetes or steroid-induced diabetes, as evidenced by improved blood glucose values or decreased insulin requirements following chromium supplementation. However, randomized trials of chromium supplementation in diabetes have not been definitive, in part because of the use of multiple formulations, varying dose ranges, and length of studies. Anderson and colleagues, who studied a non-Western population, were the first to report a significant dose-response relationship between chromium (200 or 1000 μg chromium picolinate/d) and glucose and insulin levels in diabetics *(130)*. A recent meta-analysis of 11 controlled trials concluded there was strong evidence that chromium has no effect on glucose control in healthy subjects, and the data in patients with diabetes were equivocal *(131)*. More studies are needed before chromium can be recommended as a supplement to improve serum glucose levels in patients with diabetes.

4.3. Vitamin E

There is now considerable evidence that hyperglycemia, hyperinsulinemia, and insulin resistance enhance free-radical generation, thus contributing to the oxidative stress in type 2 diabetes *(132)*. Daily supplementation with 900 mg of vitamin E was shown to improve insulin action in subjects with diabetes and in healthy mature and elderly subjects *(133,134)*. Several studies of vitamin E supplementation in diabetic individuals have demonstrated a decrease in biochemical markers of oxidative stress. One small short-term study utilizing 1800 mg vitamin E in patients with diabetes showed improvement in some surrogate markers for retinopathy and nephropathy *(135)*. In obese subjects with diabetes, however, supplementation with 600 mg/d of vitamin E for 3 mo was associated with a decline in insulin action *(136)*. An antioxidant supplement containing 24 mg of β-carotene, 1000 mg of vitamin C, and 800 IU of vitamin E was shown to significantly decrease the oxidation of LDL cholesterol in 20 diabetic men who consumed this supplement for 12 wk compared to a nonsupplemented control group *(137)*. Interpretation and application of these results are difficult as the preparation and dose of vitamin E used in these studies has been widely variable. Chronic administration of pharmacologic doses of vitamin E (600 mg/d) have been shown to improve the cardiac autonomic nervous system in patients with type 2 diabetes *(138)*. It is postulated that intervention with vitamin E therapy to inhibit atherogenesis might be more effective in patients with diabetes than in nondiabetics. However, at this time, there are insufficient data on which to propose a recommendation of vitamin E supplementation in diabetes *(50)*.

4.4. Omega-3 Fatty Acids

As noted earlier, treatment with omega-3 fatty acids, but not vitamin E, significantly lowered the risk of death, nonfatal myocardial infarction, and stroke for patients enrolled in the GISSI Prevenzione Study. In a subgroup analysis of 1600 diabetic subjects from GISSI, diabetics benefited in significant risk reduction to the same extent as the nondiabetic patients from supplementation with 850 mg of omega-3 fatty acid/d. Although concern exists regarding the worsening of glycemic control in diabetics consuming fish oil supplements, the most recent meta-analysis (which included 12 trials) concluded that fish oil supplementation in diabetes mellitus has no statistically significant effect on glycemic control *(139)*. Recently, long-term fish oil supplementation in patients with diabetes mellitus with hypertriglyceridemia has shown beneficial effects in lowering total LDL without altering the distribution of particles within the LDL subfraction *(140)*. Although it is premature to issue a public health recommendation regarding the use of omega-3 fatty acid supplements in diabetic patients with cardiovascular disease, the scientific rationale and safety profile for this supplement looks very promising.

5. DIETARY SUPPLEMENTS IN THE MANAGEMENT OF OSTEOPOROSIS

5.1. Calcium and Vitamin D

It is estimated that over 25 million adults in the United States have or are at risk of developing osteoporosis, a disease characterized by compromised bone strength that increases the risk of fracture *(141)*. Nutritional factors can significantly influence bone density, which accounts for as much as 80% of bone strength. The NIH Consensus Development Panel on Osteoporosis Prevention, Diagnosis, and Therapy concluded that adequate calcium and vitamin D intake is crucial for the development of and maintenance of bone mass throughout life and that supplementation with both nutrients may be necessary when dietary intake is inadequate *(142)*.

Optimal calcium intake is the amount that promotes strong bones and leads to the fewest osteoporotic fractures later in life *(143)*. The optimal intake of calcium is not known, but the current recommended adequate intake (AI) for men and women over age 50 is set at 1200 mg daily *(143)*. Supplemental calcium and vitamin D have been associated with reduced fracture rate and increased bone density in numerous studies. Daily supplementation of 1200 mg calcium, and 800 IU vitamin D significantly reduced nonvertebral fracture rates in 3000 retirement home residents with a mean age of 84 yr *(144)*. Researchers demonstrated that calcium supplementation could prevent seasonal changes in bone turnover in 60 postmenopausal women without osteoporosis who were randomized to a placebo, 4, 8-oz glasses of milk per day, or 500 mg of calcium carbonate twice per day with meals. Calcium intake increased stepwise, from 699 mg + 49 mg in the placebo group to 1052 + 118 mg/d in the dietary group to 1678 mg + 57 mg/d in the supplement group. After 2 yr, women who took calcium supplements experienced a significant increase in lumbar bone mineral density (+3.7 ± 1.9%) whereas women in the placebo, and dietary groups experienced no change. During winter months, women taking supplements did not lose bone, whereas placebo and dietary-treated subjects experienced slight bone loss *(145)*. In a randomized controlled trial, Reid et al. demonstrated a reduced rate of loss of bone density in 86 postmenopausal women who were treated with 1 g elemental calcium daily for 4 yr *(146)*. Efforts should always be made to promote an adequate dietary intake of calcium, but available evidence suggests that calcium supplementation can play an important role in helping the elderly maintain bone health.

Vitamin D deficiency, most often defined by blood levels of 25-hydroxyvitamin D < 30.0 nmol/L, is characterized by inadequate mineralization or demineralization of bone *(143,145)*. Vitamin D deficiency occurs more often in postmenopausal women and older Americans *(143,147–150)* and has been associated with a greater incidence of hip fractures *(10)*. A greater vitamin D intake from diet and supplements has been associated with less bone loss in older women *(147)*. Because bone loss increases the risk of fractures, vitamin D supplementation may help prevent fractures resulting from osteoporosis. In a group of women with osteoporosis hospitalized for hip fractures, 50% were found to have signs of vitamin D deficiency *(141)*. Treatment of vitamin D deficiency can result in decreased incidence of hip fractures, and daily supplementation with 20 µg (800 IU) of vitamin D has been shown to reduce the risk of osteoporotic fractures in elderly individuals who have low blood levels of vitamin D *(11)*.

More than 90% of fractures occur as a result of falls. Decreased femoral bone density, increased body sway, and impaired muscle strength are major predictive factors for nonvertebral fractures. Pfeifer et al. demonstrated that supplementation with calcium and vitamin D in community-dwelling women over 70 yr reduced body sway and mean number of falls, suggesting the benefit of such supplementation *(151)*. Evidence suggests that vitamin D supplementation may benefit the bone status of older adults, but dosage must be carefully chosen to prevent toxicity from excessive intake of vitamin D supplements.

5.2. Magnesium

Magnesium deficiency also may be a risk factor for postmenopausal osteoporosis *(143)*. The evidence available is not as extensive as for calcium and vitamin D, but it is known that magnesium deficiency results in hypocalcemia and altered vitamin D metabolism *(152)*. Seventy-one percent of postmenopausal women experienced a rise in radial bone density when supplemented with 2–6 tablets daily, each containing 125 mg magnesium hydroxide, for 6 mo followed by two tablets per day for another 18 mo *(148)*. It is difficult to identify the individual contribution of magnesium to the development of osteoporosis and bone health in studies combining several supplements, but in postmeno-pausal women, the provision of 600 mg magnesium, 500 mg calcium, and a multivitamin-mineral product increased calcaneous bone mineral density after 1 yr *(149)*. It is safe to say that magnesium plays a role in maintaining bone health, but sufficient evidence is not available to confidently recommend magnesium supplementation for the prevention of osteoporosis. The prevalence of inadequate magnesium intake among older adults sug-gested by the National Health and Nutrition Examination Survey III (NHANES III) *(150)* indicates the importance of making dietary changes to increase magnesium intake or considering the use of supplemental magnesium in individuals unable or unwilling to make appropriate dietary changes.

5.3. Vitamin K

Vitamin K (phylloquinone) has also been associated with bone mineral density and risk of hip fracture. Mechanisms involved in this association are poorly understood, but may be related to the activity of specific vitamin K-dependent proteins that are important to bone mineralization *(153)*.

Low dietary intake of vitamin K-1 (the most common dietary form of vitamin K) was associated with increased risk of hip fractures among women participating in the Nurses' Health Study *(154)*. In a cohort of the Framingham Heart Study, there were no significant associations between dietary phylloquinone intake and bone mineral density, but the range in vitamin K intake between the highest and lowest quartiles may not have been significant enough to detect differences. Men and women in the highest quartile of vitamin K intake, however, had a significantly lower related risk of hip fracture than those in the lowest quartile *(153)*. In some cases, subjects with lower vitamin K intakes also had lower caloric and calcium intakes, making the studies more difficult to interpret. This is a new area of research, and much work is needed before researchers can make conclusive recommendations on the role of dietary vitamin K in bone health.

6. DIETARY SUPPLEMENTS FOR MENTAL AND COGNITIVE FUNCTION

Rates of dementia and cognitive impairment increase exponentially with advancing age, starting at about age 65 and doubling every 5–7 yr until at least age 90. Long-term oxidative stress is believed to be one of the major contributing factors to the decline of cognitive function observed with aging *(155,156)*.

6.1. B Vitamins

Poorer cognitive function has been reported in individuals with lower serum concen-trations of B12, folate and vitamin C *(157–162)*. Lindenbaum and colleagues *(163)* demonstrated significant improvement in neuropsychiatric functions among B_{12}-deficient patients after vitamin B_{12} supplementation. Similarly, Martin et al. *(164)* repleted 18 subjects on B_{12} given intramuscularly over the course of 1 yr. Patients who had experienced cognitive decline for less than 12 mo performed better than those patients who had experienced cognitive decline for greater than 12 mo, suggesting that interventions may be time-sensitive. Serum vitamin B_{12}, C and folate concentrations were measured in a sample of 883 elderly Hispanics and non-Hispanic whites age 65 and older participating in the New Mexico Elder Health survey to examine the associations between multivitamin and vitamin C use and measures of cognitive and depressive functions. Significant associations were seen for serum folate concentrations and measures of cognitive function, but were lacking for the other vitamins *(165)*. Depressive symptoms have been reported to be the most common neuropsychiatric manifestation of folate deficiency *(166)*.

High plasma homocysteine concentrations are associated with impaired cognitive abilities and lower total life satisfaction in healthy elderly *(157,167,168)*. The relationship between Alzheimer's disease and elevated levels of homocysteine is of particular interest because blood levels of homocysteine can be reduced by increasing intake of folic acid (or folate) and vitamins B_6 and B_{12}. Data collected from participants of the Framingham Study showed that elevated homocysteine levels (>14 mmol/L) doubled the chance that a participant would develop Alzheimer's disease and each 5 mmol/L elevation was shown to increase the risk of Alzheimer's disease by 40% *(169)*. The National Institute of Aging at the NIH in cooperation with The Alzheimer's Disease Cooperative Study have launched a multicenter trial to test whether reducing homocysteine levels with high doses of folic acid, vitamins B_6 and B_{12} can slow the rate of cognitive decline in people diagnosed with Alzheimer's disease. Expected total enrollment is 400 with an estimated completion date of February 2006.

6.2. Antioxidants

Dietary antioxidants may play an important role in retarding several cognitive disorders associated with neuronal diseases, including Alzheimer's disease, Parkinson's disease, and vascular dementia *(170)*. Correlational studies in healthy older people suggest that lower serum vitamin C might be associated with poorer mental function *(171)*; however, these studies failed to demonstrate any benefit from antioxidant vitamin supplementation. Perrig and colleagues found a positive correlation between plasma vitamin C and β-carotene concentrations and memory performance in 442 elderly aged 65 and older living in Basel, Switzerland *(162)*. The Honolulu-Asia Aging Study is a longitudinal study of Japanese-American men living in Hawaii. In 1998, 3385 men, age 71–93 yr provided data on dietary intake and supplement use to determine whether vitamin E and C protect against the development of dementia or poor cognitive functions. In the reference group, 39% of subjects reported taking vitamin E and C supplements, and most were taking both. Higher rates of use (49%) were seen among subjects with Alzheimer's disease. No significant associations of cognitive measures were found for vitamin E and C supplement use with Alzheimer's disease. However, use of vitamin E and C was associated with a reduction of 88% in the frequency of subsequent vascular dementia. The authors hypothesize that antioxidant vitamins may protect against vascular dementia by limiting the extent of neuronal injury that persists after an ischemic event, rather than by decreasing the frequency of events *(172)*. Results from intervention studies are mixed. Feeding a high-dose vitamin and mineral supplement for 1 yr to 10 elderly nonvitamindeficient females showed no improvement in cognitive function *(173)*. On the other hand, Sano and colleagues tested the efficacy of daily intake of 2000 IU of vitamin E, 10 mg selegiline (a monoamine oxidase inhibitor used as adjunct therapy for Parkinson's disease), or both on the progression of Alzheimer's disease in a double-blind placebo-controlled randomized trial in 342 patients. They found that both vitamin E and selegiline, alone or in combination, significantly delayed the onset of either death, institutionalization, loss of the ability to perform basic activities of daily living, or severe dementia *(174)*. The findings from this study are encouraging. Ongoing clinical trials will further confirm vitamin E's efficacy in the prevention of the sequelae of Alzheimer's disease. However, the combined evidence does not yet support the routine use of higher than RDA supplement doses of B_{12}, folate, vitamin C or E to protect against cognitive dysfunction during aging. At very high doses, folate has been reported to cause altered sleep patterns, irritability, nausea, and pruritis and so should be used with caution.

6.3. Herbal Supplements

A number of herbal supplements are marketed to enhance mood or memory or to decrease anxiety and stress. Among some of the herbal medicines with psychiatric indications are: St. John's wort, *Ginkgo biloba*, melatonin, evening primrose, valerian, kava, German chamomile, lemon balm, and black cohosh. The most studied of the herbals are St. John's wort and *Ginkgo biloba*, both of which are now being investigated in NIH-funded multicenter clinical trials in the United States. These herbals are described below or in Table 3.

6.3.1. St. John's Wort (Hypericum)

A number of earlier studies conducted in Germany support the use of St. John's wort as an antidepressant. The active ingredient(s) of St. John's wort remain unidentified and the mechanism of action is not completely understood. Recent research suggests that the substance hyperforin may play a significant role in the herb's antidepressant effects *(175–177)*. More than 30 clinical studies have been published evaluating the efficacy of St. John's wort in patients with mild-to-moderate depression. The duration of treatment in these trials was usually 6 wk. All of these studies have confirmed that the efficacy of St. John's wort is superior to placebo and equivalent to other prescription antidepressants *(178–180)*. In 1999, the Agency for Healthcare Research and Quality conducted a systematic review of the literature on St. John's wort and depression and concluded that hypericum appears to be more effective than placebo for short-term treatment of mild-to-moderately severe depressive disorders *(181)*. However, more recent reviews and laboratory studies have raised questions about the efficacy *(182,183)* and safety *(184–187)* of St. John's wort for the treatment of mild-to-moderate depression. The studies collectively indicate that St. John's wort appears to be more effective than placebo for short-term treatment of mild-to-moderately severe depressive disorders. However, health care professionals should note that St. John's wort interacts extensively with a number of pharmaceuticals (e.g., protease inhibitors); its use is contraindicated for individuals with HIV disease, polar disorders, and schizophrenia.

6.3.2. Ginkgo Biloba

Ginkgo biloba is one of the most popular medicines in Germany and France, where physicians prescribe it for memory lapses, dizziness, anxiety, headaches, tinnitus, and other problems. Ginkgo leaf and its extracts, or GBE, contain several constituents including flavonoids, terpenoids, and organic acids. Each of these chemicals should exist in a specific amount in clinical quality GBE, representing a standard for assessing ginkgo products. Although many of ginkgo's constituents have intrinsic pharmacological effects individually, there is some evidence that the constituents work synergistically to produce more potent pharmacological effects than any individual constituent. The pharmacological actions that are most clinically relevant for ginkgo include antiischemic, antiedema, antihypoxic, free-radical scavenging and hematologic effects and inhibition of platelet aggregration and adhesion. It is not known to what extent any of these effects contribute to the clinical effectiveness of ginkgo in dementias. Results from two independent meta-analyses *(188,189)* concluded that ginkgo biloba extract in doses of 120–240 mg/d for treatment periods, ranging from 4 wk to 12 mo significantly improved objective measures of cognitive function when compared to placebo. Ginkgo has the potential to cause bleeding, especially in combination with anticoagulants *(187)*. The NIH is currently funding a 5-yr multicenter clinical trial to evaluate *ginkgo biloba* (240 mg daily) in 3000 subjects over the age of 75 to determine if ginkgo prevents dementia or Alzheimer's disease. Another NIH clinical trial is also being funded to study the effect of *ginkgo biloba* extract on preventing or delaying cognitive decline in people age 85 or older.

6.3.3. VALERIAN (*VALERIANA OFFICINALIS*)

Valerian is marketed in most countries as an over-the-counter remedy for insomnia. Dietary supplements made with valerian are generally prepared from the root (or rhizomes) of the plant. *Valeriana officinalis*, the most commonly used species, has GRAS status and is approved for food use in the United States. Valerian's exact mechanism of action has not been determined, but it is believed that valerian root extract induces an increase in γ-aminobutyric acid (GABA) levels in neuronal synapses in the brain. Improvement in sleep with valerian was evaluated in a recent systematic review of nine studies. Results were mixed, with five of the nine demonstrating clinical effectiveness *(190)*. Clinical studies have used a variety of valerian root extracts, including some standardized to contain 0.4–0.6% valerenic acid. Adverse effects of valerian are infrequent, but have included headache, restless sleep, allergic reaction, and digestive symptoms.

Because of the lack of standardization, adequate data on safety and efficacy, particularly for products formulated in the United States, it is premature for health care professionals to recommend use of valerian as a sleep aid or sedative over established conventional treatments.

7. DIETARY SUPPLEMENTS FOR SUPPORT OF IMMUNE FUNCTION

7.1. Micronutrients

An adequate nutrient intake may help maintain immunologic function in aging adults. For example, micronutrients may modulate macrophage function, and the antioxidant vitamins may enhance various steps involved in phagocytosis. Vitamin D_3 stimulates the maturation of monocytes to macrophages *(191)*. Vitamin A deficiency can result in fewer natural killer cells, which are part of an early defense system against cancer and infectious disease. Vitamin E deficiency may also impair natural killer cell activity.

To examine the effect of physiologic amounts of randomly given vitamin and trace element supplements on the immunocompetence and rate of infectious illnesses, Chandra studied 96 independently living, healthy elderly individuals. He found that subjects receiving supplements were less likely than those receiving placebo to develop an infectious illness, had higher numbers of natural killer cells, increased natural killer cell activity, and possessed higher numbers of certain types of T-cells. The micronutrient supplement also enhanced lymphocyte proliferative response, natural killer cell activity, and antibody responses to influenza vaccine *(192)*. However, a 10-wk double-blind study in 31 elderly women administered an over-the-counter multivitamin supplement failed to show an improvement in measured indices of immune system function as indicated by changes in T-cell or B-cell numbers or lymphocyte proliferative response to mitogen *(193)*.

Evidence supporting the immune enhancing effects of micronutrient supplementation in the elderly is lacking, and the data currently available regarding supplementation are not convincing.

7.2. Use of Herbal Supplements to Support Immune Function

Species of two botanical genera stand out among the immune-stimulant herbs: coneflower (*Echinacea* spp.) discussed below and mistletoe (*Viscum album*); *see* Table 3.

7.2.1. ECHINACEA

There is some evidence that *Echinacea* may help reduce the symptoms of the common cold bronchitis, influenza, bacterial and viral infections of the respiratory tract, but it does not appear to help prevent these conditions. Commerical *Echinacea* products are manufactured from three *Echinacea* species, *Echinacea purpurea* (root or herb), *E. angustifolia* (roots), and *E. pallida* (roots). The active chemical constituents of interest in these *Echinacea* species fall into five groups: alkamides, polyalkenes, polyalkynes, caffeic acid derivatives, and polysaccharides. *Echinacea* extracts appear to enhance immune function through multiple mechanisms, including activation of phagocytosis and stimulation of fibroblasts, increasing cellular respiration, and increasing the mobility of leukocytes *(194,195)*. Barrett and colleagues performed an extensive review of the literature and found that eight out of nine clinical trials on the treatment of colds and other respiratory infections reported *Echinacea* was beneficial, whereas three out of four trials on the prevention of colds reported that *Echinacea* was only marginally beneficial. These findings led the authors to conclude that *Echinacea* products may be beneficial in the early treatment of colds, but there is little evidence to support long-term use for prevention of colds *(196)*. However, clinical recommendations are lacking because of the diversity of products tested and the moderate-to-poor quality of these studies. The part of the plant used, type of preparation used, and the amount given are factors that may affect the outcome of clinical studies on *Echinacea*. The majority of clinical studies have been conducted using a preparation of the expressed juice from the tops of *E. purpurea*.

8. HERBAL SUPPLEMENTS FOR THE MANAGEMENT OF MENOPAUSAL SYMPTOMS

It has been estimated that 30% of women use acupuncture, natural estrogens, herbal supplements, or plant estrogens to treat symptoms and discomforts related to menopause *(197)*. Herbs used to treat gynecologic conditions or symptoms cannot replace sex hormones, anti-infectious agents, or antispasmodic drugs that are medically indicated *(198)*. Commonly used herbs for the relief of vasomotor symptoms or menstrual disorders associated with menopause include soy products, black cohosh, red clover, evening primrose, dong quai, chasteberry, and wild yam. These supplements are described below or in Table 3.

8.1. Soy

In addition to soy's beneficial effects in lowering plasma cholesterol levels, soy isoflavone supplements given to postmenopausal women have demonstrated improvements in vascular arterial compliance almost identical to that achieved by estrogen replacement therapy *(199)*. Some data support the efficacy of soy isoflavones (40–80 mg/d) for reducing the incidence and severity of hot flashes, but in general, the randomized controlled clinical trials demonstrate only slight reductions in these symptoms in women who consume soy or isoflavones as compared to control subjects *(200)*. A recent study found that 150 mg of soy isoflavones taken orally did not allieviate hot flashes in breast cancer survivors, 68% of whom were receiving concurrent adjuvant endocrine therapy *(201)*. At this time, few recommendations can be made with confidence regarding these products because of the general lack of their standardization, the relatively short duration of study associated with use and follow-up, and difficulty in interpreting the available clinical data. Soy and its isoflavone constituents may be helpful in the short-term treatment of vasomotor symptoms associated with menopause. However, researchers caution that these compounds may interact with endogenous estrogens and, therefore, should not be considered to be free of potential harm in women with estrogen-dependent cancers *(78)*. Research has shown both protective and stimulatory effects of soy and soy isoflavones on breast cancer, based on epidemiology, as well as in vitro, and in vivo studies *(200)*. Although isoflavones may have beneficial effects at some ages or circumstances, this cannot be assumed to be true at all ages. Isoflavones are like other estrogens in that they are two-edged swords, conferring both benefits and risks *(202)*.

8.2. Black Cohosh (Cimicifuga racemosa)

Black cohosh has been used in Germany since the mid-1950s to manage vasomotor symptoms of menopause. Although some study results suggest that black cohosh may help relieve menopausal symptoms, other study results do not *(203–206)*. Interpretation of these studies is complicated by the lack of rigor in study design, short duration, choice of formulation, and outcome measures to be studied. The pharmacologically active ingredients of black cohosh are prepared from the rhizome and root. Extracts of black cohosh are standardized by their saponin content of 26-deoxyactein. The mechanism of action of black cohosh has not been defined and laboratory evidence regarding the presence of estrogenic activity has been conflicting. Concomitant use with hormone replacement therapy has not been studied, and it is yet to be determined if black cohosh is safe for use in women with a history of breast cancer, as the effect on breast tissue is not well understood. However, recent randomized clinical trial addressed the efficacy, side effects, and safety of black cohosh among breast cancer survivors. Eighty-five women were randomized to either black cohosh (20 mg twice daily for 2 mo) or placebo, and stratified by tamoxifen use and followed for a 2-mo period. Both treatment and placebo groups reported declines in the number and intensity of hot flashes, as well as an improvement in other menopausal symptoms, but differences were not statistically significant between groups. Blood levels of follicle-stimulating hormone (FSH) and luteinizing hormone (LH) did not differ in the two groups.

The authors concluded that black cohosh was not significantly more efficacious than placebo against most menopausal symptoms in this study of short duration with a high drop-out rate of 19% *(207)*. Much of the published clinical evidence for the safety and efficacy of black cohosh is based on the utilization of a commercial extract, approved in Germany, known as Remifemin. It has been used in clinical studies lasting up to 6 mo. It is still unclear whether or not black cohosh exhibits estrogenic activity, which could cause endometrial or breast tissue stimulation, and studies have been mixed on whether black cohosh affects vaginal epithelium. Women taking black cohosh long-term should consult with their physician regarding the need for periodic vaginal ultrasound.

8.3. Red Clover (Trifolium repens)

Red clover is another botanical used extensively by women to treat menopausal symptoms. Although promoted as a phytoestrogen source similar to soybeans, red clover is a medicinal herb, not a food, and traditionally has not be used long-term. Although red clover appears to be safe, its efficacy for treatment of menopausal symptoms has not been conclusively demonstrated. Two trials of red clover extract found no effect on hot flashes or other menopausal symptoms and three of four trials examining the effect of red clover on lipids found no benefit. Potential estrogenic effects on breast and endometrium have not been adequately assessed *(208)*.

9. HERBAL SUPPLEMENTS FOR THE MANAGEMENT OF MALE UROLOGIC CONDITIONS

Among the herbals purported for relief of symptoms for male urologic conditions are saw palmetto, nettle root, and yohimbine.

9.1. Saw Palmetto (Serenoa repens)

Of the 30 herbal compounds available for the relief of symptoms related to benign prostatic hyperplasia (BPH), a nonmalignant enlargement of the prostate, saw palmetto has been most widely used. The majority of men over the age of 60 are considered to have urinary symptoms attributable to BPH. In the United States, treatment of BPH accounts for approx 1.7 million physician visits *(209)* and results in more than 300,000 prostatectomies annually *(210)*. Saw palmetto, which has been gaining in popularity for the past several years, has been advocated as an alternative therapy for treating the symptoms associated with BPH. The mechanism of action by which saw palmetto works is not known. Saw palmetto has been shown to have antiandrogenic, antiproliferative, and antiinflammatory properties that seem to be responsible for improving BPH. Evidence from a recent systematic review of 18 randomized clinical trials *(211)* suggest that saw palmetto improves urologic symptoms and flow measures when compared with placebo and was noted to be comparable to the drug finasteride with fewer reported adverse events. Additional information on herbs for the management of male urologic conditions is presented in Table 3.

10. DIETARY SUPPLEMENT INTERACTIONS

Concern exists for potential supplement–drug interactions, as an estimated 15 million adults in 1997 took prescription medications concurrently with herbal remedies and/or high-dose vitamins *(17)*. The elderly may have a higher risk of physical harm from the use of dietary supplements because they have a greater prevalence of chronic diseases and conditions and consume a disproportionate share of prescription medications when compared to younger adults. An additional concern is that individuals with potentially serious health conditions may seek alternative therapies in lieu of conventional therapies and may do so without consulting their physician.

Herb–drug interactions can increase or decrease the bioavailability of a drug, protect against a drug's adverse effects, enhance the effect of the drug, or produce an additive effect or an antagonistic effect incompatible with the drug's effect *(212)*. Among the specific types of reactions that can occur are those that modify the intestinal absorption of medicines, potentiate cardiotonic medicines, modify blood sugar in diabetes mellitus, modify the effects of anticoagulants, as well as interactions that are incompatible with medications for the gastrointestinal tract *(212)*. Patients with clotting disorders, those awaiting surgery, or those on anticoagulant therapy should be discouraged about concurrent use of herbals with conventional medications that alter bleeding and clotting functions. Herbs such as ginkgo, danshen, dong quai, papaya, or garlic interfere with platelet function, not the coagulation cascade, and thus will not affect prothrombin time, partial thromboplastin time, or the international normalized ratio (INR). Many other herbs also contain anticoagulant substances and as a precaution, INRs should be monitored periodically in these high-risk patients *(187)*.

A number of publications have systematically documented herb–drug interactions and are a valuable reference source for the health professional, and a selected collection of these are presented in Table 5. Pharmacopeias contain guidelines for the therapeutic use and/or assessment of the quality of medicines and health products (e.g., herbs). The texts are comprised of individual monographs (treatises) for each drug or therapeutic ingredient.

11. GUIDELINES FOR SAFE USE OF DIETARY SUPPLEMENTS

Dietary supplementation remains a controversial topic. There is strong evidence that dietary intake and nutritional status will influence overall health of aging adults. Determining the benefit of specific dietary supplements is complicated by the fact that there likely is a range of optimal intakes. For many products, these ranges have not yet been determined. On the other hand, there is also a lack of substantive scientific data regarding the effect of many herbal and alternative dietary supplements on specific outcome measures, safety, standard dosage, side effects, and interactions with medications and foods. The Food and Nutrition Board of the Institute of Medicine, National Academy of Sciences, in their recently published series of the DRIs, has for the first time identified functional endpoints for each nutrient that can be used to investigate the effect of supplements. It is important for health professionals to develop recommendations for supplement use based on results of well-designed scientific studies that are published in peer-reviewed journals and that address such endpoints.

11.1. Ten Guidelines for Health Professionals
When Recommending Dietary Supplements

1. Health professionals should consider whether dietary changes, such as the use of whole foods or fortified foods could satisfy the need for additional nutrient intake before recommending a dietary supplement. Also assess diet and current conditions for need of supplements (*see* Section 12).

Table 5
Reference Sources for Information on Dietary Supplements and Herb–Drug Interactions

Monographs

- American Herbal Pharmacopeia and Therapeutic Compendium (AHP)
  Monographs are available through their website by writing the American Herbal Pharmacopoia, PO Box 5159, Santa Cruz, CA 95063. Phone: 831-461-6318, e-mailing: ahpadmin@got.net. Website address: http://www.herbal-ahp.org.

- ESCOP Monographs on the Medicinal Use of Plant Drugs
  European Scientific Cooperative on Phytotherapy (ESCOP) "Monographs on the Medicinal Uses of Plant Drugs" Fascicles 1 through 6, published by ESCOP, Argyle House, Grandy Street, Exeter, EX4 3LS, UK 1996–1999, ISBN numbers 1 901964-00-0, -01-9, -02-7, -03-5, -04-3, -06-X.

- The Complete German Commission E Monographs
  Blumentahl M, Goldberg A, Brinkmann J, eds.
  Herbal Medicine-Expanded Commission E Monographs.
  American Botanical Council, Austin, TX, 1999.
  The American Botanical Council, P.O. Box 201660 Austin, TX 78720.
  Phone: 512-331-8868, and website address: www.herbalgram.org

- WHO Monographs on Selected Medicinal Plants,
  The World Health Organization (WHO) monographs are published in "WHO Monographs on Selected Plants," vol. 1, by WHO, Geneva, Switzerland, 1999, ISBN 92 4154517 8.
  The WHO website is http://www.who.org.

Books and Publications

- ADA/APhA Special Report from the Joint Working Group on Dietary Supplements
  A Healthcare Professional's Guide to Evaluating Dietary Supplements, 2000
  Available at: http://www.aphanet.org.

- Brinker FJ. Herb Contraindications and Drug Interactions, 2nd ed. Electic Medical Publications, Sand, OR, 1998.

- Foster S, Tyler VE. Tyler's Honest Herbal: A Sensible Guide to the Use of Herbs and Related Remedies. 3rd ed., Haworth Herbal Press, Binghamton, NY, 1993.

- McGuffin M, Hobbs C, Upton R, and Goldberg A, eds. Botanical Safety Handbook: Guidelines for Safe Use and Labeling for Herbs in Commerce. American Herbal Product Association. CRC Press, New York, NY, 1997.

- Newall CA, Anderson LA, Philpson JD. Herbal Medicines—A Guide for Health-Care Professionals. The Pharmaceutical Press, London, UK, 1996.

- Sarubin A. The Health Professionals Guide to Popular Dietary Supplements. American Dietetic Association, Chicago, IL, 2000.

- Schultz V, Hansel R, Tyler VE. Rational Phytotherapy: A Physician's Guide to Herbal Medicine. Springer, New York, NY, 1998.

CD-ROM Databases

- HealthNotes Clinical Essentials, Portland, OR is a comprehensive database containing science-based information on complementary and alternative medicine (website address: www.healthnotes.com)

- Natural Medicines Comprehensive Database. The Pharmacist's Letter/The Prescriber's Letter; 1999, updated yearly. Web address: www.NaturalDatabase.com.

2. Health professionals should alert their patients to the importance of investigating supplements before purchasing them. The most reliable information about supplements is developed by government agencies and trained experts. Be prepared to recommend reliable internet sites on dietary supplements, such as those developed by experts with national credentials, such as MD (medical doctor), RD (registered dietitian) and Pharm D (Doctor of Pharmacy).

3. Consumers should be aware that, in most cases, there is no known benefit to consuming more than the RDA (or AI) of a particular nutrient.

4. Consumers should be aware of the importance of limiting intake of any supplement to less than or equal to the upper level (UL) suggested by the Institute of Medicine, unless prescribed or recommended by a physician for a specific physiologic reason. A physician should consider normal physiological changes associated with aging, dietary intake data, and the results of individual nutritional and physical assessments before recommending an intake greater than the UL.

5. When possible, consumers should purchase dietary supplements standardized and certified by an accredited source. For example, US pharmacopoeia National Formulary products labeled with the USP/NF NSF notation indicate that the manufacturer adhered to prescribed standards for identity and purity established by the US Pharmacopoeia for quality, strength, purity, packaging, and labeling. Additionally, there are a number of reputable independent testing organizations such as consumerlab.com that are actually testing products and providing this service.

6. Consumers should be made aware about the potential harm from using multiple dietary supplements often referred to as "polypharmacy." Many consumers do not add up the amounts of nutrients in various supplements taken, thus increasing the risk of consuming more than the UL of an individual nutrient.

7. Health professionals should caution their patients who take multiple supplements to introduce only one product at a time and to be alert to adverse side effects. Any products that result in nausea, vomiting, diarrhea, constipation, severe headaches, rash, restlessness, or anxiety should be stopped and the reaction reported to a physician.

8. Consumers should be educated to select for product freshness by evaluating the expiration date on dietary supplements whenever possible. Also alert clients that the reputation of the manufacturer may be important. Herbal products and other supplements manufactured by nationally recognized companies are more likely to have been made under tighter quality control.

9. Consumers should read all labeling carefully and to follow all cautionary directions and dosage limits on the label. The label term "natural" doesn't guarantee that a product is safer or more effective than synthetic products. Also, consumers should be wary of any product claiming to cure a condition or disease.

10. It is very important for pregnant women *not* to take a dietary supplement unless prescribed or approved by their obstetrician.

The FDA requires that all dietary supplement labels include the following information *(213)*:

- Statement of identity (e.g., "ginseng").
- Net quantity of contents (e.g., "60 capsules").
- Structure–function claim and the statement, "This statement has not been evaluated by the Food and Drug Administration. This product is not intended to diagnose, treat, cure, or prevent any disease."
- Directions for use (e.g., "Take one capsule daily.").

- Supplement Facts panel (lists serving size, amount, and active ingredients).
- Other ingredients in descending order of predominance and by common name or proprietary blend.
- Name and place of business of manufacturer, packer, or distributor. This is the address to write for more product information.

Health professionals should also know the scientific or species names of the most popular supplements on the market, as this will help in assessing ingredient labels. In addition, for herbals, FDA requires that the scientific name of the plant or common or usual name if it is accepted for commercial use, the plant part used, and the weight of single ingredients (except for proprietary blends) also be listed on the label. It is important to understand the dose requirements of the various formulations of supplements and be alert to the potential for allergic reactions in patients sensitive to certain plants, pollen, or flowers.

12. NEED ASSESSMENT FOR DIETARY SUPPLEMENTS

Given the prevalence of inadequate dietary intake of many vitamins and minerals, as well as the potential for inappropriate use of supplements among older adults, it is important for health providers to routinely screen elderly clients for their potential need for dietary supplementation and for the risk of excessive supplement intake. The following questions can identify conditions, symptoms, or situations that suggest the need to consider counseling on the use of fortified foods and/or dietary supplements in addition to advising older adults to make appropriate dietary changes.

1. Has the older client been diagnosed with physical conditions or does he/she display symptoms that may indicate a need for fortified foods and/or dietary supplements?
   - Osteoporosis: calcium, vitamin D
   - Alcohol abuse: "B" vitamins, magnesium
   - Gastrointestinal abnormalities including diarrhea, fat malabsorption, and atrophic gastritis: vitamin B_{12}, fat soluble vitamins (A, D, E, K)
   - Renal insufficiency: vitamin D
   - Cardiovascular disease: vitamin E, folic acid
   - Nutritional anemia: iron, vitamin B_{12}, folic acid
   - Weight loss, nausea, or other symptom indicative of an inadequate intake: general multivitamin supplement

2. Does the older client have intake behaviors that place him/her at high risk for nutritional deficiency or excess?
   - Eats fewer than 2 complete meals per day
   - Drinks 1 or more (women) or 2 or more (men) alcoholic beverages per day
   - Dietary intake profile is inconsistent with the Food Guide Pyramid
   - Eats < 2 servings vegetables per day
   - Eats < 2 servings of fruits per day
   - Takes multiple dietary supplements per day
   - Takes doses of vitamin and mineral supplements that exceed the RDA unless recommended by a physician (pay particular attention to intakes greater than the UL)
   - Is unaware of doses of supplements taken

3. Do body composition changes or physical limitations suggest potential for nutrient deficiencies?

- BMI < 21
- Has unintentionally lost or gained 10 lbs in the last 6 mo
- Has difficulty chewing or swallowing

4. Are there lifestyle habits or conditions that may impair normal intake?

- Is housebound
- Has clinical evidence of depressive illness
- Needs assistance with self-care
- Demonstrates mental/cognitive impairment

Once a needs assessment has been completed, the following approach can be used to focus recommendations (*see* Fig. 2).

13. RECOMMENDATIONS FOR CLINICIANS

Most nutritionists, physicians, and health care organizations advise consumers to meet their nutritional needs via a healthful diet as suggested in science-based guidelines, such as the USDA Food Guide Pyramid. There is agreement that foods provide compounds that are essential to optimal health (although some of these remain to be identified or convincingly demonstrated), and that making dietary changes to meet current nutrient recommendations should be the first step toward improving dietary intake. However, these same organizations concede that there are times when nutritional needs exceed normal dietary intake, or when needed nutrients cannot be obtained by food or retained by the body because of impaired absorption or other physiologic limitations. In these instances, dietary supplements play a valuable role in maintaining health. The following list summarizes general considerations about dietary supplements and older adults.

13.1. General Multivitamin/Mineral Supplements

Recommendation: It is wise to limit intake of general multivitamin/mineral supplements to products providing 100% of the daily value (DV) per day. Multivitamin/mineral preparations formulated at 100% of the DV may be a very effective way to safely maintain desirable blood micronutrient levels and help promote good health. Such products are generally considered to be safe because they provide considerably less than defined upper levels. They also help maintain adequate nutrient intakes during periods of illness when food intake is less than optimal. Preparations chosen should include 100% of the DV for vitamins B_{12}, B_6, D, and folic acid, because these are key nutrients for the elderly and surveys suggest inadequate dietary intake among older persons.

13.2. Calcium

Recommendation: Unless contraindicated, older adults may benefit from supplemental intake of 500 mg calcium per day from a supplement or fortified food, or 1000 mg/d for older persons who consume inadequate calories and cannot consume milk and dairy foods.

The current AI for calcium for adults age 50 and over is 1200 mg/d. This is an increase over the 1989 RDA, but this still may not be adequate for those older adults at greatest risk of developing osteoporosis or who may already have osteoporosis. The National Institutes of Health Consensus Development Conference on Optimal Calcium Intake

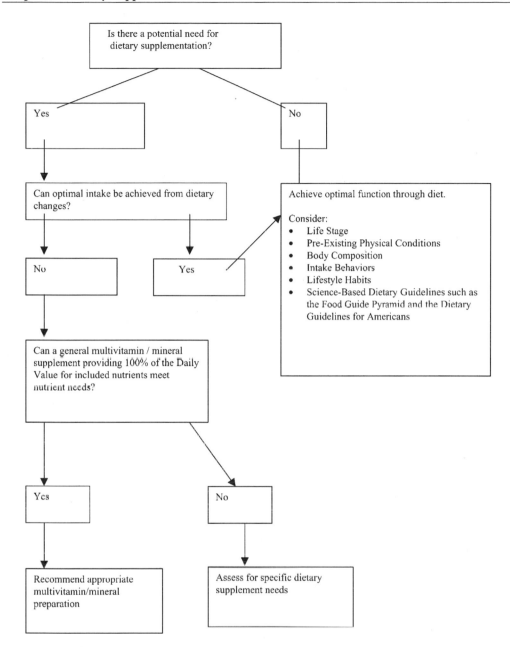

Fig. 2. Needs assessment algorithm for dietary supplement use in aging individuals. Adapted from ref. *214*.

suggested 1500 mg of calcium per day for postmenopausal women who are not on estrogen therapy and for all men and women over 65 yr (NIH Consensus Statement 1994). However, the Institute of Medicine determined that there are insufficient data to increase the AI to this level. The many studies that suggest using calcium supplements to maintain bone density, and dietary surveys indicate that significant numbers of older adults do not consume adequate dietary calcium, also support a potential role for calcium supplements.

Researchers continue to examine this issue, and nutritionists and the public await those studies that put all questions to rest. However, sufficient valid data have been assembled to state that all adults ages 50 and over should consult with their physician, registered dietitian, or pharmacist about their need for calcium supplements. At this time, it may be safest to advise those in this age group to consume 500 mg calcium from a supplement or from fortified foods daily unless otherwise contraindicated. For those who are unable or have difficulty consuming any milk or dairy products, particularly those older adults who have difficulty consuming adequate calories, 1000 mg calcium from supplements, ideally in two doses of 500 mg each, may be appropriate unless otherwise contraindicated. Calcium carbonate is adequately absorbed and is the least expensive form of calcium supplement. It is not as well absorbed as calcium citrate, but the large size of the calcium citrate molecule results in the need for much larger pills for an equal amount of calcium. The upper level (UL) for calcium, or maximum level associated with no adverse health effects, is 2500 mg consumed in foods and supplements.

13.3. Vitamin D

Recommendation: Older persons who do not consume vitamin D-fortified milk may benefit from consuming 400 IU/d from a supplement unless otherwise contraindicated. This level of supplementation is often available in basic multivitamin preparations that provide 100% of the DV for vitamin D. The current AI for vitamin D is 400 IU/d. Dietary surveys indicate that an inadequate intake and the physiologic changes that occur because of aging limit conversion of vitamin D to its most active form. Therefore vitamin D supplements may be beneficial for adults age 50 and over. It is important to limit supplementation to the AI of 400 IU because of the risk of toxicity associated with excess intakes of vitamin D.

13.4. Vitamin B$_{12}$

Recommendation: Adults age 50 and older should obtain most of their vitamin B$_{12}$ from supplements or fortified food. The RDA for vitamin B$_{12}$ is 2.4 µg. This level of supplementation is available in multivitamin preparations that provide 100% of the DV.

The evidence supporting the benefit of supplemental vitamin B$_{12}$ for older adults is so strong that in 1998, the Institute of Medicine advised all adults age 50 and over to obtain their vitamin B$_{12}$ from dietary supplements or fortified foods. The 2001 RDA for vitamin B$_{12}$ is 2.4 µg for all those over 18, and this level of supplementation via pills or fortified foods is appropriate. Crystalline vitamin B$_{12}$, the form that is used in supplements, does not require gastric acid for absorption, so a multivitamin can ensure that intake is adequate for most people. There is no evidence supporting a need for higher supplemental intake vitamin B$_{12}$ does not have an UL because higher intakes are not associated with adverse health events.

13.5. Folic Acid

Recommendation: Older persons may benefit from consuming 400 µg/d from a dietary supplement or from fortified foods. This level of supplementation is available in basic multivitamin preparations that provide 100% of the DV.

The concern over inadequate intakes of folic acid by most age groups was so strong that the FDA now requires fortification of grain products with folic acid. A primary goal of this policy is to reduce the incidence of neural tube defects in newborns. Older adults will also benefit from this program because of the association between adequate folate intake and reduced risk of cardiovascular disease. The level of supplementation recommended for women of childbearing age is also appropriate for older adults: 400 µg of folic acid per day from supplements or fortified foods. The UL for folic acid is 1000 µg (or 1 mg) because of the potential for folic acid to mask vitamin B_{12} deficiency. This is particularly important for older persons because at least 30% are likely to have difficulty absorbing vitamin B_{12} from food, and are therefore at higher risk of developing a vitamin B_{12} deficiency. Older persons should not take any supplement providing more than 400 µg of folic acid without first consulting with their physician about their vitamin B_{12} status.

13.6. Vitamin E

Recommendation: Older persons at high risk of developing cardiovascular disease or who have existing cardiovascular disease should discuss the benefit of taking a supplement of vitamin E, not to exceed 800 IU/d, with their cardiologist or primary physician. This level of supplementation is not available in most multivitamin preparations and usually requires a separate vitamin E supplement. There are various forms of vitamin E. Alpha-tocopherol is considered the most active form. Unlike other vitamins, the form of α-tocopherol made in the laboratory and found in many supplements (all Rac-α-tocopherol) is not identical to the natural form (RRR-α-tocopherol), and is not quite as active as the natural form. The RDA of 15 mg equals 22 IU of natural and 33 IU of synthetic vitamin E. The potential physiologic benefit of vitamin E and lack of known adverse health effects in doses ranging from 200–800 IU/d may be a reasonable choice for adults who are at high risk of developing heart disease or who have pre-existing cardiovascular disease. The UL for vitamin E is 1000 mg/d.

13.7. Selenium

Recommendation: There is insufficient evidence to support supplementing a diet that already provides the recommended intake for selenium. However, selenium's antioxidant properties and the potential benefit for decreasing mortality from cancer (especially from prostate cancer) suggest that supplementation at levels consistent with the DRIs, 55 µg/d, is acceptable for adults age 50 and over. The UL for selenium is 400 µg.

13.8. Zinc

Recommendation: There is no evidence to support routine supplementation with zinc beyond levels usually found in general multivitamin-mineral preparations, which generally limit zinc intake to the DV.

Research has not indicated a benefit of routine zinc supplementation in individuals whose diets already meets the recommended intake level. Zinc supplementation may be indicated for certain medical circumstances, such as for macular degeneration and wound healing, but a medical team would evaluate the need and make specific recommendations. Unless under physician guidance, zinc supplementation should be limited to the RDA because pharmacologic doses have the ability to impair immunity. The RDA for zinc for adult women is 8 mg. The RDA for zinc for adult men is 11 mg. The UL for zinc for adult men and women is 40 mg.

13.9. Magnesium

Recommendation: There is no evidence to support routine supplementation with magnesium beyond levels usually found in general multivitamin-mineral preparations. In general, aging is associated with magnesium depletion. Decreases in dietary intake, coupled with decreases in intestinal magnesium absorption and increases in urinary magnesium losses, place older adults at risk for magnesium deficiency. Older adults are also more likely to take medication that promotes urinary loss of magnesium such as some diuretics. Diabetes, which is seen with increased frequency in older adults, can result in increased magnesium excretion when poorly controlled and can also contribute to decreased levels of magnesium. On the other hand, some older adults are more likely to take magnesium-containing laxatives than younger adults, a habit that could result in excess magnesium intake and possible toxicity. This may be especially significant if there is pre-existing renal insufficiency, which can impair the kidney's ability to excrete excess magnesium.

The amount of magnesium in a general multivitamin-mineral supplement is considered safe for older adults, but it is crucial for older adults to seek medical consultation before taking individual oral magnesium supplements. A multivitamin and mineral supplement is unlikely to contain 100% of a day's recommended dose of magnesium. Thus, those needing oral supplemental magnesium will need to take a separate magnesium supplement recommended by a medical doctor. Currently it is thought that all forms of magnesium supplements are absorbed equally well, however, some forms of oral supplements may result in diarrhea. The RDA for magnesium for adult women (>31 yr of age) is 320 mg. The RDA for magnesium for adult men (>31 yr of age) is 420 mg. The UL for magnesium represents intake from drugs and supplements only. It does not include intake from food and water. The UL for magnesium for older men and women from supplements is 350 mg.

13.10. Omega-3 Fatty Acids

Recommendation: All older adults are advised to increase their dietary intake of DHA and EPA forms of omega-3 fatty acids by consuming at least 2 servings/wk of natural food sources, such as salmon, trout, swordfish, and mackerel, and by including natural sources of α-linolenic acid omega-3 fatty acids in their diet, such as flax seed (ground), flax oil, canola oil, and some nuts. If there are contraindications for including these foods, a fish oil supplement that would provide approx 900 mg/d should be considered. For control of hypertriglyceridemia, 2–4 g of EPA and DHA per day in capsule form may be beneficial. A registered dietitian could make individual dietary recommendations for increasing intake of omega-3 fats, and if still indicated, the individual should discuss the benefits and potential contraindications (e.g., the use of blood thinners, such as warfarin) of taking fish oil supplements with a physician.

REFERENCES

1. U.S. Dept of Health and Human Services, The Surgeon General's Report on Nutrition and Health. Government Printing Office, Washington, DC, 1996.
2. National Research Council Food and Nutrition Board Commission on Life Sciences Implication for reducing chronic disease risk, Report of the Committee on Diet and Health. National Academy Press, Washington, DC, 1989.

3. Ames B, Shigenaga MK, Hagen TM. Oxidants, antioxidants and the degenerative diseases of aging. Proc Natl Acad Sci USA 1993;90:7915–7922.

4. Bronstrup A, Hages M, Pietrzik K, Lowering of homocysteine concentrations in elderly men and women. Int J Vitam, Nutr Res 1999;69:187–193.

5. Brouwer I, Van Dusseldorp M, Thomas C, Duran M, Hautvast J, Eskes T, Steegers-Theunissen R. Low-dose folic acid supplementation decreases plasma homocysteine concentrations: a randomized trial. Am J Clin Nutr 1999;69:99–104.

6. Selhub J, Jacques PF, Wilson PF, Rush D, Rosenberg IH. Vitamin status and intake as primary determinants of homocysteinemia in an elderly population. J Am Med Assoc 1993;270:2693–2698.

7. Bostom A, Selhub J. Homocysteine and arteriosclerosis: subclinical and clinical disease associations. Circulation 1999;99:2361–2363.

8. La Croix A., Newton KM, Leveille SG, Wallace J. Healthy aging. A women's issue. West J Med, 1997; 167:220–232.

9. Refsum H, Ueland PM, Nygard O, Vollset SE. Homocysteine and cardiovascular disease. Annu Rev Med 1998;49:31–62.

10. Reid I. The roles of calcium and vitamin D in the prevention of osteoporosis. Endocrinol Metab Clin North Am 1998;27:389–398.

11. Reid I. Therapy of osteoporosis: Calcium, vitamin D, and exercise. Am J Med Sci 1996;312:278–286.

12. O'Brien K. Combined calcium and vitamin D supplementation reduces bone loss and fracture incidence in older men and women. Nutr Rev 1998;56:148–158.

13. Duke J. The Green Pharmacy New Discoveries in Herbal Remedies for Common Diseases and Conditions from the World's Foremost Authority on Healing Herbs. Rodale Press, Emmaus, PA, 1997.

14. Oubre A, Carlson TJ, King SR, Reaven GM. Diabetologia, From plant to patient: an ethnomedical approach to the identification of new drugs for the treatment of NIDDM. Diabetologia 1997;40:614–617.

15. United States Government Accounting Office, Report to the Chairman, Special Committee on Aging, US Senate. Health Products for Seniors. "Anti-Aging" Products Pose Potential for Physical and Economic Harm. GAO-01-1129. United States Government Accounting Office, 2001.

16. Ernst E. Herbal medications for common ailments in the elderly. Drugs Aging 1999;15:423–428

17. Eisenberg D, Davis RB, Ettner SL, Appel S, Wilkey S, Rompay MV, Kessler RC. Trends in alternative medicine use in the United States, 1990–1997: Results of a follow-up national survey. J Am Med Assoc 1998;280:1569–1575.

18. Ervin R, Wright JD, Kennedy-Stephenson J. Use of dietary supplements in the United States, 1988–94. Vital Health Statistics 1999;244:1–14.

19. Foster D, Phillips RS, Hamel MB, Eisenberg DM. Alternative medicine use in older Americans. J Am Geriatr Soc 2000;48:1560–1565.

20. Lyle B, Mares-Perlman JA, Klein BEK, Klein, R, Greger JL. Supplement users differ from nonusers in demographic, lifestyle, dietary and health characteristics. J Nutr 1998;128:2355–2362.

21. Newman V, Rock CL, Faerber S, Flatt SW, Wright FA, Pierce JP. for the Women's Healthy Eating and Living Study Group. Dietary supplement use by women at risk for breast cancer recurrence. J Am Diet Assoc 1998;98:285–292.

22. Public Law 103-417, Dietary Supplement Health and Education Act of 1994. 103d Congress, 2nd session, 1994.

23. National Research Council Food and Nutrition Board Recommended dietary allowances/Subcommittee on the Tenth Edition. National Academy Press, Washington, DC, 1989.

24. Institute of Medicine, Food and Nutrition Board How should the recommended dietary allowances be revised? National Academy Press, Washington, DC, 1994.

25. Institute of Medicine, Food and Nutrition Board. Dietary Reference Intakes: Applications in Dietary Assessment. National Academy Press, Washington, DC, 2000.

26. Position of the American Dietetic Association: Food fortification and dietary supplements. J Am Diet Assoc 2001;101:115–125.

27. Report of the Dietary Guidelines Advisory Committee on the Dietary Guidelines for Americans. Agricultural Research Service, United States Department of Agriculture (USDA), 2000.

28. Foote JA, Guiliano AR, Harris RB. Older adults need guidance to meet nutritional recommendations. J Am Coll Nutr 2000;19:628–640.

29. McKay D, Perrone G, Rasmussen H, Dallal G, Hartman W, Cao G, et al. The effects of a multivitamin/mineral supplement on micronutrient status, antioxidant capacity and cytokine production in health older adults consuming a fortified diet. J Am Coll Nutr 2000;19:613–621.

30. Vitolins MZ QS, Case LD, Bell RA, Arcury TA, McDonald J. Vitamin and mineral supplement use by older rural adults. J Gerontol A Biol Sci Med Sci 2000;55:M613–M617.

31. Boushey C, Beresford SAA, Omemm GS, Motulsky AG. A quantitative assessment of plasma homocysteine as a risk factor for vascular disease. J Am Med Assoc 1995;274:1049–1057.

32. Jacques P, Selhub J, Bostom AG, Wilson PF, Rosenberg IH. The effect of folic acid fortification on plasma folate and total homocysteine concentrations. N Engl J Med 1999;340:1449–1454.

33. Homocysteine Lowering Trialists' Collaboration. Lowering blood homocysteine with folic acid based supplements. Meta-analysis of randomized trials. Br Med J 1998;316:894–898.

34. McKay D, Perrone G, Rasmussen H, Dallal G, Blumberg JB. Multivitamin/mineral supplementation improves plasma B-vitamin status and homocysteine concentration in healthy older adults consuming a folate-fortified diet. J Nutr 2000;130:3090–3096.

35. Riddell L, Chisholm A, Williams S, Mann JI. Dietary strategies for lowering homocysteine concentrations. Am J Clin Nutr 2000;71:1448–1454.

36. Schnyder G, Roffi M, Pin R, Flammer Y, Lange H, Eberli FR, et al. Decreased rate of coronary restensosis after lowering of plasma homocysteine levels. N Eng J Med 2001;345:1593–1600.

37. Bostom A, Rosenberg IH, Silbershatz H, Jacques PF, Selhub J, D'Angostino RB, et al. Nonfasting plasma total homocysteine levels and stroke incidence in elderly persons: the Framingham Study. Ann Intern Med 1999;131:352–355.

38. Lonn E, Yusuf S. Is there a role for antioxidant vitamins in the prevention of cardiovascular disease? An update on epidemiological and clinical trials data. Can J Cardiol 1997;13:957–965.

39. Traber M. Does Vitamin E decrease heart attack risk? Summary and implications with respect to dietary recommendations. J Nutr 2001;131:395S–397S.

40. Gey K. Vitamins E plus C and interacting conutrients required for optimal health. A critical and constructive review of epidemiology and supplementation data regarding cardiovascular disease and cancer. Biofactors 1998;7:113–174.

41. Stampfer M, Hennekens CH, Manson JE, Colditz GA, Rosner B, Willett WC. Vitamin E consumption and the risk of coronary disease in women. N Eng J Med 1993;328:1444–1449.

42. Stephens N, Parsons A, Schofield PM, Kelly F, Cheeseman K, Mitchinson MJ. Randomized controlled trial of vitamin E in patients with coronary disease: Cambridge Heart Antioxidant Study (CHAOS). Lancet 1996;23:781–786.

43. Yusuf S, Dagenais G, Pogue J, Bosch J, Sleight P. Vitamin E supplementation and cardiovascular events in high-risk patients. The Heart Outcomes Prevention Study Investigators. N Eng J Med 2000; 342:154–160.

44. GISSI. Prevenzione Investigators. Dietary supplementation with n-3 polyunsaturated fatty acids and vitamin E after myocardial infarction: results of the GISSI-Prevenzione trial. Lancet 1999;354: 447–455.

45. Salonen J, Nyyssonen K, Salonen R, Lakka HM, Kaikkonen J, Porkkala-Sarataho E, et al. Antioxidant Supplementation in Atherosclerosis Prevention (ASAP) study: a randomized trial of the effect of vitamins E and C on 3-year progression of carotid atherosclerosis. J Intern Med 2000;248: 377–386.

46. Collaborative Group of the Primary Prevention Project. Low-dose aspirin and vitamin E in people at cardiovascular risk: a randomized trial in general practice. Lancet 2001;357:89–95.

47. Ascherio A. Antioxidants and stroke. Am J Clin Nutr 2000;72:337–338.

48. Meydani S, Meydani M, Blumberg JB, Leka LS, Pedrosa M, Diamond R, Schaefer EJ. Assessment of the safety of supplementation with different amounts of vitamin E in older adults. Am J Clin Nutr 1998; 68:311–318.

49. Kim J, White RH. Effect of vitamin E on the anticoagulant response to warfarin. Am J Cardiol 1996;77:545–546.

50. Institute of Medicine, Food and Nutrition Board, Dietary Reference Intakes for Vitamin C, Vitamin E, Selenium, and Carotenoids. National Academy Press, Washington, DC, 2000.

51. Krauss R, Eckel RH, Howard B, Appel LJ, Daniels SR, Deckelbaum RJ, et al. AHA Dietary Guidelines: Revision 2000: A statement for healthcare professionals from the nutrition committee of the American Heart Association. Circulation 2000;102:2296–2311.

52. Pryor W. Vitamin E and heart disease: basic science to clinical intervention trials. Free Radic Biol Med 2000;28:141–164.

53. Carr A, Frei B. Toward a new recommended dietary allowance for vitamin C based on antioxidant and health effects in humans. Am J Clin Nutr 1999;69:1086–1107.

54. Ascherio A, Rimm EB, Giovanucci EL, Colditz GA, Rosner B, Willet WC, et al. A prospective study of nutritional factors and hypertension among US men. Circulation 1992;86:1475–1484.

55. Joffres M, Reed DM, Yano K. Relationship of magnesium intake and other dietary factors to blood pressure: The Honolulu Heart Study. Am J Clin Nutr 1987;45:469–475.

56. Ma J, Folsom AR, Melnick SL, Eckfeldt JH, Sharrett AR, Nabulsi AA, et al. Associations of serum and dietary magnesium with cardiovascular disease, hypertension, diabetes, insulin, and carotid arterial wall thickness: The ARIC Study. Artherosclerosis Risk in Communities Study. J Clin Epidemiol 1995; 48:927–940.

57. McCarron D. Calcium and magnesium nutrition in human hypertension. Ann Int Med 1983;98: 800–805.

58. Witteman J, Willet WC, Stampfer MJ, Colditz GA, Sacks FM, Speizer FE, et al. A prospective study of nutritional factors and hypertension among U.S. women. Circulation 1989;80:1320–1327.

59. Shechter M, Shecter M, Sharir M, et al. Oral magnesium therapy improves endothelial function in patients with coronary artery disease. Circulation 2000;2000:2353–2358.

60. Shechter M, Merz CN, Paul-Labrador M, Meisel SR, Rude RK, Molloy MD, et al. Oral magnesium supplementation inhibits platelet-dependent thrombosis in patients with coronary artery disease. Am J Cardiol 1999;84:152–156.

61. Rude R. Disorders of magnesium metabolism. Endocrinol Metab Clin North Am 1995;24:623–641.

62. Bashir Y, Sneddon JF, Staunton A. Effects of oral magnesium chloride replacement in CHF secondary to coronary artery disease. Am J Cardiol 1993;72:1156–1162.

63. Ceremuzynski L, Gebalska J, Wolk R, Makowska E. Hypomagnesemia in heart failure with ventricular arrythmias. Beneficial effects of magnesium supplementation. J Intern Med 2000;247:78–86.

64. Burr M, Fehily AM, Gibert JF, Rogers S, Holliday RM, Sweetnam PM, et al. Effects of changes in fat, fish, and fibre intakes on death and myocardial infarction trial (DART). Lancet 1989;2:757–761.

65. Singh R, Niaz MA, Sharma JP, Kumar R, Rastogi V, Moshiri M. Randomized, double-blind, placebo-controlled trial of fish oil, and mustard oil in patients with suspected acute myocardial infarction. Cardiovasc Drugs Ther 1997;11:485–491.

66. Von Schacky C, Angerer P, Kothny W, Theisen K, Mudra H. The effect of dietary w-3 fatty acids on coronary atherosclerosis. A randomized double-blind, placebo-controlled trial. Ann Intern Med 1999; 130:554–562.

67. O'Keefe J, Harris WS. Omega-3 fatty acids: time for clinical implementation? Am J Clin Cardiol 2000; 85:1239–1241.

68. Kris-Etherton PM, Harris WS, Appel LJ. Fish consumption, fish oil, Omega-3 fatty acids, and cardiovascular disease. Circulation 2002;106:2747–2757.

69. Miettinen T, Puska P, Gylling H, Vanhanen H, Vartiainen E. Reduction of serum cholesterol with sitostanol ester margarine in a mildly hypercholesterolemic population. N Eng J Med 1995;333:1308–1312.

70. Vanhanen H, Kajander J, Lehtovirta H, Miettinen TA. Serum levels, absorption efficiency, faecal elimination and synthesis of cholesterol during increasing doses of dietary sitostanol esters in hypercholesterolemic subjects. Clin Sci 1994;87:61–67.

71. Gylling H, Radhakrishnan R, Miettinen TA. Reduction of serum cholesterol in postmenopausal women with previous myocardial infarction and cholesterol malabsorption induced by dietary sitostanol ester margarine: women and dietary sitostanol. Circulation 1997;96:4226–4231.

72. Hendriks H, Weststrate JA, van Vliet T, Meijer GW. Spreads enriched with three different levels of vegetable oil sterols and the degree of cholesterol lowering in normocholesterolemic and mildly hypercholesterolemic subjects. Eur J Clin Nutr 1999;53:319–327.

73. Gylling H, Miettinen TA. Cholesterol reduction by different plant stanol mixtures and with variable fat intake. Metabolism 1999;48:575–580.

74. Westrate J, Meijer GW. Plant sterol-enriched margarines and reduction of plasma total-and LDL-cholesterol concentrations in normocholesterolaemic and mildly hypercholesterolaemic subjects. Eur J Clin Nutr 1998;52:334–343.

75. Blair, S. Capuzzi DM, Gottlieb SO, Nguyen T, Morgan JM, Cater NB. Incremental reduction of serum total cholesterol and low-density lipoprotein cholesterol with the addition of plant stanol ester-containing spread to statin therapy. Am J Cardiol 2000;86:46–52.

76. Program, NCE. National Heart, Lung, and Blood Institute. Third Report of the National Cholesterol Education Program (NCEP) Expert Panel on Detection, Evaluation, and Treatment of High Blood Cholesterol in Adults (Adult Treatment Panel III). National Heart, Lung, and Blood Institute. NIH Publication no. 02–3670, 2001.

77. Lissin L, Cooke JP. Phytoestrogens and cardiovascular health. J Am Coll Cardiol 2000;35:1403–1410.
78. Lu L, Tice JA, Bellino FL. Phytoestrogens and healthy aging: gaps in knowledge. A workshop report. Menopause: J North American Menopause Soc 2001;8:157–170.
79. Anderson J, Johnstone B, Cook-Newell M. Meta-analysis of the effects of soy protein intake on serum lipids. N Eng J Med 1995;333:276–282.
80. Baum J, Teng H, Erdman JW Jr, Weigel RM, Klein BP, Persky VW, et al. Long-term intake of soy protein improves blood lipid profiles and increases mononuclear cell low-density-lipoprotein receptor messenger RNA in hypercholesterolemic, postmenopausal women. Am J Clin Nutr 1998;68:545–551.
81. Crouse JI, Morgan T, Terry JG, Ellis J, Vitolins M, Burke GL. A randomized trial comparing the effect of casein with that of soy protein containing varying amounts of isoflavones on plasma concentrations of lipids and lipoproteins. Arch Intern Med 1999;159:2070–2076.
82. Teede H, Dalais FS, Kotsopoulos D, Liang Y-L, Davis S, McGrath BP. Dietary soy has both beneficial and potentially adverse cardiovascular effects:a placebo-controlled study in men and postmenopausal women. J Clin Endocrinol Metab 2001;86:3053–3060.
83. Garlic: Effects on cardiovascular risks and disease, protective effects against cancer, clinical adverse effects. Agency for Healthcare Research and Quality, 2000.
84. Stevinson C, Pittler MH, Ernst E. Garlic for treating hypercholeresterolemia. A meta-analysis of randomized clinical trials. Ann Int Med 2000;133:420–429.
85. Heck A, DeWitt BA, Lukes AL. Potential interactions between alternative therapies and warfarin. Am J Health Syst Pharm 2000;57:1221–1227.
86. Willett W, Trichopoulos D. Nutrition and cancer: a summary of the evidence. Cancer Causes Control 1996;7:178–180.
87. Smith-Warner S, Spiegelman D, Yaun SS, Adami HO, Beeson WL, van den Brandt PA, et al. Intake of fruits and vegetables and risk of breast cancer. A pooled analysis of cohort studies. JAMA 2001;14:799–801.
88. Heinonen O, Albanes D, Virtamo J, Taylor PR, Huttunen JK, Hartman AM, et al. Prostate cancer and supplementation with alpha-tocopherol and beta-carotene: incidence and mortality in a controlled trial. J Natl Cancer Inst 1998;18:440–446.
89. Gann PH, Ma J, Giovannucci E, et al. Lower prostate cancer risk in men with elevated plasma lycopene levels: results of a prospective analysis. Cancer Res 1999;59:1225–1230.
90. Chan JM, Stampfer MJ, Ma J, Rimm EB, Willet WC, Giovannucci EL. Supplemental vitamin E intake and prostate cancer risk in a large cohort of men in the United States. Cancer Epidemiol Biomarkers Prev 1999;59:893–899.
91. Graham S, Sielezny M, Marshall J, Priore R, Freudenheim J, Brasure J, et al. Diet in the epidemiology of postmenopausal breast cancer in the New York State cohort. Am J Epidemiol 1992;8:263–273.
92. Bostick R, Potter JD, McKenzie DR, Sellers TA, Kushi LH, Steinmetz KA, Folsom AR. Reduced risk of colon cancer with high intakes of vitamin E: The Iowa Women's Health Study. Cancer Res 1993;15:4230–4237.
93. Slattery M, Edwards SL, Anderson K, Caan B. Vitamin E and colon cancer: Is there an association? Nutr Cancer 1998;30:201–206.
94. Ross A. Vitamin A and retinoids. In: Modern Nutrition in Health and Disease. Shils ME, Olson JA, Shike M, Ross AC (eds.) Williams & Wilkins, Baltimore, MD, 1999, pp. 305–327.
95. Fotham E, Protective dietary factors and lung cancer. Int J Epidemiol 1990;19:S32–S42.
96. Zheng W, Sellers, TA, Doyle TJ, Kushi LH, Potter JD, Folsom AR. Retinol, antioxidant vitamins, and cancers of the upper digestive tract in a prospective cohort study of postmenopausal women. Am J Epidemiol 1995;142:955–960.
97. Koo L. Diet and lung cancer 20+ years later: more questions than answers? Int J Cancer 1997;(Suppl 10): 22–29.
98. Albanes D, Heinonen OP, Taylor PR, Virtamo J, Edwards BK, Rautalahti M, et al. Alpha-tocopherol and beta-carotene supplement and lung cancer incidence in the alpha-tocopherol, beta-carotene cancer prevention study: effects of baseline characteristics and study compliance. J Natl Cancer Inst 1996;88: 1560–1570.
99. The Alpha-Tocopherol, B-Carotene Cancer Prevention study group. The effect of vitamin E and beta-carotene on the incidence of lung cancer and other cancers in male smokers. N Eng J Med 1994; 330:1029–1035.
100. Redlich C, Blaner WS, Van Bennekum AM, Chung JS, Clever SL, Holm CT, Cullen MR. Effect of supplementation with beta-carotene and vitamin A on lung nutrient levels. Cancer Epidemiol Biomarkers Prev 1998;7:211–214.

101. World Cancer Research Fund. Food, Nutrition and the Prevention of Cancer: A Global Perspective. American Institute for Cancer Research, Washington, DC, 1997.
102. Mayne S, Risch HA, Dubrow R, Chow W-H, Gammon MD, Vaughan TL, et al. Nutrient intake and risk of subtypes of esophageal and gastric cancer. Cancer Epidemiol Biomarkers Prev 2001;10: 1055–1062.
103. Bergsma-Kadijk J, van't Veer P, Kampman E, Burema J. Calcium does not protect against colorectal neoplasia. Epidemiology 1996;7:590–597.
104. Martinez M, Willet WC. Calcium, vitamin D, and colorectal cancer: a review of the epidemiologic evidence. Cancer Epidemiol Biomarkers Prev 1998;7:163–168.
105. Holt P, Atillasoy EV, Gilman J, Guss J, Moss ST, Newmark H, et al. Modulation of abnormal colonic epithelial cell proliferation and differentiation by low-fat dairy foods. A randomized controlled trial. JAMA 1998;280:1074–1079.
106. Baron J, Beach M, Mandel JS, Van Stolk RU, Haile RW, Sandler RS, et al. Calcium supplements for the prevention of colorectal adenomas. N Eng J Med 1999;340:101–107.
107. Cascinu S, Ligi M, Ferro ED, Foglietti G, Cioccolini P, Staccioli MP, et al. Effects of calcium and vitamin supplementation on colon cell proliferation in colorectal cancer. Cancer Invest 2000;18:411–416.
108. Wu K, Willett WC, Fuchs CS, Colditz GA, Giovannucci E. Calcium intake and risk of colon cancer in women and men. J Nat Cancer Inst 2002;94:437–446.
109. Russo M, Murray SC, Wurzelmann JI, Woosley JT, Sandler RS. Plasma selenium levels and the risk of colorectal adenomas. Nutr Cancer 1997;281:25–29.
110. Patterson B, Levander OA. Naturally occurring selenium compounds in cancer chemoprevention trials: a workshop summary. Cancer Epidemiol Biomarkers Prev 1997;6:63–69.
111. Knekt P, Marniemi J, Teppo L, Heliovaara M, Aromaa A. Is low selenium status a risk factor for lung cancer? Am J Epidemiol 1998;148:975–982.
112. Fleet J. Dietary selenium repletion may reduce cancer incidence in people at high risk who live in areas with low soil selenium. Nutr Rev 1997;55:277–279.
113. Shamberger R. The genotoxicity of selenium. Mutat Res 1985;154:29–48.
114. Young K, Lee PN. Intervention studies on cancer. Eur J Cancer Prev 1999;8:91–103.
115. Burguera J, Burguera M, Gallignani M, Alarcon OM, Burgueera JA. Blood serum selenium in the Province of Merida, Venezuela, related to sex, cancer incidence and soil selenium content. J Trace Elem Electrolytes Health Dis 1990;4:73–77.
116. Clark L, Combs GF Jr, Turnbull BW, Slate EH, Chalker DK, Chow J, et al. Effects of selenium supplementation for cancer prevention in patients with carcinoma of the skin. A randomized controlled trial. Nutritional Prevention of Cancer Study Group. JAMA 1996;276:1957–1963.
117. Klein E, Thompson IM, Lippman SM, Goodman PJ, Albanes D, Taylor PR, et al. SELECT: The Next Prostate Cancer Prevention Trial. J Urol 2001;166:1311–1315.
118. Blount B, Mack MM, Wehr CM, MacGregor JT, Hiatt RA, Wang G, et al. Folate deficiency causes uracil misincorporation into human DNA and chromosome breakage: implications for cancer and neuronal damage. Proc Nat Acad Sci USA 1997;94:3290–3295.
119. Christensen B. Folate deficiency, cancer and congenital abnormalities. Is there a connection? Tidsskr Nor Laegeforen 1996;116:250–254.
120. Giovannucci E, Stampfer MJ, Colditz GA, Hunter DJ, Fuchs C, Rosner BA, et al. Multivitamin use, folate, and colon cancer in women in the Nurses' Health Study. Ann Intern Med 1998;129:517–524.
121. Freudenheim J, Grahm S, Marshall JR, Haughey BP, Cholewinski S, Wilkinson G. Folate intake and carcinogenesis of the colon and rectum. Int J Epidemiol 1991;20:368–374.
122. Su LJ, Arab L. Nutritional status of folate and colon cancer risk: evidence from NHANES 1 epidemiologic follow-up study. Ann Epidemiol 2001;11:65–72.
123. Zhang S, Hunter DJ, Hankinson SE, et al. A prospective study of folate intake and the risk of breast cancer. JAMA 1999;281:1632–1637.
124. Rohan TE, Jain MG, Howe GR, Miller AB. Dietary folate consumption and breast cancer. J Nat Cancer Inst 2000;92:266–269.
125. Sellers TA, Kushi LH, Cerhan JR, et al. Dietary folate intake, alcohol, and risk of breast cancer in a prospective study of postmenopausal women. Epidemiology 2001;12:420–428.
126. Wyatt G, Friedman LL, Given CW, Given BA, Beckrow KC. Complementary therapy use among older cancer patients. Cancer Pract 1999;7:136–144.
127. DiPaola R, Zhang H, Lambert GH, Meeker R, Licitra E, Rafi MM, et al. Clinical and biologic activity of an estrogenic herbal combination (PC-SPES) in prostate cancer. N Eng J Med 1998;339:785–791.

128. Paolisso G, Sgambato S, Gambardella A, Pizza G, Tesauro P, Varricchio M, D'Onofrio F. Daily magnesium supplements improve glucose handling in elderly subjects. Am J Clin Nutr 1992;55: 1161–1167.

129. American Diabetes Association Nutrition recommendations and principles for people with diabetes mellitus. Diabetes Care 1999;22:S42–S45.

130. Anderson R, Cheng N, Bryden N, Polansky MN, Cheng N, Chi J, Feng J. Elevated intakes of supplemental chromium improve glucose and insulin variables in individuals with type 2 diabetes. Diabetes Care 1997;46:1786–1791.

131. Althuis M, Jordan N, Ludington E, Wittes J. Glucose and insulin responses to dietary chromium supplements: a meta-analysis. Am J Clin Nutr 2002;76:148–155.

132. Paolisso G, Esposito R, D'Alessio MA, Barbieri M. Primary and secondary prevention of atherosclerosis: is there a role for antioxidants? Diabetes Metab 1999;25:298–306.

133. Paolisso G, D'Amore A, Giugliano D, Ceriello A, Varricchio M, D'Onofrio F. Pharmacologic doses of vitamin E improve insulin action in healthy subjects and non-insulin-dependent diabetic patients. Am J Clin Nutr 1993;57:650–656.

134. Paolisso G, Di Maro G, Galzerano D, Cacciapuoti F, Varricchio G, Varricchio M, D'Onofrio F. Pharmacological doses of vitamin E and insulin action in elderly subjects. Am J Clin Nutr 1994;59: 1291–1296.

135. Bursell S-E, Clermont AC, Aiello LP, Aiello LM, Schlossman DK, Feener EP, et al. High-dose vitamin E supplmentation normalizes retinal blood flow with creatinine clearance in patients with type 1 diabetes. Diabetes Care 1999;22:1245–1251.

136. Skrha J, Sindelk AG, Hilgertova J. The effect of fasting and vitamin E on insulin action in obese type 2 diabetes mellitus. Ann NY Acad Sci 1997;827:556–560.

137. Anderson J, Gowri MS, Turner J, Nichols L, Diwadkar VA, Chow CK, Oeltgen PR. Antioxidant supplementation effects on low-density lipoprotein oxidation for individuals with type 2 diabetes mellitus. J Am Coll Nutr 1999;1:451–461.

138. Manzella D, Barbieri M, Ragno E, Paolisso G. Chronic administration of pharmacologic doses of vitamin E improves the cardiac autonomic nervous system in patients with type 2 diabetes. Am J Clin Nutr 2001;73:1052–1057.

139. Montari W, Farmer A, Wollan PC, Dinneen SF. Fish oil supplementationin type 2 diabetes: a quantitative systematic review. Diabetes Care 2000;23:1407–1415.

140. Patti L, Maffettone A, Lovine C, Di Marino L, Annuzzi G, Riccardi G, Rivellese AA. Long-term effects of fish oil on lipoprotein subfractions and low-density lipoprotein size in non-insulin-dependent diabetic patients with hypertriglyceridemia. Atherosclerosis 1999;146:361–367.

141. LeBoff M, Kohlmeier L, Hurwitz S, Franklin J, Wright J, Glowacki J. Occult vitamin D deficiency in postmenopausal US women with acute hip fracture. J Am Med Assoc 1999;251:1505–1511.

142. Marwick C. Consensus panel considers osteoporosis. JAMA 2001;283:2093–2095.

143. Institute of Medicine, Food and Nutrition Board Dietary Reference Intakes for Calcium, Phosphorus, Magnesium, Vitamin D, and Fluoride. National Academy Press, Washington, DC, 1997.

144. Chapuy M, Arlot ME, Duboeuf F, Brun J, Crouzet B, Arnaud S, et al. Vitamin D3 and calcium to prevent hip fractures in the elderly women. N Eng J Med 1992;327:1637–1642.

145. Storm D, Eslin R, Porter ES, Musgrave K, Vereault D, Patton C, et al. Calcium supplementation prevents seasonal bone loss and changes in biochemical markers of bone turnover in elderly New England women: a randomized placebo-controlled trial. J Clin Endo Metab 1998;83:3817–3825.

146. Reid I, Ames RW, Evans MC, Gamble GD, Sharpe SJ. Long-term effects of calcium supplementation on bone loss and fractures in postmenopausal women: a randomized controlled trial. Am J Med 1995;98: 329–330.

147. Dawson-Hughes B, Harris SS, Krall EA, Dallal GE, Falconer G, Green CL. Rates of bone loss in postmenopausal women randomly assigned to one of two dosages of vitamin D. Am J Clin Nutr 1995; 61:1140–1145.

148. Stendig-Lindenberg G, Tepper R, Leichter I. Trabecular bone density in a two-year controlled trial of personal magnesium in osteoporosis. Magnes Res 1993;6:155–163.

149. Abraham G, Grewal H. A total dietary program emphasizing magnesium instead of calcium: effect on the mineral density of calcaneous bone in postmenopausal women on hormonal therapy. J Reprod Med 1990;35:503–507.

150. Alaimo K, McDowell MA, Briefel R, et al. Dietary intake of vitamins, minerals, and fiber of persons ages 2 months and over in the United States: Third National Health and Nutrition Examination Survey,

Phase 1, 1988–91. In: Vital and Health Statistics of the Center for Disease Control and Prevention/ National Center for Health Statistics, Johnson GV (ed.) Hyattsville, MD, 1994, pp. 1–28.

151. Pfeifer M, Begerow B, Minne HW, Abrams C, Nachtigall D, Hansen C. Effects of short term vitamin D and calcium supplementation on body sway and secondary hyperparathyroidism in elderly women. J Bone Miner Res 2000;15:1113–1118.

152. Ilich J, Kerstetter JE. Nutrition in bone health revisited: a story beyond calcium. J Am C Nutr 2000;19: 715–737.

153. Booth S, Tucker KL, Chen H, Hannan MT, Gagnon DR, Cupples LA, et al. Dietary vitamin K intakes are associated with hip fracture but not with bone mineral density in elderly men and women. Am J Clin Nutr 2000;71:1031–1032.

154. Feskanich D, Weber P, Willett WC, Rockett H, Booth SL, Colditz GA. Vitamin K intake and hip fractures in women: a prospective study. Am J Clin Nutr 1999;69:74–79.

155. Kalmijn S, Feskens EJ, Launer LJ, Kromhout D. Polyunsaturated fatty acids, antioxidants, and cognitive function in very old men. Am J Epidemiol 1997;145:33–41.

156. Ince P, Lowe J, Shaw PJ. Amyotrophic lateral sclerosis: current issues in classification, pathogenesis and molecular pathology. Neuropathol Appl Neurobiol 1998;24:104–117.

157. Riggs K, Spiro A III, Tucker K, Rush D. Relations of vitamin B12, vitamin B6, folate and homocysteine to cognitive performance in the Normative Aging Study. Am J Clin Nutr 1996;63:306–314.

158. Ortega RM, Manas LR, Andres P, Gaspar MJ, Agudo FR, Jimenez A, Pascual T. Functional and psychic deterioration in elderly people may be aggravated by folate deficiency. J Nutr 1996;126:1992–1999.

159. Van Goor L, Woiski MD, Lagaay AM, Meinders AE, Tak PP. Review: cobalamin deficiency and mental impairment in elderly people. Age Aging 1995;24:536–542.

160. Bernard M, Nakonezny PA, Kashner TMJ. The effect of vitamin B12 deficiency on older veterans and its relation to health. Am Geriatr Soc 1998;46:119–1206.

161. LaRue A, Koehler KM, Wayne SJ, Chiulli SJ, Haaland KY, Garry PJ. Nutritional status and cognitive functioning in a normally ageing sample: a 6-y reassessment. Am J Clin Nutr 1997;65:20–29.

162. Perrig W, Perrig P, Stahelin HB. The relation between antioxidants and memory performance in the old and very old. J Am Geriatr Soc 1997;45:718–724.

163. Lindenbaum J, Healton EB, Savage DG, Brust JC, Garrett TJ, Podell ER, et al. Neuropsychiatric disorders caused by cobalamin deficiency in the absence of anemia or macrocytosis. N Eng J Med 1988; 318:1720–1728.

164. Martin D, Francis J, Protetch J, Huff FJ. Time dependency of cognitive recovery with cobalamin replacement: report of a pilot study. J Am Geriatr Soc 1992;40:618–172.

165. Lindeman R, Romero LJ, Koehler KM, Liang HC, LaRue A, Baumgartner RN, Garry PJ. Serum Vitamin B12, C and folate concentrations in the New Mexico Elder Health Survey: correlations with cognitive and affective functions. J Am Coll Nutr 2000;19:68–76.

166. Alpert J, Fava M. Nutriton and depression: the role of folate. Nutr Rev 1997;55:145–149.

167. Duthie SJ, Whalley LJ, Collins AR, Leaper S, Berger K, Deary IJ. Homocysteine, B vitamin status, and cognitive function in elderly. Am J Clin Nutr 2002;75:908–913.

168. Jensen E, Dehlin O, Erfurth E M, et al. Plasma homocysteine in 80-year-olds; Relationships to medical, psychological, and social variables. Arch Gerontol Geriatr 1998;26:215–226.

169. Seshadri BA, Selhub J, Jaques PF, Rosenberg IH, D'Agostino RB, Wilson PWF, Wolf PA. Plasma homocysteine as a risk factor for dementia and Alzheimer's Disease. N Eng J Med 2002;346:476–483.

170. Meydani M. Antioxidants and cognitive function. Nutr Rev 2001;59:S75–S82.

171. Goodwin J, Goodwin JM, Garry, PJ. Association between nutritional status and cognitive functioning in a healthy elderly population. J Am Med Assoc 1983;249:2917–2931.

172. Masaki K, Losonczy KG, Izmirlian G, Foley DJ, Ross GW, Petrovitch H, et al. Association of vitamin E and C supplement use with cognitive function and dementia in elderly men. Neurology 2000;54:1265–1272.

173. Baker H, De Angelis B, Baker ER, Frank O, Jaslowdagger SP. Lack of effect of 1 year intake of a high-dose vitamin and mineral supplement on cognitive function in elderly women. Gerontology 1999;45: 195–199.

174. Sano M, Ernesto MS, Thomas RG, Klauber MR, Schafer K, Grundman M, et al. A controlled trial of selegiline, alpha-tocopherol, or both as treatment of Alzheimer's disease. N Eng J Med 1997;336: 1216–1222.

175. Laakmann G, Schule C, Baghai T, Kieser M. St. John's wort in mild to moderate depression: the relevance of hyperforin for the clinical efficacy. Pharmacopsychiatry 1998;31(Suppl 1):54–59.

176. Chatterjee S, Bhattacharya SK, Wonnemann M, Siinger A, Muller WE. Hyperforin as a possible antidepressant component of hypericum extracts. Life Sci 1998;63:499–510.
177. Muller W, Singer A, Wonnemann M, Hafner U, Rolli M, Schafer C. Hyperforin represents the neurotransmitter reuptake inhibiting constituent of hypericum extract. Pharmacopsychiatry 1998;31 (Suppl 1):16–21.
178. Linde K, Ramirez G, Mulrow CD, Pauls A, Weidenhammer W, Melchart D. St. John's wort for depression: an overview and meta-analysis of randomized clinical trials. BMJ 1996;313:253–258.
179. Ernst E. Second thoughts about the safety of St. John's Wort. Lancet 1999;354:2014–2015.
180. Hypericum Depression Trial Study Group, Effect of hypericum perforatum (St John's Wort) in major depressive disorder. A randomized controlled trial. JAMA 2002;287:1807–1814.
181. Williams J, Mulrow CD, Chiquette E, Noel PH, Aguilar C, Cornell J. A systematic review of newer pharmacotherapies for depression in adults: evidence report summary. Ann Int Med 2000;132: 743–756.
182. Shelton R, Keller MB, Gelenberg A, Dunner DL, Hirschfeld R, Thase ME, et al. Effectiveness of St. John's wort in major depression: a randomized control trial. J Am Med Assoc 2001;285:1978–1986.
183. Durr D, Stieger B, Kullak-Ublick GA, Rentsch KM, Steinert HC, Meier PJ, Fattinger K. St John's wort induces intestinal P-glycoprotein/MDR1 and intestinal and hepatic CYP3A4. Clin Pharmacol Ther 2000;68:598–604.
184. Piscitelli S, Burstein A, Chaitt D, Alfaro RM, Falloon J. Indinavir concentrations and St. John's wort. Lancet 2000;355:547–548.
185. Ruschitzka F, Meier P, Turina M, Luscher TF, Noll G. Acute heart transplant rejection due to Saint John's wort. Lancet 2000;355:548–549.
186. Lantz M, Buchalter E, Giambanco V. St. John's wort and antidepressant drug interactions in the elderly. J Geriatr Psychiatry Neurol 1999;12:7–10.
187. Fugh-Berman A. Herb drug interactions. Lancet 2000;355:134–138.
188. Oken B, Storzbach DM, Kaye JA. The efficacy of ginkgo biloba on cognitive function in Alzheimer's Disease. Arch Neurol 1998;55:1409–1415.
189. Ernst E, Pittler MH. Ginkgo biloba for dementia: a systematic review of double-blind placebo controlled trials. Clin Drug Invest 1999;17:301–308.
190. Stevinson C, Pittler MH, Ernst E. Valerian for insomnia: a systematic review of randomized clinical trials. Sleep Medicine 2000;1:91–99.
191. Erickson K, Medina EA, Hubbard NE. Micronutrients and Innate Immunity. J Infect Dis 2000;182: S5–S10.
192. Chandra R. Effect of vitamin and trace-element supplementation on immune responses and infection in elderly subjects. Lancet 1992;340:1124–1127.
193. Boardley D, Fahlman M. Micronutrient supplementation does not attenuate seasonal decline of immune system indexes in well-nourished elderly women: A placebo-controlled study. J Am Diet Assoc 2000; 100:356–359.
194. Bauer R, Wagner H. Echinacea species as potential immunostimulatory drugs. In: Economic and Medicinal Plants Research. Wagner H, Farnsworth NR (eds.). Economic and Medicinal Plants Research, vol. 5. Academic Press, London, England, 1991, pp. 253–321.
195. WHO. World Health Organization Monographs on Selected Medicinal Plants. Vol. 1. World Health Organization, Geneva, 1999.
196. Barrett B, Vohmann M, Calabrese C. Echinacea for upper respiratory infection. J Fam Pract 1999;48: 628–635.
197. Kaufert P, Boggs PP, Ettinger B, Woods NF, Utian WH. Women and menopause: beliefs, attitudes, and behaviors. The North American Menopause Society 1997 Menopause Survey. Menopause 1998;55: 197–202.
198. Schulz V, Hansel R, Tyler VE. A Physicians' Guide to Herbal Medicine Rational Phytotherapy. Springer-Verlag, Berlin, Germany, 1998.
199. McGrath B, Liang YL, Teede H, Shiel LM, Cameron JD, Dart A. Age-related deterioration in arterial structure and function in postmenopausal women: impact of hormone replacement therapy. Arterioscler Thromb Vasc Biol 1998;18:1149–1156.
200. Consensus opinion of the North American Menopause Society: the role of isoflavones in menopausal health. Menopause 2000;7:215–229.
201. Loprinzi C, Quella SK, Barton DL. Respone: Phytoestrogens and adjuvant endocrine treatment of breast cancer. J Clin Oncol 2000;18:2093–2094.

202. Henkel J. Soy: Health claims for soy protein, questions about other components, FDA Consumer, 2000, pp. 13–20.
203. Jacobson JS, Troxel AB, Evans J, et al. Randomized trial of black cohosh for the treatment of hot flashes among women with a history of breast cancer. J Clin Oncol 2001;19:2739–2745.
204. Lehmann-Willenbrock E, Riedel H-H. Clinical and endocrinological studies on the therapy of ovarian defunctionalization symptoms after hysterectomy sparing the adnexa (in German). Zentralblatt fur Gynakologie 1988;110:611–618.
205. Stoll W. Phytotheraphy influences atrophic vaginal epithelium—double-blind study—Cimicifuga vs. estrogenic substances (in German). Therapeutikon 1987;1:23–31.
206. Warnecke, G. Influencing of menopausal complaints with a phytodrug: successful therapy with Cimicifuga monoextract (in German). Medizinische Welt 1985;36:871–874.
207. Jacobson J, Troxel AB, Evans J, Klaus L, Vahdat L, Kinne D, et al. Randomized trial of black cohosh for the treatment of hot flashes among women with a history of breast cancer. J Clin Oncol 2001;19: 2739–2745.
208. Fugh-Berman A, Kronenberg F. Red clover (Trifolium pratense) for menopausal women: current state of knowledge. Menopause 2001;8:333–337.
209. Guess H. Benign prostatic hyperplasia: antecedents and natural history. Epidemiol Rev 1992;14: 131–153.
210. McConnell J, Barry MJ, Bruskewitz RC. Benign prostatic hyperplasia: diagnosis and treatment. Agency for Health Care Policy and Research. Clin Pract Guide, Quick Ref Guide Clin 1994;8:1–17.
211. Wilt T, Ishani A, Stark G, MacDonald R, Mulrow C, Lau J. Serenoa repens for benign prostatic hyperplasia. Cochrane Database Syst Rev 2000;2:(CD001423):1469–143X.
212. Brinker F. Herb Contraindications and Drug Interactions, 2nd Edition Eclectic Medical Publications, 1998.
213. Kurtzweil P. An FDA Guide to Dietary Supplements. FDA Consumer, Publication no. (FDA) 99 2323 Sep-Oct, Vol. 32, 1998.
214. Zeisel S, Is there a metabolic basis for dietary supplementation? Am J Clin Nutr 2000;72(Suppl): 507S–511S.
215. Jellin JM, Batz GP, Hitchens K, et al. Pharmacist's Letter/Prescriber's Letter Natural Medicines Comprehensive Database. 3rd ed. Therapeutic Research Faculty, Stockton, CA, 2000.
216. IOM (Institute of Medicine) Dietary Reference Intakes for Thiamin, Riboflavin, Niacin, Vitamin B_6, Folate, Vitamin B_{12}, Pantothenic Acid, Biotin, and Choline. National Academy Press, Washington, DC, 1998.
217. IOM (Institute of Medicine) Dietary Reference Intakes for Vitamin A, Vitamin K, Arsenic, Boron, Chromium, Copper, Iodine, Iron, Manganese, Molybdenum, Nickel, Silicon, Vanadium, and Zinc. National Academy Press, Washington, DC, 2001.
218. American Cancer Society's Guide to Complementary and Alternative Cancer Methods. American Cancer Society, 2000.
219. Ang-Lee MK, Moss J, Yuan CS. Herbal medicines and perioperative care. JAMA 2001;286:208–216.
220. Blumenthal M. Interactions between herbs and conventional drugs: introductory considerations. HerbalGram 2000;49:52–63.
221. Ernst E. Possible interactions between synthetic and herbal medicinal products. Part 1: a systematic review of the indirect evidence. Perfusion 2000;13:4–15.
222. Mahady GB, Fong HHS, Farnsworth NR. Botanical Dietary Supplements: Quality, Safety and Efficacy. Swetz Zeitlinger, Exton, PA, 2001.
223. Miller LG. Herbal Medicinals. Selected clinical considerations focusing of known or potential drug-herb interactions. Arch Intern Med 1998;158:2200–2211.
224. Pennachio DL. Herb-drug interactions: how vigilant should you be? Patient Care 2000;19:41–68.

III GERIATRIC SYNDROMES: NUTRITIONAL CONSEQUENCES AND POTENTIAL OPPORTUNITIES

8

Nutrition and the Aging Eye

Elizabeth J. Johnson

1. INTRODUCTION

Vision loss among the elderly is an important health problem. Approximately one person in three has some form of vision-reducing eye disease by the age of 65 *(1)*. Age-related cataract and age-related macular degeneration (AMD) are the major causes of visual impairment and blindness in the aging US population. Approximately 50% of the 30–50 million cases of blindness worldwide result from unoperated cataracts *(2–4)*. A clinically significant cataract is present in about 5% of Caucasian Americans aged 52–64 yr and the incidence rises to 46% in those aged 75–85 yr *(5)*. In the United States, cataract extraction accompanied by ocular lens implant is currently the most common surgical procedure done in Medicare beneficiaries *(6)*. Lens implantation is highly successful in restoring vision; however, the procedure is costly, accounting for 12% of the Medicare budget and more than $3 billion in annual health expenditures *(6,7)*. For these reasons, there is much interest in the prevention of cataracts as an alternative to surgery. The prevalence of AMD also increases dramatically with age. Nearly 30% of Americans over the age of 75 have early signs of AMD and 7% have late-stage disease, whereas the respective prevalence among people 43–54 yr are 8 and 0.1% *(8,9)*. AMD is the leading cause of blindness among the elderly in industrialized countries *(8,10)*. Because there are currently no effective treatment strategies for most patients with AMD, attention has focused on efforts to stop the progression of the disease or to prevent the damage leading to this condition *(11)*.

Cataract and AMD share common modifiable risk factors, such as light exposure and smoking *(11,12)*. Of particular interest is the possibility that nutritional counseling or intervention might reduce the incidence or retard the progression of these diseases. The components of the diet that may be important in the prevention of cataract and AMD are vitamins C and E and the carotenoids, lutein and zeaxanthin. Given that the lens and retina suffer oxidative damage, these nutrients are thought to be protective through their role as antioxidants. Additionally, lutein and zeaxanthin may provide protection as filters against light damage, i.e., absorbers of blue light.

From: *Handbook of Clinical Nutrition and Aging*
Edited by: C. W. Bales and C. S. Ritchie © Humana Press Inc., Totowa, NJ

2. PHYSIOLOGICAL BASIS OF CATARACTS AND AMD

The role of the lens is to transmit and focus light on the retina. Therefore, for optimal performance the lens must be transparent. The lens is an encapsulated organ without blood vessels or nerves (*see* Fig. 1). The anterior hemisphere is covered by a single layer of epithelial cells containing subcellular organelles. At the lens equator the epithelial cells begin to elongate and differentiated to become fiber cells. Fully differentiated fiber cells have no organelles but are filled with proteins called crystallins organized in a repeating lattice. The high density and repetitive spatial arrangement of crystallins produce a medium of nearly uniform refractive index with dimensions similar to light wavelengths *(13)*. Cataracts result when certain events (e.g., light exposure) cause a loss of order, which results in abrupt fluctuations in refractive index causing increased light scattering and loss in transparency in the lens. It is proposed that lens opacity results from damage to lens enzymes, proteins, and membranes by activated oxygen species, e.g., hydrogen peroxide, superoxide anion, and hydroxyl free radicals, resulting from exposure to light and other types of radiation. For these reasons dietary antioxidants may be important in the prevention of cataracts.

AMD is a disease affecting the central area of the retina (macula) (Fig. 1) resulting in loss of central vision. In the early stages of the disease, lipid material accumulates in deposits underneath the retinal pigment epithelium (RPE). This is believed to arise after failure of the RPE to perform its digestive function adequately. These lipid deposits are known as drusen, and can be seen as pale yellow spots on the retina. The pigment of the RPE may become disturbed with areas of hyperpigmentation and hypopigmentation. In the later stages of the disease, the RPE may atrophy completely. This loss can occur in small focal areas or can be widespread. In some cases, new blood vessels grow under the RPE and occasionally into the subretinal space (exudative or neovascular AMD). Hemorrhage can occur, which often results in increased scarring of the retina. In general, the early stages of AMD are asymptomatic. In the later stages, there may be considerable distortion of vision and complete loss of visual function, particularly in the central area of vision *(11)*. Although the specific pathogenesis of AMD is still unknown, chemical- and light-induced oxidative damage to the photoreceptors is thought to be important in the dysfunction of the RPE. The retina is particularly susceptible to oxidative stress because of its high consumption of oxygen, its high proportion of polyunsaturated fatty acids, and its exposure to visible light. Currently, there is no treatment that can restore vision in AMD. Therefore, efforts have focused on its prevention. As with cataracts, dietary antioxidants have been suggested to play an important role in the prevention of AMD.

The antioxidants, vitamins C and E, lutein, and zeaxanthin are common components of our diet that are most often implicated as protective against eye disease. These antioxidants may prevent damage in the lens by reacting with free radicals produced in the process of light absorption. Photoreceptors in the retina are subject to oxidative stress throughout life because of combined exposures to light and oxygen.

Vitamin E and carotenoids are lipid-soluble oxidant scavangers that protect biomembranes. Vitamin C is an important water-soluble antioxidant, which also promotes the regeneration of vitamin E. Both vitamins C and E are found in the lens *(14–16)*. Of the 20–30 carotenoids found in human blood and tissues *(17)*, only lutein and zeaxanthin are found in the lens and retina *(14,18)*. Lutein and zeaxanthin are concentrated in the macula or central region of the retina and are referred to as macular pigment. In

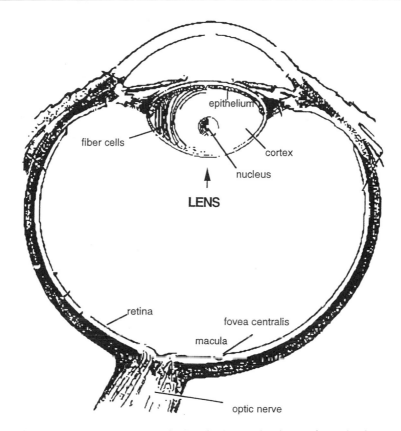

Fig. 1. The human eye showing typical organization and terminology.

addition to their role as antioxidants, lutein and zeaxanthin are believed to limit retinal oxidative damage by absorbing incoming blue light and/or quenching reactive oxygen species. Many putative risk factors for AMD have been linked to a lack of macular pigment, including female gender, lens density, smoking, light iris color, and reduced visual sensitivity *(11)*. Of these risk factors, only diet and smoking are modifiable.

3. HUMAN STUDIES ON DIETARY INTAKE AND BLOOD LEVELS OF ANTIOXIDANTS AND EYE DISEASE

Studies with human subjects provide information on the strength of associations between nutritional factors and the frequency of a disease. Such studies can be a valuable means of identifying and evaluating risk factors. Although there are limitations to such studies, consistency of findings among studies lends to the credibility of nutritional and disease associations.

3.1. Cataract

3.1.1. VITAMIN C

Several studies have found a relationship between increased dietary vitamin C and decreased risk of cataract *(see* Table 1) *(19–21)*. For example, it was observed that the prevalence of nuclear cataract was lower for men with total vitamin C intakes in the

Table 1
Summary of Epidemiologic Studies of Dietary Vitamin C* and Cataract

Data analysis method	Result	Reference
Positive outcome		
Highest vs lowest quintile (men, 104 vs 33 mg/d)	Lower prevalence of cataract in highest quintile	*19*
>490 mg/d vs <125 mg/d	Lower prevalence of cataract with high intake	*20*
Highest vs lowest quintile	Lower prevalence of cataract in highest quintile	*21*
Null outcome		
Highest vs lowest quintile (women, 171 vs 34 mg/d)	No difference in prevalence of cataract between groups	*19*
Highest vs lowest quintile (705 vs 70 mg/d) (women)	No difference in prevalence of cataract between groups	*22*
Highest vs lowest quintile between groups	No difference in prevalence of cataract extraction	*23*
Highest vs lowest quartile (261.1 vs 114.4 mg/d)	No difference in prevalence or nuclear or cortical cataract between groups	*24*
Multiple logistic regression	No association of dietary vit C with nuclear or cortical cataract	*25*

*RDA: 75 and 90 mg/d, women and men, respectively.

highest quintile category relative to the lowest intake quintile *(19)*. It has also been observed that the prevalence of cataract was approx 75% lower in persons with vitamin C intakes >490 mg/d that in those with intakes <125 mg/d *(20)*. However, such a relationship was not always observed *(19,22–25)* (Table 1).

When compared to diet, serum concentrations of a nutrient are considered to be a better measure of nutrient status. Therefore, an evaluation of serum vitamin C relationships with cataract may be useful. Serum ascorbic acid levels have been reported to be inversely associated with the prevalence of cataracts (*see* Table 2) *(20,26)*. However, Vitale et al. *(24)* observed that plasma vitamin C concentrations were not associated with risk of nuclear or cortical cataract. In contrast to these studies, one study found an increased prevalence of cataract with increased plasma vitamin C *(27)* (Table 2).

3.1.2. VITAMIN E

A protective effect of dietary vitamin E has been observed in several studies (*see* Table 3). Persons in the highest quintile for vitamin E intake were reported to be 50% less

Table 2
Summary of Epidemiologic Studies of Plasma Vitamin C* and Cataract

Data analysis method	Result	Reference
Positive outcome		
Multiple logistic regression	Serum vit C inversely associated with prevalence of cataract	26
>90 µmol/L vs <40 µmol/L	Lower prevalence of cataract with high plasma levels	20
Null outcome		
Highest vs lowest quartile	Plasma vit C levels were not associated with risk of cortical or nuclear cataract	24
Negative outcome		
	Higher prevalence of cataract with increased plasma vit C	27

*Reference range: 23–125 µmol/L (Nutrition Evaluation Laboratory, Tufts University, 2003).

Table 3
Summary of Epidemiologic Studies of Dietary Vitamin E* and Cataract

Data analysis method	Result	Reference
Positive outcome		
Highest vs lowest quintile	Lower cataract extraction in highest quintile	23
Highest vs lowest quintile (men, 12.8 vs 4.0 mg/d)	Lower prevalence of nuclear cataract in highest quintile	19
Highest vs lowest quintile quintile	40% Lower prevalence of cataract in highest	21
Null outcome		
>35.7 mg/d vs <8.4 mg/d	No difference between groups	20
Highest vs lowest quintile	No difference between groups	19
(women, 19.9 vs 5 mg/d)	No relationship between dietary vit E and cataract extraction in women	22

*RDA for adults: 15 mg/d.

Table 4
Summary of Epidemiologic Studies of Plasma Vitamin E* and Cataract

Data analysis method	Result	Reference
Positive outcome		
Highest vs lowest quartile	Decrease in cortical cataract progression in highest quintile	*28*
>30 µmol/L vs <19 µmol/L	Less nuclear cataract in high plasma vit E group	*24*
>20 µmol/L vs <20 µmol/L	Higher plasma levels of vit E had 1/2 the amount of cataract surgery	*29*
Highest vs lowest quintile	Lower prevalence of nuclear cataract in highest quintile	*30*
Regression model	High plasma vit E related to decreased prevalence of nuclear cataract	*31*
Null outcome		
>30 µmol/L vs <19 µmol/L	No difference in cortical cataract progression	*24*
Multivariate logistic regression	No relationship between plasma vit E and cataract prevalence	*25*
Negative outcome		
Highest vs lowest quintile Men, 37.8 vs 16.9 µmol/L women, 46.5 vs 18.2 µmol/L	Increased prevalence of nuclear cataract in highest	*32*

*Reference range: 12.0–43.2 µmol/L (Nutrition Evaluation Laboratory, Tufts University, 2003).

likely to undergo cataract extraction when compared to those in the lowest quintile for vitamin E intake *(23)*. Mares-Perlman et al. *(19)* observed a lower prevalence of nuclear cataract in men in the highest quintile category of total vitamin E intake relative to those in the lowest vitamin E intake. Similarly, Leske et al. *(21)* reported that those with vitamin E intakes in the highest quintile category had an approx 40% lower prevalence of cataract relative to persons with intakes in the lowest quintile category. Jacques and Chylack *(20)* reported that although persons with vitamin E intake >35.7 mg/d had a 55% lower prevalence of cataract than did persons with intakes <8.4 mg/d, a significant difference was not found. Two other studies also reported no difference in cataract prevalence between persons with high and low vitamin E intake *(19,22)* (Table 3). In the first of these two studies, the null relationship was in women only (in men, dietary vitamin E was protective). In the second study, only women were studied.

As with dietary vitamin E, results from studies reporting relationships between plasma vitamin E and cataracts have been mixed (*see* Table 4). In five of eight studies examining this issue, increased plasma vitamin E was observed to be protective against the risk of cataract *(24,28–31)* (Table 4). However, one study observed that the prevalence of cataracts was not related to plasma vitamin E concentrations *(25)*, and one study observed that the prevalence of cortical cataract did not differ between those with high and low plasma vitamin E concentrations *(24)*. In contrast, one study found increased levels of plasma vitamin E to be a risk factor for cataract *(32)*. In this study, there was a significantly increased prevalence of nuclear cataract among women and men in the highest serum vitamin E quintile relative to those in the lowest quintile (Table 4).

3.1.3. LUTEIN AND ZEAXANTHIN

Few studies have specifically examined the relationship between lutein and zeaxanthin with cataract risk. In a recent report, Chasen-Taber et al. *(33)* observed in women that those with the highest intake of lutein and zeaxanthin had a 22% decreased risk of cataract extraction when compared with those in the lowest quintile. Brown et al. *(34)* also observed that there was a lower risk of cataract extraction in men with higher intakes of lutein and zeaxanthin but not other carotenoids. Men in the highest fifth of lutein and zeaxanthin intake had a 19% lower risk of cataract relative to men in the lowest fifth. Mares-Perlman et al. *(32,35)* observed in women a significant inverse trend across quintiles of lutein intake. Women in the highest quintile of lutein intake (median 0.95 mg/d) had a 27% lower prevalence of nuclear cataract than women in the lowest lutein intake quintile (median 0.28 g/d). The trend was in the same direction in men, but did not reach statistical significance. Hankinson et al. *(22)* reported that the rate of cataract surgery was associated with lower intakes of lutein-rich foods, such as spinach and other green veg etables. Although the data are few, the studies suggest that dietary lutein and zeaxanthin play a role in cataract prevention.

3.2. AMD

3.2.1. VITAMIN C

Only one epidemiologic study has evaluated the role of dietary vitamin C and AMD risk *(see* Table 5). Seddon et al. *(36)* observed that persons in the highest and lowest intake quintiles for vitamin C had the same prevalence of advanced AMD. However, results examining relationships between plasma levels of vitamin C and AMD suggest that increased plasma vitamin C may decrease the risk of AMD. West et al. *(37)* reported that individuals with plasma vitamin C concentrations >80 µmol/L had a 45% lower prevalence of AMD compared with individuals who had concentrations <60 µmol/L. Others have reported that individuals with serum vitamin C concentrations ≥91 µmol/L had a 30% lower prevalence of AMD when compared with those who had concentrations <40 µmol/L *(38)* (Table 5).

3.2.2. VITAMIN E

The one study that has evaluated the role of dietary vitamin E and AMD risk reported no difference in prevalence of advanced AMD between individuals in the highest and lowest vitamin E intake quintiles *(see* Table 6) *(36)*. A protective effect of increased plasma vitamin E against AMD has been found in some studies *(37,38)*, but not in others *(32,39)* (Table 6).

3.2.3. LUTEIN AND ZEAXANTHIN

Results of a multicenter case-control study suggest that high intakes of carotenoids, particularly lutein and zeaxanthin, are related to lower risk of advanced neovascular AMD *(36)*. This is consistent with earlier findings from the First Health and Nutrition

Table 5
Summary of Epidemiologic Studies of Dietary and Plasma Vitamin C* with AMD

Data analysis method	Result	Reference
Dietary vitamin C		
Highest vs lowest quintile for vit C intake (1039 vs 65 mg/d)	No difference in prevalence of advanced AMD between groups	36
Plasma vitamin C		
>80 μmol/L vs <60 μmol/L	Lower prevalence of AMD in high plasma vit C group	37
>91 μmol/L <40 μmol/L	Lower prevalence of AMD in high plasma vit C group	38

*RDA for adults: 60 mg/d. Reference range 23–125 μmol/L (Nutrition Evaluation Laboratory, Tufts University, 2001).

Table 6
Summary of Epidemiologic Studies of Dietary and Plasma Vitamin E* with AMD

Data analysis method	Result	Reference
Dietary vitamin E		
Highest vs lowest quintile for vit E intake (405 vs 3.4 mg/d)	No difference in prevalence of advanced AMD between groups	36
Plasma vitamin E		
>30 μmol/L vs <19 μmol/L	Lower prevalence of AMD with high plasma vit E	37
>43 μmol/L vs <25 μmol/L	Lower prevalence of AMD with high plasma vit E	38
>23 μmol/L vs <23 μmol/L	No difference between groups in prevalence of AMD	32
Patients with AMD vs age-, sex- matched controls	No difference in plasma concentration of vit E between groups	39

*RDA: 8 and 10 mg/d, women and men, respectively. Reference range: 12.0–43.2 μmol/L (Nutrition Evaluation Laboratory, Tufts University).

Examination Survey, in which low intakes of fruits and vegetables providing vitamin A were related to higher rates of all types of advanced AMD *(40)*. The Eye Disease Case-Control Study *(38)* found, after adjusting for other risk factors, that people in the highest fifth of carotenoid intake had a 43% lower risk for neovascular AMD compared to those in the lowest fifth. Among the specific carotenoids, lutein and zeaxanthin, which are primarily obtained from dark green, leafy vegetables, were most strongly correlated with a reduced risk for age-related macular degeneration. However, a nested case-control study as part of the Beaver Dam Eye Study, found no association with serum levels of lutein and zeaxanthin in 167 cases of (largely) early age-related macular degeneration and age-, sex-, and smoking-matched controls *(32)*.

In summary, the studies examining nutrient and eye disease relationships are not entirely consistent. Methodology differences among studies may, in part, explain the inconsistencies. Also, there are limitations to such studies that examine relationships between a nutrient and disease because calculations from dietary recall may not always accurately estimate nutrient intakes because of limitations of the database or recall abilities of the subjects. Furthermore, a single blood value for a nutrient may not always be an accurate indicator of long-term status. In addition, the high degree of correlation in intake among the various dietary micronutrients makes it difficult to determine which specific nutrient or nutrients are related to the observed relationships. Despite these drawbacks, a possible protective role of vitamins C and E and the carotenoids lutein and zeaxanthin cannot be dismissed given the number of studies that found a protective effect and the very few studies that found a negative effect. In some cases, it may be difficult to measure an outcome if nutrient intake levels are at those found in diet alone. That is, dietary and plasma levels may not be sufficiently high to see an effect. In this regard, review of studies that have examined the relationship between supplemental nutrient intake with cataracts and AMD risk may be useful.

4. THE EFFECT OF NUTRIENT SUPPLEMENTS ON EYE DISEASE RISK

Supplemental vitamins C and E have long been available to the general public. Currently, there are a variety of supplement products available in health food stores that contain lutein in amounts of 6–25 mg/capsule. At this point, lutein is found in only one multivitamin product in much smaller amounts (0.25 mg/capsule).

4.1. Cataract

Jacques et al. *(41)* observed a >75% lower prevalence of early opacities in women who used vitamin C supplement for ≥10 yr *(see* Table 7). None of the 26 women who used vitamin C supplements for ≥10 yr had more advanced nuclear cataracts. Hankinson et al. *(22)* observed that women who reported use of vitamin C supplements for ≥10 yr had a 45% reduction in rate of cataract surgery. The study of Robertson et al. *(42)* observed that the prevalence of cataracts in persons who consumed a vitamin C supplement of >300 mg/d was approximately one-third the prevalence in persons who did not consume vitamin C supplements. However, Chasan-Tabar et al. *(43)* prospectively examined the association between vitamin supplement intake and the incidence of cataract extraction during 12 yr of follow-up in a cohort of 73,956 female nurses. After adjusting for cataract risk factors, including cigarette smoking, body mass index, and diabetes mellitus, there

Table 7
Summary of Epidemiologic Studies of Supplemental Vitamin C* and Cataract

Data analysis method	Result	Reference
Positive outcome		
Usage ≥10 yr vs usage <10 yr	Decrease in cataract in long-term users of vit C supplements	*41*
Usage ≥10 yr vs usage <10 yr	Decrease in cataract surgery with increase usage of vit C supplement	*22*
>300 mg/d vs nonusers of vit C supplements	Lower prevalence of cataract in vit C supplement users	*42*
Null outcome		
Usage ≥10 yr vs nonusers	No difference between groups	*33*

*RDA for adults: 60 mg/d.

Table 8
Summary of Epidemiologic Studies of Supplemental Vitamin E* and Cataract

Data analysis method	Result	Reference
Positive outcome		
Vit E supplement users vs nonusers	Decrease in cortical cataract in users of vit E supplements	*44*
Vit E supplements users vs nonusers	Decrease in nuclear cataract in users	*31*
Vit E supplements users vs nonusers	Decrease in cataract in users	*42*
Null outcome		
Vit E supplement users vs nonusers	No difference in nuclear cataract	*44*
Vit E supplements users vs nonusers	No difference in prevalence of cataract between users and nonusers	*22*

*RDA: 8 and 10 mg/d, women and men, respectively.

was no difference in the incidence of cataract between users of vitamin C supplements for 10 yr or more and nonusers (Table 7).

Nadalin et al. *(44)* cross-sectionally examined the association between prior supplementation with vitamin E and early cataract changes in volunteers (*see* Table 8). Of 1111 participants, 26% reported prior supplementation with vitamin E. Only 8.8% of these participants took supplementation greater than the recommended daily intake (10 mg/d).

A statistically significant association was found between prior supplementation and the absence of cortical opacity, after adjusting for age. However, the levels of nuclear opacity were not statistically different between those who reported intake and those with no prior vitamin E supplementation. Leske et al. *(31)* examined the association of antioxidant nutrients and risk of nuclear opacification in a longitudinal study. The risk of nuclear opacification at follow-up was decreased in regular users of multivitamin supplements and vitamin E supplements and in persons with higher plasma levels of vitamin E. The investigators concluded that in regular users of multivitamin supplements, the risk of nuclear opacification was reduced by one-third. They also reported that in regular users of vitamin E supplement and persons with higher plasma levels of vitamin E, the risk was reduced by approx one half. These results are confirmed by Robertson et al. *(42)* who reported that the prevalence of cataracts was 56% lower in persons who consumed vitamin E supplement than in persons not consuming supplements. One study observed no relation between risk of cataract and vitamin E supplements *(22)* (Table 8).

To date, there are few data from intervention trials of vitamins and cataract risk. In a recent study, it was reported that a high-dose combination of antioxidants (vitamins C and E, beta-carotene, and zinc) had no significant effect on the development or progression of cataracts *(45)*. The LINXIAN trial *(46)* examined the role of antioxidants in prevention of cataract, and the effect is not clear. The intervention was a combination dose of 14 vitamins and 12 minerals. Therefore, a specific role of any one nutrient could not be accurately evaluated. The multivitamin component demonstrated that nutrition can modify the risk of nuclear cataract, but specific nutrients were not evaluated. Also, the population examined had suboptimal nutritional intakes at the study start and the effect may have been from a correction of certain nutrient deficiencies.

4.2. AMD

A recent study reported that high levels of antioxidants and zinc significantly reduce the risk of AMD and its associated vision loss *(45)*. It was found that people at high risk for developing advanced stages of AMD (people with intermediate AMD or advanced AMD in one eye but not the other eye) lowered their risk by about 25% when treated with a high-dose combination of vitamins C and E, beta-carotene, and zinc. In the same high-risk group the nutrients reduced the risk of vision loss caused by advanced AMD by about 19%. For those subjects who had either no AMD or early AMD, the nutrients did not provide a measured benefit. Because single nutrients were not evaluated, specific effects could not be determined.

It has been reported that the prevalence of AMD in persons who consumed vitamin C supplement for >2 yr was similar to those who never took vitamin C supplements *(38)* (*see* Table 9). In a study conducted by Seddon et al. *(36)* the prevalence of AMD was also similar between those who took vitamin E supplement for >2 yr and those who never took vitamin E supplements. One primary prevention trial has been published on age-related macular degeneration *(47)* (Table 9). This trial evaluated the effect of nutritional antioxidants on AMD. Overall there were 728 people randomized to any antioxidant and 213 to placebo. The results of this study found that there was no association of a treatment group with any sign of maculopathy. There were 216 cases of the disease in the antioxidant groups and 53 in the placebo group. The majority of these cases were early age-related maculopathy. The findings are similar when each of the antioxidant groups—vitamin E, beta-carotene, and vitamin E and beta-carotene—are compared with placebo. Although

Table 9
Summary of Epidemiologic Studies of Supplement Use and AMD*

Data analysis method	Result	Reference
Null outcome		
Vit C supplement users (>2 yr) vs nonusers	No difference between groups in AMD prevalence	*38*
Vit E supplement users (>2 yr) vs nonusers	No difference between groups in AMD prevalence	*36*
Intervention trial vit E, β-carotene, or both supplements vs placebo	No association of treatment group with any sign of maculopathy	*47*

this was a large, high-quality study there were few cases of late AMD (14 cases in total) which means that the study had limited power to address the question of whether supplementation prevents AMD. There was no association with the treatment group and development of early stages of the disease. This study was conducted in Finnish male smokers, and caution must be taken when extrapolating the findings to other geographical areas, people in other age groups, women, and nonsmokers. However, the incidence of AMD, particularly neovascular disease, is likely to be higher in smokers *(48)*, which means that they provide a good population to demonstrate any potential protective effects of antioxidant supplementation.

Lutein and zeaxanthin supplements have recently become available to the general public. Therefore, time has not allowed for the adequate study of the effect of these nutrient supplements of the prevalence of either cataract or AMD.

In summary, of the studies that have examined nutrient supplement use versus the risk of eye disease, it is difficult to determine if supplements provide any added protection against eye disease. The number of studies reporting a positive outcome, i.e., a decreased risk, was about the same as the number of null outcomes. Therefore, the data are inconsistent. Certainly, it appears that nutrient supplementation does not cause an increase risk to eye disease.

5. CLINICAL RECOMMENDATIONS/TREATMENT GUIDELINES

The inconsistencies among studies in terms of the amount of nutrient required for protection against eye disease makes it difficult to make specific recommendations for dietary intakes of these antioxidants. Thus, it may be more practical to recommend specific food choices rich in vitamins C and E, lutein, and zeaxanthin, thereby benefiting from possible effects of the components in food that may also be important. This necessitates an awareness of dietary sources of nutritional antioxidants for both the patient and clinician. Good sources of vitamin C include citrus fruit, berries, tomatoes, and broccoli

Table 10
Vitamin C Content of Foods* (51)

Food	Amount	Milligrams
Orange juice	1 cup	12
Green peppers	1/2 cup	96
Grapefruit juice	1 cup	94
Papaya	1/2/med	94
Brussel sprouts	4 sprouts	73
Broccoli, raw	1/2/cup	70
Orange	1 medium	70
Cantaloupe	1/4 melon	70
Turnip greens, cooked	1/2 cup	50
Cauliflower	1/2 cup	45
Strawberries	1/2 cup	42
Grapefruit	1/2 medium	41
Tomato juice	1 cup	39
Potato, boiled with peel	2 1/2" diam.	19
Cabbage, raw, chopped	1/2/cup	15
Blackberries	1/2 cup	15
Spinach, raw, chopped	1/2/cup	14
Blueberries	1/2 cup	9

*Edible portion.

Table 11
Vitamin E Content of Foods* (52)

Food	Amount	Milligrams (α tocopherol equivalents)
Wheat germ oil	1 tb	26.2
Sunflower seeds	1/4 cup	16.0
Almonds	1/4 cup	14.0
Safflower oil	1 tb	4.7
Peanuts	1/4 cup	4.2
Corn oil	1 tb	2.9
Peanut butter	2 tb	4.0
Soybean oil	1 tb	2.0
Pecan, halves	1/4 cup	2.0

*Edible portion.

(see Table 10). Good sources of vitamin E are vegetable oils, wheat germ, whole grain cereals, nuts, and legumes (see Table 11). The two foods that were found to have the highest amount of lutein and zeaxanthin are kale and spinach (see Table 12). Other major sources include broccoli, peas, and brussel sprouts.

Table 12
Lutein/Zeaxanthin Content of 1/2 Cup Servings of Vegetables* *(53)*

Food	Lutein/zeaxanthin (mg)
Kale, cooked	8.7
Spinach, raw	6.6
Spinach, cooked	6.3
Broccoli, cooked	2.0
Corn, sweet, cooked	1.5
Peas, green, cooked	1.1
Brussels Sprouts, cooked	0.9
Lettuce, raw	0.7

*Edible portion.

A healthy diet including a variety of fresh fruit and vegetables, legumes, and nuts will have many benefits, will not do any harm, and will be a good source of the antioxidant vitamins and minerals implicated (but not proven) in the etiology of cataract and age-related macular degeneration. There is no evidence that nutrient-dense diets high in these foods, which provide known and unknown antioxidant components, are harmful. In fact, intake of fruits and vegetables is associated with reduced risk of death from cancer, cardiovascular disease, and all causes. Thus, recommendations such as consuming a more nutrient-dense diet, i.e., lower in sweets and fats, and increasing levels of fruit and vegetable intake do not appear to be harmful and may have other benefits despite their unproven efficacy in preventions or slowing disease. Until the efficacy and safety of taking supplements containing nutrients can be determined, current dietary recommendations *(49)* are advised.

In addition to antioxidant vitamins, patients ask about a wide variety of unproven and often untested nutritional supplements. These include bilberries, shark cartilage, and Ginko biloba extract. Unfortunately, little is known about the effect of these products on cataract or AMD; no clinical trials have been conducted. Patients with eye disease who are offered these often expensive and sometimes risky treatments are given little information as to their benefit or risk. Patients should be advised to avoid unproven treatments.

6. SUMMARY

The hypothesis that antioxidant nutrients may protect against cataracts and AMD is a plausable one given the role of oxidative damage in the etiology of these diseases. It is not known at what stage the protective effect may be important. The question that needs to be addressed is whether people who begin to consume antioxidant vitamins in their 60s and 70s alter their risk of age-related macular degeneration. Although data regarding the use of nutrient supplements suggests protection from cataracts, the data are less convincing for AMD. The research to date has not sufficiently evaluated the effectiveness vs safety of nutrient supplements. But advocating the use of nutrient supplementation must be done with a cautionary note given that there have been trials which have suggested that supplementation with beta-carotene may have an adverse effect on the incidence of lung cancer in smokers and workers exposed to asbestos *(47,50)*. Clearly, further trials are warranted to address the usefulness of nutrient supplementation in eye disease prevention.

It is likely that cataract and AMD develops over many years and the etiology of these diseases is due to many factors. There are likely to be differences in the potential protective effect of antioxidant supplementation depending on the stage of the disease. Future research needs to take into account the stage at which oxidative damage, and therefore antioxidant supplementation, may be important.

7. CONCLUSIONS AND RECOMMENDATIONS FOR CLINICIANS

1. Studies of diet and eye disease relationships are not yet sufficiently consistent (resulting from differences in methodology, limitations in diet recall accuracy, and equivocal blood level measurements) to permit definitive clinical recommendations about the use of specific nutrients to protect against cataract and AMD.
2. There is convincing preliminary evidence suggesting that vitamins C and E and the carotenoids lutein and zeaxanthin play a protective role. Therefore, all adults are encouraged to consume generous amounts of foods rich in vitamin C (citrus fruit, berries, tomatoes, broccoli), vitamin E (vegetable oils, wheat germ, whole grain cereals, nuts, legumes) and lutein and zeaxanthin (kale, spinach).
3. Geriatric patients whose medical, mental, or social condition makes them unable to consume a diet adequate in these nutrients (Vitamins C, E, lutein, zeazanthin) may benefit from taking a supplemental amount equal to the daily recommendations (refer to table or reference). However, caution should be used with regards to supplemental nutrients—supplementation with beta-carotene has been shown to have an adverse effect on the incidence of lung cancer in smokers and asbestos workers.
4. Patients should be advised to avoid unproven treatments, including (to date) bilberries, shark cartilage, and Ginko biloba extract, because of their unclear benefit and their cost.

REFERENCES

1. Quinlan DA. Common causes of vision loss in elderly patient. Am Fam Physician 1999;60:99–108.
2. Thylefors B, Negrel AD, Pararajasegaram R, Dadzie KY. Global data on blindness. Bull World Health Organ 1995;73:115–121.
3. World Health Organization. Use of intraocular lenses in cataract surgery in developing countries. Bull World Health Organ 1991;69:657–666.
4. Schwab L. Cataract blindness in developing nations. Intern Ophthalmol Clin 1990;30:16–18.
5. Kahn HA, Leibowitz HM, Ganley JP, et al. The Framingham eye study. I. Outline and major prevalence findings. Am J Epidemiol 1977;106:17–32.
6. Javitt JC. Who does cataract surgery in the United States? Arch Ophthalmol 1993;111:1329.
7. Steinberg EP, Javitt JC, Sharkey PD, Zuckerman A, Legro MW, Anderson GF, et al. The content and cost of cataract surgery. Arch Ophthalmol 1993;111:1041–1049.
8. Klein R, Klein BEK, Linton KL. Prevalence of age-related maculopathy. The Beaver Dam Eye Study. Ophthalmology 1992;99:933–943.
9. Leibowitz H, Krueger D, Maunder C, et al. The Framingham Eye Study Monograph. Surv Ophthalmol 1980;24S:335–610.
10. National Advisory Eye Council, Report of the Retinal and Choroidal Diseases Panel. Vision Research—A National Plan: 1983–1987. US Dept. of Health and Human Services, Bethesda, MD, 1984. NIH Pub 83–2471.
11. Snodderly DM. Evidence for protection against age-related macular degeneration by carotenoids and anti-oxidants. Am J Clin Nutr 1995;62S:1448S–1461S.
12. Taylor HR. Epidemiology of age-related cataract. Eye; 1999;13:445–448
13. Benedek GB. Theory of transparency of the eye. Appl Opt 1971;10:459–473.

14. Yeum KJ, Taylor A, Tang G, Russell RM. Measurement of carotenoids, retinoids, and tocopherols in human lenses. Invest Opthalmol Vis Sci 1995;3:2756–2761.
15. Yeum KJ, Shang F, Schalch W, Russell RM, Taylor A. Fat-soluble nutrient concentrations in different layers of human cataractous lens. Curr Eye Research 1999;19:502–505.
16. Taylor A, Jacques PF, Nadler S, Morrow F, Sulsky SI, Shepard D. Relationship in humans between ascorbic acid consumption and levels of total and reduced ascorbic acid in lens, aqueous humor and plasma. Current Eye Res 1991;10:751–759.
17. Parker RS. Bioavailability of carotenoids. Eur J Clin Nutr 1997, 51:S86–S90
18. Bone RA, Landrum JT, Tarsis SL. Preliminary identification of the human macular pigment. Vision Research 1985;25:1531–1535.17.
19. Mares-Perlman JA, Brady WE, Klein BEK, Klein H, Palta GJ, Ritter LL, Sloff SM. Diet and nuclear lens opacities. Am J Epidemiol 1995;141:322–334.
20. Jacques PF, Chylack LT Jr. Epidemiologic evidence of a role for the antioxidant vitamins and carotenoids in cataract prevention. Am J Clin Nutr 1991;53:353S–355S.
21. Leske MC, Chylack LT Jr, Wu S. The lens opacities case-control study risks factors for cataract. Arch Ophthalmol 1991;109:244–251.
22. Hankinson SE, Stampfer MJ, Seddon JM, Colditz GA, Rosner B, Speizer FE, Willett WC. Nutrient intake and cataract extraction in women: a prospective study. Br Med J 1992;305:335–339.
23. Tavani A, NegriE, laVecchia C. Food and nutrient intake and risk of cataract. Am Epidemiol 1996;6: 41–46.
24. Vitale S, West S, Hallfrisch J, Alston CM, Wang F, Moorman C, et al. Plasma antioxidants and risk of cortical and nuclear cataract. Epidemiology 1993;4:195–203.
25. The Italian-American Cataract Study Group. Risk factors for age-related cortical, nuclear and posterior subcapsular cataracts. Am J Epidemiol 1991;133:541–553.
26. Simon JA, Hudes ES. Serum ascorbic acid and other correlates of self-reported cataract among older Americans. J Clin Epid 1999;52:1207–1211.
27. Mohan M, Sperduto RD, Angra SK, et al. Indian-US case-control study of age-related cataracts India-US case-control Study Group. Arch Ophthalmology 1989;107:670–676.
28. Rouhiainen P, Rouhiainen H, Salonen JT. Association between low plasma vitamin E concentrations and progression of early cortical lens opacities. Am J Epidemiol 1996;114:496–500.
29. Knekt P, Heliovaara M, Rissenen A, Aromaa A, Aaran R. Serum antioxidant vitamins and risk of cataract. BMJ 1992;304:1392–1294.
30. Leske MC, Wu SY, Hyman L, et al., and the Lens Opacities Case Control Study Group. Biochemical factors in the Lens Opacities Case-Control Study. Arch Ophthalmol 1995;113;1113–1119.
31. Leske MC, Chylack LT Jr, He Q, et al. Antioxidant vitamins and nuclear opacities: the longitudinal study of cataract. Ophthalmology 1998;105:831–836.
32. Mares-Perlman JA, Brady WE, Klein R, et al. Serum antioxidants and age-related macular degeneration in a population-based case-control study. Arch Ophthalmol 1995;113:1518–1523.
33. Chasen-Taber L, Willett WC, Seddon JM, et al. A prospective study of carotenoid and vitamin A intakes and risk of cataract extraction in US women. Am J Clin Nutr 1999;70:509–516.
34. Brown L, Rimm EB, Seddon JM, et al. A prospective study of carotenoid intake and risk of cataract extraction in US men. Am J Clin Nutr 1999;70:517–524.
35. Mares-Perlman JA, Klein BEK, Klein J, Ritter LL. Relationship between lens opacities and vitamin and mineral use. Ophthalmology 1994;101:315–325.
36. Seddon JM, Ajani VA, Sperduto RD, et al. Dietary carotenoids , vitamins A, C, and E and advanced age-related macular degeneration. JAMA 1994;272:1413–1420.
37. West SK, Vitale S, Hallfrisch J, et al. Are antioxidants or supplements protective for age-related macular degeneration? Arch Ophthalmol 1994;112:222–227.
38. Eye Disease Case-control Study Group (EDCCSG). Antioxidant status and neovascular age-related macular degeneration. Arch Ophthalmol 1993;11:104–109.
39. Sanders TAB, Haines AP, Wormald R, Wright LA, Obeid O. Essential fatty acids, plasma cholesterol, and fat-soluble vitamins in subjects with age-related maculopathy and matched control subjects. Am J Clin Nutr 1993;57:428–433.
40. Goldberg J, Flowerdew G, Tso MOM, Brody JA. Age-related macular degeneration and cataract: are dietary antioxidants protective? Am J Epidemiol 1998;128:904–905.
41. Jacques PF, Taylor A, Hankinson SE, Lahav M, Mahnken B, Lee Y, et al. Long-term vitamin C supplement and prevalence of age-related opacities. Am J Clin Nutr 1997;66:911–916.

42. Robertson JM, Donner AP, Trevithick JR. Vitamin E intake and risk for cataracts in humans. Ann NY Acad Aci 1989;570:373–382.
43. Chasen-Taber L, Willett WC, Seddon JM, et al. A prospective study of vitamin supplement intake and cataract extraction among US women. Epidemiology 1999;10:679–684.
44. Nadalin G, Robman LD, McCarty CA, Garrett SK, McNeil JJ, Taylor HR. The role of past intake of vitamin E in early cataract changes. Ophthalmic Epidemiology 1999;6:105–112.
45. Age-Related Eye Disease Study Research Group. A randomized, placebo-controlled, clinical trial of high-dose supplementation with vitamins C and E, beta carotene, and zinc for age-related macular degeneration and vision loss. Arch Ophthalmol 2001;119:1417–1436.
46. Sperduto RD, Hu TS, Milton RC, et al. The Linxian cataract studies. Two nutrition intervention trials. Arch Ophthalmol 1993;111:1246–1253.
47. The Alpha-Tocopherol Beta-Carotene Prevention Study Group. The effect of vitamin E and beta-carotene on the incidence of lung cancer and other cancers in male smokers. N Eng J Med 1994;3309:1029–1035.
48. Solberg Y, Posner M, Belkin M. The association between cigarette smoking and ocular diseases (review). Surv Ophthalmol 1998;42:535–547.
49. US Department of Agriculture and US Department of Health and Human Services. Nutrition and Your Health: Dietary Guidelines for Americans. 3rd ed. US Government Printing Office, Washington, DC, Home and Garden Bulletin 232–1, 1990.
50. Omenn GS, Goodman GE, Thornquist, et al. Risk factors for lung cancer and for intervention effects in CARET, the beta-carotene and retinol efficiency trial. J Natl Cancer Inst 1996;88:1550–1559.
51. US Department of Agriculture, Agriculture Research Service. Nutritive value of American Foods in common units. Agriculture Handbook No. 456. US Government Printing Office, Washington DC, 1975.
52. US Department of Agriculture, Agricultural Research Service, 1999. USDA Nutrient Database for Standard Reference, Release 13. Nutrient Data Laboratory, http://www.nal.usda.gov./fnic/foodcomp
53. Mangels AR, Holden JM, Beecher GR, Forman MR, Lanza E. Carotenoid content of fruits and vegetables: an evaluation of analytic data. J Am Diet Assoc 1993;93:284–296.

9

Loss of Taste, Smell, and Other Senses with Age

Effects of Medication

Susan S. Schiffman, Mamie O. Rogers, and Jennifer Zervakis

1. INTRODUCTION

There is an increasing awareness of the potential for maintaining functional status and quality of life to very old age. Integral to that aim is retaining the function of the senses, which are vital for learning, interacting, taking pleasure from the outside world, and overall health. All sensory modalities (including taste, smell, vision, hearing, and touch) undergo age-related declines, although the time of onset and degree of loss for a particular sensory modality varies among individuals. Many changes in the senses are not an inevitable consequence of aging, but rather are influenced by such factors as disease, medication use, and environmental factors including nutrition. Current research aims to better understand the mechanisms of age-related sensory losses and to develop methods that compensate for these changes so that the elderly can maximize their remaining abilities.

This chapter provides an overview of the decrements in taste, smell, vision, hearing, and touch in elderly persons, as well as how these sensory changes impact nutritional status. The role of medications in these losses will be addressed. In addition, the relationship of nutritional factors to sensory health are examined.

2. CHEMOSENSORY LOSSES WITH AGE

Alterations in taste and smell occur with advancing age, and this can lead to poor appetite *(1)*, inappropriate food choices *(2)*, and/or lower nutrient intake *(3)*. Decreased appetite is one cause of lower energy consumption in the elderly *(4–6)*, which can ultimately impact protein and micronutrient status and may induce subclinical deficiencies that directly affect health status *(4,5,7)*. Loss of appetite is of special concern for elderly with critical illnesses who are at a higher risk to develop protein-energy malnutrition, as well as micronutrient deficiencies *(8)*.

From: *Handbook of Clinical Nutrition and Aging*
Edited by: C. W. Bales and C. S. Ritchie © Humana Press Inc., Totowa, NJ

Taste and smell affect appetite, food choices, and nutrient intake in the following ways. First, these chemosensory (e.g., taste and smell) signals initiate cephalic phase responses including salivary, gastric, pancreatic, and intestinal secretions that prepare the body to digest food *(9,10)*. Second, taste and smell provide sensory information that allows us to detect and discriminate among foods in the face of fluctuating nutritional requirements. This is accomplished in part by changes in the activity in taste neurons in response to physiological needs *(11–14)*. Third, taste and smell sensations enable us to select a nutritious diet. Learned associations between the taste and smell of a food and its postingestive effects *(10,15)* allow an individual to modulate food intake in anticipation of its nutritional consequences. That is, taste sensations serve as an indicator of a food's nutritional value. Fourth, taste and smell signals play a role in initiating, sustaining, and terminating ingestion, and thus influence the quantity of food that is eaten and the size of meals *(10)*. Fifth, taste and smell sensations induce feelings of satiety and are primary reinforcers of eating *(10,16,17)*. Thus, impairments of taste and smell can alter food choices and intake and subsequently exacerbate disease states, impair nutritional status and immunity, and produce weight loss *(16,18)*.

2.1. Taste Losses with Age

2.1.1. PHYSIOLOGY OF THE TASTE SYSTEM

In order to understand the perceptual changes in taste with age, it is helpful to describe the anatomy and physiology of the taste system. Taste sensations occur when chemicals in foods and beverages contact taste cells in the oral cavity that are clustered into buds scattered on the dorsal surface of the tongue, the soft palate, pharynx, larynx, epiglottis, uvula, and first third of the esophagus *(16,19,20)*. Taste receptor-like cells have even been identified in the lining of the stomach and intestines *(21)*. Taste buds are structures that consist of 50–100 specialized cells arranged somewhat like segments in a tangerine. Taste cells replicate constantly with a turnover time of approx 10–10.5 d. This continuous renewal renders the sense of taste vulnerable to nutritional deficiencies that impair reproduction of taste cells *(16,18)*.

Taste buds on the tongue are found in elevated structures called papillae. Papillae on the anterior two thirds of the tongue are called fungiform papillae and usually contain 1–18 taste buds. Foliate papillae consist of folds arranged vertically on the posterior lateral sides of the tongue. Taste cells in foliate papillae are especially sensitive to sour tastes. Circumvallate papillae, which are surrounded by "moats," are located on the posterior third of the tongue arranged in a V-shaped form pointing caudally. Biochemical components in taste cells transduce taste signals related to quality (e.g., salty), as well as intensity. These components include sodium channels, potassium channels, and two second messenger systems, the adenylate cyclase system and the phosphatidylinositol system *(22,23)*.

Taste signals are transmitted from taste receptor cells to the medulla in the brain stem along three cranial nerves *(17,20)*. Taste buds located on the anterior two-thirds of the tongue are innervated by one branch of the seventh cranial nerve (the chorda tympani nerve). Another branch of the seventh cranial nerve (the greater superficial petrosal nerve) innervates most of the taste buds on the soft palate. The remaining taste buds located on the soft palate are innervated by a branch of the ninth cranial nerve (the deep petrosal branch). Taste buds on the posterior third of the tongue are innervated by the ninth (glossopharyngeal) nerve. Taste buds on the far posterior tongue, the epiglottis, the larynx, and the esophagus are innervated by the tenth nerve (specifically the superior laryngeal branch of the vagus nerve). The seventh, ninth, and tenth nerves project to the rostral portion of the nucleus of the solitary tract (NST) in the dorsal medulla of the brainstem (17,20). The NST also receives information from visceral sensory fibers originating in the esophagus, stomach, intestines, and liver, as well as olfactory information via the first cranial nerve (10). Hence, the NST is the first neural processing area in which taste information signals can impact ingestive and digestive activity by producing gastric secretion, increased pancreatic exocrine secretion, and increased secretion of insulin. This processing area is important for cephalic phase responses to taste stimuli associated with food. The gustatory portion of the NST projects to the ventroposteromedial nucleus of the thalamus (20) and ultimately to the taste cortex in the brain. The NST also sends information to the hypothalamus, which also regulates feeding behavior.

Pungent qualities in the oral cavity (such as those from red and black pepper or from carbonation) are transduced by the trigeminal nerve as well as free nerve endings of the chorda tympani nerve, the glossopharyngeal nerve, and the vagus nerves (24). Pungency in the oral cavity is generally not regarded as a taste, but rather a different sense related to nociception (or pain).

2.1.2. Physiological Changes in the Taste System with Age

Studies of the anatomical changes of the taste system in older individuals have yielded conflicting results (19). Although some studies have found significant reductions in the number of papillae and taste buds per papillae with age, others have not. The equivocal results are partly because there is wide individual variation in the number of papillae and taste buds in normal individuals, and cross-sectional rather than longitudinal studies have been used to count the number of taste papillae and buds. Mistretta (25) suggested that taste losses in the elderly are the result of changes at the level of the taste cell membranes (e.g., altered functioning of ion channels and receptors) rather than losses of taste buds. This situation is complicated by the fact that medications, radiation, and disease can reduce the number of taste buds/papillae as well as alter transduction mechanisms at the cell membranes. Furthermore, the frequent turnover of taste buds makes them vulnerable to metabolic, hormonal, and nutritional disturbances. Degenerative changes in the central taste pathways may also alter taste perception in the elderly. Overall, the degree and type of physiological changes of taste perception in the elderly have not yet been fully characterized.

2.1.3. Perceptual Changes in the Sense of Taste with Age

Changes in taste perception are found in older individuals at both threshold and suprathreshold levels. Losses in sensitivity have been reported for both detection and recognition thresholds. A detection threshold is the lowest concentration of a tastant that is discriminated from water. A recognition threshold is the lowest concentration that is correctly identified. Age-related declines in taste sensitivity do not appear to be uniform across stimuli, but vary by molecular structure (26). For example, although most studies report changes in salt and bitter detection, some studies do not find age-related changes for sucrose (sweet) or sour detection (27). However, careful testing with repeated measures has found declines in sweet taste (28). Determining true age-related changes for chemosensory perception is complicated by the fact that most studies have not controlled for medication use. Schiffman *(26)* found that community-dwelling elderly taking an average of 3.4 medications exhibited higher detection thresholds than young individuals for basic taste compounds: sodium salt thresholds were 11.6 times higher, thresholds for acids 4.3 times higher, bitter compound thresholds 7 times higher, amino acid thresholds 2.5 times higher, glutamate salts 5 times higher, and sweeteners 2.7 times higher. However, a study of unmedicated healthy individuals ranging from 10–77 yr of age indicated that losses at the threshold levels were small *(29)*. Elderly in assisted-living or nursing facilities are likely to have even more elevated detection thresholds *(18)*. Thus, at the threshold level, medications (and medical conditions) may account for a significant proportion of loss in taste sensitivity.

Suprathreshold taste losses include reductions in the magnitude of perceived intensity *(30–38)*, loss in the ability to identify foods on the basis of taste and smell *(39,40)*, and inability to judge the presence of salt and monosodium glutamate in foods *(41)*. The elderly also require a greater difference in concentration between two tastants to detect a change in intensity (i.e., they have greater difference thresholds). When both young and elderly compare differences between pairs of food items, elderly perceive foods as more similar to each other *(39,42)*. Although young subjects perceived the taste of foods to have a number of dimensions or qualities, the elderly scaled food tastes on a single pleasant/unpleasant dimension. Although food tastes are often different to elderly persons as a result of normal aging, diseases, and medications, older individuals often attribute the altered perception to the food itself, stating the food does not taste as good as or flavorful as it used to in "the good old days" (when they were young).

2.1.4. EFFECT OF MEDICATIONS AND DISEASE ON TASTE PERCEPTION

There are many diseases or medical conditions that potentially affect the sense of taste (Table 1). Medical conditions such as Bell's palsy, multiple sclerosis, and head injury may impair the sense of taste by affecting nerves that transmit taste information to the brain. Other diseases may affect the sense of taste through nutritional or metabolic disturbances, such as nutritional deficiencies of B vitamins or zinc, cancer, renal failure, and liver disease. Cancer and its treatments (radiation and chemotherapy) can often cause profound effects on taste and appetite. Changes in both detection and recognition thresholds have been observed in patients with cancer as well as many other medical conditions *(16,18)*. Changes in recognition thresholds can be due either to hypogeusia, in which taste stimuli are perceived as being weaker in intensity, or to dysgeusia, in which the taste is distorted or changed. Patients with cancer who experience taste changes are more likely to lose weight, experience food aversions, and have tumor progression *(43)*. Although cancer patients of all ages experience these changes, elderly cancer patients are more affected by taste side effects because of lower nutritional and body mass reserves. Decreases in the taste intensity of food and food ingredients can also have medical consequences for certain subsets of the population including diabetic and hypertensive patients. A common response to not perceiving sweet or salty aspects of food is to add more sugar or salt to compensate. This can reduce compliance with a carbohydrate-controlled or low-sodium diet.

Over 250 medications are associated with taste side effects (Table 2). This is the most complete compilation of medications that affect taste (along with other sensory side-effects) with which we are familiar. Medications that frequently have taste side effects include those with sulfydryl groups (e.g., captopril), medications used to treat HIV infec-

Table 1
Representative Medical Conditions That Have
Been Reported to Affect the Senses of Taste and/or Smell

Classification	Disorder
Nervous	Alzheimer's Disease, Bell's palsy, damage to chorda tympani, Down's syndrome, epilepsy, Guillain-Barré syndrome, familial dysautonomia, head trauma, Korsakoff's syndrome, multiple sclerosis, Parkinson's Disease, Raeder's paratrigeminal syndrome, tumors and lesions
Nutritional	Cancer, chronic renal failure, liver disease including cirrhosis, niacin (vitamin B_3) deficiency, thermal burn, vitamin B_{12} deficiency, zinc deficiency
Endocrine	Adrenal cortical insufficiency, congenital adrenal hyperplasia, Cretinism, Cushing's syndrome, diabetes mellitus, hypothyroidism, gonadal dysgenesis (Turner's syndrome), Kallman's syndrome, pseudohypoparathyroidism
Local	Allergic rhinitis, atopy, and bronchial asthma, glossitis and other oral disorders, leprosy, oral aspects of Crohn's disease, radiation therapy, Sjögren's syndrome, sinusitis, and polyposis
Viral and infectious	Acute viral hepatitis, HIV infections, influenza-like infections
Other	Amyloidosis and sarcoidosis, cystic fibrosis, high altitude, hypertension, laryngectomy, psychiatric disorders

Adapted from ref. *16*.

tion, and antibiotics. The main categories of complaints include distorted taste (e.g., taste perversion, taste alteration), an unpleasant taste (e.g., metallic, bitter, medicinal, acid, salty), and loss of taste (e.g., decreased taste, hypogeusia, ageusia). Dry mouth is the most common oral side effect and is sometimes but not always associated with decreased salivation. Oral side effects of drugs including dry mouth have been reviewed by Smith and Burtner *(44)* and Sreebny and Schwartz *(45)*. Other oral complaints from drugs include inflammation and ulceration (e.g., glossitis, gingivitis, stomatitis), as well as oral bleeding.

The potential for medication-induced taste disorders in an elderly population is immense owing to the extensive use of prescription drugs. Epidemiological studies suggest that that the mean number of medications used by community-dwelling elderly

Table 2
Drugs That Interfere with the Taste System

Classification/drug	Side effects						
	Taste	Smell	Other oral/nasal conditions	Vision	Hearing	Somathesis sense	Cognitive
AIDS- & HIV-related therapeutic drugs							
Didanosine (Videx) (95,137)	Distorted[a]	–	Dryness	Dry eyes Opthalmologic disorder Other	Inflammation	Peripheral neuropathy	–
Lamivudine (Epiver) (95,137)	Distorted[a]	–	Other	–	–	Abnormal touch sensation Peripheral neuropathy	Clinical psychiatric disorder Dizziness/vertigo Insomnia
Nevirapine (Viramune) (95,137)	Distorted[a]	–	Inflammation	–	–	Abnormal touch sensation Peripheral neuropathy	–
Stavudine (Zerit) (95,137)	Distorted[a]	–	–	–	–	Abnormal touch sensation Peripheral neuropathy	Insomnia

216

Drug	Taste	Smell	Mouth	Vision	Hearing	Peripheral neuropathy	Clinical psychiatric disorder
Zalcitabine (Hivid) (95)	Distorted; Loss	Distorted	Bleeding, Dryness, Inflammation, Saliva, Other	Abnormal vision, Blurred vision/pupil dilation, Dry eyes, Inflammation, Loss, Other	Loss, Tinnitus, Other	Peripheral neuropathy	Clinical psychiatric disorder, Disorientation/confusion, Dizziness/vertigo, Memory loss, Other
Zidovudine (Retrovir and Retrovir IV) (95,137)	Distorted[b]	—	Bleeding, Inflammation	Abnormal vision	Loss	Abnormal touch sensation	Clinical psychiatric disorder, Confusion, Dizziness, Vertigo, Insomnia, Memory loss, Other
AIDS- & HIV-related therapeutic drugs: Protease Inhibitors							
Indinavir (Crixivan) (95,138)	Distorted[b]	—	Dryness	—	—	—	Dizziness, Vertigo, Insomnia, Other
Nelfinavir (Viracept) (95,138)	Distorted[a]	—	Inflammation	Inflammation, Other	—	Abnormal touch sensation	Clinical psychiatry disorder, Dizziness/vertigo, Insomnia, Other

(continued)

[a] Indicates that the taste was distorted when the drug was applied directly to the tongue.

[b] Indicates that taste was distorted both when applied directly to the tongue or given by mouth. The term "other" in the tables refers to sensory losses that are not easily categorized as loss or distortion.

Table 2 (*Continued*)
Drugs That Interfere with the Taste System

Classification/drug	Side effects						
	Taste	Smell	Other oral/nasal conditions	Vision	Hearing	Somathesis sense	Cognitive
Ritonavir (Norvir) (95,138)	Loss; Distorted[a]	Distorted	Dryness Inflammation Other	Abnormal vision Blurred vision/ pupil dilation Inflammation Loss Other	Loss Tinnitus Other	Abnormal touch sensation Peripheral neuropathy	Clinical psychiatric disorder Disorientation/ confusion Dizziness/vertigo Insomnia Memory loss Other
Saquinavir (Invirase) (95,138)	Distorted	—	Dryness Inflammation Other	Abnormal vision Dry eyes Inflammation Other	Inflammation Loss Tinnitus Other	Abnormal touch sensation Peripheral neuropathy	Clinical psychiatric disorder Disorientation/ confusion Dizziness/vertigo Insomnia Memory loss Other
Amebicides and anthelmintics							
Metronidazole (Metrogel-vaginal, Protostat, Flagyl, Flagyl IV) (95,139,140)	Distorted	—	Dryness Inflammation Other	—	—	Abnormal touch sensation Peripheral neuropathy	Clinical psychiatric disorder Disorientation/ confusion

218

Drug						
Niclosamide (Niclocide) (95)	Other	Other	—	—	Abnormal touch sensation	Dizziness/vertigo Insomnia Other
Niridazole (141)	Distorted	—	—	—	—	Dizziness/vertigo Other
Anesthetics Benzocaine (Americaine) (95)	—	—	—	—	Abnormal touch sensation	—
Dibucaine hydrochloride (142)	Distorted	—	—	—	—	—
Euprocin (142)	Distorted	—	—	—	—	—
Lidocaine (Elamax cream) (95,143)	—	—	Blurred vision/pupil dilation	Tinnitus	Abnormal touch sensation	Clinical psychiatric disorder Disorientation/confusion Dizziness/vertigo Other
Procaine hydrochloride (Novocain) (95,142)	—	—	Blurred vision/pupil dilation	—	—	Dizziness/vertigo
Propofol (Diprivan) (95)	Distorted	Dryness Saliva	Abnormal vision Other	Inflammation Tinnitus Other	Abnormal touch sensation Peripheral neuropathy	Clinical psychiatric disorder Disorientation/confusion Dizziness/vertigo Insomnia Other

(continued)

Table 2 (*Continued*)
Drugs That Interfere with the Taste System

Classification/drug	Side effects						
	Taste	Smell	Other oral/nasal conditions	Vision	Hearing	Somathesis sense	Cognitive
Tropacocaine (142)	Distorted	—	—	—	—	—	—
Anticholesteremic and antilipidemics							
Atorvastatin calcium (Lipitor) (95)	Distorted Loss	Distorted	Bleeding Dryness Inflammation	Abnormal vision Dry eyes Inflammation Ophthalmologic disorder	Loss Tinnitus	Abnormal touch sensation Peripheral neuropathy	Clinical psychiatric disorder Dizziness/vertigo Insomnia Memory loss Other
Cholestyramine (Questran and Questran Light) (95)	Distorted	—	Bleeding Other	Inflammation	Tinnitus	Abnormal touch sensation	Clinical psychiatric disorder Dizziness/vertigo Other
Clofibrate (Atromid-S) (95,144)	Loss	—	Inflammation	Blurred vision/ pupil dilation	—	Abnormal touch	Dizziness/vertigo Other sensation
Fluvastatin sodium (Lescol) (95)	Distorted	—	Dryness Inflammation Other	Ophthalmologic disorder Other	—	Abnormal touch sensation Peripheral neuropathy	Clinical psychiatric disorder Dizziness/vertigo Insomnia Memory loss

Drug						
Gemfibrozil (Lopid) (95)	Distorted	—	—	Blurred vision	—	Abnormal touch sensation Peripheral neuropathy	Clinical psychiatric disorder Disorientation/confusion Dizziness/vertigo Other
Lovastatin (Mevacor) (95)	Distorted	—	Dryness	Abnormal vision Ophthalmologic disorder Blurred vision Other	—	Abnormal touch sensation Peripheral neuropathy	Clinical psychiatric disorder Dizziness/vertigo Insomnia Memory loss Other
Pravastatin sodium (Pravachol) (95)	Distorted	—	Dryness Inflammation	Ophthalmologic disorder Other	—	Abnormal touch sensation Peripheral neuropathy	Clinical psychiatric disorder Dizziness/vertigo Insomnia Memory loss Other
Probucol (Lorelco) (95)	Loss	Loss	—	Blurred vision/pupil dilation Inflammation	Tinnitus	Abnormal touch sensation Peripheral neuropathy	Dizziness/vertigo Insomnia
Simvastatin (Zocor) (95)	Distorted	—	Dryness	Ophthalmologic disorder Other	—	Abnormal touch sensation Peripheral neuropathy	Clinical psychiatric disorder Dizziness/vertigo Insomnia Memory loss Other

(continued)

221

Table 2 (*Continued*)
Drugs That Interfere with the Taste System

				Side effects			
Classification/drug	Taste	Smell	Other oral/nasal conditions	Vision	Hearing	Somathesis sense	Cognitive
Anticoagulants							
Phenindione (145)	Distorted	–	–	–	–	–	–
Warfarin sodium (Coumadin) (95)	Distorted	–	–	–	–	Abnormal touch sensation	Dizziness Other
Antihistamines							
Chlorpheniramine maleate (Atrohist) (16)	–	–	Dryness	Abnormal vision Blurred vision/ pupil dilation	Tinnitus	–	Dizziness/vertigo Insomnia Other
Loratadine (Claritin) (95)	Distorted	–	Dryness Inflammation Saliva Other	Blurred vision/ pupil dilation Inflammation Other	Tinnitus Other	Abnormal touch sensation	Clinical psychiatric disorder Disorientation/ confusion Dizziness/vertigo Insomnia Memory loss Other
Terfenadine and pseudoephedrine (Seldane-D) (95)	Distorted	–	Dryness Inflammation	Blurred vision	–	–	Clinical psychiatric disorder Dizziness/vertigo Disorientation/ confusion Insomnia Other

222

Antimicrobial agents

Drug							
Amphotericin B (Abelcet) (95,146)	Loss, Distorted	—	—	—	—	—	Dizziness/vertigo
Ampicillin (Omnipen) (95,147)	Loss	—	Inflammation	—	—	—	—
Atovaquone (Mepron) (95)	Distorted	—	Inflammation, Other	—	—	Abnormal touch sensation	Clinical psychiatric disorder, Dizziness/vertigo, Insomnia
Aztreonam (Azactam) (95)	Distorted	—	Inflammation, Other	Abnormal vision	Tinnitus	Abnormal touch sensation	Disorientation/confusion, Dizziness/vertigo, Insomnia
Bleomycin (Blenoxane) (95,148)	Loss	—	Inflammation	—	—	—	Disorientation/confusion
Carbenicillin indanyl sodium (Geocillin) (95)	Distorted	—	Dryness, Inflammation, Other	Other	—	—	—
Cefamandole (Mandol) (95,149)	Distorted	—	—	—	—	—	—
Cefpodoxime proxetil (Vantin) (95)	Distorted	—	Inflammation, Saliva	Other	Tinnitus	—	Clinical psychiatric disorder, Dizziness/vertigo, Insomnia, Other
Ceftriaxone sodium (Rocephin) (95)	Distorted	—	—	—	—	Abnormal touch sensation	Dizziness/vertigo
Cefuroxime axetil (Ceftin) (95)	Other	—	Inflammation	—	Inflammation	Abnormal touch sensation	Dizziness/vertigo, Other

(*continued*)

Table 2 (*Continued*)
Drugs That Interfere with the Taste System

				Side effects				
Classification/drug	Taste	Smell	Other oral/nasal conditions	Vision	Hearing	Somathesis sense	Cognitive
Cinoxacin (Cinobac) (95)	Distorted	—	—	Abnormal vision	Tinnitus	Abnormal touch sensation	Dizziness/vertigo Insomnia Other
Ciprofloxacin (Cipro, Cipro IV, Cipro IV Pharmacy Bulk, Ciloxan) (95,139)	Distorted Loss	Loss	Dryness Inflammation Other	Abnormal vision Blurred vision/ pupil dilation Loss Other	Loss Tinnitus	Abnormal touch sensation	Clinical psychiatric disorder Disorientation/ confusion Dizziness/vertigo Insomnia Other
Clarithromycin (Biaxin) (95)	Distorted	Distorted	Inflammation Other	—	Loss Tinnitus	Abnormal touch sensation	Clinical psychiatric disorder Disorientation/ confusion Dizziness/vertigo Insomnia Other
Clindamycin phosphate (Cleocin phosphate) (95)	Distorted	—	—	—	—	Abnormal touch sensation	Dizziness/vertigo

224

Drug						
Clofazimine (Lamprene) (95)	Other	—	Dry eyes Loss Other	—	Abnormal touch sensation Peripheral neuropathy	Clinical psychiatric disorder Dizziness/vertigo Other
Dapsone (95)	Distorted	—	Blurred vision/pupil dilation Opthalmologic disorder	Tinnitus	Peripheral neuropathy	Clinical psychiatric disorder Dizziness/vertigo Insomnia
Enoxacin (Penetrex) (95)	Distorted	Dryness Inflammation	Abnormal vision Inflammation	Tinnitus	Abnormal touch sensation	Clinical psychiatric disorder Disorientation/confusion Dizziness/vertigo Insomnia Memory loss Other
Ethambutol hydrochloride (Myambutol) (95,146)	Distorted	—	Loss Ophthalmologic disorder	—	Abnormal touch sensation Peripheral neuropathy	Clinical psychiatric disorder Disorientation/confusion Dizziness/vertigo Other
Griseofulvin (Fulvicin) (95,150)	Loss	Other	—	—	Abnormal touch sensation	Disorientation/confusion Dizziness/vertigo Insomnia Other

(continued)

Table 2 (*Continued*)
Drugs That Interfere with the Taste System

Classification/drug	Side effects						
	Taste	Smell	Other oral/nasal conditions	Vision	Hearing	Somathesis sense	Cognitive
Imipenem-cilastatin sodium (Primaxin IM, Primaxin IV) (95)	Distorted	—	Inflammation Saliva Other	—	Loss Tinnitus	Abnormal touch sensation	Clinical psychiatric disorder Disorientation/ confusion Dizziness/vertigo Other
Lincomycin HCl (95,144)	Loss	—	Inflammation	—	Tinnitus	—	Dizziness/vertig
Lomefloxacin HCl (Maxaquin) (95	Distorted	—	Dryness Inflammation Saliva Other	Abnormal vision Dry eyes Inflammation Other	Tinnitus Other	Abnormal touch sensation	Clinical psychiatric disorder Disorientation/ confusion Dizziness/vertigo Insomnia Other
Mezlocillin sodium (Mezlin, Mezlin Bulk) (95)	Distorted	—	—	—	—	Abnormal touch sensation	Other
Norfloxacin (Chibroxin, Noroxin) (95)	Distorted	—	Dryness Inflammation	Abnormal vision Blurred vision/ pupil dilation Other	Loss Tinnitus	Abnormal touch sensation Peripheral neuropathy	Clinical psychiatric disorder Disorientation/ confusion

226

							Dizziness/vertigo Insomnia Other
Ofloxacin (Floxin Floxin IV) *(95)*	Distorted	Distorted	Dryness Other	Abnormal vision Blurred vision/ pupil dilation Other	Loss Tinnitus	Abnormal touch sensation Peripheral neuropathy	Clinical psychiatric disorder Disorientation confusion Dizziness/vertigo Insomnia Memory loss Other
Pentamidine isethionate (NebuPent, Pentam 300) *(95)*	Distorted Loss	Loss	Dryness	Blurred vision/ pupil dilation Inflammation Other	–	Peripheral neuropath	Disorientation/ confusion Dizziness/vertigo
Piperacillin and tazobactam sodium (Zosyn, Zosyn Pharmacy Bulk) *(95)*	Distorted	–	Inflammation Other	Abnormal vision Inflammation	Loss Tinnitus Other	Abnormal touch sensation	Clinical psychiatric disorder Disorientation/ confusion Dizziness/vertigo Insomnia Other
Pyrimethamine (Daraprim) *(95,151)*	Distorted[a]	–	Inflammation	–	–	–	
Rifabutin (Mycobutin) *(95)*	Distorted	–	–	Inflammation	–	Abnormal touch sensation	Disorientation/ confusion Dizziness/vertigo Insomnia

(*continued*)

Table 2 (*Continued*)
Drugs That Interfere with the Taste System

Classification/drug	Side effects						
	Taste	Smell	Other oral/nasal conditions	Vision	Hearing	Somathesis sense	Cognitive
Sulfamethoxazole (Bactrim, Septra) (95,151)	Distorted[a]	—	Inflammation	—	Tinnitus	Abnormal touch sensation Peripheral neuropathy	Clinical psychiatric disorder Disorientation/confusion Dizziness/vertigo Insomnia Other
Tetracyclines (Achromycin V) (16,95,152,153)	Distorted	—	Inflammation	Abnormal vision	Tinnitus	—	Dizziness/vertigo
Ticarcillin disodium and clavulanate potassium (Timentin) (95)	Distorted	Distorted	Inflammation	—	—	Abnormal touch sensation	Other
Tyrothricin (154)	Distorted	—	—	—	—	—	—
Antiproliferative, including immuno-suppressive agents Azathioprine (95,146)	Distorted Loss	—	—	—	—	—	—
Carmustine (BiCNU, Gliadel Wafer) (95,155)	Distorted Other	—	—	Abnormal vision Loss Other	—	—	Clinical psychiatric disorder Disorientation/confusion

228

Drug					
Cisplatin (Platinol) (95,151)	Distorted	—	Abnormal vision Blurred vision/ pupil dilation Loss Ophthalmologic disorder	Loss Tinnitus	Peripheral neuropathy — Dizziness/vertigo Insomnia Memory loss Other
Carboplatin (Paraplatin) (95,151)	Distorted	Inflammation	—	Other	Peripheral neuropathy	—
Cyclosporine (Neoral) (95)	Distorted	Bleeding Dryness Inflammation Other	Abnormal vision Inflammation Ophthalmologic disorder Other	Loss Tinnitus	Abnormal touch sensation Peripheral neuropathy	Clinical psychiatric disorder Disorientation/ confusion Dizziness/vertigo Insomnia Other
Doxorubicin and methotrexate (156,157)	Distorted Loss	—	—	—	—	—
Fluorouracil (Efudex) (95)	Distorted	Inflammation Other	Dry eyes Inflammation Other	—	Abnormal touch sensation	Insomnia Other
Interferon alfa-2a (recombinant) (Roferon-A) (95)	Distorted	Bleeding Inflammation Other	Abnormal vision Inflammation Loss Other	Tinnitus Other	Abnormal touch sensation Peripheral neuropathy	Clinical psychiatric disorder Disorientation/ confusion Dizziness/vertigo Insomnia Memory loss Other

(continued)

Table 2 (*Continued*)
Drugs That Interfere with the Taste System

Classification/drug				Side effects			
	Taste	Smell	Other oral/nasal conditions	Vision	Hearing	Somathesis sense	Cognitive
Interferon alfa-2b (recombinant) (Intron A) (95)	Distorted Loss	Distorted	Dryness Inflammation	Abnormal vision Blurred vision/ pupil dilation Dry eyes Inflammation Other	Inflammation Loss Tinnitus	Abnormal touch sensation Peripheral neuropathy	Clinical psychiatric disorder Disorientation/ confusion Dizziness/vertigo Memory loss Other
Vincristine sulfate (Onocovin) (95,158)	Other	—	Inflammation	Loss Ophthalmologic disorder Other	Inflammation Loss	Abnormal touch sensation	Dizziness/vertigo
Antirheumatic, antiarthritic, analgesic-anti-pyretic, and anti-inflammatory							
Auranofin (Ridaura) (95)	Distorted	—	Inflammation	Inflammation Other	—	Peripheral neuropathy Abnormal touch sensation	Dizziness/vertigo
Aurothioglucose (Solganal) (95)	Distorted	—	Inflammation	Inflammation Other	—	Abnormal touch sensation Peripheral neuropathy	Other

230

Benoxaprofen (*139*)	Distorted	—	—	—	—	—	—	—
Butorphanol tartrate (Stadol, Stadol NS) (*95*)	Distorted	—	Dryness Inflammation Other	Blurred vision/ pupil dilation	—	Tinnitus Other	Abnormal touch sensation	Clinical psychiatric disorder Disorientation/ confusion Dizziness/vertigo Insomnia Other
Choline magnesium tri-salicylate (Trilisate) (*95,151*)	Distorted	—	—	—	—	Loss Tinnitus	Abnormal touch sensation	Disorientation/ confusion Dizziness/vertigo Other
Colchicine (ColBENEMID) (*95,159*)	Loss	—	Inflammation	—	—	—	Peripheral neuropathy Abnormal touch sensation	Dizziness/vertigo
Dexamethasone (Decadron) (*95,160*)	Distorted	—	—	Ophthalmologic disorder Other	—	—	—	Clinical psychiatric disorder Dizziness/vertigo
Diclofenac potassium/ diclofenac sodium (Cataflam/ Voltaren) (*95*)	Distorted	—	Dryness Inflammation	Abnormal vision Blurred vision/ pupil dilation Loss Other	—	Loss Tinnitus	Abnormal touch sensation	Clinical psychiatric disorder Dizziness/vertigo Insomnia Memory loss Other
Dimethyl sulfoxide (Rimso-50) (*95*)	Distorted	—	—	—	—	—	—	—

(*continued*)

Table 2 (*Continued*)
Drugs That Interfere with the Taste System

				Side effects			
Classification/drug	Taste	Smell	Other oral/nasal conditions	Vision	Hearing	Somathesis sense	Cognitive
Etodolac (Lodine) (95)	Distorted	—	Dryness Inflammation	Abnormal vision Blurred vision/ pupil dilation Inflammation	Tinnitus Loss	Abnormal touch sensation	Clinical psychiatric disorder Disorientation/ confusion Dizziness/vertigo Insomnia Other
Fenoprofen calcium (Nalfon) (95)	Distorted	—	Dryness Inflammation Other	Abnormal vision Blurred vision/ pupil dilation Ophthalmologic disorder	Loss Tinnitus	Abnormal touch sensation	Clinical psychiatric disorder Disorientation/ confusion Dizziness/vertigo Other
Flurbiprofen (Ansaid) (95)	Distorted	Distorted	Dryness Inflammation	Abnormal vision Inflammation Ophthalmologic disorder Other	Loss Tinnitus Other	Abnormal touch sensation	Clinical psychiatric disorder Disorientation/ confusion Dizziness/vertigo Insomnia Memory loss Other

Drug	Taste		Smell/Nasal	Eyes	Ears	Touch	CNS/Mental
Gold (146) Gold sodium thiomalate (Myochrysine) (95)	Distorted	—	Inflammation	Inflammation Other	—	Peripheral neuropathy Abnormal touch sensation	Disorientation/ confusion Dizziness/vertigo Other
Hydrocortisone (Hydrocortone) (95,160)	Loss	—	—	Ophthalmologic disorder Other	—	—	Clinical psychiatric disorder Dizziness/vertigo
Hydromorphone HCl (Dilaudid, Dilaudid-HP) (95)	Distorted	—	Dryness	Abnormal vision Blurred vision/ pupil dilation Other	—	Abnormal touch sensation	Clinical psychiatric disorder Dizziness/vertigo Insomnia Memory loss Other
Ibuprofen (Motrin) (95,151)	Distorted[a]	—	Dryness Inflammation	Abnormal vision Dry eyes Inflammation Loss Ophthalmologic disorder	Loss Tinnitus	Abnormal touch sensation	Clinical psychiatric disorder Disorientation/ confusion Dizziness/vertigo Insomnia Other
Ketoprofen (Orudis) (95)	Distorted	—	Dryness Inflammation	Abnormal vision Inflammation Ophthalmologic disorder Other	Loss Tinnitus	Abnormal touch sensation	Clinical psychiatric disorder Disorientation/ confusion Dizziness/vertigo Memory loss Other

(continued)

Table 2 (*Continued*)
Drugs That Interfere with the Taste System

Classification/drug	Side effects						
	Taste	Smell	Other oral/nasal conditions	Vision	Hearing	Somathesis sense	Cognitive
Ketorolac tromethamine (Toradol) (95)	Distorted	—	Dryness Inflammation	Abnormal vision Blurred vision/ dilation of pupil	Loss Tinnitus	Abnormal touch sensation	Clinical psychiatric disorder Dizziness/vertigo Insomnia Other
Morphine sulfate (MS Contin, MSIR, Oramorph SR) (95)	Distorted	—	Dryness	Abnormal vision Blurred vision/ pupil dilation Other	—	Abnormal touch sensation	Clinical psychiatric disorder Disorientation/ confusion Dizziness/vertigo Insomnia Other
Nabumetone (Relafen) (95)	Distorted	—	Dryness Inflammation	Abnormal vision	Tinnitus	Abnormal touch sensation	Clinical psychiatric disorder Disorientation/ confusion Dizziness/vertigo Insomnia Other
Nalbuphine HCl (Nubain) (95)	Distorted	—	Dryness	Blurred vision/ pupil dilation	—	Abnormal touch sensation	Clinical psychiatric disorder Disorientation/ confusion

Oxycodone HCl (OxyContin) (95)	Distorted	—	Dryness Inflammation	Abnormal vision	Tinnitus	Abnormal touch sensation	Dizziness/vertigo Other Clinical psychiatric disorder Disorientation/confusion Dizziness/vertigo Insomnia Memory loss Other
Oxaprozin (Daypro) (95)	Distorted	—	Inflammation	Blurred vision/pupil dilation Inflammation	Loss Tinnitus	Abnormal touch sensation	Clinical psychiatric disorder Disorientation/confusion Other
D-penicillamine and penicillamine (Cuprimine, Depen) (95,139,161,162)	Loss	—	Inflammation	Abnormal vision Ophthalmologic disorder	Tinnitus	Abnormal touch sensation Peripheral neuropathy	Clinical psychiatric disorder
Pentazocine HCl (Talwin) (95,151)	Distorted	—	—	Blurred vision/pupil dilation	Tinnitus	Abnormal touch sensation	Clinical psychiatric disorder Disorientation/confusion Dizziness/vertigo Insomnia Other

(continued)

Table 2 (*Continued*)
Drugs That Interfere with the Taste System

Classification/drug	Side effects							
	Taste	Smell	Other oral/nasal conditions	Vision	Hearing	Somathesis sense	Cognitive	
Phenylbutazone (*146*)	Distorted	–	–	–	–	–	–	
Piroxicam (Feldene) (*95,139*)	Other	–	Dryness Inflammation	Blurred vision/ pupil dilation Inflammation Other	Loss Tinnitus	Abnormal touch sensation	Clinical psychiatric disorder Disorientation/ confusion Dizziness/vertigo Insomnia Other	
Salicylates (*163,164*)	Other	–	–	–	–	–	–	
Sulindac (Clinoril) (*95*)	Distorted Loss		Dryness Inflammation	Abnormal vision Blurred vision/ pupil dilation Ophthalmologic disorder	Loss Tinnitus	Abnormal touch sensation Peripheral neuropathy	Clinical psychiatric disorder Dizziness/vertigo Insomnia Other	
Sumatriptan succinate (Imitrex) (*95*)	Distorted	Distorted	Bleeding Inflammation Saliva Other	Abnormal vision Blurred vision/ pupil dilation Dry eyes Inflammation Loss Ophthalmologic disorder Other	Inflammation Loss Tinnitus Other	Abnormal touch sensation Peripheral neuropathy	Clinical psychiatric disorder Disorientation/ confusion Dizziness/vertigo Memory loss Other	

236

5-thiopyridoxine (165)	Loss	—	—	—	—	—	—	—	—
Antiseptics									
Hexetidine (166)	Distorted	—	—	—	—	—	—	—	—
Antispasmodics, irritable bowel syndrome									
Dicyclomine HCl (Bentyl) (95)	Loss	—	Dryness	Abnormal vision/Blurred vision/pupil dilation/Ophthalmologic disorder/Other	—	—	Abnormal touch sensation	—	Disorientation/confusion, Dizziness/vertigo, Insomnia, Other
Oxybutynin Chloride (Ditropan) (95,139)	Distorted	—	Dryness	Abnormal vision/Blurred vision/pupil dilation/Other	—	—	—	—	Dizziness/vertigo, Insomnia, Other
Phenobarbital + hyoscyamine SO_4 + atropine SO_4 + Scopolamine hydrobromide (Donnatal, Donnatal Extentabs) (95)	Loss	—	Dryness	Blurred vision/pupil dilation/Ophthalmologic disorder	—	—	—	—	Dizziness/vertigo, Insomnia, Other
Antithyroid agents									
Carbimazole (167)	Distorted	—	—	—	—	—	—	—	—
Methimazole (Tapazole) (95,167,168)	Loss	—	—	—	—	—	Abnormal touch sensation, Peripheral neuropathy	—	Dizziness/vertigo, Other

(continued)

Table 2 (*Continued*)
Drugs That Interfere with the Taste System

Classification/drug	Side effects						
	Taste	Smell	Other oral/nasal conditions	Vision	Hearing	Somathesis sense	Cognitive
Methylthiouracil (*169*)	Distorted	–	–	–	–	–	–
Propylthiouracil (*170*)	Distorted	–	–	–	–	–	–
Thiouracil (*146*)	Distorted	–	–	–	–	–	–
Antiulcerative							
Clidinium bromide (Quarzan) (*95*)	Loss	–	Dryness	Blurred vision/pupil dilation Ophthalmologic disorder	–	–	Disorientation/confusion Dizziness/vertigo Insomnia Other
Famotidine (Pepcid) (*95*)	Distorted	–	Dryness	Inflammation	Tinnitus	Abnormal touch sensation	Clinical psychiatric disorder Disorientation/confusion Dizziness/vertigo Insomnia Other
Glycopyrrolate (Robinul) (*95*)	Loss	–	Dryness	Blurred vision/pupil dilation Ophthalmologic disorder Other	–	–	Clinical psychiatric disorder Disorientation/confusion Dizziness/vertigo Insomnia Other

Hyoscyamine sulfate (Levsin, Levsinex) (95)	Loss	—	Dryness	Blurred vision/pupil dilation; Ophthalmologic disorder; Other	—	—	Disorientation/confusion; Dizziness/vertigo; Insomnia; Other
Mesalamine (Asacol) (95)	Distorted	—	Dryness; Inflammation	Abnormal vision; Blurred vision/pupil dilation; Inflammation; Other	Tinnitus; Other	Abnormal touch sensation; Peripheral neuropathy	Clinical psychiatric disorder; Disorientation/confusion; Dizziness/vertigo; Insomnia; Other
Misoprostol (Cytotec) (95)	Distorted	—	Inflammation	Abnormal vision; Inflammation	Loss; Tinnitus; Other	Peripheral neuropathy	Clinical psychiatric disorder; Disorientation/confusion; Dizziness/vertigo; Insomnia; Other
Omeprazole (Prilosec) (95)	Distorted	—	Dryness; Inflammation; Other	—	Tinnitus	Abnormal touch sensation	Clinical psychiatric disorder; Disorientation/confusion; Dizziness/vertigo; Insomnia; Other
Propantheline bromide (Pro-Banthine) (95)	Loss	—	Dryness	Blurred vision/pupil dilation; Ophthalmologic disorder; Other	—	—	Disorientation/confusion; Dizziness/vertigo; Insomnia; Other

(continued)

Table 2 (*Continued*)
Drugs That Interfere with the Taste System

Classification/drug	Side effects						
	Taste	Smell	Other oral/nasal conditions	Vision	Hearing	Somathesis sense	Cognitive
Sulfasalazine (Azulfidine) (95,146)	Distorted	–	–	–	–	–	–
Antiviral							
Acyclovir (Zovirax) (95,151)	Distorted[a]	–	–	Abnormal vision	–	Abnormal touch sensation	Disorientation/confusion Dizziness/vertigo Other
Foscarnet sodium (Foscavir) (95)	Distorted	–	Dryness Inflammation	Abnormal vision Inflammation Other	–	Abnormal touch sensation Peripheral neuropathy	Clinical psychiatric disorder Disorientation/confusion Dizziness/vertigo Insomnia Memory loss Other
Idoxuridine (171)	Distorted	–	–	–	–	–	
Interferon alfa-n3 (Alferon N) (95)	Distorted	–	Dryness Inflammation Saliva Other	Abnormal vision Blurred vision/pupil dilation Other	Tinnitus	Abnormal touch sensation	Clinical psychiatric disorder Disorientation/confusion Dizziness/vertigo Insomnia Other

240

Drug	Taste	Mouth	Eyes	Ears	Touch	CNS/Psychiatric
Interferon beta-1b (Betaseron) (95)	Distorted Loss	Dryness Inflammation Saliva Other	Abnormal vision/ Blurred vision/ pupil dilation Dry eyes Inflammation Loss Ophthalmologic disorder Other	Inflammation Loss Other	Abnormal touch sensation Peripheral neuropathy	Clinical psychiatric disorder Disorientation/confusion Dizziness/vertigo Memory loss Other
Rimantadine HCl (Flumadine) (95)	Distorted Loss	Dryness Inflammation	Other	Tinnitus	Abnormal touch sensation	Clinical psychiatric disorder Disorientation/confusion Dizziness/vertigo Insomnia Other
Agents for dental hygiene						
Sodium fluoride (Florical) (95,172)	Distorted	—	—	—	—	—
Sodium lauryl sulfate (146,173)	Distorted	—	—	—	—	—
Chlorhexidine digluconate mouthrinses (Peridex) (95,174)	Distorted	—	—	—	—	—
Bronchodilators and anti-asthmatic drugs						
Albuterol sulfate (Ventolin, Volmax, Proventil) (95)	Distorted	Dryness Inflammation Other	—	Tinnitus	—	Clinical psychiatric disorder Dizziness/vertigo Insomnia Other

(continued)

Table 2 (*Continued*)
Drugs That Interfere with the Taste System

Classification/drug	Side effects						
	Taste	*Smell*	*Other oral/nasal conditions*	*Vision*	*Hearing*	*Somathesis sense*	*Cognitive*
Beclomethasone dipropionate (Beconase) (95,139)	Distorted Loss	Distorted Loss	Dryness Inflammation Other	Ophthalmologic disorder	–	Abnormal touch sensation	Clinical psychiatric disorder Dizziness/vertigo
Bitolterol mesylate (Tornalate) (95, 151)	Other	–	Inflammation	–	–	Abnormal touch sensation	Dizziness/vertigo Insomnia
Cromolyn sodium (Gastrocrom, Intal, Nasal-com) (95)	Distorted	–	Bleeding Inflammation Other	–	Inflammation Tinnitus	Abnormal touch sensation	Clinical psychiatric disorder Dizziness/vertigo Insomnia Other
Ephedrine HCl + phenobarbitol + potassium iodide + theophylline calcium salicylate (Quadrinal) (95)	Distorted	–	Saliva Other	Other	–	–	Clinical psychiatric disorder Disorientation/confusion Dizziness/vertigo Insomnia Other
Flunisolide (AeroBid, AeroBid-M, Nasalide) (95)	Distorted Loss	Loss	Dryness Inflammation Saliva Other	Blurred vision/pupil dilation Inflammation Other	Inflammation Other	Abnormal touch sensation	Clinical psychiatric disorder Dizziness/vertigo Insomnia Other

Drug						
Metaproterenol sulfate (Metaproterenol, Arm-a-Med, Alupent, Metaprel) (95)	Distorted	—	Dryness, Inflammation	—	Blurred vision/pupil dilation	Abnormal touch sensation	Dizziness/vertigo, Insomnia, Other
Nedocromil (Tilade) (95)	Distorted	—	Inflammation, Saliva	—	Inflammation	—	Dizziness/vertigo
Pirbuterol acetate inhalation aerosol (Maxair autohaler & inhaler) (95)	Distorted	Distorted	Dryness, Inflammation, Other	—	—	Abnormal touch sensation	Clinical psychiatric disorder, Disorientation/confusion, Dizziness/vertigo, Insomnia, Other
Terbutaline sulfate (Brethine) (95)	—	—	—	—	—	—	Dizziness/vertigo, Other
Diuretics, antiarrhythmic, antihypertensive, and antifibrillatory agents							
Acetazolamide (Diamox, Diamox Sequels) (95,175)	Distorted	—	—	Loss, Tinnitus	—	Abnormal touch sensation	Disorientation/confusion, Other
Adenosine (Adenocard) (95)	Distorted	—	—	—	Blurred vision/pupil dilation	Abnormal touch sensation	Dizziness/vertigo, Other
Amiodarone HCl (Cordarone) (95)	Distorted	Distorted	Saliva	—	Abnormal vision, Dry eyes, Loss, Ophthalmologic disorder, Other	Abnormal touch sensation, Peripheral neuropathy	Dizziness/vertigo, Insomnia, Other

(continued)

Table 2 (*Continued*)
Drugs That Interfere with the Taste System

| Classification/drug | Side effects | | | | | | | |
	Taste	Smell	Other oral/nasal conditions	Vision	Hearing	Somathesis sense	Cognitive	
Amiloride and its analogs (Moduretic) (95,139,176,177)	Distorted	—	Dryness Other	Abnormal vision Ophthalmologic disorder	Tinnitus	Abnormal touch sensation	Clinical psychiatric disorder Disorientation/ confusion Dizziness/vertigo Insomnia Other	
Amlodipine besylate (Norvasc) (95)	Distorted	Distorted	Dryness Other	Abnormal vision Inflammation Other	Tinnitus	Abnormal touch sensation	Clinical psychiatric disorder Dizziness/vertigo Insomnia Other Dizziness/vertigo	
Benazepril HCl and hydrochlorothia- zide (Lotensin HCT) (95)	Distorted	—	Inflammation Dryness Other	Abnormal vision Inflammation Blurred vision/ pupil dilation	Tinnitus	Abnormal touch sensation Abnormal touch sensation	Clinical psychiatric disorder Dizziness/vertigo Insomnia Other Dizziness/vertigo	

244

Betaxolol HCl (Kerlone) (95)	Distorted Loss	—	Dryness Inflammation Saliva	Abnormal vision Blurred vision/ pupil dilation Dry eyes Inflammation Loss Ophthalmologic disorder Other	Loss Tinnitus Other	Abnormal touch sensation Peripheral neuropathy	Clinical psychiatric disorder Disorientation/ confusion Dizziness/vertigo Insomnia Memory loss Other
Bisoprolol fumarate and bisoprolol fumarate with hydrochlorothiazide (Zebeta, Ziac) (95)	Distorted	—	Dryness Inflammation	Abnormal vision Ophthalmologic disorder Other	Tinnitus Other	Abnormal touch sensation	Clinical psychiatric disorder Disorientation/ confusion Dizziness/vertigo Insomnia Memory loss Other
Captopril and Captopril/ hydrochlorothiazide (Capoten, Capozide) (95,139,178–180)	Loss	—	Dryness Inflammation	Blurred vision/ pupil dilation	—	Abnormal touch sensation	Clinical psychiatric disorder Disorientation/ confusion Dizziness/vertigo Insomnia Other

(continued)

245

Table 2 (*Continued*)
Drugs That Interfere with the Taste System

				Side effects			
Classification/drug	Taste	Smell	Other oral/nasal conditions	Vision	Hearing	Somathesis sense	Cognitive
Clonidine (Catapres-TTS) (95)	Distorted	–	Dryness	Blurred vision/ pupil dilation Dry eyes Other	–	Abnormal touch sensation	Clinical psychiatric disorder Disorientation/ confusion Dizziness/vertigo Insomnia Other
Diazoxide (Hyperstat IV) (16,95)	Distorted	–	Dryness Saliva	Blurred vision/ pupil dilation Other	Inflammation Loss Tinnitus	–	Disorientation/ confusion Dizziness/vertigo Other
Diltiazem (Cardizem, Cardizem CD and SR) (95,181)	Distorted	–	Dryness Other	Abnormal vision Ophthalmologic disorder Other	Tinnitus	Abnormal touch sensation	Clinical psychiatric disorder Disorientation/ confusion Dizziness/vertigo Insomnia Memory loss Other
Doxazosin mesylate (Cardura) (95)	Distorted	Distorted	Dryness Inflammation	Abnormal vision Inflammation Other	Tinnitus Other	Abnormal touch sensation	Clinical psychiatric disorder Disorientation/ confusion Dizziness/vertigo Insomnia Memory loss Other

Drug	Distorted	Loss	Dryness / Inflammation	Abnormal vision	Tinnitus / Loss	Abnormal touch sensation	Clinical psychiatric disorder
Enalapril (95,139,178) Enalapril maleate (95) (Vaseretic) Enalaprilat (95) (Vasotec IV) Enalapril maleate (95) (Vasotec)	Distorted	Loss — — —	Dryness Inflammation — —	Abnormal vision Blurred vision/pupil dilation Dry eyes Inflammation Other	Tinnitus — — —	Abnormal touch sensation Peripheral neuropathy	Clinical psychiatric disorder Disorientation/confusion Dizziness/vertigo Insomnia Other
Esmolol HCl (Brevibloc) (95)	Distorted	—	Dryness Other	Abnormal vision	Tinnitus —	Abnormal touch sensation	Clinical psychiatric disorder Disorientation/confusion Dizziness/vertigo Other
Ethacrynic acid (Edecrin) (95,182)	Other	—	—	Blurred vision/pupil dilation Other	Loss Tinnitus	—	Disorientation/confusion Dizziness/vertigo Other
Flecainide acetate (Tambocor) (95)	Distorted	—	Inflammation Dryness	Abnormal vision Other	Tinnitus	Abnormal touch sensation Peripheral neuropathy	Clinical psychiatric disorder Disorientation/confusion Dizziness/vertigo Insomnia Memory loss Other
Fosinopril sodium (Monopril) (95)	Distorted	—	Dryness Inflammation Other	Abnormal vision Other	Tinnitus	Abnormal touch sensation	Clinical psychiatric disorder Disorientation/confusion Dizziness/vertigo Insomnia Memory loss Other

(continued)

Table 2 (*Continued*)
Drugs That Interfere with the Taste System

Classification/drug	Taste	Smell	Other oral/nasal conditions	Vision	Hearing	Somathesis sense	Cognitive
Guanfacine HCl (Tenex) (95)	Distorted	—	Dryness Inflammation	Abnormal vision Blurred vision/pupil dilation Inflammation	Tinnitus	Abnormal touch sensation	Clinical psychiatric disorder Disorientation/confusion Dizziness/vertigo Insomnia Memory loss Other
Hydrochlorothiazide (HydroDIURIL) (95,139)	Loss Distorted	—	—	Abnormal vision Blurred vision/pupil dilation	—	Abnormal touch sensation	Dizziness/vertigo Other
Labetalol HCl (Trandate, Normodyne) (95)	Distorted	—	Other	Abnormal vision Dry eyes	—	Abnormal touch sensation	Clinical psychiatric disorder Dizziness/vertigo Memory loss Other
Metolazone (Mykrox) (95)	Distorted	—	Dryness Inflammation Bleeding Other	Blurred vision/pupil dilation Other	Tinnitus	Abnormal touch sensation Peripheral neuropathy	Clinical psychiatric disorder Dizziness/vertigo Other
Mexiletine HCl (Mexitil) (95)	Distorted	—	Dryness Saliva Other	Blurred vision/pupil dilation	Tinnitus	Abnormal touch sensation	Clinical psychiatric disorder Disorientation/confusion Dizziness/vertigo Memory loss

Side effects

Drug							
Moricizine HCl (Ethmozine) (95)	Distorted	—	Dryness Inflammation	Abnormal vision Blurred vis on/pupil dilation Inflammation Other	Tinnitus	Abnormal touch sensation	Clinical psychiatric disorder Disorientation/confusion Dizziness/vertigo Memory loss Other
Nifedipine (Procardia XL) (95,183)	Distorted	—	Dryness Inflammation Other	Abnormal vision Blurred vision/pupil dilation Inflammation Loss Other	Tinnitus	Abnormal touch sensation	Clinical psychiatric disorder Dizziness/vertigo Insomnia Other
Procainamide HCl (Procanbid) (95)	Distorted	—	—	—	—	Abnormal touch sensation	Clinical psychiatric disorder Dizziness/vertigo Other
Propafenone HCl (Rythmol) (95)	Distorted	Distorted	Dryness	Abnormal vision Blurred vision/pupil dilation Other	Tinnitus	Abnormal touch sensation	Clinical psychiatric disorder Disorientation/confusion Dizziness/vertigo Insomnia Memory loss Other
Propranolol HCl (Inderal) (95,139)	Loss Distorted	—	—	Abnormal vision Dry eyes	—	Abnormal touch sensation	Clinical psychiatric disorder Dizziness/vertigo Insomnia Memory loss Other

(continued)

Table 2 (*Continued*)
Drugs That Interfere with the Taste System

Classification/drug	Side effects							
	Taste	Smell	Other oral/nasal conditions	Vision	Hearing	Somathesis sense	Cognitive
Ramipril (Altace) (*95*)	Distorted	–	Dryness Saliva	Abnormal vision	Loss Tinnitus	Abnormal touch sensation Peripheral neuropathy	Clinical psychiatric disorder Dizziness/vertigo Insomnia Memory loss Other
Spironolactone (Aldactazide) (*95,139*)	Loss	–	–	Abnormal vision	–	Abnormal touch sensation	Disorientation/ confusion Dizziness/vertigo Other
Tocainide HCl (Tonocard) (*95*)	Distorted	Distorted	Dryness Inflammation	Abnormal vision Blurred vision/ pupil dilation Other	Loss Tinnitus Other	Abnormal touch sensation	Clinical psychiatric disorder Disorientation/ confusion Dizziness/vertigo Insomnia Memory loss Other

Triamterene/hydro-chlorothiazide (Maxzide) (95)	Distorted	—	Dryness	Abnormal vision Blurred vision/pupil dilation	—	Abnormal touch sensation	Clinical psychiatric disorder Dizziness/vertigo Insomnia Other
Hyper- and Hypoglycemic drugs							
Diazoxide (Hyperstat, Proglycem) (95)	Distorted Loss	—	Dryness Saliva	Blurred vision/ pupil dilation Other Blurred vision/ pupil dilation Ophthalmologic disorder	Inflammation Loss Tinnitus	Abnormal touch sensation	Clinical psychiatric disorder Disorientation/ confusion Dizziness/vertigo Other Clinical psychiatric disorder Dizziness/vertigo Insomnia
Glipizide (Glucotrol) (95,184)	Loss	—	—	—	—	Abnormal touch sensation	Dizziness/vertigo Other
Phenformin and derivatives (146,185)	Distorted	—	—	—	—	—	—

(continued)

251

Table 2 (*Continued*)
Drugs That Interfere with the Taste System

Classification/drug	Side effects						
	Taste	*Smell*	*Other oral/nasal conditions*	*Vision*	*Hearing*	*Somathesis sense*	*Cognitive*
Hypnotics and Sedatives							
Estazolam (ProSom) (95)	Distorted	—	Dryness Inflammation	Abnormal vision Inflammation Loss Other	Loss Tinnitus Other	Abnormal touch sensation Peripheral neuropathy	Clinical psychiatric disorder Disorientation/ confusion Dizziness/vertigo Memory loss Other
Flurazepam HCl (Dalmane) (95,139)	Distorted	—	Dryness Saliva	Blurred vision/ pupil dilation Other	—	Abnormal touch sensation	Clinical psychiatric disorder Disorientation/ confusion Dizziness/vertigo Other
Midazolam HCl (Versed) (95)	Distorted	—	Saliva Other	Abnormal vision Blurred vision/ pupil dilation Other	Other	Abnormal touch sensation	Clinical psychiatric disorder Disorientation/ confusion Dizziness/vertigo Insomnia Memory loss Other

Prochlorperazine (Compazine) (95,151)	Distorted[a]	—	Dryness Other	Blurred vision/ pupil dilation Other	—	—	Clinical psychiatric disorder Dizziness/vertigo Insomnia Other
Promethazine HCl (Phenergan) (95,151)	Distorted[a]	—	Dryness	Blurred vision/ pupil dilation	—	—	Clinical psychiatric disorder Disorientation/ confusion Dizziness/vertigo Other
Quazepam (Doral) (95)	Distorted	—	Dryness	Abnormal vision Ophthalmologic disorder	—	Abnormal touch sensation	Clinical psychiatric disorder Disorientation/ confusion Dizziness/vertigo Memory loss Other
Triazolam (Halcion) (95,139)	Distorted	—	Dryness Inflammation Other	Abnormal vision	Tinnitus	Abnormal touch sensation	Clinical psychiatric disorder Disorientation/ confusion Dizziness/vertigo Insomnia Memory loss Other

(continued)

Table 2 (*Continued*)
Drugs That Interfere with the Taste System

Classification/drug	Taste	Smell	Other oral/nasal conditions	Side effects Vision	Hearing	Somathesis sense	Cognitive
Zolpidem tartrate (Ambien) (95)	Distorted	Distorted	Dryness Inflammation Saliva Other	Abnormal vision Inflammation Ophthalmologic disorder Other	Inflammation Tinnitus	Abnormal touch sensation	Clinical psychiatric disorder Dizziness/vertigo Disorientation/ confusion Insomnia Memory loss Other
Zoplicone (139) *Muscle relaxants and drugs for treatment of Parkinson's disease*	Distorted	–	–	–	–	–	–
Baclofen (Lioresal, Lioresal Intrathecal) (95,146)	Distorted	–	Dryness Other	Abnormal vision Blurred vision/ pupil dilation Other	Tinnitus	Abnormal touch sensation	Clinical psychiatric disorder Disorientation/ confusion Dizziness/vertigo Insomnia Other

254

Drug						
Chlormezanone (Trancopal) (95,146)	Loss Distorted	—	—	—	—	Clinical psychiatric disorder Disorientation/confusion Dizziness/vertigo Other
Cyclobenzaprine HCl (Flexeril) (95)	Distorted Loss	Dryness Inflammation Other	Abnormal vision Blurred vision/ pupil dilation	Inflammation Tinnitus	Abnormal touch sensation Peripheral neuropathy	Clinical psychiatric disorder Disorientation/confusion Dizziness/vertigo Insomnia Other
Dantrolene sodium (Dantrium) (95)	Distorted	—	Abnormal vision Other	—	—	Clinical psychiatric disorder Disorientation/confusion Dizziness/vertigo Insomnia Other
Levodopa (Atamet, Dopar, Larodopa) (95,186)	Distorted	Dryness Other	Abnormal vision Blurred vision/ pupil dilation Other	—	—	Clinical psychiatric disorder Disorientation/confusion Dizziness/vertigo Insomnia Other
Methocarbamol (Robaxin) (95,151)	Distorted Other	—	Abnormal vision Blurred vision/ pupil dilation Inflammation	—	Abnormal touch sensation	Clinical psychiatric disorder Dizziness/vertigo Other

(continued)

Table 2 (*Continued*)
Drugs That Interfere with the Taste System

Classification/drug	Side effects						
	Taste	Smell	Other oral/nasal conditions	Vision	Hearing	Somathesis sense	Cognitive
Pergolide mesylate (Permax) (95)	Distorted	–	Dryness Inflammation Saliva Other	Abnormal vision Inflammation Loss Ophthalmologic disorder Other	Inflammation Tinnitus Loss Other	Abnormal touch sensation Peripheral neuropathy	Clinical psychiatric disorder Disorientation/confusion Dizziness/vertigo Insomnia Memory loss Other
Selegiline HCl (Eldepryl) (95)	Distorted	–	Dryness Other	Abnormal vision Blurred vision/pupil dilation	Tinnitus	–	Clinical psychiatric disorder Disorientation/confusion Dizziness/vertigo Insomnia Memory loss Other
Psychopharmacologic including antiepileptic							
Alprazolam (Xanax) (95)	Distorted	–	Dryness Saliva Other	Abnormal vision Blurred vision/pupil dilation	Tinnitus	Abnormal touch sensation	Clinical psychiatric disorder Disorientation/confusion Dizziness/vertigo Insomnia Memory loss Other

Drug						
Amitriptyline HCl (Elavil, Endep) (95)	Distorted Loss	—	Dryness Inflammation Other	Abnormal vision Blurred vision/ pupil dilation Ophthalmologic disorder	Inflammation Tinnitus	Abnormal touch sensation Peripheral neuropathy	Clinical psychiatric disorder Disorientation/ confusion Dizziness/vertigo Insomnia Other
Amoxapine (Asendin) (95)	Distorted	—	Dryness Inflammation Other	Abnormal vision Blurred vision/ pupil dilation Other	Inflammation Tinnitus	Abnormal touch sensation	Clinical psychiatric disorder Insomnia Disorientation/ confusion Dizziness/vertigo Other
Buspirone HCl (BuSpar) (95)	Distorted	Distorted	Dryness Inflammation Saliva Other	Abnormal vision Blurred vision/ pupil dilation Inflammation Loss Ophthalmologic disorder Other	Tinnitus Other	Abnormal touch sensation	Clinical psychiatric disorder Disorientation/ confusion Dizziness/vertigo Insomnia Memory loss Other
Carbamazepine (Carbarol) (95,187)	Loss Distortion	—	Dryness Inflammation	Abnormal vision Blurred vision/ pupil dilation Inflammation Other	Tinnitus Other	Abnormal touch sensation Peripheral neuropathy	Clinical psychiatric disorder Disorientation/ confusion Dizziness/vertigo Other

(continued)

257

Table 2 (*Continued*)
Drugs That Interfere with the Taste System

Classification/drug	Side effects						
	Taste	Smell	Other oral/nasal conditions	Vision	Hearing	Somathesis sense	Cognitive
Chlordiazepoxide + Amitriptyline HCl (Limbitrol) (95)	Distorted	–	Dryness Inflammation Other	Abnormal vision Blurred vision/ pupil dilation	Inflammation	Abnormal touch sensation	Clinical psychiatric disorder Disorientation/ confusion Dizziness/vertigo Other
Clomipramine HCl (Anafranil) (95)	Distorted Loss	Distorted	Bleeding Dryness Inflammation Saliva Other	Abnormal vision Blurred vision/ pupil dilation Inflammation Loss Ophthalmologic disorder Other	Inflammation Loss Tinnitus Other	Abnormal touch sensation Peripheral neuropathy	Clinical psychiatric disorder Disorientation/ confusion Dizziness/vertigo Insomnia Memory loss Other
Clozapine (Clozaril) (95)	Distorted	–	Bleeding Dryness Inflammation Saliva Other	Abnormal vision Blurred vision/ pupil dilation Inflammation Other	Other	Abnormal touch sensation	Clinical psychiatric disorder Disorientation/ confusion Dizziness/vertigo Insomnia Memory loss Other

258

Drug						
Desipramine HCl (Norpramin) (95)	Distorted	—	Dryness Inflammation Other	Abnormal vision Blurred vision/ pupil dilation Ophthalmologic disorder	Inflammation Tinnitus	Abnormal touch sensation Peripheral neuropathy	Clinical psychiatric disorder Disorientation/confusion Dizziness/vertigo Insomnia Other
Doxepin HCl (Sinequan) (95)	Distorted	—	Dryness Inflammation	Blurred vision/ pupil dilation	Tinnitus	Abnormal touch sensation	Disorientation/confusion Dizziness/vertigo Other
Felbamate (Felbatol) (95)	Distorted	Distorted	Bleeding Dryness Inflammation Other	Abnormal vision Inflammation Loss Other	Inflammation Loss	Abnormal touch sensation	Clinical psychiatric disorder Disorientation/confusion Dizziness/vertigo Insomnia Other
Fluoxetine HC (Prozac) (95)	Distorted Loss	Distorted	Bleeding Dryness Inflammation Saliva	Abnormal vision Dry eyes Blurred vision/ pupil dilation Inflammation Loss Ophthalmologic disorder Other	Loss Tinnitus Other	Abnormal touch sensation Peripheral neuropathy	Clinical psychiatric disorder Disorientation/confusion Dizziness/vertigo Insomnia Memory loss Other

(continued)

Table 2 (*Continued*)
Drugs That Interfere with the Taste System

				Side effects			
Classification/drug	Taste	Smell	Other oral/nasal conditions	Vision	Hearing	Somathesis sense	Cognitive
Imipramine HCl and Imipramine pamoate (Tofranil-PM) (95)	Distorted	–	Dryness Inflammation Other	Abnormal vision Blurred vision/ pupil dilation	Inflammation Tinnitus	Abnormal touch sensation Peripheral neuropathy	Clinical psychiatric disorder Disorientation/ confusion Dizziness/vertigo Insomnia Other
Lithium carbonate (Eskalith, Lithium Carbonate, Lithionate/ Lithotabs) (95,188,189)	Distorted	–	Dryness Inflammation Saliva Other	Blurred vision/ pupil dilation Loss Other	Tinnitus	Abnormal touch sensation	Disorientation/ confusion Dizziness/vertigo Memory loss Other
Maprotiline HCl (Ludiomil) (95)	Distorted	–	Inflammation Dryness Other	Abnormal vision Blurred vision/ pupil dilation	Tinnitus	Abnormal touch sensation Peripheral neuropathy	Clinical psychiatric disorder Disorientation/ confusion Dizziness/vertigo Insomnia Memory loss Other

Drug	Taste	Smell	Mouth	Eyes	Ears	Touch/Nerve	CNS
Nortriptyline HCl (Pamelor) (95)	Distorted	—	Dryness Inflammation Other	Abnormal vision Blurred vision/pupil dilation	Inflammation Tinnitus	Abnormal touch sensation Peripheral neuropathy	Clinical psychiatric disorder Disorientation/confusion Insomnia Other
Paroxetine HCl (Paxil) (95)	Distorted Loss	Distorted	Bleeding Dryness Inflammation Saliva Other	Abnormal vision Blurred vision/pupil dilation Inflammation Loss Ophthalmologic disorder Other	Inflammation Loss Tinnitus Other	Abnormal touch sensation Peripheral neuropathy	Clinical psychiatric disorder Disorientation/confusion Dizziness/vertigo Insomnia Memory loss Other
Perphenazine-amitriptyline HCl (Triavil, Etrafon) (95)	Distorted	—	Dryness Inflammation Other	Abnormal vision Blurred vision/pupil dilation Ophthalmologic disorders Other	Inflammation Tinnitus	Abnormal touch sensation Peripheral neuropathy	Clinical psychiatric disorder Disorientation/confusion Dizziness/vertigo Insomnia Other
Phenytoin (Dilantin-125) (16,95)	Distorted	—	Inflammation Other	Other	—	—	Disorientation/confusion Dizziness/vertigo Insomnia Other
Pimozide (Orap) (95)	Distorted	—	Dryness Saliva Other	Abnormal vision Blurred vision/pupil dilation Inflammation Loss Ophthalmologic disorder	—	—	Insomnia Dizziness/vertigo Clinical psychiatric disorder Other

(continued)

Table 2 (*Continued*)
Drugs That Interfere with the Taste System

Classification/drug	Side effects						
	Taste	Smell	Other oral/nasal conditions	Vision	Hearing	Somathesis sense	Cognitive
Protriptyline HCl (Vivactil) (95)	Distorted	–	Dryness Inflammation Other	Abnormal vision Blurred vision/ pupil dilation Ophthalmologic disorder	Inflammation Tinnitus	Abnormal touch sensation Peripheral neuropathy	Clinical psychiatric disorder Disorientation/ confusion Dizziness/vertigo Insomnia Other
Psilocybin (190)	Distorted	–					–
Risperidone (Risperdal) (95)	Distorted	–	Inflammation Dryness Saliva Other	–	Loss Tinnitus Other	Abnormal touch sensation	Clinical psychiatric disorder Disorientation/ confusion Dizziness/vertigo Insomnia Memory loss Other
Sertraline HCl (Zoloft) (95,151)	Distorted	–	Dryness Inflammation Saliva Other	Abnormal vision Blurred vision/ pupil dilation Dry eyes Inflammation Loss Ophthalmologic disorder Other	Tinnitus Other	Abnormal touch sensation	Clinical psychiatric disorder Disorientation/ confusion Dizziness/vertigo Insomnia Memory loss Other

Drug							
Trazodone HCl (Desyrel) (95,151)	Other	—	Dryness Saliva Other	Abnormal vision Blurred vision/ pupil dilation Inflammation	Tinnitus	Abnormal touch sensation	Clinical psychiatric disorder Disorientation/ confusion Dizziness/vertigo Insomnia Memory loss Other
Trifluoperazine HCl (Stelazine) (95,190)	Loss	—	Dryness Other	Blurred vision/ pupil dilation Other	—	Abnormal touch sensation	Dizziness/vertigo Insomnia Other
Trimipramine maleate (Surmontil) (95)	Distorted	—	Dryness Inflammation Other	Abnormal vision Blurred vision/ pupil dilation	Inflammation Tinnitus	Abnormal touch sensation Peripheral neuropathy	Clinical psychiatric disorder Disorientation/ confusion Dizziness/vertigo Insomnia Other
Venlafaxine HC (Effexor) (95)	Distorted Loss	Distorted	Dryness Inflammation Saliva Other	Abnormal vision Blurred vision/ pupil dilation Dry eyes Inflammation Loss Ophthalmologic disorder Other	Inflammation Loss Tinnitus Other	Abnormal touch sensation Peripheral neuropathy	Clinical psychiatric disorder Disorientation/ confusion Dizziness/vertigo Insomnia Other
Sympathomimetic drugs Amphetamine (Biphetamine) (95,191)	Distorted	—	Dryness	—	—	—	Dizziness/vertigo Insomnia Other

(continued)

Table 2 (*Continued*)
Drugs That Interfere with the Taste System

				Side effects				
Classification/drug	Taste	Smell	Other oral/nasal conditions	Vision	Hearing	Somathesis sense	Cognitive	
Benzphetamine HCl (Didrex) (95)	Distorted	—	Dryness	—	—	—	Clinical psychiatric disorder Dizziness/vertigo Insomnia Other	
Dextroamphetamine sulfate (Dexedrine) (95)	Distorted	—	Dryness	—	—	—	Clinical psychiatric disorder Dizziness/vertigo Insomnia Other	
Fenfluramine HCl (Pondimin) (95)	Distorted	—	Dryness	Blurred vision/ pupil dilatio Other	—	—	Clinical psychiatric disorder Dizziness/vertigo Insomnia Other	
Mazindol (Sanorex) (95)	Distorted	—	Dryness	Blurred vision/ pupil dilation	—	Abnormal touch sensation	Clinical psychiatric disorder Dizziness/vertigo Insomnia Other	

264

Methamphetamine HCl (Desoxyn) (95)	Distorted	—	Dryness	—	—	—	Clinical psychiatric disorder, Dizziness/vertigo, Insomnia, Other
Phendimetrazine tartrate (Prelu-2) (95)	Distorted	—	Dryness	—	—	—	Clinical psychiatric disorder, Dizziness/vertigo, Insomnia, Other
Phentermine resin (Ionamin) (95)	Distorted	—	Dryness	—	—	—	Clinical psychiatric disorder
Phentermine HCl Adipex-P, Fastin) (95)	Distorted	—	Dryness	—	—	—	Dizziness/vertigo, Insomnia, Other
Vasodilators							
Bamifylline hydrochloride (146)	Distorted	—	—	—	—	—	—
Dipyridamole (Persantine) (95,192)	Distorted	—	—	—	—	Abnormal touch sensation	Dizziness/vertigo
Isosorbide mononitrate (Monoket) (95)	Distorted	—	Dryness, Inflammation	Abnormal vision	—	Abnormal touch sensation	Clinical psychiatric disorder, Dizziness/vertigo, Insomnia, Other
Nitroglycerin patch (Deponit) (95,193)	Loss	—	—	—	—	—	Dizziness/vertigo
Oxyfedrine (194,195)	Distorted	—	—	—	—	—	—

(continued)

Table 2 (*Continued*)
Drugs That Interfere with the Taste System

Classification/drug	Side effects						
	Taste	Smell	Other oral/nasal conditions	Vision	Hearing	Somathesis sense	Cognitive
Others (indication)							
Allopurinol (reduces serum and urinary uric acid) (Zyloprim) (95,146)	Distorted Loss	–	Inflammation	Abnormal vision Inflammation Ophthalmologic disorder	Tinnitus	Abnormal touch sensation Peripheral neuropathy	Clinical psychiatric disorder Disorientation/ confusion Dizziness/vertigo Insomnia Memory loss Other
Antihemophilic factor (recombinant) (clotting factor-hemophilia) (Kogenate) (95)	Distorted	–	Inflammation	–	–	Abnormal touch sensation	Dizziness/vertigo
Antithrombin III (human) (antithrombin III deficiency) (Thrombate III) (95)	Distorted	–	–	Other	–	–	Dizziness/vertigo
Bepridil HCl (antianginal/anti-spasmodic) (Vascor) (95)	Distorted	–	Dryness Inflammation	Blurred vision/ pupil dilation	Tinnitus	Abnormal touch sensation	Clinical psychiatric disorder Dizziness/vertigo Insomnia Other

Drug							
Calcitonin (Paget's Disease, hypercalcemia, osteoporosis) (Miacalcin, Cibacalcin) (95)	Distorted	Distorted	Bleeding Dryness Inflammation Other	Blurred vision/pupil dilation Inflammation Other	Loss Tinnitus Other	Abnormal touch sensation	Clinical psychiatric disorder Dizziness/vertigo Insomnia
Etidronate (hypercalcemia, antipsoriatic) (Didronel) (95,196)	Distorted Loss	—	Inflammation	—	—	Abnormal touch sensation	Clinical psychiatric disorder Disorientation/confusion Other
Gadodiamide (diagnostic imaging product) (Omniscan) (95)	Distorted Loss	—	Dryness Inflammation	Abnormal vision	Tinnitus	Abnormal touch sensation Other	Clinical psychiatric disorder Dizziness/vertigo
Germine monoacetate (Eaton-Lambert syndrome) (197)	Distorted	—	—	—	—	—	—
Granisetron HCl (antiemetic/antinauseant) (Kytril) (95,151)	Other	—	—	—	—	—	Clinical psychiatric disorder Insomnia Dizziness/vertigo Other
Histamine phosphate (control for allergic skin testing) (Histratrol) (95)	Distorted	—	—	—	—	—	—

(continued)

267

Table 2 (*Continued*)
Drugs That Interfere with the Taste System

Classification/drug	Side effects						
	Taste	Smell	Other oral/nasal conditions	Vision	Hearing	Somathesis sense	Cognitive
Iohexol (diagnostic imaging product) (Omnipaque) (95)	Distorted	—	Dryness Inflammation Other	Abnormal vision Blurred vision/ pupil dilation	Tinnitus	Abnormal touch sensation	Clinical psychiatric disorder Disorientation/ confusion Dizziness/vertigo Insomnia Memory loss Other
Iron sorbitex (hematinic) (198)	Distorted	—	—	—	—	—	—
Leuprolide acetate (inhibits gonadotropin secretion/prostatic cancer) (Lupron, Lupron Depot) (95)	Distorted	—	Dryness Inflammation Other	Blurred vision/ pupil dilation Inflammation Ophthalmologic disorders	Loss	Abnormal touch sensation Peripheral neuropathy	Clinical psychiatric disorder Disorientation/ confusion Dizziness/vertigo Insomnia Memory loss Other

Drug							
Levamisole HCl (immunomodulator-restores depressed immune function) (Ergamisol) (95)	Distorted	Distorted	Inflammation	Abnormal vision/ Blurred vision/ pupil dilation Inflammation Other	—	Abnormal touch sensation	Clinical psychiatric disorder Disorientation/ confusion Dizziness/vertigo Insomnia Memory loss Other
Mesna (detoxifying agent) (Mesnex) (95)	Distorted	—	—	—	—	—	—
Methylergonovine maleate (prevent post-partum hemorrhage) (Methergine) (95)	Distorted	—	Inflammation	Tinnitus	—	—	Dizziness/vertigo Other
Pentoxifylline (blood viscosity modulator) (Trental) (95	Distorted	—	Dryness Inflammation Saliva Other	Blurred vision/ pupil dilation Inflammation Loss	Other	Abnormal touch sensation	Clinical psychiatric disorder Disorientation/ confusion Dizziness/vertigo Insomnia Other
Potassium iodide (expectorant) (Pima, SSKI) (95)	Distorted	—	—	—	—	—	—
Sermorelin acetate (diagnostic) (Geref) (95)	Distorted	—	—	—	—	—	Dizziness/vertigo Other

(continued)

Table 2 (*Continued*)
Drugs That Interfere with the Taste System

Classification/drug	Side effects						
	Taste	Smell	Other oral/nasal conditions	Vision	Hearing	Somathesis sense	Cognitive
Succimer (lead poisoning) (Chemet) (95	Distorted	Distorted	Other	Other	Inflammation Other	Abnormal touch sensation	Dizziness/vertigo Other
Terbinafine (Lamisil) (95,139)	Distorted Loss	–	–	Abnormal vision	–	Abnormal touch sensation	–
Ursodiol (gall stone dissolution) (Actigall) (95,151)	Other	–	Inflammation	–	–	–	Dizziness/vertigo Insomnia
Vitamin D/Calcitriol (hypocalcemia) (Calcijex, Roxaltrol) (16,95,146)	Distorted	–	Dryness Other	Abnormal vision Inflammation	–	Abnormal touch sensation	Clinical psychiatric disorder Other
Vitamin K₁/Phytona-dione (coagulation disorders) (Aqua-MEPHYTON, Mephyton) (95)	Distorted	–	–	–	–	–	Dizziness/vertigo

over the age of 65 ranges from 2.9 to 3.7 medications *(46)*, and this number increases to 6 or more drugs for elderly living in retirement and nursing homes *(18)*. One of the best predictors of adverse drug reactions is the absolute number of drugs taken by an individual patient *(47,48)*. For anticholinergic medications that have prominent oral side-effects, it is the total burden of anticholinergic drug activity that determines the likelihood of adverse events *(49)*, with older individuals more sensitive to these effects than young adults *(49–51)*. Over 600 drugs have been reported to have anticholinergic effects *(52)*, and nearly 60% of 5902 nursing home residents and 23% of ambulatory elderly controls were taking medications with anticholinergic properties *(53)*.

Neither the site nor mode of action for most pharmaceutical compounds that induce taste losses is known, but medications can exert effects at several levels including peripheral receptors, chemosensory neural pathways, and/or the brain. Drugs secreted into the saliva can modify taste transduction mechanisms or produce a taste of their own. Drugs can also diffuse from the blood to the basolateral side of taste cells to affect taste. Medications, such as cancer drugs, can impair turnover of taste cells. The relative frequencies with which drugs alter taste has not yet been determined using prospective testing procedures.

2.2. Smell Losses with Age

2.2.1. Physiology of the Olfactory System

Olfactory receptor cells are bipolar neurons that are located in the olfactory epithelium in the upper nasal cavity.

Bony structures in the nose called turbinates create airflow patterns that allow volatile compounds to reach the olfactory cells. These volatile compounds bind to receptors on the olfactory receptor cells. Olfactory cells, like taste cells, undergo continual renewal, but with an average turnover time of approx 30 d. The axons of the receptor cells are then threaded through holes in the cribiform plate to connect to the olfactory bulb in bushy masses called "glomeruli." The glomeruli are structures that atrophy with age, taking on a "moth-eaten" appearance as fibers degenerate and disappear. The axons of the secondary neurons converge into the lateral olfactory tract and connect to the primary olfactory cortex. Other olfactory bulb neurons connect to the olfactory tubercle, the corticomedial nuclei of the amygdala, and the prepyriform cortex. Many of these structures comprise the so-called "limbic system" of the brain, which also processes emotions and memories. This neuroanatomical overlap between olfaction and emotions may be the basis by which odors invoke hedonic responses. Olfactory information is ultimately transmitted to the hypothalamus, which is a feeding center in the brain.

2.2.2. Physiological Changes in the Olfactory System with Age

Olfactory losses in the elderly result from one or more causes that include normal aging, diseases, medications, viral insult, malnutrition, accumulated exposure to toxic fumes (and other environmental agents), surgical interventions, and head trauma (Tables 1 and 2). Noninvasive neuroimaging studies suggest that olfactory dysfunction after trauma is associated with damage primarily in the olfactory bulbs and tracts and the inferior frontal lobes *(54)*. Anatomical and physiological changes occur with age in the structure of the upper airway, olfactory epithelium, olfactory bulb and nerves, hippocampus and amygdaloid complex, and hypothalamus, including reductions in cell number, damage to cells, and diminished levels of neurotransmitters *(16,18)*. In certain disease states, such as Alzheimer's disease and Parkinson's disease, the losses can be profound *(55)*.

Because of the exposed location of the olfactory receptors, viral and environmental insults, such as sinusitus, viral infection, and exposure to toxic compounds, can damage or kill olfactory receptors. Head trauma can sever the olfactory nerves that course through the cribriform plate. Falls are common among the elderly and account for some of the odor losses they experience.

2.2.3. PERCEPTUAL CHANGES IN THE SENSE OF SMELL WITH AGE

Most research suggests that the sense of smell is more impaired by normal aging than the sense of taste as a result of the profound anatomical and physiological changes. Losses in odor perception occur at both threshold and suprathreshold levels *(56–58)*. Suprathreshold odor studies indicate elderly persons experience a reduction in the magnitude of perceived intensity *(59–62)*. Older adults also have impairments in odor identification *(39,40,57,63–65)* and odor discrimination *(42,66,67)*. In addition, there are age-related losses in the ability to perceive nasal pungency (e.g., CO_2, which stimulates the trigeminal nerve) *(61)*. The disorders and drugs that can affect smell (along with taste) are given in Tables 1 and 2.

2.3. Consequences of Chemosensory Losses for Nutrition

Losses in taste and smell sensations can have profound effects on appetite, food choices, nutrient intake, and, ultimately, health status. Taste and smell losses can interfere with the ability to select appropriate foods and to modulate intake as nutritional requirements vary with aging. If there is also a reduction in the variety of foods that are eaten, this may further reduce that probability of getting a balanced diet. Persons with chemosensory impairments lose the motivation to eat, which can reduce nutrient intake and hence exacerbate disease states, impair nutritional status/immunity, and produce weight loss. Because chemosensory signals initiate responses that prepare the body for food, cephalic phase responses including salivary, gastric, pancreatic, and intestinal secretions are blunted. This can potentially affect digestion of food and absorption of nutrients.

The inability to detect noxious tastes and odors renders the elderly vulnerable to poisoning from spoiled foods (e.g., mayonnaise or fish). Elderly with decrements in memory and chemical senses are especially at risk for foodborne illnesses because they may leave food on the table or in the refrigerator too long. Importantly, loss in taste and smell sensations interferes with quality of life. Odor is an integral aspect of flavor in foods, and in fact most "flavor" of food is derived from retronasal stimulation (through the back of the throat) of the olfactory receptors by food odors when chewing. Loss of odor sensations also deprives the elderly of pleasant odor-evoked memories, such as Christmas cookies baking in the oven. Overall, chemosensory dysfunction can impair nutritional status and reduce the pleasure from food.

3. LOSSES IN VISION WITH AGE

3.1. Physiology of the Visual System

Functionally, important structures of the eye include the cornea (the clear part of the front of the eye that admits light), the iris (the structure that gives color to the eye), the pupil (the opening in the iris that controls light being admitted), the lens (which is used to focus light), and the retina (the back of the eye which contains the receptors for vision, cones and rods). The aqueous humor is the thin, watery fluid that occupies the space between the cornea and the iris. The vitreous humor is the gel-like medium between the lens and the back of the eye. Each eye has a set of six extrinsic muscles that are attached at one end to the tissues of the eyeball and at the other end to the bony eye socket. Information from the cones and rods is transmitted to visual processing areas of the brain by the second cranial nerve (optic nerve).

3.2. Physiological Changes in the Visual System with Age

The visual system undergoes a number of physiological changes that are associated with aging. Physiological losses occur both at the peripheral (e.g., eye) and central (neurons and brain) levels.

3.2.1. CORNEA

The most significant age-related change that impacts the cornea is decreased tear production (68). The lacriminal fluids provide a smooth surface for refraction and also protect the eye. Decreased tear production can decrease clarity of vision, cause discomfort, and predispose the cornea to infection and corneal disease (69).

3.2.2. IRIS AND PUPIL

With age, individuals experience "senile miosis," a smaller pupil diameter during normal light conditions, and decreased ability to fully dilate the pupil during low-light conditions (70,71). Although small pupil size may be helpful for increasing focus under bright-light conditions, older individuals are not able to fully adjust to low-light conditions.

3.2.3. LENS

The lens consists of epithelial cells that continue to grow throughout the lifespan. As a consequence, cells become packed in the center of the lens, and the lens becomes increasingly dense, yellowed, and inflexible with advanced age. The diminished transparency of the lens attenuates (or filters) available light, especially for short wavelengths (blue and violet) (72). The lens also becomes more resistant to deformation, and accommodation for near distances becomes impaired (73). This condition, termed presbyopia, usually becomes noticeable by the 40s or 50s. The lens may also lose its clarity and develop opacities. When these opacities are clinically significant, they are termed a cataract (Chapter 8).

3.2.4. AQUEOUS AND VITREOUS HUMOR

The aqueous humor that flows out of the iris and between the cornea and lens delivers nutrients and removes waste products from the anterior chamber of the eye. However, in older individuals, the drainage network for the aqueous humor can become blocked (74), leading to increased ocular pressure and potential damage to the eye. With age, the vitreous humor tends to liquefy, contract, and separate from the retina, creating floaters in front of the retina. These changes, in addition to alterations in the iris and lens, have the consequence of increasing light scatter and reducing the amount of focused light reaching the retina. This both reduces contrast of visual images and increases glare. A person in his or her 70s is estimated to have one-third as much light reaching the retina as a 20-yr-old (75), and these losses account in part for the decreased visual performance found with age.

3.2.5. Retina

Retinal changes may also occur with age, particularly in the macula. The macula is the central portion of the retina and includes the fovea, the area of the macula used for fine detail and color vision. Macular degeneration is an age-related pathological condition involving the photoreceptors and the supporting retinal pigment epithelium. Results from the Framingham study suggest that 6.4% of people aged 65–74 yr have macular degeneration with visual acuity 20/30 or worse; this increases to 19.7% of individuals 75 yr or more *(76)*. Even greater percentages of elderly have lesser degrees of macular degeneration. It is hypothesized that macular degeneration begins at the level of the retinal pigment epithelium, a metabolically active layer that supports the retina and is characterized by deposits of drusen and other waste products, atrophy, and increased new vessel formation *(77)*. Small tears or breaks may occur in the retina as a consequence of changes in the composition of the vitreous humor, such as liquefaction and decreased volume. The resulting lack of structure may allow the retina to pull away from the back of the eye. The choroid (layer of blood vessels that nourishes the back of the eye) thickens, and blood vessels become more torturous and dilated.

3.2.6. Eye Muscles

There is a significant and progressive limitation in upward gaze with advancing age *(78)*. Vertical or upward gaze for children and adolescents was 40° which decreased to 16° for persons 75 yr or more. This may be due to atrophy of the elevator muscles of the eyeball from reduced use of upper field vision with advancing age.

3.2.7. Central Changes

The occipital (visual) cortex exhibits less degenerative changes compared to other areas of the brain with age. However, not all changes in vision with age can be attributed to losses at the periphery. Age-related changes in visual perception are found even when elderly participants are fitted with optical correction and are considered free of eye disease *(71)* suggesting that some losses may occur along the visual pathways. Decrements have been reported in the number of optic nerve fibers and neurons in the visual cortex *(71)*. Disagreement exists in estimating the relative contribution of neural factors to visual decline *(79,80)*, with estimates ranging from 0.1 log *(79)* to 1.0 log per decade *(81)*.

3.3. Perceptual Changes in the Sense of Vision with Age

Virtually all aspects of vision undergo changes with age. Far visual acuity (resolution of spatial detail) and contrast sensitivity are relatively preserved until around age 65, at which time performance decreases, even in the absence of any eye disease *(82,83)*. The largest change in contrast sensitivity is seen at high spatial frequencies (e.g., thin bars close together) and low contrast. Peripheral vision decreases, with the visual field shrinking to two-thirds by age 75, and to half by age 90 *(84,85)*. There are age-related declines in the rate and maximum level of dark adaptation. Measures performed under ideal conditions of high contrast and bright light underestimate age-related impairments because elderly vision is especially impaired in conditions of reduced illumination or contrast *(82)*. Other changes found with age are decreased ability to discriminate colors *(86,87)*, especially blue and green colors *(87)*, lower threshold for flicker fusion (flashing lights fuse at lower temporal frequencies due to increased persistence of images) *(83)*, decreased perception of motion *(88,89)*, decreased depth perception *(90,91)*, and decreased brightness contrast *(83)*.

3.4. Effect of Medications and Disease on Visual Perception

3.4.1. AGING AND EYE DISEASE

Although not considered a part of normal aging, the incidence of ocular diseases such as cataracts, glaucoma, macular degeneration, and circulatory problems increases with age so that a significantly higher proportion of elderly have vision problems compared to other age groups. Age is a risk factor for both cataract and age-related macular degeneration *(92,93)*. Cataracts are divided into three types: nuclear sclerosis (a yellowing of entire lens), posterior subcapsular (cells forming between the back of the lens and the capsule holding the lens), and cortical (opacities developing along the periphery of the lens and radiating like spokes to the center of the lens). Risk factors for cataracts include age, trauma to the eye, sun exposure, malnutrition, and smoking. In glaucoma, an imbalance of the inflow to outflow of the aqueous humor in the ocular media occurs increasing intraocular pressure and eventually destroying the nerve fibers in the optic disk and optic nerve, causing permanent damage to vision. As glaucoma initially causes no symptoms and affects the peripheral visual field first, vision loss can be quite advanced before being noticed by the individual. Regular eye check ups in which eye pressure is recorded and the back of the eye are viewed are the only methods to prevent blindness from glaucoma.

The most common retinal problem in older individuals is macular degeneration, in which the central portion of the retina (the macula) is damaged by accumulation of waste products, presumably due to abnormal processes in the supporting blood vessels in the retinal pigment epithelium (choroid). Macular degeneration destroys the central portion of the retina that contains the cones, receptors that are necessary for color vision and detailed vision such as used in reading, sewing, and driving. Currently 25–30 million people worldwide are blind due to age-related macular degeneration *(94)*. Additionally, problems of the retina occurring with aging are retinopathy, the growth of abnormal and weak blood vessels, and leakage of blood vessels.

3.4.2. EFFECT OF HEALTH STATUS ON VISION

The retina is highly dependent on a healthy blood supply to provide oxygen and remove waste products. In general, elderly individuals with poor health or circulation problems such as arteriosclerosis are more likely to have retinal problems. Diabetes increases risk for a number of eye problems including cataracts, retinopathy (proliferation of abnormal blood vessels), and retinal hemorrhage. The risk of diabetic retinopathy is directly related to the length of time of diabetes, and can cause partial to total blindness in the eye *(71,93)*.

3.4.3. OPTHAMOLOGICAL SIDE EFFECTS OF DRUGS

Many medications cause visual or opthamological side effects. Table 2 gives the visual side effects of drugs known to affect taste. Many more drugs have visual side effects without taste effects *(95)*. Although some studies screen for eye disease when measuring age-related decrements of vision, few screen for medication use, so that the relative contribution of medications to age-related visual changes is not known. Medications can cause both perceptual changes such as blurred vision, double vision, and vision loss, and physiological changes, such as optic neuritis, cataracts, and retinopathy as shown in the tables. Representative classes of medications with visual side effects include those with anticholinergic activity, antihistamines, certain nonsteroidal anti-inflammatory drugs (NSAIDS), and thiazide diuretics. Steroid use is associated with cataract formation. Many medications decrease production of tears so that eyes become dry, itchy, and painful. Some medication side effects are temporary and may remit with discontinued use; others may cause permanent changes to sight.

3.4.4. RISK FACTORS FOR VISION LOSS

It is believed that age-related changes in the visual system are due in part to environmental and nutritional factors such as light exposure, cigarette smoking, and antioxidant levels (96). Exposure to UV (A and B) and blue light exacerbates the progression of cataract formation and incidence of macular degeneration; in particular, there is association between UV B light exposure and cortical cataracts. Cigarette smoking is associated with an increased risk of macular degeneration and nuclear sclerosis cataracts. Nutritional factors, in particular antioxidant status, appear to play a role in cataract formation (Chapter 8).

The association is strongest in nutritionally deprived countries, with mixed results in developed countries in which some studies show an effect, others not, and some an effect only for smokers. The specific nutrients that are responsible for a protective effect have not been determined. Nutrients that are being investigated for protective benefits for eye disease include selenium, zinc, and antioxidants such as vitamin C, E, and carotenoids (97–99).

Nutritional supplementation with antioxidants has been recommended for the elderly as this population may have both increased need for antioxidant defense mechanisms, as a result of lower reserves of antioxidants, and increased production of free radicals because of disease states and medication use (97,100). The lens and retina are particularly vulnerable to cumulative oxidative damage because they are subjected to light energy (radiation), and the high metabolic demands of the retina. Elderly individuals have been found to have reduced levels of antioxidants in blood plasma (101). Some antioxidants are enzymes, such as superoxide dismutase (SOD), glutathione peroxidase, and some are smaller antioxidant molecules such as vitamin C, vitamin E, and carotenoids, such as lutein and zeaxanthin. The lens and retina are particularly vulnerable to cumulative oxidative damage because they are subjected to light energy (radiation).

3.5. Consequences of Visual Losses for Nutrition

Loss of vision can impact nutritional status because it interferes with activities of daily living, including mobility, food preparation, and use of utensils (102). Driving restrictions, especially for those living alone, can make individuals more isolated and less likely to participate in social activities such as cooking and dining out. If one cannot drive, grocery shopping trips are less frequent or performed by other individuals, so that the elderly have less access to preferred foods, fresh produce, and perishable items. Diminished vision increases the risk for falls and car accidents (103,104) and thus serves as a disincentive for obtaining meals. Reduced upper field vision resulting from atrophy of the elevator muscle of the eyeball limits food choices while shopping in the supermarket. Inability to distinguish between colors because of yellowed lenses may make it difficult to read labels. In the extreme case, visual loss from macular degeneration may interfere with the identification of food.

Visual losses reduce the motivation to eat, which is especially problematic in persons who also have chemosensory deficits. Visual cues from food stimulate appetite as well as provide information about monitoring food safety. Color, arrangement, doneness, and apparent quality of food play a major role in the quality and enjoyment of the eating experience. Hence, loss of these visual cues in the elderly can affect intake and ultimately nutritional status.

4. LOSSES IN AUDITION WITH AGE

There are clear age-related declines in hearing with aging. It is estimated that hearing problems are the second most common chronic condition (after arthritis) affecting the elderly (Chapter 10).

4.1. Physiology of the Auditory System and Changes with Age

The outer ear, the pinna is used to direct sound waves to the tympanic membrane. The outer ear demonstrates a number of physical changes with age but they have minimal impact on hearing quality or ability. The middle ear consists of the tympanic membrane (ear drum), three bones (the ossicular chain), and the oval window. The three bones, called the malleus (mallet), the incus (anvil), and the stapes (stirrup), transmit the force of the sound waves impinging on the ear drum to deform the oval window. Arthritic changes can affect these bones so that the bones become more fixed and less likely to transmit sound (105).

The important organ of the inner ear is the cochlea, which contains the receptors for hearing (the hair cells). It is a coiled structure that is divided into three lengthwise chambers and has two membranes that run along its length, the basilar membrane and Reissner's membrane. The organ of Corti is a mechanism that is attached lengthwise along the basilar membrane and holds the auditory receptor cells (hair cells). Receptor cells are spaced along the basilar membrane and consist of inner hair cells and outer hair cells. Sound is transmitted by two processes. In transmission, the energy at the oval window is transferred to the outer hair cells via a traveling wave along the basilar membrane. Displacement of the basilar membrane bends the cilia of the fixed outer hair cells and generates an action potential. In transduction, acoustic energy in the organ of Corti is translated into electrical action potentials, hypothetically by the change in velocity and displacement of the fluid surrounding the free cilia of the inner hair cells. Neural degeneration along the auditory pathway and auditory cortex of the brain is found with aging (106).

Presbycusis, or age-related losses in hearing, is classified into four categories (107). Sensory presbycusis is due to degeneration and atrophy of hair and supporting cells in the basilar membrane. Neural presbycusis is the loss of neurons in the cochlea and auditory pathway. Metabolic presbycusis is the atrophy of the stria vascularis. This atrophy affects metabolic processes in the cochlea, particularly the fluid surrounding the hair cells (endolymph), leading to hair cell loss. Mechanical or conductive presbycusis is the atrophy of the vibratory structures of the cochlea. Typically, elderly persons experiencing presbycusis suffer from a combination of losses, rather than an isolated form of degeneration (107).

There are some conditions that are not strictly age-related but also occur in older individuals. Otosclerosis occurs when bone forms in the cochlear capsule. Hearing can be restored by performing a stapedectomy in which the stapes is removed and replaced with a wire prosthesis. Another condition that affects individuals of all ages is ear infections, causing both pain and hearing loss. Antibiotics are necessary to resolve the infection, although some losses in hearing may be permanent.

Another consideration of hearing loss in elderly is the accumulation of wax in the outer ear. Wax becomes harder and less likely to be shed so that it may become hardened and embedded to the extent it causes conductive hearing loss. Wax can be removed by squirting warm water into the ear canal to allow the wax to be softened and removed.

4.2. Perceptual Changes in the Sense of Hearing with Age

Age-related changes in audition occur at both threshold (sensitivity) and suprathreshold levels. Both cross-sectional and longitudinal studies have found decreases in sensitivity to pure tones with age, with losses most pronounced for high frequencies (from 2 to 8 kHz) (108,109). Older individuals require larger changes to detect a change in the pitch of tones or locate sound in space. Elderly may experience problems with loudness recruitment, i.e., sounds of low intensity may be difficult to hear but higher intensity sounds may become painfully loud. The most disruptive impairment for the elderly is the decreased ability to comprehend speech. Decreased ability to comprehend speech is in part the result of a disproportionate loss in high frequencies needed to distinguish consonants (108). Elderly individuals are also more disrupted by background noise, or alterations in the speech signal, such as interrupted speech, speeded speech, and/or speech without supporting semantic context. The cause of these age-related changes is not fully understood, but is assumed to be largely neural in nature, because of both damage to auditory receptors and degenerative changes along the auditory pathway (110).

4.3. Effect of Medications, Disease, and Environmental Factors on Auditory Perception

Over 130 medications have potential hearing effects, although certain drug classes such as aminoglycoside antibiotics, NSAIDS such as aspirin, loop diuretics, and the chemotherapeutic medication cisplatin are known for drug-induced ototoxicity. Table 2 gives the auditory side effects of drugs that also impact the sense of taste. The mechanism by which medications damage hearing is not fully understood, but evidence suggests at least some of these medications cause ototoxicity via free radical damage (111). Aminoglycosides and the drug cisplatin are hypothesized to cause hair cell death due to iron-induced free radical formation (112); iron chelators prevent hearing damage in the animal model (113). Antioxidant levels in the blood are lower in patients on cisplatin or cisplatin-related drugs (114). Concurrent treatment with the antioxidant glutathione has been found to reduce ototoxic side effects of these medications (115) and allow higher doses to be used. Ethacrynic acid and furosemide also affect hearing at the level of the cochlea. Adverse effects may occur over long-term administration, or may occur acutely. Overall, elderly are at increased risk for medication-related adverse events. Current research is underway to investigate whether use of antioxidants or other compounds can prevent medication ototoxicity.

Although some hearing loss is a consequence of age, diseases, and medications, other environmental factors like noise can induce hearing loss noise (e.g., occupational noise or proximity to instruments like guns, chainsaws, or loud motors.) Vibrations, head injury, viral and bacterial infections, and cigarette smoking may also affect hearing *(116)*. As many forms of hearing loss are permanent, prevention is more effective than treating existing symptoms.

4.4. Consequences of Hearing Losses for Nutrition

Studies have found that hearing loss and deafness are associated with an increased risk of social isolation, depression, and dementia. Both social isolation and depression are associated with increased risk of malnutrition in the elderly *(117)*. Part of the enjoyment of a meal is sharing meals with other people both as a social act and to converse about the food served at the meal.

5. LOSSES IN SOMESTHESIS WITH AGE

5.1. Physiology of the Somatosensory System and Changes with Age

The somatosensory system consists of various receptors in the skin that transmit the perception of touch, temperature, pressure, and pain. Cauna *(118)* divided skin receptors into two main types: free nerve endings and encapsulated nerve endings, such as Meissner's corpuscles, pacinian corpuscles, and Merkel's disks. Researchers have measured reduced numbers of various touch receptors in the skin with age *(119,120)* with Meissner and pacinian corpuscles showing the greatest change in both numbers and morphology, and free nerve endings the least. Kenshalo *(121)* found a correlation between the loss of Meissner's corpuscles and loss of skin sensitivity with aging. Other physical changes that impact somatosensory sensitivity in the elderly is a wrinkling and loss of elasticity of the skin, and neuronal losses along the cutaneous pathways and somatosensory area of the brain.

5.2. Perceptual Changes in the Somatosensory System with Age

Decrease in touch sensitivity has been found using the two-point discrimination task *(119)*, orientation of line grating *(122,123)*, point localization, detection of a gap in a disk, line length discrimination, and line or point orientation *(124,125)*. Although these tasks measure different aspects of touch ability and have different thresholds, they decline about the same rate (1% per yr) with age, with acuity declining faster at the fingertip than at the forearm or lip *(126)*. Elderly persons show decreased sensitivity to vibratory stimulation, with preferential loss at higher frequencies *(127)*. Thermal sensitivity also declines with age, with virtually no age-related reduction at the lips and face and the highest decline at the extremities such as the toe, sole of foot, and finger *(128)*. Disorders like reduced circulation and warmth in the extremities, diabetes, and peripheral neuropathies exacerbate age-related somatosensory declines. Medications have been associated with somatosensory losses. Table 2 gives somatosensory side effects for drugs that alter taste perception. There have been no prospective studies of the role of medications in somatosensory losses.

5.3. Consequences of Somatosensory Losses for Nutrition

Losses in the ability to perceive heat can reduce the appeal of foods and become a safety issue if foods are served at boiling temperatures. Oral burns can occur from eating and drinking foods that are too hot just as burns over the entire body can occur from bathing in excessively hot water. Inability to perceive heat in the fingers may also lead to burns during cooking. Tactile losses make it more difficult to prepare food and to manipulate utensils. Impairments in tactile feedback can interfere with balance, and thus older individuals may restrict themselves from food-making activities as they may accidentally injure themselves. Persons with tactile impairment may also avoid public transport (buses, trains), as well as escalators and moving walkways. This reduces the range of food shopping opportunities for a variety of foods.

6. PRACTICAL SUGGESTIONS FOR PERSONS WITH SENSORY LOSSES

6.1. Assessment of Taste and Smell Dysfunction

There are no universal measures to assess taste and smell function that are standardized across laboratories. When performing an assessment of a patient with a taste or smell complaint, one should first attempt to characterize the taste or smell disturbance through patient interview and by the use of psychophysical measures. Commonly used measures of taste and smell function are detection thresholds (the concentration at which a stimulus is first detected), recognition thresholds (the concentration at which the stimulus is recognized or identified), and identification tasks. Inclusion of an identification task is useful because individuals experiencing impairments may be able to detect the presence or absence of a taste or smell, yet not be able to discriminate among them. Identification tasks are also helpful for identifying dysgeusia (distortion of taste).

One should next attempt to identify the cause of the impairment. Again, the medical history of the patient, as well as details of the onset and characteristics of the disturbance should be recorded. Impairments of taste are often due to medication use, disease states and nutritional/metabolic changes. Disturbances in olfaction are commonly due to viral infections, nasal obstructions, head injury, environmental exposure, and also the aging process. A clinician should first search for any local injury to the receptors (resulting from physical or chemical trauma), and damage to the projecting cranial nerves. Second, any conditions that impair regeneration of taste and smell receptors should be investigated. Metabolic/endocrine changes, nutritional deficiencies, disease states, medications, and radiation can all affect taste receptor growth cycles.

6.2. Treatment of Taste and Smell Dysfunction

There are no standard pharmacological methods to treat age-related chemosensory decrements, and the prognosis for recovery of smell and taste sensation is poor. Clinical observations suggest, however, that a small percentage of chemosensory disorders associated with medical conditions and medications are self-limited. Acute dysfunction is reversed when the concomitant medical conditions are treated or the offending drugs removed, although full recovery may take several months. For elderly individuals who experience hypogeusia or hyposmia, cooking techniques and food presentation that enhance the visual and textural qualities of the food improve food enjoyment. Hyposmia (reduced, but not absent odor acuity) can be "treated" by adding simulated food flavors to meats, vegetables, and nutritious foods to amplify the odor intensity. Flavors are mixtures of odorous molecules that are extracted from natural products or are synthesized after chromatographic analysis of the target food. They are analogous to aromas found in frozen concentrated orange juice or extract of vanilla. Flavors have an advantage over spices in that they have the same odor quality as foods themselves, do not add extra salt and sugar, and do not irritate the stomach like spices. Food technologists have employed both artificial and natural flavors to increase flavor in commercial frozen entrees targeted at older populations (e.g., meatloaf). However, simulated flavor enhancers such as produced by Manheimer Inc. *(129)* are not currently available for public use. The flavor of foods can also be amplified by the use of concentrated juices such as apricot nectar, bouillon cubes, concentrated stocks, and butter sprinkles. The addition of simulated food flavors to meats, vegetables, and other nutritious foods to compensate for chemosensory losses has been shown to improve a variety of nutritional parameters in an elderly population, including improved appetite, increased total number of lymphocytes (including T and B cells), increased secretion rate of salivary IgA, and improved functional status *(130–133)*. Interestingly, improved immunity and functional status were found even when macro- and micronutrient intakes were not changed *(130)*. The addition of meat flavors along with monosodium glutamate (MSG) to entrees containing protein has been found to increase protein consumption in the elderly *(133)*. The addition of smoked bacon flavor can increase consumption of vegetables *(130)*. Enhanced tastes and odors also elevate cephalic phase responses including salivation in elderly persons *(132)*. Food technologists often add both artificial and natural flavors to commercial frozen entrees that are targeted at older populations (e.g., meatloaf). The additional use of flavor enhancement in home-cooked meals to compensate for chemosensory losses could improve appetite and nutritional status for a large segment of the elderly population.

Other techniques for helping persons with diminished chemosensory acuity obtain more flavor from a meal include thorough chewing of food, as well as rotation among different foods on the plate. Mastication breaks down tissue in food to release compounds that stimulate taste and smell receptors. Rotating the order of foods eaten during a meal (i.e., switching from meat to potatoes to vegetables) helps counteract sensory fatigue in which subsequent bites of the same food are perceived as less intense than the preceding bite. Serving a variety of foods that vary in texture, color, and temperature is also helpful. Adding crunchy components, such as almonds, to foods can also increase the auditory component of eating.

Choosing foods that differ in color can be helpful for persons with modest loss in vision. For example, a vegetable plate could consist of foods with contrasting colors such as green beans, beets, carrots, eggplant with the skin, and potatoes. The color of plates should contrast sharply with the color of the table cloth (e.g., both should not be white). Use of ready-to-serve foods, such as finger foods and prepackaged salads, may improve intake in persons whose diminished vision limits food preparation.

For persons with decrements in temperature and tactile sensations, there are no known methods for enhancement. Although massages may improve blood circulation, there is no convincing evidence that it restores losses in somesthesis. However, it is important that the elderly become aware of their reduced ability to perceive heat so that they do not burn themselves. Food that is soft but adhesive and easy to manipulate may improve intake. Shopping can also be made easier by walking more slowly, wearing low-heeled nonslip shoes, keeping one hand free to take hold of banisters, or using a cane to prevent falls. It should also be mentioned that eating and meal time has a psychological/emotional dimension. Making meal time pleasant in other ways, such as eating with company, setting attractive place settings, or providing other cues for eating can improve food intake and meal enjoyment.

7. SUMMARY

Busse *(134)* classified aging into two divisions: primary aging; representing age-related maturational declines in function, and secondary aging; which is the influence of disease, medications, and the environment on changes associated with age. Although changes in primary aging may be unavoidable, preventing or compensating for other factors, such as medication side effects, disease, and other risk factors will go a long way towards preserving the sensory abilities of the aged. However, the degree to which these losses result from normal aging or from medication use (and other factors) is not known at this time. This gap in our knowledge results from the fact that most studies of sensory functioning in the elderly have not controlled for the use of medications. Clinical reports by physicians suggest that prescription medications play a major role in sensory decline in the elderly, but this has not been addressed in prospective studies. Of the over 250 drugs associated clinically with taste and smell disorders, 87% were reported to cause alterations in other sensory modalities (Table 2). Persons with losses in multiple sensory functions have increased mortality when compared to those with a single deficit *(135)*, as well as greater impairment in functional status *(136)*.

Elderly individuals should be viewed as an entire system with strengths and weaknesses, rather than an isolated set of problems. Optimal nutrition can help maintain the health of the sensory systems; conversely, decrements in the senses of smell, taste, vision, and hearing can have both direct and indirect effects on nutrition. Awareness of the relationship between the senses and overall health and nutrition will lead to strategies to best preserve elderly functional status and quality of life into later life.

8. RECOMMENDATIONS FOR CLINICIANS

1. Clinicians should recognize that prescription medications can play a major role in sensory losses. Taste and smell disorders may occur as well as alterations in vision, hearing, and sense of touch. All of these changes can impede the consumption of an adequate diet.
2. A thorough assessment of sensory function, including potential effects of medications, should be included in the evaluation of any patient with food intake deficit or reported taste or smell impairments.
3. In cases of permanent chemosensory loss, when poor food intake and weight loss threaten long-term health, the addition of simulated food flavors (flavor amplification) to meats, vegetables, and other nutritious foods may improve nutritional status.
4. Other suggestions for helping persons with diminished chemosensory acuity include serving foods that vary in texture, color, and temperature, and instructing the patient to chew foods thoroughly and to rotate tastes of food on the plate to reduce sensory fatigue.
5. Make patients and caregivers aware of safety issues when temperature or tactile sensations are blunted. Adaptive changes, such as thermometer checks of food and beverage temperature would be useful when temperature perception is reduced. In the case of somatosensory system impairments, low-heeled shoes, banisters, and cane use may help prevent falls and thus enhance confidence in the ability to shop for food.

ACKNOWLEDGMENT

Taste and smell research in this paper was supported in part by NIA Grant AG00443.

REFERENCES

1. de Jong N, Mulder I, de Graaf C, van Staveren WA. Impaired sensory functioning in elders: the relation with its potential determinants and nutritional intake. J Gerontol A Biol Sci Med Sci 1999;54: B324–B331.
2. Duffy VB, Backstrand JR, Ferris AM. Olfactory dysfunction and related nutritional risk in free-living, elderly women. J Am Diet Assoc 1995;95:879–884.
3. Griep MI, Verleye G, Franck AH, Collys K, Mets TF, Massart DL. Variation in nutrient intake with dental status, age and odour perception. Eur J Clin Nutr 1996;50:816–825.
4. Chapman KM, Nelson RA. Loss of appetite: managing unwanted weight loss in the older patient. Geriatrics 1994;49:54–59.
5. Morley JE. Anorexia of aging: physiologic and pathologic. Am J Clin Nutr 1997;66:760–773.
6. Morley JE, Thomas, DR. Anorexia and aging: Pathophysiology. Nutrition 1999;15:499–503.
7. Blumberg J. Nutritional needs of seniors. J Am Coll Nutr 1997;16:517–523.
8. Opper FH, Burakoff R. Nutritional support of the elderly patient in an intensive care unit. Clin Geriatr Med 1994;10:31–49.
9. Giduck SA, Threatte RM, Kare MR. Cephalic reflexes: their role in digestion and possible roles in absorption and metabolism. J Nutr 1987;117:1191–1196.
10. Schiffman SS, Warwick ZS. The biology of taste and food intake. In: The science of food regulation: food intake, taste, nutrient partitioning, and energy expenditure. Bray GA, Ryan DH (eds.), Pennington Center Nutrition Series, vol. 2.: Louisiana State University Press, Baton Rouge, LA, 1992, pp. 293–312.
11. Contreras RJ, Frank M. Sodium deprivation alters neural responses to gustatory stimuli. J Gen Physiol 1979;73:569–594.
12. Giza BK, Scott TR, Vanderweele DA. Administration of satiety factors and gustatory responsiveness in the nucleus tractus solitarius of the rat. Brain Res Bull 1992;28:637–639.
13. Giza BK, Deems RO, Vanderweele DA, Scott TR. Pancreatic glucagon suppresses gustatory responsiveness to glucose. Am J Physiol 1993;265:R1231–1237.
14. Jacobs KM, Mark GP, Scott TR. Taste responses in the nucleus tractus solitarius of sodium-deprived rats. J Physiol 1988;406:393–410.
15. Booth DA. Food-conditioned eating preferences and aversions with interoceptive elements: conditioned appetites and satieties. Ann NY Acad Sci 1985;443:22–41.
16. Schiffman SS. Taste and smell in disease. N Eng J Med 1983;308:1275–1279, 1337–1343.
17. Scott TR. Taste: the neural basis of body wisdom. World Rev Nutr Diet 1992;67:1–39.
18. Schiffman SS. Taste and smell losses in normal aging and disease. JAMA 1997;278:1357–1362.
19. Bradley RM. Effects of aging on the anatomy and neurophysiology of taste. Gerodontics 1988;4: 244–248.
20. Pritchard TC. The primate gustatory system. In: Smell and Taste in Health and Disease. Getchell TV, Doty RL, Bartoshuk LM, Snow JB (eds.), Raven, New York ,1991, pp. 109–125.
21. Höfer D, Puschel B, Drenckhahn D. Taste receptor-like cells in the rat gut identified by expression of alpha-gustducin. Proc Natl Acad Sci USA 1996;93:6631–6634.
22. Kinnamon SC, Margolskee RF. Mechanisms of taste transduction. Curr Opin Neurobiol 1996;6:506–513.
23. Spielman AI, Huque T, Whitney G, Brand JG. The diversity of bitter taste signal transduction mechanisms. Soc Gen Physiol Ser 1992;47:307–324.
24. Green BG. Chemesthesis: pungency as a component of flavor. Trends Food Sci Technol 1996;7:415–420.
25. Mistretta CM. Aging effects on anatomy and neurophysiology of taste and smell. Gerodontology 1984;3:131–136.
26. Schiffman SS. Perception of taste and smell in elderly persons. Crit Rev Food Sci Nutr 1993;33:17–26.
27. Weiffenbach JM, Baum BJ, Burghauser R. Taste thresholds: Quality specific variation with human aging. J Gerontol 1982;37:372–377.
28. Stevens JC, Cruz LA, Hoffman JM, Patterson MQ. Taste sensitivity and aging: high incidence of decline revealed by repeated threshold measures. Chem Senses 1995;20:451–459.
29. Schiffman SS. The role of taste and smell in appetite and satiety: impact of chemosensory changes due to aging and drug interactions. In: Nutrition in a Sustainable Environment (Proceedings of the XV

International Congress of Nutrition: IUNS Adelaide). Wahlqvist ML, Truswell AS, Smith R, Nestel PJ (eds.), Gordon; London; Niigata-Shi, Nishimura, Japan, 1994, pp. 728–731.

30. Bartoshuk LM, Rifkin B, Marks LE, Bars P. Taste and aging. J Gerontol 1986;41:51–57.

31. Cowart BJ. Direct scaling of the intensity of basic tastes: a life span study. Paper presented at the annual meeting of the Association of Chemoreception Sciences, Sarasota 1983.

32. Little AC, Brinner L. Taste responses to saltiness of experimentally prepared tomato juice samples. J Am Diet Assoc 1984;21:1022–1027.

33. Murphy C. The effect of age on taste sensitivity. In: Special Senses in Aging: A Current Biological Assessment. Han SS, Coons DH (eds.), University of Michigan Institute of Gerontology, Ann Arbor, 1979, pp. 21–33.

34. Murphy C, Gilmore MM. Quality–specific effects of aging on the human taste system. Percept Psychophys 1989;45:121–128.

35. Schiffman SS, Clark TB. Magnitude estimates of amino acids for young and elderly subjects. Neurobiol Aging 1980;1:81–91.

36. Schiffman SS, Lindley MG, Clark TB, Makino C. Molecular mechanism of sweet taste: relationship of hydrogen bonding to taste sensitivity for both young and elderly. Neurobiol Aging 1981;2:173–185.

37. Schiffman SS, Gatlin LA, Frey AE, Heiman SA, Stagner WC, Cooper DC. Taste perception of bitter compounds in young and elderly persons: relation to lipophilicity of bitter compounds. Neurobiol Aging 1994;15:743–750.

38. Weiffenbach JM, Cowart BJ, Baum BJ. Taste intensity perception in aging. J Gerontol 1986;41:460–468.

39. Schiffman S. Food recognition by the elderly. J Gerontol 1977;32:586–592.

40. Schiffman S. Changes in taste and smell with age: Psychophysical aspects. In: Sensory Systems and Communication in the Elderly, vol. 10. Ordy JM, Brizzee K (eds.), Raven, New York, 1979, pp. 227–246.

41. Schiffman SS, Sattely-Miller EA, Zimmerman IA, Graham BG, Erickson RP. Taste perception of monosodium glutamate (MSG) in foods in young and elderly subjects. Physiol Behav 1994;56:265–275.

42. Schiffman S, Pasternak M. Decreased discrimination of food odors in the elderly. J Gerontol 1979;34:73–79.

43. DeWys WD, Walters K. Abnormalities of taste sensation in cancer patients. Cancer 1975;36:1888–1896.

44. Smith RG, Burtner AP. Oral side-effects of the most frequently prescribed drugs. Spec Care Dentist 1994;14:96–102.

45. Sreebny LM, Schwartz SS. A reference guide to drugs and dry mouth. Gerodontology 1986;5:75–99.

46. Lewis IK, Hanlon JT, Hobbins MJ, Beck JD. Use of medications with potential oral adverse drug reactions in community-dwelling elderly. Spec Care Dentist 1993;13:171–176.

47. Atkin PA, Veitch PC, Veitch EM, Ogle SJ. The epidemiology of serious adverse drug reactions among the elderly. Drugs Aging 1999;14:141–152.

48. Dawling S, Crome P. Clinical pharmacokinetic considerations in the elderly. An update. Clin Pharmacokinet 1989;17:236–263.

49. Moore AR, O'Keeffe ST. Drug-induced cognitive impairment in the elderly. Drugs Aging 1999;15:15–28.

50. Feinberg M. The problems of anticholinergic adverse effects in older patients. Drugs Aging 1993;3:335–348.

51. Molchan SE, Martinez RA, Hill JL, et al. Increased cognitive sensitivity to scopolamine with age and a perspective on the scopolamine model. Brain Res Brain Res Rev 1992;17:215–226.

52. Tollefson GD, Montague-Clouse J, Lancaster SP. The relationship of serum anticholinergic activity to mental status performance in an elderly nursing home population. J Neuropsychiatry Clin Neurosci 1991;3:314–319.

53. Blazer DG II, Federspiel CF, Ray WA, Schaffner W. The risk of anticholinergic toxicity in the elderly: a study of prescribing practices in two populations. J Gerontol 1983;38:31–35.

54. Yousem DM, Geckle RJ, Bilker WB, McKeown DA, Doty RL. Posttraumatic olfactory dysfunction: MR and clinical evaluation. AJNR Am J Neuroradiol 1996;17:1171–1179.

55. Doty RL. Olfactory capacities in aging and Alzheimer's disease: psychophysical and anatomic considerations. Ann NY Acad Sci 1991;640:20–27.

56. Cain WS, Gent JF. Olfactory sensitivity: reliability, generality, and association with aging. J Exp Psychol Hum Percept Perform 1991;17:382–391.

57. Doty RL, Shaman P, Applebaum SL, Giberson R, Siksorski L, Rosenberg L. Smell identification ability: changes with age. Science 1984;226:1441–1443.

58. Stevens JC, Cain WS. Age-related deficiency in the perceived strength of six odorants. Chem Senses 1985;10:517–529.

59. Murphy, C. Age-related effects on the threshold, psychophysical function, and pleasantness of menthol. J Gerontol 1983;38:217–222.

60. Schiffman SS, Warwick ZS. Changes in taste and smell over the lifespan: Effects on appetite and nutrition in the elderly. In: Chem Senses, vol. 4: Appetite and Nutrition. Friedman MI, Tordoff MG, Kare MR (eds.), Marcel Dekker, New York, 1991, pp. 341–365.

61. Stevens JC, Plantinga A, Cain WS. Reduction of odor and nasal pungency associated with aging. Neurobiol Aging 1982;3:125–132.

62. Stevens JC, Bartoshuk LM, Cain WS. Chemical senses and aging: taste versus smell. Chem Senses 1984;9:167–179.

63. Anand MP. Accidents in the home. In: Current Achievements in Geriatrics. Anderson WF, Isaacs B (eds.) Cassell, London, 1984, pp. 239–245.

64. Murphy C. Cognitive and chemosensory influences on age-related changes in the ability to identify blended foods. J Gerontol 1985;40:47–52.

65. Schemper T, Voss S, Cain WS. Odor identification in young and elderly persons: sensory and cognitive limitations. J Gerontol 1981;36:446–452.

66. Schiffman SS, Leffingwell JC. Perception of odors of simple pyrazines by young and elderly subjects: A multidimensional analysis. Pharmacol Biochem Behav 1981;14:787–798.

67. Stevens DA, Lawless HT. Age related changes in flavor perception. Appetite 1981;2:127–136.

68. Van Haeringen NJ. Aging and the lacrimal system. Brit J Ophthalmol 1997;81:824–826.

69. Tseng SC, Tsubota K. Important concepts for treating ocular surface and tear disorders. Am J Opthalmol 1997;124:825–835.

70. Weale RA. The ageing eye. Scientific basis of medicine: Annual Reviews. Athlone, London, 1971, 224–260.

71. Owsley C, Sloane ME. Vision and aging. In: Handbook of Neuropsychology, vol. 4. Boller F, Grafman J (eds.), Elsevier Science Publishers, New York, 1990, pp. 229–249.

72. Hood BD, Garner B, Truscott RJ. Human lens coloration and aging. Evidence for crystallin modification by the major ultraviolet filter, 3-hydroxy-kynurenine O-beta-D-glucoside. J Biol Chem 1999;274: 32,547 32,550.

73. Fisher RF, Pettet BE. Presbyopia and the water content of the human crystalline lens. J Physiol. 1973; 234:443–447.

74. Toris CB, Yablonski ME, Wang YL, Camras CB. Aqueous humor dynamics in the aging human eye. Am J Ophthalmol 1999;127:407–412.

75. Weale RA. Retinal illumination and age. Trans Illumin Eng Soc 1961;26:95–100.

76. Leibowitz HM, Krueger DE, Maunder LR, et al. The Framingham Eye Study monograph: An ophthalmological and epidemiological study of cataract, glaucoma, diabetic retinopathy, macular degeneration, and visual acuity in a general population of 2631 adults, 1973–1975. Surv Ophthalmol 1980;24 (suppl):335–610.

77. Zarbin MA. Age-related macular degeneration: review of pathogenesis. Eur J Ophthalmol 1998;8: 199–206.

78. Chamberlain W. Restriction in upward gaze with advancing age. Trans Am Ophthalmol Soc 1970;68: 234–244.

79. Burton KB, Owsley C, Sloane ME. Aging and neural spatial contrast sensitivity: photopic vision. Vision Res 1993;33:939–946.

80. Elliott D, Whitaker D, MacVeigh D. Neural contribution to spatiotemporal contrast sensitivity decline in healthy ageing eyes. Vision Res 1990;30:541–547.

81. Morrison JD, McGrath C. Assessment of the optical contributions to the age-related deterioration in vision. Quart J Exper Physiol 1985;70:249–269.

82. Haegerstrom-Portnoy G, Schneck ME, Brabyn JA. Seeing into old age: Vision function beyond acuity. Optom Vis Sci 1999;76:141–158.

83. Owsley C, Sekuler R, Siemsen D. Contrast sensitivity throughout adulthood. Vision Res 1983;23: 689–699.

84. Burg A. Lateral visual field as related to age and sex. J Appl Psych 1968;52:10–15.

85. Wolf E. Studies on the shrinkage of the visual field with age. Highway Res Rec 1967;167:1–7.

86. Fiorentini A, Porciatti V, Morrone MC, Burr DC. Visual ageing: unspecific decline of the responses to luminance and colour. Vision Res 1996;36:3557–3566.

87. Knoblauch K, Saunders F, Kusuda M, et al. Age and illuminance effects in Farnsworth-Munsell 100-hue test. Appl Optics 1987;26:1441–1448.
88. Gilmore GC, Wenk HE, Naylor LA, Stuve TA. Motion perception and aging. Psychol Aging 1992;7: 654–660.
89. Burg A. Visual acuity as measured by dynamic and static tests: a comparative evaluation. J Appl Psychol 1966;50:460–466.
90. Jani SN. The age factor in stereopsis screening. Am J Optom Arch Am Acad Optometry 1966;43: 653–657.
91. Bell B, Wolf E, Bernholz CD. Depth perception as a function of age. Aging Hum Develop 1972;3: 77–81.
92. Marsh G.R. Perceptual changes with aging. In: Handbook of Geriatric Psychiatry. Busse EW, Blazer DG (eds.) Van Nostrand Reinhold Co, New York, 1980, pp. 147–168.
93. Marsh GR. Aging and the impact of environmental hazards on sensory function. In: Aging and Environmental Toxicology: Biological and behavioral perspectives. Cooper RL, Goldman JM, Harbin TJ (eds.), Johns Hopkins University Press, Baltimore, 1991.
94. Verma L, Das T, Binder S, et al. New approaches in the management of choroidal neovascular membrane in age-related macular degeneration. Indian J Ophthalmol 2000;48:263–278.
95. Physicians' Desk Reference. Medical Economics Company, Montvale, NJ, 2001.
96. Hodge WG, Whitcher JP, Satariano W. Risk factors for age-related cataracts. Epidemiol Rev 1995;17: 336–346.
97. Brown NA, Bron AJ, Harding JJ, Dewar HM. Nutrition supplements and the eye. Eye 1998;12: 127–133.
98. Seddon JM, Ajani UA, Sperduto RD, et al. Dietary carotenoids, vitamins A, C, and E, and advanced age-related macular degeneration. Eye Disease Case-Control Study Group. JAMA 1994;272:1413–1420.
99. Sperduto Rd, Hu TS, Milton RC. The Linxian Cataract Studies: two nutrition intervention trials. Arch Opthalmol 1993;111:1246–1253.
100. Kasapoglu M, Ozben T. Alterations of antioxidant enzymes and oxidative stress markers in aging. Exper Gerontol 2001;36:209–220.
101. Cai J, Nelson KC, Wu M, Sternberg P Jr, Jones DP. Oxidative damage and protection of the RPE. Prog Retinal Eye Res 2000;19:205–221.
102. Keller BK, Morton JL, Thomas VS, Potter JF. The effect of visual and hearing impairments on functional status. J Am Geriatr Soc 1999;47:1319–1325.
103. Owsley C, Ball K, McGwin G Jr, Sloane ME, Roenker DL, White MF, Overley ET, Visual processing impairment and risk of motor vehicle crash among older adults. JAMA 1998;279:1083–1088.
104. Klein BE, Klein R, Lee KE, Cruickshanks KJ. Performance-based and self-assessed measures of visual function as related to history of falls, hip fractures, and measured gait time. The Beaver Dam Eye Study. Ophthalmology 1998;105:160–164.
105. Etholm B, Belal A Jr. Senile changes in the middle ear joints. Ann Otol Rhinol Laryngol 1974;83: 49–54.
106. Hansen CC, Reske-Nielsen E. Pathological studies in presbycusis. Arch Otolaryngol 1965;82: 115–132.
107. Schuknecht HF, Igarashi M. Pathology of slow progressive sensori-neural deafness. Trans Am Acad Opthalmol Ototolaryngol 1964;68:222–224.
108. Brandt JL, Fozard JL. Age changes in pure-tone hearing thresholds in a longitudinal study of normal human aging. J Acoust Soc Am 1990;88:813–820.
109. Spoor A. Presbycusis values in relationship to noise-induced hearing loss. Intern Audiol 1967;6: 48–57.
110. Marsh GR. Perceptual changes with aging. In: Busse EW, Blazer DG, eds. Textbook of Geriatric Psychiatry. The American Psychiatric Press, Washington, 1996, pp. 49–59.
111. Evans P, Halliwell B. Free radicals and hearing. Cause, consequence and criteria. Ann NY Acad Sci 1999;884:19–40.
112. Humes HD. Insights into ototoxicity. Analogies to nephrotoxicity. Ann NY Acad Sci 1999;884:15–18.
113. Schacht J. Aminoglycoside ototoxicity: prevention in sight? Otolaryngol–Head Neck Surg 1998;118:674–677.
114. Weijl NI, Hopman GD, Wipkink-Bakker A, et al. Cisplatin combination chemotherapy induces a fall in plasma antioxidants of cancer patients. Ann Oncol 1998;9:1331–1337.

115. Bohm S, Oriana S, Spatti G, et al. Dose intensification of platinum compounds with glutathione protection as induction chemotherapy for advanced ovarian carcinoma. Oncology 1999;57:115–120.

116. Mills JH, Going JA. Review of environmental factors affecting hearing. Environ Health Perspect 1982;44:119–127.

117. Casper RC. Nutrition and its relationship to aging. Exp Gerontol 1995;30:299–314.

118. Cauna N. Light and electron-microscopal structures of sensory end-organs in human skin. In: The Skin Senses. Kenshalo DR (ed.) Charles C. Thomas, Springfield, IL, 1968, pp. 15–28.

119. Bolton CF, Winkelman RK, Dyck PJ. A quantitative study of Meissner's corpuscles in man. Neurology 1965;16:1–9.

120. Cauna N. The effects of aging on the receptor organs of the human dermis. In: Advances in Biology of Skin, vol. 6. Montagna W (ed.), Pergamon Press, Elmsford NY, 1965, pp. 63–96.

121. Kenshalo DR. Somesthetic sensitivity in young and elderly humans. J Gerontol 1986;41:732–742.

122. Van Boven RW, Johnson KO. A psychophysical study of the mechanisms of sensory recovery following nerve injury in humans. Brain 1994;117:149–67.

123. Van Boven RW, Johnson KO. The limit of tactile spatial resolution in humans: grating orientation discrimination at the lip, tongue, and finger. Neurology 1994;44:2361–2366.

124. Stevens JC, Choo KK. Spatial acuity of the body surface over the life span. Somatosens Mot Res 1996; 13:153–166.

125. Stevens JC, Cruz LA. Spatial acuity of touch: ubiquitous decline with aging revealed by repeated threshold testing. Somatosens Mot Res 1996;13:1–10.

126. Stevens JC, Patterson MQ. Dimensions of spatial acuity in the touch sense: Changes over the life span. Somatosens Mot Res 1995;12:19–47.

127. Verrillo RT. Age related changes in the sensitivity to vibration. J Gerontol 1980;35:185–193.

128. Stevens JC, Choo KK. Temperature sensitivity of the body surface over the life span. Somatosens Mot Res 1998;15:13–28.

129. Manheimer Flavors (flavor division), J. Manheimer, Inc. Teterboro, New Jersey, www.manheimer.com.

130. Schiffman SS, Warwick ZS. Effect of flavor enhancement of foods for the elderly on nutritional status: food intake, biochemical indices and anthropometric measures. Physiol Behav 1993;53:395–402.

131. Schiffman SS, Wedral E. Contribution of taste and smell losses to the wasting syndrome. Age Nutr 1996;7:106–120.

132. Schiffman SS, Miletic ID. Effect of taste and smell on secretion rate of salivary IgA in elderly and young persons. J Nutr Health Aging 1999;3:158–164.

133. Schiffman SS, Graham, BG. Taste and smell perception affect appetite and immunity in the elderly. Eur J Clin Nutr 2000;54(suppl):S54–S63.

134. Busse EW. In: Behaviour and Adaptation in Later Life. Busse EW, Pfeiffer E (eds.), Little, Brown, Boston, 1969, pp. 11–32.

135. Appollonio I, Carabellese C, Magni E, Frattola L, Trabucchi M. Sensory impairments and mortality in an elderly community population: a six-year follow-up study. Age Ageing 1995;24:30–36.

136. Tinetti ME, Inouye SK, Gill TM, Doucette JT. Shared risk factors for falls, incontinence, and functional dependence. Unifying the approach to geriatric syndromes. JAMA 1995;273:1348–1353.

137. Schiffman SS, Zervakis J, Shaio E, Heald AE. Effect of the nucleoside analogs zidovudine, didanosine, stavudine and lamivudine on the sense of taste. Nutrition 1999;15:854–859.

138. Schiffman SS, Zervakis J, Heffron S, Heald AE. Effect of protease inhibitors on the sense of taste. Nutrition 1999;15:767–772.

139. Griffin JP. Drug-induced disorders of taste. Adverse Drug React Toxicol Rev 1992;11:229–239.

140. Strassman HD, Adams B, Pearson AW. Metronidazole effect on social drinkers. Q J Stud Alcohol 1970;31;394–398.

141. Prata A. Clinical evaluation of niridazole in Schistosoma mansoni infections. Ann NY Acad Sci. 1969; 160:660–669.

142. von Skramlik E. The fundamental substrates of taste. In: Zotterman, Y. ed. Olfaction and taste. Pergamon, Oxford, 1963, pp. 125–132.

143. Yamada Y, Tomita H. Influences on taste in the area of chorda tympani nerve after transtympanic injection of local anesthetic (4% lidocaine). Auris Nasus Larynx 1989;16 (suppl):S41–S46.

144. Henkin RI. Griseofulvin and dysgeusia: Implications? Ann Intern Med 1971;74:795–796.

145. Scott PJ. Glossitis with complete loss of taste sensation during Dindevan treatment: Report of a case. NZ Med J 1960;59:296.

146. Rollin H. Drug-related gustatory disorders. Ann Otol Rhinol Laryngol 1978;87:37–42.

147. Jaffe IA. Ampicillin rashes. Lancet 1970;1:245.

148. Soni NK, Chatterji P. Gustotoxicity of bleomycin. Orl J Otorhinolaryngol 1985; Relat Spec 1985;47: 101–104.

149. Hodgson TG. Bad taste from cefamandole. Drug Intell Clin Pharm 1981;15:136.

150. Fogan L. Griseofulvin and dysgeusia: implications? Ann Intern Med 1971; 74:795.

151. Schiffman SS, Zervakis J. Taste and smell perception in the elderly: effect of medications and disease. Adv Food Nutr Res 2002;44:247–346.

152. Magnasco LD, Magnasco AJ. Metallic taste associated with tetracycline therapy. Clin Pharm 1985;4: 455–456.

153. Soni NK, Chatterji P. Abnormalities of taste. Br Med J 1976;2:198.

154. Seydell EM, McKnight WP. Disturbances of olfaction resulting from intranasal use of tyrothricin: A clinical report of seven cases. Arch Otolaryngol 1948;47:465–470.

155. Reyes ES, Talley RW, O'Bryan RM, Gastesi RA. Clinical evaluation of 1,3-Bis(2-chloroethyl)-1-nitrosourea (BCNU: NSC-409962) with fluoxymesterone (NSC-12165) in the treatment of solid tumors. Cancer Chemother Rep 1973;57:225–230.

156. Guthrie D, Way S. Treatment of advanced carcinoma of the cervix with adriamycin and methotrexate combined. Obstet Gynecol 1974;44:586–589.

157. Duhra P, Foulds IS. Methotrexate-induced impairment of taste acuity. Clin Exper Dermatol 1988;13: 126–127.

158. State FA, Hamed MS, Bondok AA. Effect of vincristine on the histological structure of taste buds. Acta Anat 1977;99:445–449.

159. Beidler LM, Smallman, RL. Renewal of cells within taste buds. J Cell Biol 1965;27:263–272.

160. Fehm-Wolfsdorf G, Scheible E, Zenz H, Born J, Fehm HL. Taste thresholds in man are differentially influenced by hydrocortisone and dexamethasone. Psychoneuroendocrinology 1989;14:433–440.

161. Sternlieb I, Scheinberg IH. Penicillamine therapy for hepatolenticular degeneration. JAMA 1964;189: 748–754.

162. Keiser HR, Henkin RI, Bartter FC, Sjoerdsma, A. Loss of taste during therapy with penicillamine. JAMA 1968;203:381–383.

163. Bourliere F, Cendron H, Rapaport A. Action de l'acide acetylsalicylique sur la sensibilite au gout amer chez l'homme. Rev Fr Etudes Clin Biol 1959;4:380–382.

164. Hellekant G, Gopal V. Depression of taste responses by local or intravascular administration of salicylates in the rat. Acta Physiol Scand 1975;95:286–292.

165. Huskisson EC, Jaffe IA, Scott J, Dieppe PA. 5-Thiopyridoxine in rheumatoid arthritis: Clinical and experimental studies. Arthritis Rheum 1980;23:106–110.

166. Plath P, Otten E. Untersuchungen uber die Wirksamkeit von Hexetidine bei akuten Erkrankungen des Rachens und der Mundhohle sowie nach Tonsillektomie. Therapiewocke 1969;19:1565–1566.

167. Erikssen J, Seegaard E, Naess K. Side-effect of thiocarbamides. Lancet 1975;1:231–232.

168. Hallman BL, Hurst JW. Loss of taste as toxic effect of methimazole (Tapazole) therapy: Report of three cases. JAMA 1953;152:322.

169. Schneeberg NG. Loss of sense of taste due to methylthiouracil therapy. JAMA 1952;149:1091–1093.

170. Grossman S. Loss of taste and smell due to propylthiouracil therapy. NY State J Med 1953;53:1236.

171. Simpson JR. Idoxuridine in the treatment of herpes zoster. Practitioner 1975;215:226–229.

172. Thumfart W, Plattig KH, Schlict N. Smell and taste thresholds in older people. Zeit fur Gerontol 1980; 13:158–188.

173. DeSimone JA, Heck GL, Bartoshuk LM. Surface active taste modifiers: A comparison of the physical and psychophysical properties of gymnemic acid and sodium lauryl sulfate. Chem Senses 1980;5:317–330.

174. Lang NP, Catalanotto FA, Knopfli RU, Antczak AA. Quality-specific taste impairment following the application of chlorhexidine digluconate mouthrinses. J Clin Periodonol 1988;15:43–48.

175. Dahl H, Norskov K, Peitersen E, Hilden J. Zinc therapy of acetazolamide-induced side-effects. Acta Ophthalmolgica 1984;62:739–745.

176. Schiffman SS, Lockhead E, Maes FW. Amiloride reduces the taste intensity of Na+ and Li+ salts and sweeteners. Proc Natl Acad Sci USA 1983;80:6136–6140.

177. Schiffman SS, Frey AE, Suggs MS, Cragoe EJ Jr, Erickson RP. The effect of amiloride analogs on taste responses in gerbil. Physiol Behav 1990;47:435–441.

178. McFate-Smith W, Davies RO, Gabriel MA, et al. Tolerance and safety of enalapril. Br J Clin Pharmacol 1984;18:2(suppl), 249S–255S.

179. McNeil JJ, Anderson A, Christophidis N, Jarrott B, Louis WJ. Taste loss associated with oral captopril treatment. Br Med J 1979;2:1555–1556.
180. Vlasses PH, Ferguson RK. Temporary ageusia related to captopril. Lancet 1979;2:526.
181. Berman JL. Dysosmia, dysgeusia, and diltiazem [letter] Ann Intern Med 1985;102:717.
182. Gifford RW. Ethacrynic acid alone and in combination with methyldopa in management of mild hypertension: A report of 23 patients. Int Z Klin Pharmakol Ther Toxik 1970;3:255–260.
183. Levinson JL, Kennedy K. Dysosmia, dysgeusia, and nifedipine [letter]. Ann Intern Med 1985;102:135–136.
184. Lahon HFJ, Mann RD. Glipizide: Results of a multicentre clinical trial. J Int Med Res 1973;1:608–615.
185. Ferguson AW, de la Harpe PL, Farquhar JW. Dimethyldiguanide in the treatment of diabetic children. Lancet 1961;1:1367–1369.
186. Siegfried J, Zumstein H. Changes in taste under L-DOPA therapy. Z Neurol 1971; 200:345–348.
187. Halbreich U. Tegretol dependency and diversion of the sense of taste. Isr Ann Psychiatry 1974;12:328–332.
188. Bressler B. An unusual side-effect of lithium. Psychosomatics 1980;21:688–689.
189. Duffield JE. Side effects of lithium carbonate. Br Med J 1973;1:491.
190. Fischer R, Griffin F, Archer RC, Zinmeister SC, Jastram PS. Weber ratio in gustatory chemoreception: An indicator of systemic (drug) reactivity. Nature 1965;207:1049–1053.
191. Mata F. Effect of dextro-amphetamine on bitter taste threshold. J Neuropsychiatry 1963;4:315–320.
192. Goy JJ, Finci L, Sigwart U. Dysgeusia after high dose dipyridamole treatment [Short communication]. Arzneimittelforschung 1985;35:854.
193. Ewing RC, Janda SM, Henann NE. Ageusia associated with transdermal nitroglycerin. Clin Pharm 1989;8.146–147.
194. Rabe F. Isolierte ageusie: Ein neues Symptom als Nebenwirkung von Medikamenten. Nervenarzt 1970;41:23 27.
195. Whittington J, Raftery EB. A controlled comparison of oxyfedrine, isosorbide dinitrate and placebo in the treatment of patients suffering attacks of angina pectoris. Br J Clin Pharmacol 1980;10:211–215.
196. Jones PB, McCloskey EV, Kanis JA. Transient taste-loss during treatment with etidronate [letter]. Lancet 1987;2:637.
197. Cherington M. Guanidine and germine in Eaton-Lambert syndrome. Neurology (Minneap) 1976;26:944–946.
198. McCurdy PR. Parenteral iron therapy. II. A new iron-sorbitol citric acid complex for intra-muscular injection. Ann Intern Med 1964;61:1053–1064.

10   Hearing Loss and Nutriton
in Older Adults

Mary Ann Johnson, Albert R. DeChicchis,
James F. Willott, Kelly J. Shea-Miller,
and Robert J. Nozza

1. INTRODUCTION

This chapter focuses on selected medical, metabolic, and nutritional factors that may impair auditory function in older adults. The relationship of hearing loss and nutritional status is a relatively new area of investigation with many potential opportunities in basic research, primary prevention, and clinical practice. More in-depth discussions of age-related hearing loss and geriatric audiology are available (*1,2*).

2. HEARING LOSS IN OLDER ADULTS

Effective communication is essential in our modern society. One of every six Americans has a communication disorder such as hearing impairment, dizziness, balance problems, smell and taste disorders, voice, speech, or language disturbances. These disorders impair social, emotional, and vocational aspects of people's lives, and have enormous costs related to poor quality of life. With the aging of our population and improved survival rates for medically fragile infants and individuals who have sustained injury, the prevalence of communication disorders will continue to increase (*3*).

Approximately 28 million people in the United States are deaf or hard of hearing and nearly 1.5 million people aged 3 yr or older are deaf in both ears (*4–6*). Genetic factors, noise or trauma, sensitivity to certain drugs or medications, and viral or bacterial infections may cause deafness or hearing impairment. Hearing impairment occurs in more than 300 inherited syndromes. Advances in molecular genetics will improve identification of people at risk for late-onset or progressive hearing loss so that appropriate treatment or rehabilitation options can be initiated. People are losing hearing earlier in life, largely as a result of noise exposure.

Hearing loss in elderly people is a major concern (*5,6*). Presbycusis, the loss of hearing associated with aging, affects 30–35% of people aged 65–75 yr and 40–50% of people aged 75 and older. The risk of hearing loss is increased greatly with age and is greater in

From: *Handbook of Clinical Nutrition and Aging*
Edited by: C. W. Bales and C. S. Ritchie © Humana Press Inc., Totowa, NJ

men than in women *(7)*. Hearing impairment, along with heart problems, hypertension, and arthritis, is one of the top four chronic conditions experienced by elderly people *(8)*. Only about 1 in 4 older adults requiring a hearing aid actually use one.

Presbycusis is associated with a proportionately greater loss of high-pitched sounds (e.g., ringing of a telephone). Individuals with presbycusis may experience a variety of difficulties such as the speech of others seems mumbled, slurred, unclear and low in volume; high-pitched sounds such as "s" and "th" are difficult to hear and distinguish; conversations are difficult to understand, particularly with background noise; higher pitched women's voices are more difficult to hear than men's voices; and some sounds seem annoying or overly loud *(5,6)*. Some older adults also experience tinnitus, a ringing, roaring and/or hissing sound in one or both ears. Hearing problems can make it difficult for an older adult to understand and follow health advice from their physician and other health professionals. Hearing loss has a very negative influence on the lives of elderly people—even mild hearing loss is associated with impaired quality of life and functional disabilities and adversely affects physical, cognitive, emotional, behavioral, and social function *(9)*. Mental and emotional problems associated with hearing loss include fear, anger, depression, frustration, embarrassment, anxiety, withdrawal, emotional lability, aloofness, paucity of speech, and confusion or dementia *(10)*. Thus, hearing impairment in the older adult can lead to frustrating, embarrassing, and even dangerous situations *(5,6)*.

2.1. Rehabilitation, Amplification, and Hearing Aids

There are a variety of strategies to assist people with presbycusis including hearing aids and assistive listening devices (e.g., telephones with amplifiers, TV listening systems, FM systems for use in auditoriums, churches, and movie theaters *[5,6]*). Recent advances in technology are markedly improving hearing aids and for those individuals who cannot benefit from conventional hearing aids, cochlear implants are available. Cochlear implants are most often used in young children, but some older adults can benefit from these implants. Consultation with an otolaryngologist and audiologist is essential for maximum success of rehabilitation. Audiologic services should be available to residents of long-term care facilities, such as nursing homes and adult day care *(2)*. An audiologist should also provide regular and periodic inservices in long-term care to assist all staff members to optimize the communication potential of the older adults they serve *(2)*.

Proper care of hearing aids is essential for their optimal performance. The following are some suggestions for maintenance of hearing aids *(2)*:

- Keep hearing aids dry (preferably in a hearing-aid dehumidifier at night).
- Do not wear hearing aids in the shower, when applying hair spray or when sleeping.
- Battery should be removed when hearing aid is taken out of the ear and checked before reinserting.
- Hearing aid should be stored in a safe place and in the same place each night (e.g., in a drawer).
- Prior to inserting hearing aid, check for wax build-up. If present, it should be removed by a health professional.
- The earmold from behind-the-ear hearing aids should be disconnected from the hearing aid, washed, and dried regularly using a blower supplied by the audiologist.

2.2. Communication Tips for Older Adults with Hearing Loss

These strategies can be used by speakers in health care settings, long term-care, and with family, friends, and colleagues to assist the hearing impaired listener (5).

- Face the listener who has a hearing loss so that the listener can see the face of the speaker.
- Be sure there is adequate lighting in front of the speaker. This helps the listener with hearing impairment, see facial expressions, gestures, and lip and body movements that provide communication clues.
- Turn off the radio or television during conversations.
- The speaker should avoid talking while chewing gum or food or covering their mouth with their hands.
- Speak slightly louder than normal, but don't shout. Shouting may distort speech.
- Speak at a normal rate, and do not exaggerate sounds.
- Clue the listener with the hearing loss about the topic of the conversation whenever possible.
- Rephrase statements into short simple sentences if it appears that the listener does not understand.
- At social gatherings and in restaurants, sit away from crowded or noisy areas.

3. BIOLOGICAL BASIS OF AGE-RELATED HEARING LOSS

The progressive loss of hearing sensitivity with age is attributed largely to disorders of the peripheral auditory system; specifically, abnormalities within the cochlea (Fig. 1) (5,6,9,11).

The cochlea is the auditory portion of the inner ear that rests within a bony spiral canal containing fluid-filled membranous channels (12). Although the nature of the impairment associated with age-related hearing loss has been well documented and some areas within the auditory system that are affected have been identified, the causes remain unknown. It is likely that the accumulation of years of exposure to noise and other environmental agents (e.g., toxic substances, drugs) we encounter in our daily lives contribute to hearing loss in at least some older people (13–15). Less frequently, age-related hearing loss may be a conductive hearing disorder caused by abnormalities of the outer ear and/or middle ear, such as reduced function of the tympanic membrane (the eardrum) or the ossicles of the middle ear that carry sound waves from the tympanic membrane to the inner ear. There may be a genetic link predisposing certain individuals to hearing losses with age (11,14,16,17). Nevertheless, further investigation is needed concerning other risk factors that either have been suggested by previous research or have theoretical support for a role in age-related hearing loss.

4. MEDICAL CONDITIONS AND HEARING LOSS

Hearing loss has been associated to varying degrees with many conditions, such as ototoxicity, noise exposure, acoustic neuroma, dementia, cardiovascular disease, and metabolic disorders (e.g., diabetes and kidney disease) (2). These disorders have been discussed in detail by others (1,2). Ototoxic medications and cardiovascular disease, as well as nutritional status, will be discussed in more detail.

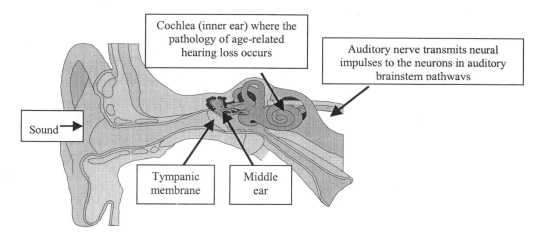

Fig. 1. Peripheral auditory system.

4.1. Medications and Hearing Loss

Ototoxic medications have the potential to temporarily or permanently aggravate existing sensorineural hearing loss (inner ear) and/or damage inner ear structures *(18)*. These effects depend on the type, amount and duration of medication use. Both over-the-counter and prescription medications can have ototoxic effects. Older adults should be encouraged to tell their physician that they have hearing loss and to consider ototoxic side effects when prescribing medications (*see also* Chapter 9). Older adults should also read the labels and ask their pharmacist about potential ototoxic effects. Some signs of ototoxicity that should be immediately reported to the physician are *(18)*:

- Development of tinnitus in one or both ears;
- Intensification of existing tinnitus;
- Fullness or pressure in the ears—other than being secondary to an upper respiratory infection;
- Awareness of a hearing loss in an unaffected ear or progression or fluctuation of an existing loss; and
- Development of vertigo or spinning sensation possibly aggravated by motion and/or accompanied by nausea.

Below is a partial list of potentially ototoxic medications. Older adults should consult their physician and pharmacist for more information about the ototoxic effects of these and other medications that they are taking *(2,18)*.

- Salicylates (aspirin and aspirin-containing products).
- Antibiotics (e.g., aminoglycosides and the "mycin" family).
- Loop diuretics (e.g., Lasix).
- Chemotherapeutic agents (e.g., Cisplatin).
- Quinine (e.g., for treatment of malaria).

Several studies in animals suggest that nutritional status may influence the ototoxicity of some medications *(19–21)*. The potential for nutritional interventions to ameliorate the ototoxic effects of certain medications in humans awaits further investigation.

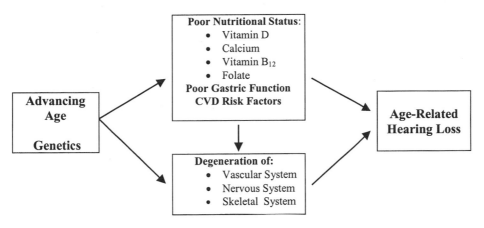

Fig. 2. Working model for hypothesized relationships of nutrition with age-related hearing loss.

5. NUTRITION AND HEARING LOSS

The hypothesis that nutrition may play a causal role in hearing loss is based on evidence from two converging bodies of knowledge: previous research has shown that auditory dysfunction is linked to vascular disease, skeletal disorders, and neural degeneration or disorders *(22–26)*, and knowledge that the vascular, skeletal, and neural systems rely on certain nutrients for optimal structure and function. Despite the contribution of diet and genes to many age-related chronic health conditions, such as cardiovascular disease, cancer, osteoporosis, diabetes, cataracts, and age-related macular degeneration *(27)*, there has been no comprehensive and systematic research effort directed toward understanding the possible interactions among poor diet, genetic disorders, and age-related hearing loss. Thus, there is a profound gap in our knowledge concerning the role of these factors in hearing loss in older adults.

Research on the relationships of age-related hearing loss with nutritional status may lead to identification of risk factors for age-related hearing loss and possibly to prevention and treatment strategies aimed at reducing the prevalence and progression of this devastating disorder. Our working model for exploring the associations of nutrition and age-related hearing loss is illustrated in Fig. 2.

5.1. Cardiovascular Disease Risk Factors and Hearing Loss

Research that suggests a relationship of cardiovascular disease risk factors and hearing loss extends back more than 30 yr. Rosen et al. *(28)* reported that low fat diets when compared to a normal diet (relatively high in saturated fat) were associated with a slower rate of decline in hearing levels in prisoners. More recently, Gates et al. *(23)* reported that certain cardiovascular disease events and cardiovascular disease risk factors were associated with hearing loss in men and women in the Framingham Study. Low-frequency hearing loss was related to cardiovascular disease events in both genders, but somewhat more so in women. Among the risk factors, hypertension and systolic blood pressure were related to hearing thresholds in both genders, whereas the blood glucose level was related to the pure-tone average in women. Brant et al. *(13)* examined the relationship of cardiovascular disease risk factors in participants of the Baltimore Longitudinal Study of Aging.

They found that men who were borderline hypertensive with a systolic blood pressure of 140 have a 32% greater risk of developing hearing loss than normotensive men. Men with hypertension (systolic pressure of 160) had a 74% greater risk of hearing loss than the borderline hypertensive group. Smoking has also been associated with hearing loss *(7)*. Associations of cardiovascular risk factors with hearing loss are not seen in all studies (e.g., in adults aged 50 or less *[29]*), and perhaps are not detectable until later ages. Although these epidemiological studies cannot prove cause and effect, it is possible that management of cardiovascular disease (CVD) risk factors may slow the progression of age-related hearing loss.

5.2. Micronutrients and Auditory Function

Auditory dysfunction occurs in experimental animals with vitamin and/or mineral deficiencies and in humans with nutritional disorders *(30)* (*see* Table 1). Interpretation of human studies is difficult because the subjects had a variety of types of hearing loss, other metabolic disorders, and the etiology and type of nutritional disorder varied (dietary deprivation, gastrointestinal disorders, alcoholism, or drug–nutrient interactions). Most of the research in animals suffers from limitations including poor formulation of diets, no report of body weight during micronutrient deficiencies, and lack of biochemical confirmation of nutrient deficiencies. Despite these limitations, evidence is growing that nutritional deficiencies may play a causal role in hearing loss. We discuss in detail the relationship of auditory function with vitamin D and vitamin B_{12} because these are two of the most common micronutrient problems in older adults *(31)*.

5.2.1. VITAMIN B_{12} AND AUDITORY FUNCTION

Auditory dysfunction and severe vitamin B_{12} deficiency in rhesus monkeys were examined over a 5-yr period *(32)*. Although peripheral hearing levels were not monitored, the auditory nerve and other nerves had active lesions associated with vitamin B_{12} deficiency. Despite the profound influence of vitamin B_{12} deficiency on the nervous system *(33)* and the key role of the nervous system in auditory function *(26)*, complete audiological evaluations are generally not included in neurological assessments of vitamin B_{12}-deficient patients *(33)*. Vitamin B_{12} deficiency has been associated with impaired auditory brainstem response (ABR) in some but not all human patients *(34–36)*. Tinnitus or "ringing in the ears" *(37)* and auditory hallucinations *(38)* have been recorded as symptoms of vitamin B_{12} deficiency.

Shemesh et al. *(39)* examined serum vitamin B_{12} in 113 noise-exposed men with a mean age of 39 yr. Those with both chronic tinnitus (ringing in the ears) and noise-induced hearing loss were about 2.6 times more likely to be vitamin B_{12} deficient (defined by serum vitamin B_{12} < 250 pg/mL) when compared to those with normal hearing. Shemesh et al. suggested that inadequate vitamin B_{12} may be associated with myelin damage in those with repeated noise exposure. Subjective improvement in tinnitus was observed in 12 patients following 4 mo of vitamin B_{12} replacement therapy (1 mg/wk, parenteral). Although subjects were primarily middle-aged and dietary patterns were not assessed, this study does provide some evidence that vitamin B_{12} status may influence auditory function.

Relationships between the ABR and vitamin B_{12} deficiency have been examined in human subjects *(34–36)*. However, the lack of control groups and the small sample sizes make it difficult to derive meaningful conclusions regarding the role of vitamin B_{12}

deficiency in the ABR [$n = 7$, *(34)*; $n = 3$, *(35)*; $n = 10$, *(36)*]. In total, these studies involved 20 subjects, 3 of whom had abnormal ABR results (prolonged I–V interpeak latencies). In 2 of these 3 subjects, I–V interpeak latencies were within normal limits when they were retested after repletion with vitamin B_{12}, suggesting that vitamin B_{12} supplementation may improve some indices of auditory function in vitamin B_{12} deficient people.

We reported that poor vitamin B_{12} and folate status was associated with hearing loss in older women ($n = 55$, age 60–71 yr) *(40)*. These data were collected in 1996 prior to FDA-mandated fortification of the food supply with folic acid. Hearing function was determined by the mean of pure tone thresholds at 0.5, 1, 2, and 4 kHz pure-tone average (PTA_4) and was categorized into two groups for statistical analyses: normal hearing (<20 dB hearing loss [HL]; n = 44) and impaired hearing (≥20 dB [HL]; $n = 11$). Mean pure tone thresholds were significantly correlated with serum vitamin B_{12} ($r = -0.58$, $p = 0.0001$) and red cell folate ($r = -0.37$, $p = 0.01$). Compared to women with normal hearing, women with impaired hearing *(40)*:

- Had 38% lower serum vitamin B_{12} (236 vs 380 pmol/L, $p = 0.008$);
- Had 31% lower red cell folate (425 vs 619 nmol/L, $p = 0.02$);
- Consumed 43% less dietary vitamin B_{12} (2.4 vs 4.2 μg/d, $p = 0.02$);
- Consumed 41% less dietary folate (195 vs 332 μg/d, $p = 0.01$);
- Had 47% lower serum pepsinogen I, suggesting a higher prevalence of gastric problems that might interfere with the absorption of vitamin B_{12} and other nutrients (44 vs 83 ng/mL, $p = 0.01$).

These relationships remained statistically significant when controlled for age in logistic regression analyses. Decreases in red blood cell folate might have been associated with poor vitamin B_{12} nutriture *(41)*. There was also a trend in a subsample of these women for hearing impairment to be associated with high-serum homocysteine ($n = 20$, 8.3 vs 7.6 μM, $p = 0.18$) and methylmalonic acid (275 vs 243 nM, $p = 0.16$; analyses performed by Dr. Sally P. Stabler, University of Colorado Health Sciences Center, Boulder, CO).

Berner et al. *(42)* reported that hearing thresholds were not related to vitamin B_{12}, folate, or homocysteine in older men and women ($n = 91$, median age = 78). However, all subjects had >25 dB hearing loss (PTA_4, 0.5–4 kHz); thus, there was no control group. In contrast, our study had a hearing impaired group (≥20 dB HL; PTA_4, 0.5–4 kHz) and two normal hearing control groups (<10 dB HL and ≥10 to <20 dB HL); a dose-response relationship between hearing loss and nutritional status occurred at <20 dB HL. Control groups are essential for studying the hypothesis that people with normal hearing tend to have better nutritional status and people with impaired hearing tend to have poorer nutrition *(40)*. Both Berner et al. *(42)* and Houston et al. *(40)* found that their hearing impaired older adults had similar serum vitamin B_{12} concentrations (237 and 236 pmol/L, respectively). Nonetheless, animal studies, as well as prospective and/or intervention studies in humans, are needed to demonstrate a causal role for vitamin B_{12} and other nutrients in hearing loss.

5.2.2. VITAMIN D DEFICIENCY AND AUDITORY DYSFUNCTION

Vitamin D deficiency may have direct and indirect effects on auditory function by altering calcium metabolism, fluids and nerve transmission, and bone structure. Vitamin D deficiency directly or indirectly through its role in calcium homeostasis, may cause *(43–51)*:

Table 1
Micronutrients Associated with Auditory Dysfunction in Human and Animal Studies

Nutrient, species	Findings	Reference
Vitamin B12 and/or folate, humans	Vitamin B12 deficiency associated with abnormal auditory brainstem responses in some, but not all patients	(34–36,39,40,42,65)
	Moderate hearing impairment associated with lower serum vitamin B12 and lower red cell folate	
	Epidemic of sensorineural hearing loss suspected to be related to inadequate intake of folate and possibly other B vitamins	
Vitamin B12 deficiency, rhesus monkeys	Vitamin B12 deficiency associated with lesions in the auditory nerve	(32)
Thiamine deficiency, rats	Middle ear infections, alterations in ganglion cells and myelin sheath	(52)
Riboflavin deficiency, rats	Middle ear infections, alterations in ganglion cells and myelin sheath	(52)
Vitamin B6 deficiency, rats	External hair cells normal, but abnormalities in the spiral ganglion cells and myelin sheath	(52,66–69)
	Abnormal auditory brainstem responses	
	Reduced reactions to acoustic stimuli	
	Strain differences in auditory changes in response to vitamin deficiency	
Vitamin B6 deficiency, cats	Abnormal auditory brainstem responses	(70)
B vitamin combinations, guinea pigs	B vitamin treatment protected against cisplatin-induced ototoxicity as assessed by transient evoked otoacoustic emission	(20)
Vitamin A deficiency, rats	Epithelial metaplasia of lining with keratinization and secondary infection; degeneration of external sulcus cells, cells of stria vascularis; scattered spiral ganglion cells; demyelinization of distal part of nerve	(52)

Vitamin C deficiency, guinea pigs	Disorders in organ of Corti, external sulcus, stria vascularis, endolymphatic duct, and areas near spiral ligament and bony wall	(52)
Vitamin C supplementation, rats	Improved auditory brainstem responses	(17)
Vitamin D deficiency, rats	Middle ear infections, formation of osteoid in the periosteal and enchondral layers of the capsule and degenerative changes in cochlear nerve	(45,52)
	Decreased calcium concentration of calcium in the perilymph and prolonged latency of the cochlear potentials	
Vitamin D, humans	Attempts made to link vitamin D status, as assessed by serum 1,25-dihydroxyvitamin D and 25-hydroxyvitamin D, in people in relatively good health, as well as those with a variety of disorders in hearing	(22,30,53–59,71)
	Additional evidence needed to confirm relationships of vitamin D status with auditory function in humans	
Vitamin E, guinea pigs	Vitamin E supplements suppress cisplatin-induced ototoxicity as assessed by auditory thresholds, lipid peroxidation, hair cell counts, and DNA-fragmentation in cochlear hair cells	(21)
Vitamin E deficiency, rats	Hemorrhage, middle ear inflammation, formation of small irregularities in the periosteal layer and degeneration of muscle fibers in the inner ear	(52)
Vitamin E supplements, rats	Improved auditory thresholds	(17)

continued

Table 1 (*continued*)
Micronutrients Associated with Auditory Dysfunction in Human and Animal Studies

Nutrient, species	Findings	Reference
Copper deficiency, rats	Deficiency caused an irreversible decrease in the auditory startle response	(72)
Iron deficiency, rats	Abnormalities in outer and inner hair cells, atrophy of ganglion cells, decreased activity of iron enzymes such as cochlear succinic dehydrogenase, and impaired auditory thresholds	(73–76)
Iron deficiency, humans	Iron deficient infants had abnormal auditory brainstem responses and slowed conduction. Benefits of iron supplementation on reversing auditory abnormalities not clear	(77–79)
Magnesium deficiency, guinea pigs	Abnormalities in auditory thresholds	(19,80)
Magnesium deficiency, rats	Magnesium deficiency exacerbates noise-induced hearing loss and audiogenic seizures	(81,82)
Magnesium and zinc deficiency, rats	Magnesium, but not zinc deficiency impaired auditory evoked potentials Deficiency of either nutrient exacerbated ototoxicity of various medications	(83)
Zinc deficiency, rats	Both zinc deficiency and pair feeding were associated with delayed maturation of the auditory startle response, thus low energy intake rather than zinc deficiency may account for the auditory disorder Zinc deficiency was not related to abnormal auditory brainstem responses or abnormalities of the cochlea or stria vascularis	(84,85)

- Alterations in the calcium concentration in the essential fluids, hair cells, and nervous tissue of the inner ear;
- Degeneration of auditory structures including the spiral ligament, stria vascularis, and cochlear hair cells;
- Sensitization of the cochlea to the effects of chronic ischemia;
- Imbalance in lysosomal enzymes leading to cell destruction and deafness; and
- Cochlear demineralization and changes in bone remodeling of the otic capsule.

Vitamin D deficiency may cause disruption of the calcium concentration in the essential fluids, hair cells, and nervous tissue of the inner ear. Calcium-binding proteins, such as parvalbumin and calbindin, are present in auditory nervous tissue. The endolymph, perilymph, and intrastrial fluids of the cochlea each have a unique ionic composition that must be maintained for proper auditory function *(51)*. The intracellular concentration of free calcium (Ca^{+2}) modulates inner ear and hair cell function. Inner ear Ca^{+2} concentration influences pH, protein phosphorylation, cell volume regulation, and neurotransmitter release; thus, alterations in intracellular Ca^{+2} concentrations may disrupt the inner ear and might be associated with otologic damage in many inner ear disorders *(43,46,51)*. Alterations in intracellular Ca^{+2} concentrations could damage the inner ear because excess Ca^{+2} is linked to excessive free radical production, membrane damage, DNA fragmentation and ultimately Ca^{+2}-mediated cell death *(51)*. With increasing age, there may be altered calcium homeostasis in the central auditory system *(11)*. Dietary factors, such as vitamin D deficiency, have been associated with cochlear dysfunction and disruption in calcium homeostasis in the cochlea of rats *(45)*.

A variety of approaches have been used to investigate vitamin D and auditory function:

- Vitamin D-depletion studies in rats *(45,52)*;
- Supplementation with vitamin D and other nutrients in people with poor vitamin D status and hearing loss (conductive deafness, cochlear deafness, otosclerosis, chronic suppurative otitis media, Meniere's disease, early progressive sensorineural hearing loss, senile deafness, noise exposure) *(53–58)*;
- Examination of populations with metabolic disorders associated with impaired calcium and/or vitamin D status (metabolic bone disease, hypoparathyroidism or abnormal blood indices of calcium, phosphate, or alkaline phosphatase) *(58,59)*;
- Assessment of vitamin D status in case-control studies comparing hearing impaired vs normal hearing older adults *(22,30,60)*.

Although these studies provide some evidence that vitamin D status is associated with auditory dysfunction, they have several weaknesses and limitations. Limitations in the animals studies included incomplete information on dietary formulation and composition; strong possibility that control and experimental diets differed in composition and were lacking in other essential nutrients; limited information of food intake, body weight, and body weight gain; and lack of biochemical confirmation of nutrient deficiencies. Also, one of the earliest studies on nutritional deficiencies and hearing loss in animals was published in 1940 *(52)* before some essential nutrients were discovered, and the methods used to assess auditory function were less sophisticated than those available today.

To overcome these difficulties, we examined the effects of vitamin D deficiency on auditory function in DBA/2J (DBA) mice, which have severe progressive hearing loss of early onset *(61,62)*. The DBA mice have the *Ahl* gene and are homozygous for other genes responsible for age-related decrease in auditory sensitivity *(61,63,64)*. Auditory function was assessed by presenting brief tone bursts at each of five test frequencies and recording responses electrophysiologically via ABR measurements. The ABR is an electrical response generated by the auditory nerve and nerve fibers within the auditory brainstem pathways that results from an auditory stimulus presented to the ear. The inner ear (cochlea) responds to the stimulus, and, subsequently, the auditory nerve and nerves within the auditory brainstem pathway generate electrical signals in response to the auditory stimulus. The ABR correlates well with hearing function. In the DBA mouse, cochlear pathology is evident yielding an impaired ABR.

ABR thresholds were measured at 35 and 45 d of age which corresponds to 10 and 20 d of vitamin D depletion, respectively (Fig. 3). The higher the ABR threshold, the louder the sound must be for the animal to have an ABR response. Although vitamin D deprivation was only for a brief period, these preliminary data provided some interesting findings. At 35 d of age (10 d of vitamin D depletion), vitamin D-deficient mice had worse hearing at all frequencies ($P < 0.05$ at 8 kHz). Thus, even in mice that have a severe progressive hearing loss of early onset, it was shown that a vitamin D-deficient diet accelerates the rate of hearing loss. Because the rate of hearing loss is so rapid in this strain, the effect of vitamin D deficiency on hearing loss appears to be lost after 20 d of vitamin D deprivation (45-d-old DBA mice); that is, these animals have profound hearing loss by 45 d of age and the effects of nutritional deprivation may no longer be evident. Serum 25-hydroxyvitamin D [25(OH)D] was significantly lower in mice given vitamin D-deficient rather than vitamin D-adequate diet (<5 ng/mL vs 18.4 ng/mL, 45 d of age, 20 d of vitamin D depletion; analyses courtesy of Ms. Elaine W. Gunter, Centers for Disease Control and Prevention, Atlanta, GA). There were no differences in mean body weight in the two dietary treatments during the course of this experiment. These data suggest that the DBA mouse, and perhaps other animal models, can be used to explore nutrient–gene interactions that influence auditory function over the life cycle.

The relationship of vitamin D and auditory function has also been examined in humans (*see* Table 1). In most of the human studies, participants had a variety of hearing, metabolic, and/or chronic disorders, and may have been deficient in other nutrients in addition to vitamin D. Frequently, factors related to age, gender, ethnicity, medications and disease history were not reported. Many human studies had no control group, lacked well-defined inclusion and exclusion criteria, and had no statistical treatment of the data. The amounts of vitamin D and calcium used in the supplementation trials were not always reported. The small sample sizes and case studies are difficult to generalize to the general population. Research conducted by this lab *(30,60)* and others *(22)* suggests that poor vitamin D status may be linked to auditory function in healthy older adults who have age-related hearing loss, without excessive noise exposure, otosclerosis, Meniere's disease, or other types of hearing loss.

We examined the relationships of vitamin D and calcium status in older women (age 60–69: $n = 98$; age 70–80: $n = 96$) *(30,60)*. Age-related hearing loss was defined as hearing loss $\geq$ 20 dB HL with onset after age 50 yr with no other known etiology, (PTA$_4$ of the relevant speech frequencies: 0.5–4 kHz). Compared to those with normal hearing, those with hearing loss consumed less calcium (diet plus supplements: 1423 vs 1209 mg/d, $p = 0.006$) and were less likely to meet the Adequate Intake (AI) for calcium (AI, 1200 mg/d: 63 vs 43%, $p = 0.01$), but had similar intakes of energy ($p = 0.98$) and protein ($p = 0.36$).

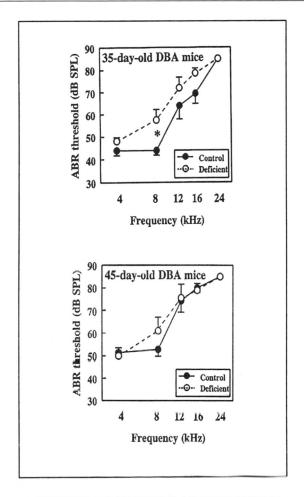

ABR thresholds (mean ±SEM) as a function of frequency in DBA/2J mice fed vitamin D-deficient diets (o, n=10) and vitamin D-adequate diets (•, n = 9) starting at 25 days of age for 10 to 20 days.

Fig. 3. Vitamin D deprivation accelerates hearing loss in DBA/2J mice.

Serum 25-hydroxyvitamin D was higher in women with normal hearing when compared to impaired hearing in the subgroup of women aged 70–80 yr (<20 ng/mL: 13% vs 32%, $p = 0.04$). All 3 women with vitamin D deficiency had hearing loss (25(OH)D < 10 ng/mL; age 75–77). In the total sample, the relationship of vitamin D and calcium with hearing function did not appear to be related to overall dietary quality because the intakes of energy and protein were not significantly different between the groups and were not associated with hearing loss. These findings suggest that calcium and vitamin D status may be associated with age-related hearing loss even in women with relatively good calcium and vitamin D status. However, the causal role of vitamin D and calcium status in hearing loss remains to be established.

It is intriguing, yet disappointing, that vitamin D repletion improved hearing function in only a small percentage of people with both vitamin D deficiency and hearing loss *(55–57)*. Possible explanations for the apparently low rate of improvement include the possibility that vitamin D deficiency indeed causes permanent hearing loss, or perhaps vitamin D deficiency occurred coincidentally with other nutritional deficiencies, metabolic disorders, and/or other irreversible forms of hearing loss.

6. SUMMARY AND RECOMMENDATIONS FOR CLINICIANS

In summary, a variety of approaches are being used to investigate the relationship of vitamin D deficiency with hearing loss. Animal models are needed to explore the biological plausibility and the temporal relationships of these associations. Studies in animals can also be used to determine if vitamin D deficiency causes a reversible or irreversible form of hearing loss by conducting depletion-repletion studies of vitamin D deficiency. In the meantime, it is prudent to ensure that vitamin D status is adequate in older adults by provision of vitamin D through diet and/or supplements.

Much of the hearing loss caused by noise exposure can be prevented by reducing the amount of time exposed to loud noises at home and at work. It is also possible that improved prevention and management of a variety of metabolic, medical, and nutritional factors may also delay the onset of age-related hearing loss as well. Health professionals must be sensitive to the communication problems that occur frequently in older adults and implement methods to improve communication. The following are specific recommendations.

1. Precautions should be taken to reduce noise exposure at home and in the workplace.
2. Because medical and nutritional factors may precipitate hearing loss, good wellness practices, and adequate nutritional status could be important factors for preserving the sense of hearing in old age. In particular, the prevention of cardiovascular disease may indirectly benefit hearing status.
3. Nutrients of particular importance for hearing include vitamin B_{12}, folacin, vitamin D and calcium; thus, generous dietary intakes of these nutrients is encouraged for older adults. In the cases of vitamin B_{12} (which may be poorly absorbed if achlorhydria is present) and vitamin D (which is difficult to obtain from food sources), a supplement may be necessary for some individuals to achieve adequacy.

REFERENCES

1. Hull RH. Hearing in Aging. Danhauer JL (ed.) Singular Publishing Group, Inc., San Diego, CA, 1995.
2. Weinstein B. Geriatric Audiology. Seils A (ed.) Thieme Medical Publishers, Inc., New York, 2000.
3. National Institute on Deafness and other Communication Disorders, National Institutes of Health. National Strategic Research Plan. US Dept. of Health and Human Services, Bathesda, MD, 2000. http://www.nidcd.nih.gov/strategic/strategic.htm
4. Healthy People 2010: Understanding and Improving Health. Vision and Hearing, Chapter 28, Department of Health and Human Services, 1999. http://www.health.gov/healthypeople/Document/HTML/Volume2/28Vision.htm
5. National Institute of Communication Sciences and Disorders. Presbycusis. NIDCD Health Information, 2001. http://www.nidcd.nih.gov/textonly/health/pubs_hb/presbycusis.htm

6. National Institute of Communication Sciences and Disorders. Hearing Loss and Older Adults. NIDCD Health Information, 2001. http://www.nidcd.nih.gov/textonly/health/pubs_hb/older.htm.

7. Cruickshanks KJ, Klein R, Klein BE, Wiley TL, Nondahl DM, Tweed TS. Cigarette smoking and hearing loss: the epidemiology of hearing loss study. JAMA 1998;279:1715–1719.

8. National Vital Statistics Report. Number of selected reported chronic conditions per 1,000 persons, by sex and age: United States, 1995, Table 58, page 79, Series 10, no. 199, 1998. http://www.cdc.gov/nchs/products/pubs/pubd/hus/00tables.htm# Determinants and Measures of Health.

9. Jerger J, Chmiel R, Wilson N, Luchi R. Hearing impairment in older adults: new concepts. J Am Geriatr Soc 1995;43:928–935.

10. Mader S. Hearing impairment in elderly persons. J Am Geriatr Soc 1984;32:548–553.

11. Moscicki EK, Elkins EF, Baum HM, McNamara PM. Hearing loss in the elderly: an epidemiologic study of the Framingham Heart Study Cohort. Ear Hear 1985;6:184–190.

12. Stach BA. Comprehensive Dictionary of Audiology. Williams & Wilkins, Baltimore, MD, 1997, p. 291.

13. Brant L, Gordon-Salant S, Pearson J, Klein L, Morrell C, Metter E, Fozard J. Risk factors related to age-associated hearing loss in the speech frequencies. Ear Hear 1996;7:152–161.

14. Gates GA, Cooper JC, Kannel WB, Miller NJ. Hearing in the elderly: the Framingham cohort 1980–1985. Ear Hear 1990;11:247–256.

15. Rosenhall U, Sixt E, Sundh V, Svanborg A. Correlations between presbyacusis and extrinsic noxious factors. Audiology 1993;32:234–243.

16. Gates GA, Couropmitree NN, Myers RH. Genetic associations in age-related hearing thresholds. Arch Otolaryngol Head Neck Surg 1999;125:654–659.

17. Seidman MD. Effects of dietary restriction and antioxidants on presbyacusis. Laryngoscope 2000;110:727–738.

18. Epstein S. What You Should Know About Ototoxic Medications. International Federation of Hard of Hearing People, 1995. http://www.ifhoh.org/Epstein.htm.

19. Cevette MJ, Franz KB, Brey RH, Robinette MS. Influence of dietary magnesium on the amplitude of wave V of the auditory brainstem response. Otolaryngol Head Neck Surg 1989;101:537–541.

20. Güneri EA, Serbetcioglu B, Ikoz AO, Güneri A, Ceryan K. TEOAE monitoring of Cisplatin induced ototoxicity in guinea pigs: the protective effect of vitamin B treatment. Auris Nasus Larnyx 2001;28:9–14.

21. Teranishi M, Nakashima T, Wakabayashi T. Effects of alpha-tocopherol on cisplatin-induced ototoxicity in guinea pigs. Hear Res 2001;151:61–70.

22. Clark K, Sowers MR, Wallace RB, Jannausch ML, Lemke J, Anderson CV. Age-related hearing loss and bone mass in a population of rural women aged 60 to 85 yr. Ann Epidemiol 1995;5:8–14.

23. Gates G, Cobb J, D'agostino R, Wolf P. The relation of hearing in the elderly to the presence of cardiovascular disease and cardiovascular risk factors. Arch Otolaryngol Head Neck Surg 1993;119:156–161.

24. Makishima K. Arteriolar sclerosis as a cause of presbyacusis. Otolaryngology 1978;86:322–326.

25. Seidman MD, Khan MJ, Dolan DF, Quirk WS. Age-related differences in cochlear microcirculation and auditory brain stem response. Arch Otolaryngol Head Neck Surg 1996;122:1221–1226.

26. Willott JF. Aging and the inner ear of animals. In: Aging and the Auditory System. Singular Publishing Group, Inc., San Diego, CA, 1991:18–55.

27. Bendich A, Deckelbaum RJ. Preventive Nutrition. Humana Press, Totowa, NJ, 1997, p. 579.

28. Rosen S, Olin P, Rosen HV. Dietary prevention of hearing loss. Acta Otolaryngol 1970;70:242–247.

29. Karlsmose B, Lauritzen T, Engberg M, Parving A. A five-year longitudinal study of hearing in a Danish rural population aged 31–50 years. Br J Audiol 2000;34:47–55.

30. Porter KH. Age related hearing loss and nutrition in older women. Dissertation, University of Georgia, 1999.

31. Russell RM. The aging process as a modifier of metabolism. Am J Clin Nutr 2000;72:529S–532S.

32. Agamanolis DP, Chester EM, Victor M, Kark JA, Hines JD, Harris JW. Neuropathology of experimental vitamin B12 deficiency in monkeys. Neurology 1976;26:905–914.

33. Healton EB, Savage MD, Brust JCM, Garrett TJ, Lindenbaum MD. Neurologic aspects of cobalamin deficiency. Medicine 1991;70:229–245.

34. Krumholz A, Weiss HD, Goldstein PJ, Harris KC. Evoked responses in vitamin B12 deficiency. Ann Neurol 1981;9:407–409.

35. Fine EJ, Hallett M. Neurophysiological study of subacute combined degeneration. J Neurol Sci 1980;45:331–336.

36. Fine EJ, Soria E, Paroski MW, Petryk D, Thomasula L. The neurophysiological profile of vitamin B_{12} deficiency. Muscle Nerve 1990;13:158–164.

37. Nexo E, Hansen M, Rasmussen K, Lindgren A, Gräsbeck R. How to diagnose cobalamin deficiency. Scand J Clin Lab Invest 1994;54:61–76.

38. Hector M, Burton JR. What are the psychiatric manifestations of vitamin B_{12} deficiency? J Am Geriatr Soc 1988;36:1105–1112.

39. Shemesh Z, Attias J, Ornan M, Shapira N, Shahar A. Vitamin B12 deficiency in patients with chronic tinnitus and noise-induced hearing loss. Am J Otolaryngol 1993;2:94–99.

40. Houston DK, Johnson MA, Nozza RJ, Gunter EW, Shea KJ, Cutler GM, Edmonds TJ. Age-related hearing loss, vitamin B_{12} and folate in elderly women. Am J Clin Nutr 1999;69:564–571.

41. Herbert V, Das KC. Folic acid and vitamin B_{12}. In: Modern Nutrition in Health and Disease. Shils ME, Olsen JA, Shike M (eds.) Lea & Febiger, Philadelphia, PA, 1994, pp. 402–425.

42. Berner B, Ødem L, Parving A. Age-related hearing impairment and B vitamin status. Acta Otolaryngol 2000;120:633–637.

43. Horner K. Review: morphological changes associated with endolymphatic hydrops. Scanning Microsc 1993;7:223–238.

44. Idrizbegovic E, Willott JF, Bogdanovic N, Canlon B. Aging and the total number of calbindin D-28k and parvalbumin immunopositive neurons in the dorsal cochlear nucleus of CBA/CaJ mice. In: Abstracts of the ARO Midwinter Meeting, 1999, p. 258. (abstract) http://www.aro.org/archives/1999/258.html

45. Ikeda K, Kusakari J, Kobayashi T, Saito Y. The effect of vitamin D deficiency on the cochlear potential and the perilymphatic ionized calcium concentration of rats. Acta Otolaryngol (Stockh) 1987A;435S: 64–72.

46. Sewell WF. Neurotransmitters and synaptic transmission. In: The Cochlea. Dallos P, Popper AN, Fay RR (eds.), Springer-Verlag, New York, 1996, pp. 501–533.

47. Sørensen MS. Temporal bone dynamics, the hard way. Acta Otolaryngol 1994;512:6–22.

48. Sørensen MS, Bretlau P, Jorgensen B. Quantum type bone remodeling in the human otic capsule. Acta Otolaryngol 1992A;496:4–10.

49. Sørensen MS, Bretlau P, Jorgensen B. Bone remodeling in the human otic capsule. Acta Otolaryngol 1992B;496:11–19.

50. Sørensen MS, Bretlau P, Jorgensen B. Fatigue microdamage in perilabyrinthine bone. Acta Otolaryngol 1992C;496:20–27.

51. Wangemann P, Schacht J. Homeostatic mechanisms in the cochlea. In: The Cochlea. Dallos P, Popper AN, Fay RR (eds.) Springer-Verlag, New York 1996;130–185.

52. Covell WP. Pathologic changes in the peripheral auditory mechanism due to avitaminosis (A, B complex, C, D, and E). Laryngoscope 1940;2:632–647.

53. Yamazaki T, Ogawa K, Imoto T, Hayashi N, Kozaki H. Senile deafness and metabolic bone disease. Am J Otol 1988;9:376–382.

54. Ikeda K, Kobayashi T, Hoh Z, Kusakari J, Takasaka T. Evaluation of vitamin D metabolism in patients with bilateral sensorineural hearing loss. Am J Otol 1989;10:11–13.

55. Brookes GB. Vitamin D deficiency—a new cause of cochlear deafness. J Laryngol Otol 1983;97:405–420.

56. Brookes GB. Vitamin D deficiency and otosclerosis. Otolaryngol Head Neck Surg 1985a;93:313–321.

57. Brookes GB. Vitamin D deficiency and deafness: 1984 update. Am J Otol 1985;6:102–107.

58. Irwin J. Hearing loss and calciferol deficiency. J Laryngol Otol 1986;100:1245–1247.

59. Ikeda K, Kobayashi T, Takasaka T, Kuskari J, Yumita S, Furukawa Y. Sensorineural hearing loss associated with hypoparathyroidism. Laryngoscope 1987B;97:1075–1079.

60. Johnson MA, Porter KH, Houston DK, Nozza RJ, Shea-Miller K, Gunter EW. Age-related hearing impairment is associated with poor calcium and vitamin D status in older women. Experimental Biology, Orlando, FL, in April 2001.

61. Erway LC, Willott JF, Archer JR, Harrison D. Genetics of age-related hearing loss in mice: Inbred and F1 hybrid strains. Hear Res 1993;65:125–132.

62. Willott JF, Erway LC. Genetics of age-related hearing loss in mice. IV. Cochlear pathology and hearing loss in 25 BXD recombinant inbred mouse strains. Hear Res 1998;119:27–36.

63. Willott JF, Erway LC, Archer JR, Harrison D. Genetics of age-related hearing loss in mice: II. Strain differences and effects of caloric restriction on cochlear pathology and evoked response thresholds. Hear Res 1995;88:143–155.

64. Johnson KR, Erway LC, Cook SA, Willott JF, Zheng Q. A major gene on chromosome 10 affecting age-related hearing loss in C57BL/6 mice. Hear Res 1997;114:83–92.

65. Román GC. An epidemic in Cuba of optic neuropathy, sensorineural deafness, peripheral sensory neuropathy and dorsolateral myeloneuropathy. J Neurol Sci 1994;127:11–28.

66. Dakshinamurti K, Singer WD, Paterson JA. Effect of pyridoxine deficiency in the neuronally mature rat. Int J Vit Nutr Res 1987;57:161–167.

67. Hoover PJ, Rice S. Physical and behavioral development in two strains of mice fed excess dietary vitamin B6. Nutr Res 1992;12:773–786.

68. Schaeffer MC. Attenuation of acoustic and tactile startle responses of vitamin B-6 deficient rats. Physiol Behav 1987;40:473–478.

69. Stephens MC, Havlicek V, Dashinamurti K. Pyridoxine deficiency and development of the central nervous system in the rat. J Neurochem 1971;18: 2407–2416.

70. Buckmaster PS, Holliday TA, Bai SC, Rogers QR. Brainstem auditory evoked potential interwave intervals are prolonged in vitamin B-6-deficient cats. J Nutr 1993;123:20–26.

71. Allen SH, Shah JH. Calcinosis and metastatic calcification due to vitamin D intoxication. Horm Res 1992;37:68–77.

72. Prohaska JR, Hoffman RG. Auditory startle response is diminished in rats after recovery from perinatal copper deficiency. J Nutr 1996;126:618–627.

73. Sun AH, Xiao SZ, Li BS, Zhao JL, Wang TY, Zhang YS. Iron deficiency and hearing loss. Experimental study in growing rats. Otorhinolaryngology and Related Spec 1987A;49:118–122.

74. Sun AH, Xiao SZ, Zheng Z, Li BS, Chao J, Wang TY. A scanning electron microscopic study of cochlear changes in iron-deficient rats. Acta Otolaryngol (Stockholm) 1987B;104:211-216.

75. Sun AH, Li JY, Xiao SZ, Li ZJ, Wang TY. Changes in the cochlear iron enzymes and adenosine triphosphatase in experimental iron deficiency. Ann Otol Rhinol Laryngol 1990;99:988–992.

76. Sun AH, Wang ZM, Xiao SZ, Li ZJ, Ding JC, et al.. Idiopathic sudden hearing loss and disturbance of iron metabolism. ORL 1992B;54:66–70.

77. Li Y, et al. The effect of iron deficiency anemia on the auditory brainstem response in infant. Nat Med J China 1994;74:392.

78. Roncagliolo M, Garrido M, Walter T, Peirano P, Lozoff TB. Evidence of altered central nervous system developments in infants with iron deficiency anemia at 6 mo: delayed maturation of auditory brainstem responses. Am J Clin Nutr 1998;68:683–690.

79. Sun AH, Wang ZM, Xiao SZ, Li ZJ, Zheng Z, Li JY. Sudden sensorineural hearing loss induced by experimental iron deficiency in rats. ORL 1992A;54:246–250.

80. Ising H, Handrock M, Gunther T, Fischer R, Dombrowski M. Increased noise trauma in guinea pigs through magnesium deficiency. Arch Otorhinolaryngol 1982;236:139–146.

81. Bac P, Tran G, Paris M, Binet P. Caracteristiques de la crise convulsive audiogene chez les souris rendues sensibles par carence magnesique. C R Acad Sci III 1993;316:676–681.

82. Joachims Z, Babisch W, Ising H. Dependence of noise-induced hearing loss upon perilymph magnesium concentration. J Acoust Soc Am 1983;74:104–108.

83. Gunther T, Rebentisch E, Vormann J. Enhanced ototoxicity of salicylate by magnesium deficiency. Magnesium Bulletin 1989;11:15–18.

84. Eberhardt MJ, Halas ES. Developmental delays in offspring of rats undernourished or zinc deprived during lactation. Physiol Behav 1987;41:309–314.

85. Wensink J, Hoever H, Mertens zur Borg I, van den Hamer CJA. Dietary zinc deficiency has no effect on auditory brainstem responses in the rat. Biol Trace Elem Res 1989;22:55–62.

11 Sarcopenia and Nutritional Frailty

Diagnosis and Intervention

Christine Seel Ritchie
and Connie Watkins Bales

1. INTRODUCTION AN DEFINITIONS

The term "frailty" is a broad one that stems from a number of possible contributing conditions (*see* Fig. 1). The definition proposed by Fried et al. *(1)* includes the presence of three or more of the following five factors:

- Unintentional weight loss
- Self-reported exhaustion
- Weakness
- Slow gait speed
- Low physical activity

In this chapter, nutritional frailty is defined as the disability that occurs in old age due to loss of lean body mass (sarcopenia) *and* rapid, unintentional loss of body weight. Sarcopenia and unintentional weight loss encompass the five domains described by Fried et al. and will be discussed here, along with the role of illness and its cachexic effects on unintentional weight and lean body mass loss (*see* Table 1). The effects of illness are also discussed in a number of other chapters in this text, including Chapters 5 (weight loss), 14 (terminal illness), 18 (chronic heart failure), 19 (chronic obstructive pulmonary disease), 20 (cancer), 24 (stroke, dysphagia), and 31 (trauma, sepsis).

Sarcopenia is the loss of muscle mass and strength that occurs with aging *(2,3)*. This loss of lean body mass, accompanied by decreases in muscle strength, efficiency (strength/unit of muscle mass), and protein synthesis *(4–6)*, can occur in overweight individuals (sarcopenic–obese), as well as normal and underweight individuals.

Weight loss, a decrease in body cell mass, can occur in the presence or absence of a cytokine-mediated response. Those with a cytokine-mediated inflammatory/injury response are defined as having *cachexia*, those without such a response are defined as experiencing *wasting (7)*.

From: *Handbook of Clinical Nutrition and Aging*
Edited by: C. W. Bales and C. S. Ritchie © Humana Press Inc., Totowa, NJ

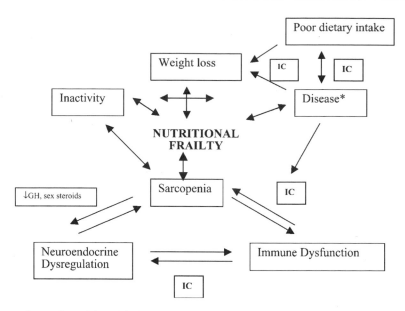

Fig. 1. Dimensions of nutritional frailty. *Disease includes dysphoria, cognitive impairment, pain syndromes, vascular disease, gait and balance disorders. Gh, growth hormone; IC, inflammatory cytokines.

Table 1
Glossary of Terms Related to Weight Loss and Frailty

Frailty: The presence of three or more of the following: unintentional weight loss, self-reported exhaustion, weakness, slow gait speed, and low physical activity *(1)*.

Nutritional Frailty: The disability that occurs in old age due to loss of lean body mass (sarcopenia) and rapid, unintentional weight loss. Food intake is reduced and loss of body weight and lean mass is precipitous.

Sarcopenia: The loss of muscle mass and strength that occurs with aging, defined by a value for appendicular muscle mass that is 2 standard deviations or more below the mean for young healthy adults.

Cachexia: Weight loss due to a cytokine-mediated response, which can involve anorexia, increased lipolysis, muscle protein breakdown, and nitrogen loss.

Wasting: Weight loss that occurs in the absence of cytokine effects.

Saropenic-lean: Individuals with sarcopenia who have a percent body fat below sex-specific cutoff values and an approximate BMI of <27 kg/m^2.

Sarcopenic-obese: Individuals with sarcopenia who have a pecent body fat greater than sex-specific cutoff values, approximate BMI of ≥27 kg/m^2.

Weight loss is commonly the result of a reduction in food intake; both physiologic and nonphysiologic causes may be responsible. Semi-starvation may occur in response to changes in cognition, affective status, appetite, medications, psychosocial support, and/or functional status. As noted previously, inflammatory cytokines released during chronic illness promote frailty because of their anorectic effect, as well as their contribution to lipolysis, muscle protein breakdown, and nitrogen loss. Frailty results from a combination of factors and is eventually expressed as an overall decline in function. Although functional decline can occur apart from sarcopenia and weight loss (e.g., in the case of myocardial infarction, hip fracture, or stroke), it often develops progressively along with these two factors, ultimately resulting in a cycle of undernourishment and deteriorating health.

2. CAUSES AND ASSESSMENT

2.1. Causes of Nutritional Frailty

2.1.1. BODY COMPOSITION CHANGE: SARCOPENIA

As humans age, their ratio of fat to muscle increases. In general, total body fat increases and lean body mass (muscle mass) decreases (8). The term for this loss of muscle mass and strength that inevitably occurs with aging has been coined sarcopenia (2,3). Along with chronic diseases, neuroendocrine dysregulation, and chronic inflammation, sarcopenia contributes significantly to the development of frailty and functional impairment in older age.

In order to better define the prevalence of severe loss of lean body mass, Baumgartner et al. (9) defined sarcopenia as values of 2 standard deviations or more below the mean for appendicular muscle mass of young healthy adults. Using this definition, 13.5%–16.9% of men under age 70 and 52.6%–57.6% of men over age 80 were sarcopenic. In women, those who were sarcopenic ranged from 23.1%–24.1% in those under 70 yr of age to 43.2%–60% in those over 80 yr. Sarcopenia was associated with functional impairment, disabilities, and falls independent of age, ethnicity, smoking, and comorbidity, but the relationships were surprisingly strongest in those with sarcopenic obesity.

The causes of sarcopenia have not been completely defined but they can include detrimental endocrine effects, release of proinflammatory cytokines, reduced alpha motor units in the spinal cord, decreased physical activity, and/or suboptimal protein intake. Reductions in testosterone and estrogen that accompany aging appear to accelerate loss of muscle mass (9,10). Estrogen and testosterone promote anabolic effects on muscle and inhibit catabolic cytokines such as IL-1 and IL-6 (11); the reduction of these hormones can be expected to have the opposite effect. Although growth hormone (GH) also declines with aging and has been hypothesized to contribute to loss of lean body mass, the relationship between GH and lean mass is confounded by fat mass. Recent studies have not borne out a close association between GH and lean body mass (12). Insulin resistance also increases with age. Given that insulin inhibits muscle breakdown, reduction of insulin action on muscle may contribute to muscle catabolism (13).

Activation of proinflammatory cytokines (interleukin-1, tumor necrosis factor, and interleukin-6) commonly occurs among older adults, after acute illness, and with chronic inflammatory conditions like rheumatoid arthritis. These cytokines can cause amino acid export from muscle and accelerated breakdown of protein *(14)*.

In older adults, there is a decrease in the number of lumbosacral motor units innervating each muscle fiber *(15)*. This results from a loss of the larger alpha motor units and relative preservation of the smaller motor units. The remaining motor units have a greater number of muscle fibers to innervate, leading to a loss of muscle efficiency and power *(16)*.

In developed countries, physical inactivity declines with age, especially among women. In the United States, only 25% of persons 65–74 yr of age and 17% of those 75 yr and older engaged in regular leisure time physical activity *(17)*. This inactivity exacerbates ongoing muscle loss *(18)*. In fact, inactive individuals may lose up to 40% of their muscle mass over the course of their adult life *(19)*.

Inadequate protein intake can also contribute to sarcopenia. Castaneda et al. *(20)* reported that consumption of inadequate dietary protein (postmenopausal women consuming 0.4 g/kg/d, which is half of the recommended dietary allowance of protein) led to deterioration in strength and lean body mass. As more than 10% of adults over age 60 yr consume less than 75% of the RDA for protein, a number of older individuals may be at risk for sarcopenia based on low protein intake alone.

2.1.2. ANOREXIA

Food intake gradually diminishes with age *(21,22)*. This finding has been noted in large-scale studies of healthy, community-dwelling elderly *(23,24)*. Between ages 20 and 80 yr, mean energy intake is reduced by up to 1200 kcal in men and 800 kcal in women *(23)*. Over time, older adults experience reduced physical activity, decreases in resting energy expenditure (REE), and/or loss of lean body mass. These changes produce a decrease in demand for calories and thus for food intake *(25,26)*. Other causes of reduced food intake may include physiologic changes, such as loss of appetite, alterations in taste and smell *(27–29)*, poor oral health *(30,31)*, gastrointestinal changes *(32,33)*, dementia *(34)*, and a reduced ability to regulate appetite in response to acute weight changes *(35–37)*. Additionally, nonphysiologic factors like social isolation *(38)*, psychological disorders *(39)*, economic limitations, and a variety of pathologic factors, such as illness and medication effects *(40)*, may contribute to a chronic progressive reduction in food intake.

In contrast to the gradual reduction in food intake seen with aging, nutritional frailty often has unexplained causes or is multifactorial in etiology. Food intake is dramatically reduced, and loss of body weight and lean body mass is precipitous. Often, the onset of this deterioration cannot be linked to a specific medical event or physical challenge; in fact, the precise trigger for the transition from gradual to precipitous weight loss is unknown, and it may occur separate from or along with cachexia (*see* Section 2.1.3.).

2.1.3. CACHEXIA

Cachexia is the involuntary loss of lean body mass with little or no weight loss. It usually occurs in the setting of underlying illnesses involving a cytokine-mediated response, which leads to anorexia, increased lipolysis, muscle protein breakdown, and nitrogen loss. Older adults are often afflicted by or are at increased risk for conditions characterized by activation of pro-inflammatory cytokines—conditions such as rheumatoid arthritis, congestive heart failure, and cancer. Pro-inflammatory cytokines commonly involved in cachexia include interleukin-1 (IL-1), interleukin-6 (IL-6), and tumor necrosis factor-α (TNF-α). IL-1 and TNF-α cause significant anorexia. Both of these cytokines increase IL-6, which has been associated with anorexia in older adults *(41)*. They also increase leptin and corticotropin releasing hormone (CRH) levels, both potent anorexigenic agents *(42,43)*. In addition to being anorectic, these cytokines also contribute to lipolysis, muscle protein breakdown, and nitrogen loss. They augment the acute phase response, upregulating the production of C-reactive protein and downregulating the transcription of albumin *(44)*.

TNF-α concentrations are often elevated in chronic congestive heart failure and in rheumatoid arthritis, especially when these conditions occur concurrently with cachexia *(45,46)*. Elevated IL-6 levels are also seen in inflammatory diseases, infections, and trauma. In a study of Framingham Heart Study participants, IL-6 levels were elevated in older subjects and correlated well with C-reactive protein concentrations *(47)*. IL-1 reduces food intake in laboratory animals. In humans, increased IL-1 levels are seen in patients with cachexia, even when infection and cancer are not present *(48)*. In summary, elevated pro-inflammatory cytokines (especially IL-1, IL-6, and TNF-α) are commonly seen in older adults, especially in those with cachexia, suggesting that targeting these cytokines may be an effective method to counter cachexia and nutritional frailty in some older adults.

2.2. Assessment

2.2.1. ASSESSMENT OF DIETARY INTAKE

The assessment of dietary intake has been addressed earlier in this book (*see* Chapters 5 and 6) but there are some unique considerations in the case of frail and seriously ill elderly individuals. Some of the more effective means of collecting information may be extremely difficult to implement for a number of reasons, including the time and effort burden on the patient or caregiver, cognitive limitations and lack of a proxy source of information, and shortage of staff time for collecting data (in-hospital or nursing home settings).

Standard methods of dietary assessment can be used, but are likely to be practical only in a research setting or a metabolic unit. Persson et al. *(49)* evaluated the effectiveness of a 7-d estimated dietary record kept by staff in five Swedish nursing home wards using the doubly labeled water method as the reference. The study found the dietary record method acceptably valid: staff overestimated the patients' energy intake by 8% and water intake by <1%. Frisoni et al. *(50)* used the direct weighing method to assess nutrient intake in 72 frail elderly subjects. Although these methods work, it is unlikely that busy caregivers or nursing home staff would be able to implement them in the clinical setting. Other methods that have been used for nutritional evaluation in the elderly *(51)* include assessment indices, such as the Mini Nutritional Assessment (MNA) *(52,53)*, a rapid assessment tool that has been cross-validated in three studies of more than 600 elderly subjects in the United States and Europe *(54)*. The MNA can be used to correctly classify nutritional status in about 75% of elderly patients *(52)*. The SCALES questionnaire (Chapter 5) *(55)* is another tool that has been used with some success; however, it requires biochemical measurements as part of the index.

In the clinical setting, the use of simple calorie counts or nursing reports of meals eaten is often employed to assess food intake, but these approaches are less than ideal. Castellanos and Andrews *(56)* found that the method of assessing the meal tray as a whole by assigning a value of 0, 25, 50, 75, or 100% consumed was not sufficiently accurate when patients were eating less than 75% of the majority of their meals. When this is the case, assessment of body weight change may be the best way to ascertain whether or not dietary needs are being met.

2.2.2. ASSESSMENT OF WEIGHT AND BODY COMPOSITION CHANGES

It is critical to detect the onset of nutritional frailty as early as possible. More advanced deterioration will be readily apparent from the clinical course then intervention will be less successful. Signs and symptoms to watch for in the clinical exam include fatigue, weakness, changes in ability to taste or smell, gastrointestinal complaints (poor appetite, oral problems, nausea, vomiting, diarrhea, constipation), and changes in mental or emotional status *(57)*. Protein deficiency may cause alopecia, edema, glossitis, desquamation of skin, and hair depigmentation. But the serial measurement of body weight is likely the single most important strategy for the evaluation of nutritional adequacy in the frail older adult. Published weight-for-height tables are of little benefit as standards for comparison because they were not developed for assessment of the ill or the very old. Careful monitoring of the rate of weight loss over time is often the best indicator of change in nutritional status. Chapter 5 provides a detailed discussion of the assessment of body weight loss and clinically significant weight-loss triggers. Fabiny and Kiel *(57)* also provide an expanded discussion of nursing home assessment (and treatment) of weight loss.

Obtaining regular body weights is not always easy, particularly in the frail patient, whether at home or in the nursing home. If the patient cannot stand on an upright balance-beam scale, a chair or bed scale should be used, and all scales should be regularly calibrated. Best practice includes weighing the patient in the same amount of clothing at the same time of day and two successive measurements at the same weighing should be within 1/4 pound or 0.1 kg. *(58)*. If weight loss is noted, the measurement should be confirmed by a repeat weighing, and the frequency of monitoring weight for that patient should be increased to weekly intervals *(57)*. Care should also be used when ascertaining height for calculation of body mass index (BMI). The patient's height before age 50 yr should be used as the reference height in order to avoid the effects of kyphosis because of osteoporosis *(54)*.

The Omnibus Budget Reconciliation Act (OBRA) of 1987 stipulates that nursing home patients are considered to have unintentional weight loss if they have lost 5% of usual body weight in 30 d or 10% in 6 mo *(59)*, using the calculation of weight change percentage as (usual weight – current weight) / (usual weight × 100). Progression of wasting may not be steady but episodic periods of undernutrition, as during times of medical stress such as infections, may contribute to the eventual loss of significant amounts of body weight *(60)*.

Measurement of body composition in the elderly is complicated by age-related shifts in body composition (*see* Chapters 5 and 6). As a result of poor reproducibility, skinfold measurements, if obtained at all, should be recorded by a single trained technician so as to limit measurement error. Bioelectrical impedence can also be used to measure fat free mass. Body composition is most accurately measured using dual X-ray absorptiometry; however, this test is often unavailable and is generally not necessary for making the diagnosis of nutritional frailty. Many clinicians rely on serum albumin levels as an index of general and protein nutritional status. The pitfalls inherent in this approach have been explained in Chapter 5. It should also be noted that inflammatory responses to infection alter albumin levels; TNF-α, IL-2, and IL-6 are known to inhibit albumin production. In these cases reduced serum albumin serves as a marker of inflammation rather than malnutrition.

2.2.3. ASSESSMENT OF UNDERLYING CONDITIONS

A host of different problems may be the cause for weight loss. They can include emotional factors like depression, malignancies (particularly of the gastrointestinal tract), oral/dental factors, and the symptoms and treatment side effects of many other chronic conditions.

Depression and dysphoria are commonly present in older adults and often remain unrecognized and undertreated. In a study of 1017 medical outpatients, depression was the cause of weight loss in 30% of the older patients evaluated *(61)*. Depression is also an important cause of weight loss in both the subacute care setting and in the nursing home *(54)*.

Depending on the case series reported and the definition of weight loss (all vs only those with unintentional weight loss), malignancy is linked to weight loss in 9–36% of elderly subjects *(61,62)*. Gastrointestinal malignancies commonly present with weight loss *(63)* due to loss of appetite, nausea, obstruction, and/or frequently being placed *non per os* (NPO) for medical testing.

A large percentage of older adults experience chewing difficulty, placing them at risk for poor food intake. In a study of community dwelling older adults in the New England area, after adjusting for gender, income, age, and baseline weight, edentulousness remained an independent risk factor for significant weight loss over a 1-yr period *(64)*. Other case studies have reported similar findings *(61)*.

Other conditions that may commonly cause weight loss include restrictive "therapeutic diets," poorly controlled diabetes, medications, thyrotoxicosis, congestive heart failure, and chronic obstructive pulmonary disease.

3. THERAPEUTIC INTERVENTIONS

3.1. Medical/Physical

The correction of the underlying cause for weight loss and functional decline is the first strategic defense against frailty. Unfortunately, this approach may not be possible, either because the condition cannot be resolved by medical treatment or because the primary

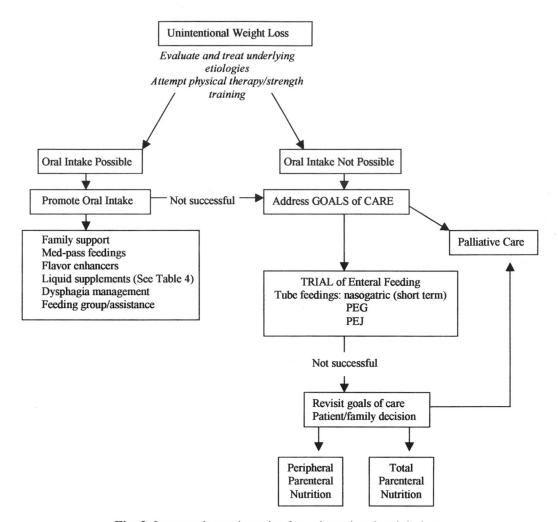

Fig. 2. Intervention trajectories for unintentional weight loss.

causal factor cannot be pinpointed. But, whenever possible, correction of known underlying causes for poor food intake such as reduced access to food, depression, social isolation, poor dentition, and overmedication should be immediately undertaken *(65)*. The Council on Nutrition has developed an evidence-based approach to nutritional surveillance and management of chronically ill patients in long-term care (Figs. 1 and 2 in Chapter 5), which serves as a good model for clinical decision making when multiple causal factors need to be addressed.

3.2. Nutritional

The fact that appropriate energy and nutrients must be consumed for nutritional status to be enhanced can sometimes be overlooked as medical interventions for frailty are undertaken. Often, calorie deficits are a major cause of weight loss and frailty. Malnu-

Table 2
Suggestions for Enhancing Self-Feeding and Assisted Feeding[a]

- Serve food in small portions and as finger foods to encourage self-feeding.
- Serve favorite and familiar foods. Encourage family to visit at mealtime.
- Serve foods at appropriate temperatures.
- Place food within visual range of patient. Place finger food in hands of functionally impaired patients.
- Reduce noise levels and provide a calm environment minimizing distractions and interruptions.
- Involve patient in the meal as active participant.
- Feeding-assisted patients may benefit from behavioral interventions such as:

    –repeating instructions;
    –frequent verbal prompting (such as when to chew and when to swallow);
    –physical demonstration of functional behaviors; and
    –frequent praise and positive reinforcement.

- Allow sufficient time for all food desired to be consumed.
- Have a consistent feeder to improve mealtime interactions, especially with demented patients.
- Whenever possible, have eat with others at a table, consider half-circle table for feeding multiple patients. Place those with impaired abilities next to self-feeders.

[a]Based, in part, on Van Ort and Phillips (79) and Lange-Alberts and Shott (80).

trition rates in nursing homes are estimated to range from 30% to over 50% (66–68). Nutritional frailty is also a concern in hospitalized elderly and in homebound elders in the community. Sullivan et al. (69) found that of 497 hospitalized elderly patients, 21% were consuming less than 50% of required calories. This undernutrition was associated with increased in-hospital and 90-d mortality. In community-based studies, the age-related progression toward frailty is also documented. Results of the National Health and Nutrition Examination Follow-up Survey (NHEFS) showed that during the time interval studied, 50% of subjects aged 65 to 74 had lost at least 5% of their body weight and 26% of women and 14% of men had lost at least 15% (70). When the gradual age-related decrease in food intake becomes more rapid and unintentional weight loss accelerates (onset of nutritional frailty), one of the most important therapeutic strategies is to take steps to maximize oral intake of calories and other essential nutrients (Fig. 2).

3.2.1. Enhancing Oral Food Intake

While enhancing oral intake cannot always be accomplished, it should be one of the first interventions attempted. The type of dietary assistance that is needed will depend upon a variety of physical, functional, economic, and psychosocial factors.

3.2.1.1. Increasing Food Acceptance. One of the most common reasons given by elderly patients for reduced food consumption intake is that the perceived quality of the food is poor. They may say that the food is tasteless or unfamiliar, or they may associate certain foods with previous gastrointestinal complaints and choose to avoid them. While the loss of taste and smell can affect the appeal of foods for some older adults

Table 3
Calorie and Protein Content of Familiar Foods and Snacks of High Caloric Density

Food	Serving size typical and (g)	Calories	Calories per g food	Protein (g)
Bagel with cream cheese	1/2 bagel (28)	72	2.6	2.5
	2 T. cream cheese (30)	100	3.3	2.0
	Total (58)	172	3.0	4.5
Eggo™ waffle with butter and syrup	1 waffle (39)	110	2.8	2.5
	2 t. butter (9.5)	68	7.2	0.08
	1 T. syrup (60)	158	2.6	0
	Total (108)	336	3.1	2.6
Cheddar cheese on crackers	2 oz cheese (57)	223	3.9	14.2
	4 Saltine squares (11)	50	4.6	1.0
	Total (68)	273	8.5	15.2
Cream soup, chicken, made with whole milk	6 oz (186)	109	0.6	5.5
Custard with egg and whole milk	1/2 cup (133)	162	1.2	5.4
Fried chicken	1 leg (62)	162	2.6	16.6
	1/2 boneless chicken breast (98)	218	2.2	31.2
Mashed potatoes with gravy	1/2 cup potatoes (105)	81	0.8	2.1
	2 T. gravy (30)	25	0.8	0.5
	Total (135)	106	1.6	2.6
Hershey™ chocolate kisses	6 (28)	145	5.1	2.0
Apple pie with ice cream	1/2 slice pie (89)	265	2.9	2.0
	1 scoop ice cream (70)	150	2.2	3.0
	Total (159)	415	2.6	5.0
Instant breakfast powder	1 packet + 8 oz whole milk (281)	280	1.0	15.4
Macaroni and cheese				
–home recipe	1/2 cup (100)	215	2.2	8.4
–box type	1/2 cup (100)	160	1.6	7.0
Milkshake, chocolate				
–fast food type	8 oz (147)	174	1.2	6.3
Nonfat dry milk powder[a]	2 T. (15)	54	3.6	5.4
Olive Oil[b]	2 T. (27)	239	8.8	0
Peanut butter sandwich	2 slices bread, wheat (50)	130	2.6	5.0
	2 T. peanut butter (32)	190	5.9	8.2
	Total (82)	320	8.5	13.2
Peanuts, dry roasted	2 T. (19)	107	5.8	4.3
Pudding, chocolate	1/2 cup (110)	160	1.4	4.0
Yogurt, full fat, flavored	8 oz (227)	253	1.1	10.7

[a]Can be used to fortify beverages, soups, puddings, and sauces.
[b]Can be added as source of calories to savory sauces and foods.

(Chapter 9), this is clearly not the only reason that food complaints occur in this population group. Hospitalized and nursing home patients of any age often find the meals that they are served "in house" to be less than desirable. Even in the best of situations, food mass-produced in an institutional kitchen and transported to patient rooms or service areas rarely tastes like a home-cooked meal. Moreover, in many cases, institutional menu choices may be unavoidably limited by resources, logistics, or the clinical situation, such that personal food preferences cannot be taken into account. Even in the home setting, loneliness, fatigue, disabilities, poor kitchen facilities and/or cooking skills, and limited shopping opportunities may combine to diminish food enjoyment at mealtime. The more frequent occurrence of gastrointestinal complaints in the elderly (Chapter 25) may also contribute to a progressively shrinking list of accepted foods as the patient gradually restricts more and more foods from the diet because they have "hurt their stomach" in the past.

Taken together, all these factors argue for increased attention to the quality of taste and appealing presentation of meals and snacks for the frail elderly patient who is losing weight. This effort could include arranging for favorite foods to be "brought in" to the patient, whether at home or in an institution, and a host of other simple tactics (Table 2). The addition of foods of high caloric content and natural food fortification can be an effective approach for getting more calories and protein into the daily regimen. Table 3 provides a list of easy-to-eat foods and snacks along with their caloric density-per-gram of food and their protein content.

Another important step in enhancing food intake is the lifting of dietary restrictions whenever possible so as to offer a wider selection of food choices. In many cases, frail, undernourished nursing home patients need not be given a special diet prescription. Coulston et al. (71) reported that in elderly chronic-care patients with noninsulin-dependent diabetes mellitus, the short-term substitution of a regular for a "diabetic diet" increased calorie consumption and did not cause gross deterioration of glycemic control. More recently, Buckler et al. (72) conducted a chart review in four chronic-care settings and linked evidence of undernutrition (average weight loss >1 pound per month, serum albumin <3.5 g/dL) with dietary restrictions. Fifty-nine percent of the patients with weight loss and 75.2% of those with hypoalbuminia were on some type of dietary restriction. Tariq et al. (73) has extended the findings of Coulston et al. (71), reporting that patients in long-term care with diabetes could be successfully managed on a regular diet. They recommend the regular monitoring of blood glucose and adjustment of medication levels rather than implementing dietary restrictions or even "no concentrated sweets" prescription.

The addition of simulated food flavors to nutritious foods in order to enhance consumption may provide benefit by improving food consumption. Schiffman and Warwick (74) used this approach and found increased food consumption when food flavors (roast beef, ham, natural bacon, maple, and cheese) were added to the diets of nursing home residents. Food flavors have also been used in hospitalized elderly patients to enhance intake (75). If these short-term changes can be maintained, an increase in body weight potentially could be achieved by adding these food flavors.

Several orexigenic drugs have been considered as a means for increasing food intake, but most have been found unsuccessful and/or have adverse side effects. These drugs are discussed in more detail in Chapter 5. A recent review by Karcic et al. *(76)* suggests that megestrol acetate, a semi-synthetic progestational steroid, is the most effective known appetite stimulant at present. Previously used in patients with cancer and acquired immunodeficiency syndrome, only a few studies have considered the applicability of this drug in malnourished older persons *(76–78)*. Yeh et al. *(78)* reported that 800 mg/d of megestrol acetate increased appetite, food intake, and (in 3 mo) body weight in nursing home patients who had lost 5% or more of their body weight. Likewise, Karcic et al. *(76)* reported improvement in nutritional parameters (including food intake and body mass index [BMI]) in 13 nursing home patients for whom other methods of nutritional support had failed. Dronabinol (tetrahydrocannabinol, a cannabis derivative with FDA approval for use in AIDS and cancer) is also being studied for applicability in elderly patients.

3.2.1.2. Feeding Assistance, Feeding Groups, and Family Support. For home-dwelling elderly persons who are undernourished, the use of community resources such as home delivery services (e.g., Meals on Wheels) and feeding programs at senior nutrition centers can help with food access and enhance the meal time experience by providing social stimulation. For both free living and institutionalized frail elders, family/caregivers should be encouraged to provide favorite foods and beverages prepared in familiar ways.

With advancing old age and especially in elderly patients with cognitive impairments, the ability to self-feed can decline markedly. The process of eating and swallowing may be physically affected by a variety of changes, including dementia. Functional feeding *(79)* emphasizes a behavioral approach that maximizes the patient's involvement in the meal and an ongoing interaction between the patient and feeder throughout the entire meal. Simple modifications by nursing staff can promote self-feeding without extending the time required for the meal (Table 2). Lange-Alberts and Shott *(80)* found that a feeding therapy program involving touch and/or verbal cueing also enhanced the nutritional intakes of severely cognitively impaired elderly patients in the hospital.

However, not all patients benefit equally from feeding assistance. Simmons et al. *(81)* provided a feeding intervention to 74 nursing home residents who were eating less than 75% of food offered for most meals. The intervention included continuous one-to-one assistance, prompting protocol to enhance self-feeding capacities, social interaction, choice of dining location, proper positioning, meal tray substitutions as desired, and extended tray access (up to 1.5 h per meal). Despite this intensive and individualized support, which required almost 20 extra minutes of staff time per meal, half of the participants showed slight or no improvement in average food intakes. The authors recommended a 1–2-d trial of feeding assistance for the purpose of identifying those individuals who are likely to be responsive to assistance. In their study, this approach was more likely to be beneficial for the more severely cognitively impaired subjects, who required a relatively greater amount of physical assistance at mealtime.

3.3.2. ORAL NUTRITIONAL SUPPLEMENTS

Table 4 lists some of the more commonly used commercial supplements and indicates their nutritional content and potential application (e.g., oral use, tube feeding). Commercially prepared supplements, mainly available in liquid form, are more expensive, but are often used instead of traditional foods to increase nutrient intake, particularly in the institutional setting. Although the expense and monotony are definite concerns, there can

Table 4
Selected Commercially Available Nutritional Supplements: Composition and Description

Name of product manufacturer nutritional description	*Boost/Mead Johnson*	*Ensure/Ross*
Kcal/mL	1.01	1.06
Protein g/L	42.27	38
Protein source	Milk protein concentrate	Calcium caseinate, soy protein isolate, whey protein concentrate
Carbohydrate g/L	173.29	169.07
Carbohydrate source	Corn syrup solids, sucrose	Sucrose, corn syrup, maltodextrin
Fat g/L total (t), saturated (s)	16.91 (t), 2.11 (s)	25.36 (t), 2.11 (s)
Fat source	Canola oil, high oleic sunflower oil, corn oil	High oleic safflower oil, canola oil, corn oil
Fiber g/mL	0	0
Osmolality	380 mOsm/L	590 mOsm/kg H_2O
Unit amount flavors	8 fl oz serving; chocolate, chocolate mocha, chocolate malt, vanilla, strawberry, and butter pecan	8 fl oz serving; vanilla, chocolate, strawberry, butter pecan, and coffee (home delivery only)
Website	http://www.meadjohnson.com/products/hcp-adultmed/boost.html	http://www.ensure.com/OurProducts/Ensure.asp
Name of product manufacturer nutritional description	*Jevity/Ross*	*Lipisorb/Mead Johnson*
Kcal/mL	1.06	1.35
Protein g/L	44.3	57
Protein source	Sodium and calcium caseinates	Calcium and sodium caseinates
Carbohydrate g/L	154.7	161
Carbohydrate source	Maltodextrin, corn syrup, soy fiber	Maltodextrin, sucrose
Fat g/L total (t), saturated (s)	34.7 (t), 8.6 (s)	57 (t)
Fat source	High oleic safflower oil, canola oil, MCT oil lecithin	MCT oil, soy oil
Fiber g/mL	14.4	N/A[b]
Osmolality	250 mOsm/L	510 mOsm/L

Unit amount flavors	8 fl oz serving; unflavored, for tube feeding	8 fl oz serving; vanilla
Website	http://www.ross.com/ productHandbook/ adultNut.asp	http://meadjohnson.com/ products/hcp-adultmed/ lipisorb.html
Name of product manufacturer nutritional description	*Osmolite/Ross*	*Promote/Ross[a]*
Kcal/mL	1.06	1
Protein g/L	37.1	62.5
Protein source	Sodium and calcium caseinates, soy protein isolate	Sodium and calcium caseinates, soy protein isolate
Carbohydrate g/L	151.1	130
Carbohydrate source	Maltodextrin	Maltodextrin, sucrose
Fat g/L total (t), saturated (s)	34.7 (t), 8.6 (s)	26 (t), 6.3 (s)
Fat source	High oleic safflower oil, canola oil, MCT oil, lecithin	High oleic safflower oil, canola oil, MCT oil, lecithin
Fiber g/mL	N/A[b]	N/A[b]
Osmolality	252 mOsm/L	285 mOsm/kg
Unit amount flavors Website	8 fl oz serving; mild taste http://www.ross.com/ productHandbook/ adultNut.asp	8 fl oz serving; vanilla http://www.ross.com/ productHandbook/ adultNut.asp
Name of product manufacturer nutritional description	*Subdue/Mead Johnson[a]*	*Replete/Nestle[a]*
Kcal/mL	1	1
Protein g/L	49.9	62.4
Protein source	Hydrolyzed whey protein concentrate	Calcium-potassium caseinates, soy lecithin
Carbohydrate g/L	126.8	113.2
Carbohydrate source	Sycrose, maltodextrin, modified corn starch	Maltodextrin
Fat g/L total (t), saturated (s)	33.8 (t)	34 (t)
Fat source	Canola oil, high oleic sunflower oil, corn oil MCT oil	MCT oil, canola oil

Fiber g/mL	0	N/A
Osmolality	330 mOsm/kg H_2O (unflavored) 525mOsm/kg H_2O (other)	300 mOsm/kg H_2O (unflavored) 350 mOsm/kg H_2O (vanilla)
Unit amount flavors	8 fl oz serving; orange, vanilla, chocolate almond, and unflavored	8.4 fl oz serving; vanilla and unflavored
Website	http://www.meadjohnson.com/products/hcp-adult-med/subdue.html	http://www.nestleclinicalnutrition.com/product_info_template.asp?ID=30
Name of product manufacturer nutritional description	*Slim Fast/Slim Fast Foods*	*Carnation Instant Breakfast/Nestle*
Kcal/mL	0.68	0.68
Protein g/L	30.7	40.6
Protein source	Calcium caseinate, casein, whey, soy lecithin	Casein, whey
Carbohydrate g/L	123	104.8
Carbohydrate source	Sucrose, fructose, maltodextrin, dextrose	Sucrose, maltodextrin, dextrose
Fat g/L total (t), saturated (s)	9.2 (t), 3.1 (s)	10.14 (t), 1.69 (s)
Fat source	Canola oil	Canola oil
Fiber g/mL	15	0
Osmolality	N/A[b]	500–620 mOsm/kg H_2O
Unit amount flavors	11 fl oz serving; banana cream, cappuccino delight, dark chocolate fudge, rich chocolate royale, dark chocolate fudge, french vanilla, strawberries in cream	10 fl oz serving; creamy milk chocolate, french vanilla, strawberry créme
Website	http://www.slim-fast.com/index.asp	http://www.carnationinstant-breakfast.com/main.asp

[a]All products as described are in liquid from, ready-to-drink and/or used in tube feedings.
[b]N/A = Information not available.

be advantages for these products, including that they (1) provide a ready source of nutrients, often including fortification with essential micronutrients, (2) help assure safety from food borne illness and inadvertent contamination during preparation (due to standardized manufacturing processes), and (3) provide easy access to nutrition, being ready to serve and suitable for long-term storage at room temperature. Johnson et al. *(65)* and others *(82,83)* make a strong case against the use of commercially prepared supplements unless absolutely necessary, citing concerns about relatively low protein content, lack of fiber and other beneficial components of natural foods, potential misuse as meal replacements, avoidance of liquid intake by elderly patients with urinary incontinence, and the chance of electrolyte and carbohydrate overload in chronic renal insufficiency and diabetes, respectively. In a recent study reported by Fiatarone Singh et al. *(83)*, the investigators found that short-term intake of nutritional supplements by elderly nursing home residents (mean age 88 yr) was mostly offset by a decrease in voluntary food intake and that the small amount of associated weight gain represented fat gain and not an accretion of lean mass. Additionally, Gray-Donald and Payette *(84)* reported that frail elderly subjects could gain weight when given a high-energy nutrient-dense commercial supplement (for 12 wk), but there were no corresponding improvements in functional status.

Not all studies have shown a lack of benefit from oral supplements, and not all clinical investigators and clinicians agree about their usefulness. Lauque et al. *(51)* supplemented elderly nursing home patients who were malnourished or at risk of being malnourished (by MNA score) with oral nutrition supplements of about 400 kcal/d and found improvements in weight (up by 1.4 ± 0.5 kg) and MNA score at the end of the 60 d study. Turic and coworkers *(85)* studied nutritional adequacy in nursing home residents who met OBRA standards for nutritional risk and offered them either snacks or medical nutritional supplements three times per day between meals. The supplemented group consumed more calories, protein, and all other nutrients measured than the snack "control" group. Even if there is no appreciable increase in weight, there may be some benefit to the judicious use of these supplements. Krondl et al. *(86)* studied the impact of having 71 community dwelling subjects (mean age 70 ± 7 yr) add six 235 mL cans of a liquid nutritional supplement per week and found improvements in SF-36 scores (improved vitality, general health perception) and General Well-Being scores (improved general well-being and reduced anxiety), in addition to improved intake of protein and selected micronutrients. In view of the particularly positive effects of nutritional supplements on the recovery of elderly patients from acute hip fracture *(87,88)*, it has been suggested *(83)* that such supplements may be more beneficial in the case of acute catabolic events or severe undernutrition than in the case of milder, chronic nutritional inadequacy.

Obviously, a balanced diet of natural foods is the optimal nutritional choice for any elderly person who is able to eat. The commercial supplement approach should be reserved for use with patients who have specific limitations in their oral food intake, such as food intolerances, inability or unwillingness to eat adequate amounts of nutritious foods, and in situations where having the patient do their own food preparation is prohibited or unsafe *(65)*. The timing and administration of the appropriate supplements is one important aspect of success. Kayser-Jones et al. *(89)* reported little measurable benefit when liquid oral supplements were administered to nursing home patients without regard to dose, diagnosis and management of underlying problems, amount of supplement consumed, and outcome. Evidence that older adults reach satiation more quickly and have slower gastric emptying *(90)* must be kept in mind. A recent study by Wilson et al. *(91)* suggests that liquid dietary supplements be administered between meals in order to optimize net energy consumption for the day.

A sidebar to this discussion is the use of micronutrient supplements to correct dietary deficiencies in the frail elderly patient whose dietary intake is dwindling. Although the main goal in treating nutritional frailty is to increase the intake of energy-yielding macronutrients (protein, carbohydrate, and fat), any inadequacy in micronutrient (vitamins and minerals) status should also be addressed. Rudman et al. *(92)* noted the low usage rates for multivitamin (35%) and trace mineral (3%) supplements in eating-dependent residents of a VA nursing home. While correcting micronutrient deficiencies will not reverse wasting in the frail patient with a poor dietary intake, it has the potential to enhance appetite, vigor, immune response, and cognition by correcting vitamin and mineral deficits *(93,94)*.

As illustrated in Fig. 2, every effort should be made to sustain and increase oral food intake. When this is not possible, other options such as enteral nutrition may be considered.

3.2.3. Nutrition Support

Enteral feedings may be considered if the patient is unable to ingest sufficient calories through other means and the patient's condition and patient/family wishes dictate such an approach. Nutritional support for the elderly patient is also discussed in Chapters 14 and 26. Although the fairly limited research literature indicates that enteral tube feeding can be used to produce modest increases in nutrient intake and body weight, ultimate health outcomes (complications, survival times) may not be improved *(95)*. Mitchell et al. *(96)* studied 1386 nursing home residents with severe cognitive impairment and compared clinical characteristics and survival data in those with and without tube feeding placement. Survival was not prolonged in the patients receiving the tube feedings. Henderson et al. *(97)* conducted a cross-sectional study of long-term-care patients who had been receiving prolonged tube feeding. Despite adequate provision of calories and protein, these patients showed weight loss and severe depletion of lean and fat mass. The authors concluded that chronic disease, immobility, and neurologic deficits may undermine attempts at long-term nutritional support.

In cases where enteral nutrition is planned, the clinical situation will dictate the use of either nasogastric, nasointestinal, percutaneous gastric (PEG), or percutaneous jejunal (PEJ) tubes for delivery of nutritional support. Because of patient discomfort and the risk for sinusitis with long-term use of nasogastric and nasointestinal tubes, a PEG or PEJ should be considered if enteral feeding is expected to continue for more than 30 d. PEG tubes are often larger than PEJ tubes and thus facilitate easier administration of medications without causing clogging. Weighted tubes have no advantage for passing into the duodenum compared with nonweighted tubes *(98)*. Norton et al. *(99)* compared PEG versus nasogastric feeding routes in 30 subjects with persistent dysphagia following acute stroke. Patients fed via PEG showed greater improvement in nutritional status by several measures, including serum albumin, and were less likely to have treatment failures. Klor and Milianti *(100)* also found a favorable outcome when PEGs were used in patients with dysphagia; when provided an individualized treatment program, the oral intakes of all patients were upgraded and 10 of the 16 eventually had their PEGs removed.

Loser et al. *(101)* followed 210 patients after PEG placement (not all were elderly) for an average of 133 d and found an increase in body weight at 1 yr in the 34.4% of the population that survived. Acceptability was excellent in 83% of the subjects and complication rates were low (3.8% severe and 20% mild). It was concluded that distinct improvements in nutritional status were achieved. However, Kaw and Sekas *(102)* studied outcomes with PEG placement in 46 nursing home patients and found no improvement in functional or nutritional status and a 34.7% complication rate. It is important that nutritional status continue to be monitored after the feeding regime is initiated as some patients may have higher nutritional requirements than provided for in the initial diet order. Serial measurements of weight over time will permit the best evaluation; this allows use of the patient as his/her own control, a wise approach since many available norms are not applicable to this population *(97)*.

Parenteral nutrition is discussed by Wilson and Morley in Chapter 5 and DeLegge and Sabol in Chapter 26 and may be considered when the enteral route cannot be used. However, very little data exist regarding the efficacy of this form of nutrition support for the elderly. Complications are multiple and include increased risk of systemic bacterial and fungal infections, hyperglycemia, and intestinal atrophy. Delivery by larger central veins is preferable to peripheral delivery if the support is expected to be needed for more than 10–14 d. Careful monitoring for tolerance, nutritional adequacy, and complications by a dedicated multidisciplinary team (including physician, nurse, nutritionist, and pharmacist) is required to reduce complications. Exclusive parenteral nutrition is generally not recommended, as there is a lack of evidence that long-term outcomes will be improved using this approach.

As already mentioned, artificial nutrition support cannot be guaranteed to provide a solution to nutritional problems for high-risk patients who can't or won't eat. Complication rates from surgical and endoscopic tube placement are high (32%–70%) *(103)*. Thus the decision to provide nutritional support via these routes must be carefully considered by the health care provider and the patient/surrogate (Chapter 14). Foregoing, withholding, or withdrawing nutrition can be an appropriate choice at the end of life *(104,105)*. However, often the issue of nutrition support is not addressed in advance directives (unless the care team brings it up), and patients may not be consulted before feeding tubes are placed *(104,106)*. In particular, decisions to provide aggressive nutritional support for patients with severe cognitive impairments need to be evaluated from an ethical standpoint (Chapter 14) and discussed in detail with the family or closest caregiver *(107,108)*. Decisions about the use of tube feedings and the potential benefits that might be expected are not straightforward. Although one-third of nursing home patients say they would choose to be fed by tube if they could no longer eat because of cognitive deficits *(109)*, this preference may be based on the potentially erroneous conclusion that a prolonged survival would be the outcome *(110)*. A sensitive, but honest, presentation of the physiological aspects of nutrition support at the end of life and expectations about its impact needs to be presented to the patient/family/caregiver by the health care team so that decisions about nutrition support can be guided by the best interest of the patient.

4. PROMISING INTERVENTIONS FOR THE FUTURE

4.1. Exercise and Food Intake

A potentially promising intervention for increasing food intake in older persons is exercise. Poehlman and Danforth *(111)* reported an increase of energy intake by 12% among older persons participating in an 8-wk endurance training program. In Fiatarone's study of very elderly adults *(112)*, a combination of strength training and protein calorie supplementation was more likely to increase calories consumed than protein calorie supplementation alone, although this trend did not reach statistical significance. More studies are needed to evaluate the impact of a combination of strength training and anabolic hormones or strength training and nutritional supplementation on nutritional frailty.

4.2. Potential Interventions Against Cachexia

A number of agents that inhibit the action of proinflammatory cytokines are being evaluated in patients with cachexia. Pentoxifylline could theoretically interfere with TNF-α production by reducing TNF-α messenger RNA transcription *(113)*. No studies have been published to date using pentoxifylline in older adults; its evaluation in AIDS patients has not demonstrated benefit in terms of weight gain *(114)*. Thalidomide also decreases TNF-α levels by increasing the breakdown of TNF-α messenger RNA. Initial trials in HIV patients have been promising for increasing weight; but no data regarding its efficacy is yet available in the geriatric population *(115)*. Megestrol acetate (megace) increases appetite and weight gain, in part through its reduction of IL-1, IL-6, and TNF-α *(116)*. In a study of nursing home residents, those receiving megace 800 mg/d demonstrated maximum weight gain at 12 wk. Individuals with elevated cytokine levels at baseline were most likely to respond to megace with increased weight gain *(78,117)*. Omega-3 fatty acids alter cyclooxygenase and lipooxygenase activity and secondarily inhibit cytokine production, but no studies to date have been reported in cachectic geriatric patients *(118)*. N-acetyl cysteine and s-adenosyl methionine (SAMe) have both been shown to modulate concentrations of pro-inflammatory cytokines such as TNF, IL-1, and IL-6. These agents have been studied in other conditions of chronic inflammation and may have promise for treatment of geriatric cachexia *(119,120)*.

5. SUMMARY AND RECOMMENDATIONS

In summary, the approach to nutritional frailty in older adults must be multidimensional, attending to both physiologic and nonphysiologic determinants. Many simple interventions, such as increasing physical activity, providing appealing favorite foods with enhanced flavoring, eliminating unnecessary medications, and providing supplemental calories in the form of calorie dense foods, may provide meaningful benefit. Decisions regarding enteral nutrition must be made carefully, with attention to the patient's underlying condition and treatment goals.

6. RECOMMENDATIONS FOR CLINICIANS

1. A balanced diet of natural foods is the optimal nutritional choice for any elderly person who is able to eat.

2. Early interventions to maintain/enhance oral intake of natural foods are strongly encouraged. These interventions could include community and family support, mealtime enhancements, the addition of food flavors, and feeding assistance with verbal cueing for eating-dependent individuals.

3. The use of commercially prepared oral nutrient supplements is the best choice when the patient has significant limitations on oral food intake or is unable to consume adequate amounts of nutrients from a natural foods diet. Micronutrient supplements (multivitamin/mineral) may also be beneficial, especially if energy intake is marginal.

4. If oral consumption of calories is not possible, feedings may be delivered by tube; potential routes may be either nasogastric, nasointestinal, percutaneous gastric (PEG), or percutaneous jejunal (PEJ). A PEG or PEJ should be considered if the enteral feeding is expected to continue for more than 30 d.

5. Complication rates with enteral nutrition support are high. Decisions to provide aggressive nutritional intervention should be weighed carefully and decisions about feeding tubes should be included in the patient's advance directives.

REFERENCES

1. Fried LP, Tangen CM, Walston J, et al. Frailty in older adults: Evidence for a phenotype. J Gerontol 2001;56:M146–M156.
2. Rosenberg IH. Epidemiologic and methodologic problems in determining nutritional status of older persons. Am J Clin Nutr 1989;50(suppl):1231–1233.
3. Roubenoff R. Origins and clinical relevance of sarcopenia. Can J Appl Physiol 2001;26:78–89.
4. Lindle RS, Metter EJ, Lynch NA, et al. Age and gender comparisons of muscle strength in 654 women and men aged 20–93 yr. J Appl Physiol 1997;83:1581–1587.
5. Nair KS. Age-related changes in muscle. Mayo Clin Proc. 2000;75(suppl):S14–S18.
6. Short KR, Nair KS. The effect of age on protein metabolism: current opinion. Clinical Nutrition and Metabolic Care 2000;3:39–44.
7. Roubenoff R, Heymsfield SB, Kehayias JJ, Cannon JG, Rosenberg IH. Standardization of nomenclature of body composition in weight loss. Am J Clin Nutr 1997;66:192–196.
8. Guo SS, Zeller C, Chumlea WC, Siervogel RM. Aging, body composition, and lifestyle: the Fels Longitudinal Study. AJCN 1999;70:402–411.
9. Baumgartner R, Koehler KM, Gallagher D, Romero L, Heymsfeld SB, Ross RR, et al. Epidemiology of sarcopenia among the elderly in New Mexico. Am J Epidemiol 1999;149:1163.
10. Poehlman ET, Toth MJ, Gardner AW. Changes in energy balance and body composition at menopause: A controlled longitudinal study. Ann Intern Med 1995;123:673–675.
11. Pottratz ST, Bellido T, Mocharla H, Crabb D, Manolaga SC. 17 α-Estradiol inhibits expression of human interleukin-6 promoter-reporter constructs by a receptor-dependent mechanism. J Clin Invest 1994;93:944–950.
12. Roubenoff R, Harris TB, Abad LW, Wilson PW, Dallal GE, Dinarello CA. Monocyte cytokine production in an elderly population: effect of age and inflammation. J Gerontol Med Sci 1998;53:M20–M26.
13. Roubenoff R, Hughes VA. Sarcopenia: current concepts. J Gerontol 2000;55A:M716–M724.
14. Warren, RS, Starnes HF, Gabrilove JL, Oettgen HF, Brennan MF. The acute metabolic effects of tumor necrosis factor administration in humans. Arch Surg 1987;122:1396–1400.

15. Galea V. Changes in motor unit estimates with aging. J Clin Neurophysiol 1996;13:253–260.

16. Roos MR, Rice CL, Vandervoort AA. Age-related changes in motor unit function. Muscle Nerve 1997; 20:679–690.

17. U.S. Dept of Health and Human Services. National Health Interview Survey, Jan.–Sept., 2002, Atlanta, GA, CDC, National Center for Chronic Disease Prevention and Health Promotion, 2002.

18. Rantanen T, Era P, Heikkinen E. Physical activity and changes in maximal isometric strength in men and women from the age of 75 to 80 years. J Am Geriatr Soc 1997;45:1439–1445.

19. Hughes V, Frontera W, Roubenoff R, Evans W, Fiatarone Singh M. 10-yr body composition changes in older men and women: role of body weight change and physical activity. Am J Clin Nutr 2002;76: 473–481.

20. Castaneda C, Charmley JM, Evans WJ, Crim MC. Elderly women accommodate to a low-protein diet with losses of body cell mass, muscle function and immune response. Am J Clin Nutr 1995;62:30–39.

21. Roberts SB. A review of age-related changes in energy regulation and suggested mechanisms. Mech Age Dev 2000;116:157–167.

22. Morley JE. Decreased food intake with aging. J Gerontol Med Sci 2001;56A:81–88.

23. Wakimoto P, Block G. Dietary intake, dietary patterns, and changes with age: An epidemiological perspective. J Gerontol: Series A. 2001;56A:65–80.

24. Vellas BJ, Hunt WC, Romero LJ, Koehler KM, Baumgartner RN, Garry PJ. Changes in nutritional status and patterns of morbidity among free-living elderly persons: A 10-year longitudinal study. Nutrition 1996;13:515–519.

25. Hunter GR, Weinsier RL, Gower BA, Wetzstein C. Age-related decrease in resting energy expenditure in sedentary white women: effects of regional differences in lean and fat mass. Am J Clin Nutr 2001; 73:333–337.

26. Klausen B, Toubro S, Astrup A. Age and sex effects on energy expenditure. Am J Clin Nutr 1997; 65:895–907.

27. Schiffman SS. Taste and smell losses in normal aging and disease. JAMA 1997,278:1357–1362.

28. Stevens JC, Cruz LA, Marks LE, Lakatos S. A multimodal assessment of sensory thresholds in aging. J Gerontol Psych Sci 1998;53B:P263–P272.

29. Murphy C, Gilmore MM, Seery CS, Salmon DP, Lasker BR. Oflactory thresholds are associated with degree of dementia in Alzheimer's disease. Neurobiol Aging 1990;11:465–469.

30. Krall E, Hayes C, Garcia R. How dentition status and masticatory function affect nutrient intake. J Am Dent Assoc 1998;129:1261–1269.

31. Sheiham A, Steele JG, Marcenes W, et al. The relationships among dental status, nutrient intake, and nutritional status in older people. J Dent Res 2001;80:408–413.

32. Clarkson WK, Pantano MM, Morley JS, Horowitz M, Littlefield JM, Burton FR. Evidence for the anorexia of aging: gastrointestinal transit and hunger in healthy elderly vs. young adults. Am J Physiol 1997;272:R243–R248.

33. MacIntosh CG, Andrews JM, Jones KL, et al. Effects of age on concentrations of plasma cholesystokinin, glucagon-like peptide I and peptide YY and their relation to appetite and pyloric mobility. Am J Clin Nutr 1999;69:999–1006.

34. White H. Weight change in Alzheimer's disease. J Nutr Health Aging 1998;2:110–112.

35. Roberts SB, Fuss P, Heyman MB, et al. Control of food intake in older men. JAMA 1994;272: 1601–1606.

36. Rolls BJ, Dimeo KA, Shide DJ. Age-related impairments in the regulation of food intake. Am J Clin Nutr 1995;62:923–931.

37. Roberts SB. Regulation of energy intake in relation to metabolic state and nutritional status. Eur J Clin Nutr 2000;54(suppl 3):S64–S69.

38. De Castro JM, de Castro ES. Spontaneous meal patterns of humans: influence of the presence of other people. Am J Clin Nutr 1989;50:237–247.

39. Katz IR, Beaston-Wimmer P, Parmelee P, Friedman E, Lawton MP. Failure to thrive in the elderly: exploration of the concept and delination of psychiatric components. J Geri Psych Neur 1994;6:161–169.

40. Morley JE. Anorexia of aging: physiologic and pathologic. Am J Clin Nutr 1997;66:760–773.

41. Martinez M, Arnalich F, Hernanz A. Alterations of anorectic cytokine levels from plasma and cere-brospinal fluid in idiopathic senile anorexia. Mech Ageing Dev 1993;72:145–153.

42. Oldenburg HS, Rogy MA, Lazarus DD, et al. Cachexia and the acute phase protein response in inflam-mation are related by interleukin-6. Eur J Immunol 1993;23:1889–1894.

43. Uehara A, Sekiya C, Takasugi Y, Namiki M, Arimura A. Anoerxia induced by interleukin 1: involve-ment of corticotrophin-releasing factor. Am J Physiol 1989;257:R613–R617.

44. Aggarwal BB, Puri RK. Human Cytokines: Their Role in Disease and Therapy. Blackwell Science, Cambridge, MA, 1995.

45. Anker SD, Chua TP, Ponikowski P, et al. Hormonal changes and catabolic/anabolic imbalance in chronic heart failure and their importance for cardiac cachexia. Circulation 1997;96:526–534.

46. Roubenoff R, Roubenoff RA, Cannon JG, et al. Rheumatoid cachexia: cytokine-driven hypermetabo-lism and loss of lean body mass in chronic inflammation. J Clin Invest 1994;93:2379–2386.

47. Roubenoff R, Rall LC, Veldhuis JD, et al. The relationship between growth hormone kinetics and sarcopenia in postmenopausal women: the role of fat mass and leptin. Clin Endocrinol Metabol 1998;83: 1502–1506.

48. Liao Z, Tu JH, Small CB, Schnipper SM, Rosenstreich DL. Increased urine IL-1 levels in aging Geron-tology 1993;39:19–27.

49. Persson M, Elmstahl S, Westerterp KR. Validation of a dietary record routine in geriatric patients using doubly labelled water. Eur J Clin Nutr 2000;54:789–796.

50. Frisoni GB, Franzoni S, Rozzini R, Ferrucci L, Boffelli S, Trabucchi M. Food intake and mortality in the frail elderly. J Gerontol A Biol Sci 1995;50:M203–M210.

51. Lauque S, Arnaud-Battandier F, Mansourian R, et al. Protein-energy oral supplementation in malnour-ished nursing-home residents: a controlled trial. Age Aging 2000;29:51–56.

52. Guigoz Y, Vellas B, Garry PJ. Mini Nutritional Assessment: a practical assessment tool for grading the nutritional state of elderly patients. Facts Res Gerontol 1994;4:15–59.

53. Guigoz Y, Vellas B, Garry PJ. Assessing the nutritional status of the elderly: the Mini Nutritional Assessment as part of the geriatric evaluation. Nutr Rev 1996;54:S59–S65.

54. Thomas DR, Zdrowski CD, Wilson MM, et al. Malnutrition in subacute care. Am J Clin Nutr 2002;75: 308–313.

55. Omran ML, Morley JE. Assessment of protein energy malnutrition in older persons, part I: history, examination, body composition, and screening tools. Nutrition 2000;16:50–63.

56. Castellanos VH, Andrews YN. Inherent flaws in a method of estimating meal intake commonly used in long-term-care facilities. J Am Dietet Assoc 2002;102:826–830.

57. Fabiny AR, Kiel DP. Assessing and treating weight loss in nursing home patients. Clin Geriatr Med 1997;4:737–751.

58. Matthews LE. Monitoring weight changes in nursing home residents. J Nutr Elderly 1989;9:67–72.

59. MDS Reference Manual, Appendix section A-4. Eliot Press, Natick, MA, 1993.

60. Prentice AM, Leavesley K, Murgatroyd PR, et al. Is severe wasting in elderly mental patients caused by excessive energy requirement? Age Aging 1989;18:158–167.

61. Wilson MMG, Vaswani S, Liu D, Morley JE, Miller DK. Prevalence and causes of undernutrition in medical outpatients. Am J Med 1998;104:56–63.

62. Thompson MP, Morris LK. Unexplained weight loss in the ambulatory elderly. J Am Geriatr Soc 1991; 39:497–501.

63. Rabinovitz M, Pitlik SD, Leifer M, et al. Unintentional weight loss: a retrospective analysis of 154 cases. Arch Intern Med 1986;146:186–187.

64. Ritchie CS, Joshipura K, Silliman RA, Miller B, Douglas CW. Oral health problems and significant weight loss among community-dwelling older adults. J Gerontol 2000;55A:M366–M371.

65. Johnson C, East JM, Glassman P. Management of malnutrition in the elderly and the appropriate use of commercially manufactured oral nutritional supplements. J Nutr Health Aging 2000;4:42–46.

66. Abbasi AA, Rudman D. Observation on the prevalence of protein-calorie undernutrition in VA nursing homes. J Am Geriatr Soc 1993;41:117–121.

67. Thomas DR, Verdery RB, Gardner L, Kant A, Lindsay J. A prospective study of outcome from protein-energy malnutrition in nursing home residents. JPEN 1991;15:400–404.

68. Blaum C, Fries B, Fiatarone MA. Factors associated with low body mass index and weight loss in nursing home residents. J Gerontol Med Sci 1992;50A:M162–M168.

69. Sullivan DH, Sun S, Walls RC. Protein-energy under-nutrition among elderly hospitalized patients. JAMA 1999;281:2013–2019.

70. Williamson DF. Descriptive epidemiology of body weight and weight change in U.S. adults. Ann Intern Med 1993;119:646–649.

71. Coulston AM, Mandelbaum D, Reaven GM. Dietary management of nursing home residents with non-insulin-dependent diabetes mellitus. Am J Clin Nutr 1990;51:67–71.

72. Buckler DA, Kelber ST, Goodwin JS. The use of dietary restrictions in malnourished nursing home patients. J Am Geriatr Soc 1994;42:1100–1102.

73. Tariq SH, Kardic E, Thomas DR, et al. The use of a no-concentrated-sweets diet in the management of type 2 diabetes in nursing homes. J Am Diet Assoc 2002;101:1463–1466.

74. Schiffman SS, Warwick ZE. Effect of flavor enhancement of foods for the elderly on nutritional status: food intake, biochemical indices, and anthropomorphic measures. Physiol Behav 1993;53:395–402.

75. Schiffman SS. Intensification of sensory properties of foods for the elderly with monosodium glutamate and flavors. Food Rev Int 1998;14:321–333.

76. Karcic E, Philpot C, Morley JE. Treating malnutrition with megestrol acetate: Literature review and review of our experience. J Nutr Health Aging 2002;6:191 200.

77. Jackobs MK. Megestrol acetate: a medical nutrition therapy tool to affect positive weight outcomes in the elderly. J Am Dietet Assoc (suppl)1999;99.

78. Yeh SS, Wu SY, Lee TP, et al. Improvement in quality-of-life measures and stimulation of weight gain after treatment with megestrol acetate oral suspension in geriatric cachexia: results of a double-blind, placebo-controlled study. J Am Geriatr Soc 2000;48:485–492.

79. Van Ort S, Phillips LR. Nursing interventions to promote functional feeding. J Gerontol Nurs 1995;10:6–14.

80. Lange-Alberts ME, Shott S. Nutritional intake: use of touch and verbal cueing. J Gerontol Nurs 1994;2:36–40.

81. Simmons SF, Osterwell D, Schnelle JF. Improving food intake in nursing home residents with feeding assistance: A staffing analysis. J Gerontol Med Sci 2001;56A:M790–M794.

82. Steigh C, Glassman P, Fajardo F. Physician and dietitian prescribing of a commercially available oral nutritional supplement. Am J Man Care 1998;4:567–572.

83. Fiatarone Singh MA, Bernstein MA, Ryan ND, O'Neill EF, Clements KM, Evans WJ. The effect of oral nutritional supplements on habitual dietary quality and quantity in frail elderly . J Nutr Health Aging 2000;4:5–12.

84. Gray-Donald K, Payette H. Randomized clinical trial of nutritional supplementation shows little effect on functional status among free living frail elderly. J Nutr 1995;125:2965–2971.

85. Turic A, Gordon KL, Craig LD, Ataya DG, Voss AC. Nutritional supplementation enables residents of long-term-care facilities to meet or exceed RDA's without displacing energy or nutrient intakes from meals. J Am Diet Assoc 1998;98:1457–1459.

86. Krondl M, Coleman PH, Bradley CL, Lau D, Ryan N. Subjectively healthy elderly consuming a liquid nutrition supplement maintained body mass index and improved some nutritional parameters and perceived well-being. J Am Diet Assoc 1999;99:1542–1548.

87. Delmi M, Rapin C-H, Bengoa J-M, Delmas DD, Vasey H, Bonjour J-P. Dietary supplementation in elderly patients with fractured neck of the femur. Lancet 1990;335:1013–1016

88. Schurch MA, Rizzoli R, Slosman D, Vadas L, Vergnaud P, Bonjour J-P. Protein supplements increase serum insulin-like growth factor-1 levels and attenuate proximal femur bone loss in patients with recent hip fracture: a randomized, double-blind, placebo-controlled trial. Ann Intern Med 1998;128:801–809.

89. Kayser-Jones J, Schell ES, Porter C, et al. A prospective study of the use of liquid oral dietary supplements in nursing homes. JAGS 1998;46:1378–1386.

90. Cook CG, Andrews JM, Jones KL, et al. The effects of small intestinal infusion on appetite and pyloric motility are modified by age. Am J Physiol 1997;273:755–761.

91. Wilson MMG, Purushothaman R, Morley JE. Effect of liquid dietary supplements on energy intake in the elderly. Am J Clin Nutr 2002;75:944–947.

92. Rudman D, Abbasi AA, Isaacson K. Observations on the nutrient intakes of eating-dependent nursing home residents: underutilization of micronutrient supplements. J Am Coll Nutr 1995;14:604–613.

93. Willett WC. Stampfer MJ. Clinical practice. What vitamins should I be taking, doctor? New Engl J Med 2001;345:1819.

94. Bales CW. Micronutrient deficiencies in nursing homes: Should clinical intervention await a research consensus? (Editorial) J Am Coll Nutr 1995;14:563–564.

95. Sanders DS, Carter MJ, D'Silva J, James G, Bolton RP, Bardhan KD. Survival analysis in percutaneous endoscopic hastrostomy feeding: A worse outcome in patients with dementia. Am J Gastroenterol 2000;95:1472–1475.

96. Mitchell SL, Kiely DK, Lipsitz LA. The risk factors and impact on survival of feeding tube placement in nursing home residents with severe cognitive impairment. Arch Intern Med 1997;157:327–332.

97. Henderson CT, Trumbore LS, Mobarhan S, Benya R, Miles TP. Prolonged tube feeding in long-term care: Nutritional status and clinical outcomes. J Am Coll Nutr 1992;11:309–325.

98. Lord LM, Wiser-Maimone A, Pulhamus M, et al. Comparison of weighted vs unweighted enteral feeding tubes for efficacy of transpyloric intubation. JPEN 1993;17:271–273.

99. Norton B, Homer-Ward M, Donnelly MT, Long RG, Holmes GKT. A randomised prospective comparison of percutaneous endoscopic gastrostomy and naso gastric tube feeding after acute dysphagic stoke. BMJ 1996;312:13–16.

100. Klor BM, Milianti FJ. Rehabilitation of neurogenic dysphagia with percutaneous endoscopic gastrostomy. Dysphagia 1999;14:162–164.

101. Loser C, Wolters S, Folsch UR. Enteral long-term nutrition via percutaneous endoscopic gastrostomy (PEG) in 210 patients. Dig Dis Sci 1998;43:2549–2557.

102. Kaw M, Sekas G. Long-term follow-up of consequences of percutaneous endoscopic gastrostomy (PEG) tubes in nursing home patients. Digest Dis Sci 1994;39:738–743.

103. Peterson TI, Kruse A. Complications of percutaneous endoscopic gastrostomy. Eur J Surg 1997;163: 351–356.

104. Langdon DS, Hunt A, Pope J, Hackes B. Nutrition support at the end of life: Opinions of Louisiana dietitians. J Am Diet Assoc 2002;102:837–841.

105. Taper LJ, Hockin DB. Life sustaining nutrition support for the terminally ill elderly: dietitians' ethical attitudes and beliefs. J Can Diet Assoc 1996;57:19–24.

106. Ackerman RJ. Withholding and withdrawing life-sustaining treatment. Am Fam Phys 2000;62: 1555–1560.

107. Gillick MR. Rethinking the role of tube feeeding in patients with advanced dementia. New Eng J Med 2000;342:206–210.

108. Finucane TE, Christmas C, Travis K. Tube feeding in patients with advanced dementia. JAMA 1999;282:1365–1370.

109. O'Brien LA, Grisso G, Maislin G, et al. Nursing home residents' preferences for life-sustaining treatments. JAMA 1995;274:1775–1779.

110. Ouslander JG, Tymchuk AJ, Krynski MA. Decisions about enteral tube feeding among the elderly. J Am Geriatr Soc 1993;41:70–77.

111. Poehlman ET, Danforth E Jr. Endurance training increases metabolic rate and norepinephrine appearance rate in older individuals. Am J Physiol 1991;261:E233–E239.

112. Fiatarone MA, O'Neill EF, Ryan ND, et al. Exercise training and nutritional supplementation for physical frailty in very elderly people. N Engl J Med 1994;330:1769–1775.
113. Doherty GM, Jensen JC, Alexancer HR, Buresch CM, Norton JA. Pentoxifylline suppression of tumor necrosis factor gene transcription. Surgery 1991;110:192–198.
114. Landman D, Sarai A, Sathe SS. Use of pentoxifylline therapy for patients with AIDS-related wasting: pilot study. Clin Infect Dis 1995;20:1069–1070.
115. Yeh SS, Schuster MW. Geriatric cachexia: the role of cytokines. Am J Clin Nutr 1999;70:1833–1897.
116. Mantovani G, Maccio A, Esu S, Lai P, et al. Medroxyprogesterone acetate reduces the in vitro production of cytokines and serotonin involved in anorexia/cachexia and emesis by peripheral blood mononuclear cells of cancer patients. Eur J Cancer 1997;33:602–607.
117. Yeh SS, Wu SY, Levine DM, et al. The correlation of cytokine levels with body weight after megestrol acetate treatment in geriatric patients. J Gerontol A Biol Sci Med Sci 2001;56:M48–M54
118. Tisdale MJ, Dhesi JK. Inhibition of weight loss by omega-3 fatty acids in an experimental cachexia model. Cancer Res 1990;50:5022–5026.
119. McClain CJ, Barve S, Deaciuc I, Kugelmas M, Hill D. Cytokines in alcoholic liver disease. Sem Liver Dis 1999;19:205–219.
120. Hill DB, Devalaraja R, Joshi-Barve S, Barve S, McClain CJ. Antioxidants attenuate nuclear factor-kappa B activation and tumor necrosis factor-alpha production in alcoholic hepatitis patient monocytes and rat Kupffer cells, in vitro. Clin Biochem 1999;32:563–570.

12 The Relationship of Nutrition and Pressure Ulcers

David R. Thomas

1. INTRODUCTION AND BACKGROUND

Wound healing is intricately linked to nutrition. Severe protein-calorie undernutrition in humans alters tissue regeneration, the inflammatory reaction, and immune function *(1)*. Undernourished patients are more likely to have postoperative complications than well-nourished patients *(2)*. After vascular surgery, hypoalbuminemia and low transferrin levels have predicted wound healing complications *(3)*. Hospitalized patients with severe undernutrition are at a higher risk for death, sepsis, infections, and increased length of stay *(4)*.

Experimental studies in animal models suggest a biologically plausible relationship between undernutrition and development of pressure ulcers. When pressure was applied for 4 h to the skin of well-nourished animals and malnourished animals, pressure ulcers occurred equally in both groups. However, the degree of ischemic skin destruction was more severe in the malnourished animals. Epithelialization of the pressure lesions occurred in normal animals at 3 d postinjury, whereas necrosis of the epidermis was still present in the malnourished animals *(5)*. This data suggests that although pressure damage may occur independently of nutritional status, malnourished animals may have impaired healing after a pressure injury.

Further indication of a relationship between nutrition and tissue damage is suggested by the finding that mitotic activity in normal epidermis is severely depressed in mice whose food intake was reduced to 70% of normal intake *(6)*. Dietary restriction to 60% of normal intake in other animal models is associated with impaired collagen crosslinking 1 wk after wounding *(7)*. Classical studies have shown that wound dehiscence occurs more commonly in dogs with chronic protein undernutrition *(8)*. Nevertheless, animal studies may not accurately reflect human wound healing. For example, collagen deposition is completed in 42 d in animal wounds when compared to 88 d in humans in human wounds *(9)*. Hypoalbuminemia is not associated with impaired wound healing in analbuminemic rats *(10)*. The effects of short-term starvation is much more severe in animals than in humans *(11)*.

From: *Handbook of Clinical Nutrition and Aging*
Edited by: C. W. Bales and C. S. Ritchie © Humana Press Inc., Totowa, NJ

2. EPIDEMIOLOGICAL ASSOCIATIONS OF NUTRITION AND PRESSURE ULCERS

Nutritional status has been thought to influence the incidence, progression, and severity of pressure sores. Most of the data derives from epidemiological studies.

Undernutrition, defined by an index of biochemical and anthropometric variables, including hemoglobin, albumin, lymphocyte count, history of weight loss, body weight, triceps skinfold thickness, and mid-arm circumference, was present in 29% of patients at hospital admission in a prospective study of high-risk patients. Using At 4 wk, 17% of the undernourished patients had developed a pressure ulcer in comparison to 9% of the nonundernourished patients. Thus, patients who were undernourished at hospital admission were twice as likely to subsequently develop pressure ulcers as nonundernourished patients (RR 2.1, 95% CI 1.1, 4.2) *(12)*.

In a long-term-care setting, 59% of residents were diagnosed as undernourished on admission, using a combination of serum albumin, total lymphocyte count, and somatic protein deficit expressed as a percentage. Among these residents, 7.3% were classified as severely undernourished. Pressure ulcers occurred in 65% of these severely undernourished residents. No pressure ulcer developed in the mild-to-moderately undernourished or well-nourished groups *(13)*.

Two epidemiological studies have correlated development of pressure ulcers with dietary intake. In a long-term care setting, the estimated percent intake of dietary protein, but not total caloric intake, predicted development of pressure ulcers. Patients with pressure ulcers ingested 93% of the recommended daily intake of protein compared to an intake of 119% of the recommended protein in the nonpressure ulcer group. Only dietary intake of protein was important in this study. The total dietary intake of calories or the calculated intake of vitamins A and C, iron and zinc did not predict ulcer development *(14)*.

Impaired nutritional intake, defined as a persistently poor appetite, meals held from gastrointestinal disease or a prescribed diet less than 1100 kcal or 50 g protein/d predicted pressure ulcer development in another long-term care setting *(14a)*. However, no other nutritional variable, including albumin, serum protein, hemoglobin, total lymphocyte count, body mass index, or body weight, was univariately significant.

Table 1 demonstrates the association of serum albumin and other nutritional variables with the development of a pressure ulcer. Pressure ulcers appear to be associated with traditional markers of nutritional status in some studies. However, serum albumin acts as an acute phase reactant *(15)*. Physiological stress (such as surgical operations), cortisol excess, and hypermetabolic states reduce serum albumin even in the presence of adequate protein intake. Decreases in serum albumin may reflect the presence of inflammatory cytokine production or comorbidity rather than nutritional status. Thus, serum albumin has not consistently been an independent predictor of pressure ulcers.

Similarly, large reductions in body weight may indicate disease associated cachexia rather than impaired intake alone. Poor nutritional status defined by these variables may indicate poor health rather than poor nutrient intake. Serum albumin and weight loss may be independent markers for poor outcome regardless of nutrient intake.

The controversy apparent in defining the relationship of pressure ulcers and nutrition may have roots in the physiological variables used to define malnutrition. There is no

Table 1
Epidemiological Association of Nutritional Markers with Development of a Pressure Ulcer (PU)

Reference	Setting	Associated with presence of PU	Not associated with presence of PU
Allman (85)	AC	Albumin	Weight, hemoglobin, TLC, nutritional assessment
Gorse (86)	AC	Albumin	Nutritional assessment score
Inman (87)	AC, ICU	Albumin (measured at 3 d)	Serum protein, hemoglobin, weight
Allman (78)	AC	BMI, TLC	Albumin, TSF, arm circumference, weight loss, hemoglobin, nitrogen balance
Hartgrink (50)	AC, orthopedic		Nocturnal enteral feeding
Anthony (88)	AC	Albumin < 32 g/L	
Moolten (89)	LTC	Albumin < 35 g/L	
Pinchcofsky-Devin (13)	LTC	Severe malnutrition	Mild-to-moderate malnutrition or normal nutrition
Berlowitz (14a)	LTC	Impaired nutritional intake	Albumin, serum protein, hemoglobin, TLC, BMI/weight
Bennett (90)	LTC		Weight, BMI, weight gain
Brandeis (91)	LTC	Dependency in feeding	BMI/weight, TSF
Trumbore (92)	LTC	Albumin, cholesterol	
Breslow (93)	LTC	Albumin, hemoglobin	Serum protein, cholesterol, zinc, copper, transferrin, body weight, BMI, TLC
Bergstrom (14)	LTC	Dietary protein intake 93% of RDA vs 119%, dietary iron	Serum protein, cholesterol, zinc, copper, transferrin, weight, BMI, TLC
Ferrell (94)	LTC		Albumin, serum protein, BMI, hematocrit
Bourdel-Marchasson (49)	LTC		Oral nutritional supplement (26%vs 20% incidence)
Guralnik (95)	Community		Albumin, BMI, impaired nutrition, hemoglobin

AC, acute care; LTC, long-term care; BMI, body mass index; TLC, total lymphocyte count; TSF, triceps skinfold thickness; ICU, intensive care unit; RDA, recommended daily allowance.

accepted gold standard for the diagnosis of undernutrition and the markers for nutritional status may reflect underlying disease rather than undernutrition in older, ill persons. The association is confounded by lack of adjustment for comorbidity or severity of illness (16). Despite a strong association, a causal relationship of poor nutritional status to pressure ulcers has not been established. The association does not confirm that one follows the other (causality), but that both undernutrition and pressure ulcers frequently coexist in the same persons.

3. GENERAL NUTRITIONAL SUPPORT FOR PERSONS WITH PRESSURE ULCERS

3.1. Protein

The hypothesized relationship between poor nutritional status and pressure ulcers forms the cornerstone of nutritional support. Table 2 summarizes the interventional trials for pressure ulcers. Greater healing of pressure ulcers has been reported with a higher protein intake irrespective of positive nitrogen balance *(17)*. Clinical trials have examined dietary interventions in the healing pressure ulcers. In 48 patients with stage II–IV pressure ulcers who were being fed enterally, undernutrition was defined as a serum albumin below 35 g/L *or* body weight more than 10% below the midpoint of the age-specific weight range. Total truncal pressure ulcer surface area showed more decrease (-4.2 cm^2 vs -2.1 cm^2) in surface area in patients fed the enteral formula containing 24% protein when compared to a formula containing 14% protein. However, changes in body weight or in biochemical parameters of nutritional status did not occur between groups. The study was limited by a small sample size (only 28 patients completed the study), nonrandom assignment to treatment groups, confounding effects of air-fluidized beds, and the use of two different feeding routes *(18)*.

In a small study of 12 enterally fed patients with pressure ulcers, the group who received 1.8 g/kg of protein had a 73% improvement in pressure ulcer surface area when compared to a 42% improvement in surface area in the group receiving 1.2 g/kg of protein, despite that the group that received the higher protein level began the study with larger surface-area pressure ulcers (22.6 cm^2 vs 9.1 cm^2) *(17)*.

The optimum dietary protein intake in patients with pressure ulcers is unknown, but may be much higher than current adult recommendation of 0.8 g/kg/d. Current recommendations for dietary intake of protein in stressed elderly patients lies between 1.2 and 1.5 g/kg/d. Stress generally includes persons with burns, pressure ulcers, cancer, infections, and other similar conditions. Yet, half of chronically ill elderly persons cannot maintain nitrogen balance at this level *(19)*. On the other hand, increasing protein intake beyond 1.5 g/kg/d may not increase protein synthesis and may cause dehydration *(20)*. The optimum protein intake for these patients has not been defined, but may lie between 1.5 and 1.8 g/kg/d.

3.2. Amino Acids

The association of dietary protein intake with wound healing has led to the investigation of the use of specific amino acids. Glutamine is essential for the immune system function, but supplemental glutamine has not been shown to have noticeable effects on wound healing *(21)*. Arginine supplementation is well tolerated but does not enhance mitogen-induced lymphocyte proliferation in elderly nursing home residents that have pressure ulcers *(22)*. No improvement in wound healing has been detected by using high supplements of branched-chain amino acid formulations *(23)*. Few studies have addressed the rate of amino acids in the healing of pressure ulcers.

3.3. Energy

Daily caloric requirements range from 25 kcal/kg/d for sedentary adults to 40 kcal/kg/d for stressed adults. In general, caloric requirements can be met at 30–35 kcal/kg/d for

Table 2
Nutritional Interventions in the Treatment of Pressure Ulcers

Reference	Setting	Intervention	Outcome
Breslow (18)	Long-term care	24% Protein vs 14% protein enteral feeding	-4.2 cm^2 vs -2.1 cm^2 decrease in surface area
Chernoff (17)	Long-term care	1.8 g/kg Protein vs 1.2 g/kg protein enteral feeding	73% vs 43% improvement in surface area
Henderson (51)	Long-term care	1.6 × Basal energy expenditure,1.4 g of protein per kg/d	65% PU at onset; 61% prevalence at 3 mo
Mitchell (52)	Long-term care	Enteral feeding	RR of death 1.49 (1.2–1.8) vs RR of death 1.06 (0.8–1.4) after 2 yr
Hartgrink (50)	Acute hip fracture patients	Enteral feeding	No difference in incidence
ter Riet (30)	Long-term care	Vitamin C 10 mg vs 1000 mg	No difference in healing rate
Taylor (31)	Acute surgical patients	Vitamin C large dose vs none	84% vs 43% (control) reduction surface area at 30 d
Norris (39)	Acute hip fracture	Zinc	No difference

RR, relative risk (95% confidence intervals).

elderly patients under moderate stress. Various formulas, including the Harris-Benedict equation, can be used to predict caloric requirements, but controversy exists over accuracy in obese or severely undernourished individuals (24). Other formulas have been adjusted for severely stressed hospitalized subjects (25). Considerable debate exists over whether to use ideal body weight or an adjusted body weight in calculations. The best instrument for predicting nutritional requirements in older, undernourished individuals in whom ideal or usual body weight if often unknown is not clear.

3.4. Vitamins

The deficiency of several vitamins has significant effects on wound healing. However, supplementation of vitamins to accelerate wound healing in the absence of a deficiency state is controversial. Vitamin C is essential for wound healing and impaired wound healing has been observed in clinical scurvy. However, in studies of clinically impaired wound healing, six months of a ascorbate-free diet is required to produce a deficient state (26). In animals who are vitamin C deficient, wound healing is abnormal at 7 d but completely normal at 14 d (27). Although essential, there is no evidence of acceleration of wound healing by vitamin C supplementation in patients who are not vitamin C deficient (28). Supertherapeutic doses of vitamin C has not been shown to accelerate wound healing (29). The recommended daily allowance (RDA) of vitamin C is 60 mg. This RDA is easily achieved from dietary sources that include citrus fruits, green vegetables, peppers, tomatoes, and potatoes.

Two clinical trials have evaluated the effect of supplemental vitamin C in the treatment of pressure ulcers. In a multicenter, blinded trial, 88 patients with pressure ulcers were randomized to either 10 mg or 500 mg twice daily of vitamin C. The wound closure rate, relative healing rate, and wound improvement score was not different between groups *(30)*. An earlier trial in acute surgical patients with pressure ulcers found a mean reduction in surface area of 84% at 1 mo in patients treated with large doses of vitamin C when compared to a reduction in surface area of 43% in the control group ($p < 0.005$) *(31)*.

Vitamin A deficiency results in delayed wound healing and increased susceptibility to infection *(32)*. Vitamin A has been shown to be effective in counteracting delayed healing in patients on corticosteroids *(33)*. Vitamin E deficiency does not appear to play an active role in wound healing *(34)*.

Zinc was first implicated in delayed wound healing in 1967 *(35)*. No study to date has shown improved wound healing in patients supplemented with zinc who were not zinc deficient *(36,37)*. Zinc levels have not been associated with development of pressure ulcers in patients with femoral neck fractures *(38)*. In a small study of patients with pressure ulcers, no effect on ulcer healing was seen at 12 wk in zinc supplemented vs nonzinc supplemented patients *(39)*. Indiscriminate or long-term zinc supplementation should be avoided because high serum zinc levels may inhibit healing, impair phagocytosis, and interfere with copper metabolism *(40–42)*. The RDA for zinc is 12–15 mg, but most elderly persons intake 7–11 mg of zinc/d *(43)*, primarily from meats and cereal.

4. NUTRITION SUPPORT AND PRESSURE ULCERS

Although correction of poor nutrition is part of total patient care and should be addressed in each patient, controversy exists about the ability of nutritional support to reduce wound complications or improve wound healing *(44,45)*.

Increasing knowledge of the complexity of wound healing has led to a hypothesis that providing hypercaloric feeding in the form of nutritional supplements to patients at risk for undernutrition might lead to reversal of undernutrition and the prevention of pressure ulcers. Several attempts have been made to improve nutritional status and thus decrease the incidence of pressure ulcers (Table 2). No nutritional intervention has shown effectiveness in prevention of pressure ulcers *(41,46,47)*.

The effect of oral nutrition supplements was observed in hospitalized, severely ill patients. Nurtritional supplements were given to 32.6% of a nonrandomized group when compared to 86.9% of subjects on another hospital ward. There was no significant difference between groups in pressure ulcer incidence (26.4% vs 20.2%), pressure ulcer prevalence at discharge (14.7% vs 10.3%), mortality (15.6% vs 14.2%), length of stay (17.3 d vs 17.4 d), or nosocomial infections (26.4% vs 19.0%) *(48)*.

The effect of higher caloric and protein intakes in nutritionally supplemented, severely ill older patients was evaluated in a prospective trial. Despite a higher caloric intake in the intervention group (1081 Kcal vs 957 Kcal, $p = 0.006$) and higher protein intake (45.9 g protein vs 38.3 g protein in the control group, $p < 0.001$), the cumulative incidence of pressure ulcers was 41% in the nutritional intervention group vs 47% in the control group *(49)*.

Attempts to prevent development of pressure ulcers in patients with hip fracture by provision of enteral nutrition has not been supported by randomized clinical trials. The effect of overnight supplemental enteral feeding in patients with a fracture of the hip and a high pressure-sore risk score has been evaluated. Of the 62 patients randomized for enteral feeding, only 25 tolerated their tube for more than 1 wk, and only 16 tolerated their tube for 2 wk. No difference was found for the development of a pressure ulcer, total serum protein, serum albumin, or the severity of pressure sores after 1 and 2 wk. Comparison of the actually tube-fed group ($n = 25$ at 1 wk, $n = 16$ at 2 wk) and the control group showed 2–3 × higher protein and energy intake ($p < 0.0001$), and a significantly higher total serum protein and serum albumin after 1 and 2 wk in the actually tube-fed group ($p < 0.001$). However, the development of pressure ulcers and severity were not significantly influenced in the actually tube-fed group *(50)*. It is possible that the lack of effect on supplemental enteral feeding was due to poor tolerance of the feedings.

A study of enteral tube feedings in patients with a pressure ulcer in a long-term care setting, observed 49 patients for 3 mo *(51)*. Patients received 1.6 × basal energy expenditure daily, 1.4 g of protein/kg/ d, and 85% or more of their total RDA. At the end of 3 mo, there was no difference in number or healing of pressure ulcers.

In a study of survival among residents in long-term care with severe cognitive impairment, 135 residents were followed for 24 mo *(52)*. The reasons for the placement of a feeding tube included the presence of a pressure ulcer. Having a feeding tube was not associated with increased survival; in fact the risk of death was slightly increased (odds ratio [OR] 1.09). There was no apparent effect on the prevalence of pressure ulcers in this group of enterally fed persons.

5. FACTORS CONTRIBUTING TO THE NUTRITIONAL PARADOX

One reason for the lack of effect in nutritional trials may be the failure to adjust for comorbidity. Involuntary weight loss, reduced appetite, and severe undernutrition are common in the geriatric population, and are often unexplained *(53)*. A common cause may be loss of appetite, due to dysregulation of a variety of psychological, gastrointestinal, metabolic, and nutritional factors *(54)*. Loss of appetite may initiate a vicious cycle of weight loss and increasing undernutrition.

Cachexia is associated with cancer *(55)*, congestive heart failure *(56)*, end-stage renal disease *(57)*, AIDS *(58)*, and rheumatoid arthritis *(59)*. Tumor necrosis factor-α (TNF) levels are elevated in patients with severe undernutrition and congestive heart failure, but not in patients with congestive heart failure who do not have severe undernutrition *(60)*. TNF can either promote wound healing or induce cascades that interfere with inflammatory resolution and foster autoimmune reactions *(61)*. Severe undernutrition occurs in both chronic infections and neoplastic disorders, suggesting that severe undernutrition develops along a common pathway and is not dependent on a specific infection or a particular neoplasm. Interleukin (IL)-1 concentrations are elevated in elderly patients with severe undernutrition of unknown etiology *(62)*, and levels of IL-1β and IL-6 can be increased in elderly persons without evidence of infection or cancer *(63)*.

Cytokines may regulate appetite directly through the central feeding drive. Significant interaction between the central feeding drive, neuropeptide Y, and IL-1β has been demonstrated in rats *(64,65)* IL-1, IL-6, TNF, interferon-γ, leukemia inhibitory factor (D-factor), and prostaglandin E_2 have all been implicated in cancer-induced severe undernutrition *(66,67)*. Leptin, a central regulator of food intake and body fat mass, increases under the stress of hip operations *(68)*, but is low in undernourished men *(69)*.

Table 3
Documented Relations Among Cytokines, Undernutrition, and Chronic Wounds

Undernutrition
  – Poor wound healing
  – Increased risk of infection
  – Increased incidence of pressure ulcers

Proinflammatory cytokines
  – Suppress appetite
  – Promote/interfere with wound healing

Chronic wounds
  – Source of cytokines
  – Increased association with undernutrition
  – Increased serum levels of cytokines

In 72 male subjects admitted to a geriatric rehabilitation unit, soluble IL-2 receptor was negatively associated with albumin $R^2 = -0.479$, $p < 0.0001$), prealbumin $R^2 = -0.520$, $p = < 0.0001$), cholesterol $R^2 = -0.487$, $p = 0.0001$), transferrin $R^2 = -0.455$, $p = 0.0002$), and hemoglobin $R^2 = -0.371$, $p = 0.002$). This suggests that inflammation increases the incidence of hypoalbuminemia and hypocholesterolemia. The use of albumin and cholesterol in these patients as nutritional markers could potentially lead to overdiagnosis of malnutrition *(70)*.

The lack of effect of hypercaloric feeding in pressure ulcers may reflect that the underlying pathophysiology is cytokine-induced cachexia, rather than simple starvation. Starvation is amenable to hypercaloric feeding in all patients, with the exception of the terminally undernourished patients. Cytokine-induced cachexia is remarkably resistant to hypercaloric feeding *(71,72)*

Cytokine mediated anorexia and weight loss are common in populations that develop pressure ulcers. The interrelationship is outlined in Table 3. However, the role of cytokines in subjects with pressure ulcers remains unclear. Serum IL-1β is elevated in patients with pressure ulcers *(73)*. Levels of IL-1α are elevated in pressure ulcers but low in acute wound fluid *(74)*. Circulating serum levels of IL-6, IL-2 and IL-2R are higher in spinal cord-injured patients compared to normal controls, and highest in subjects with pressure ulcers. The highest concentration of cytokines were in subjects with the slowest healing pressure ulcers *(75)*. In other studies, IL-6 serum levels were increased in patients with pressure ulcers, but IL-1 and TNF were not elevated *(76)*.

A preliminary study of cytokines in patients with pressure ulcers indicates that serum IL-6 was not different between subjects with and those without pressure ulcers within 5 d of acute hospitalization.

Several cytokines, particularly IL-1α, IL-1β, and IL-6, may be elevated in subjects with pressure ulcers. Whether these levels change with healing or are predictive of healing is not known. These cytokines are known to also increase in severe undernutrition. Existing studies are not clear whether the elevation is a result of the presence of a pressure ulcer or due to underlying severe undernutrition. Alternatively, the elevation of cytokine levels may be a common pathway for both conditions. The hypotheses are depicted in Fig. 1.

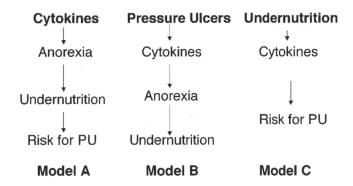

Fig. 1. Possible models for the interaction of cytokines, pressure ulcers, and nutrition.

Interventions to modulate cytokine activity are possible. Cytokine modulation has been postulated as a potential treatment for cachexia *(77–83)*. If a significant positive relationship exists between circulating cytokines and pressure ulcers, a opportunity for potential intervention to promote healing exists.

6. SUMMARY

Wound nutrition is whole body nutrition. Unquestionably, providing nutritional support can prevent the effects of starvation. Death is an inevitable consequence of starvation. Whether nutrition can improve the outcome of a disease remains disputable. Improvements in nutritional markers, such as serum protein concentrations, nitrogen balance, and weight gain, usually have not been accompanied by clinical benefits *(71,84)*.

There is no doubt that undernutrition does not have a positive effect on wound healing. However, there is no magic nutritional bullet that will accelerate wound healing. General nutritional support should be provided to persons with pressure ulcers, consistent with medical goals and patient wishes.

7. RECOMMENDATIONS FOR CLINICIANS

1. Optimize protein intake with a goal of 1.5–1.8 g/kg/d of protein.
2. In general, caloric requirements can be met at 30–35 kcal/kg/d for elderly patients under moderate stress (most patients with pressure ulcers are under moderate stress).
3. Consider vitamin A supplements in patients on corticosteriods.
4. There is no data to support the *routine* use of vitamin C and zinc in patients with pressure ulcers.

REFERENCES

1. Young ME. Malnutrition and wound healing. Heart Lung 1988;17:60–67.
2. Detsky AS, Baker JP, O'Rourke K, et al. Predicting nutrition-associated complications for patients undergoing gastrointestinal surgery. JPEN 1987;11:440–446.
3. Casey J, Flinn WR, Yao JST, et al. Correlation of immune and nutritional status with wound complications in patients undergoing vascular operations. Surgery 1983;93:822–827.
4. Dempsey DT, Mullen JL, Buzby GP. The link between nutritional status and clinical outcome: can nutritional intervention modify it? Am J Clin Nutr 1988;47(suppl):352–356.

5. Takeda T, Koyama T, Izawa Y, et al. Effects of malnutrition on development of experimental pressure sores. J Dermatol 1992;19:602–609.
6. Bullough WS, Eisa EA. The effects of a graded series of restricted diets on epidermal mitotic activity in the mouse. Br J Cancer 1950;4:321–328.
7. Reiser KM. Nonenzymatic glycations and enzymatic crosslinking in a model of wound healing. J Ger Dermotol 1993;1:90–99.
8. Thompson W, Ravdin IS, Frank IL. The effect of hypoproteinemic on wound disruption. Arch Surg 1938;26:500.
9. Levenson SM. Some challenging wound healing problems for clinicians and basic scientists. In: Repair and Regeneration: the Scientific Basis for Surgical Practice. Dunphy JE, Van Winkle W Jr (eds.), McGraw-Hill, New York, 1969, pp 309–337.
10. Felcher A, Schwartz J, Schechter C, et al. Wound healing in normal and analbuminemic rates. J Surg Res 1987;43:546.
11. Barbul A, Purtill WA. Nutrition in wound healing. Clinics in Dermatol 1994;12:133–140.
12. Thomas DR, Goode PS, Tarquine PH, Allman R. Hospital acquired pressure ulcers and risk of Death. J Am Geriatr Soc 1996;44:1435–1440.
13. Pinchcofsky-Devin GD, Kaminski MV Jr. Correlation of pressure sores and nutritional status. J Am Geriatr Soc 1986;34:435–440.
14. Bergstrom N, Braden B. A prospective study of pressure sore risk among institutionalized elderly. J Am Geriatr Soc 1992;40:747–758.
14a. Berlowitz DR, Wilking SV. Risk factors for pressure sores: a comparison of cross-sectional and cohort-derived data. J Am Geriatr Soc 1989;37:1043–1050.
15. Friedman FJ, Campbell AJ, Caradoc-Davies. Hypoalbuminemia in the elderly is due to disease not malnutrition. Clin Exper Gerontol 1985;7:191–203.
16. Finucane TE. Malnutrition, tube feeding and pressure sores: Data are incomplete. J Am Geriatr Soc 1995; 43:447–451.
17. Chernoff RS, Milton KY, Lipschitz DA. The effect of very high-protein liquid formula (Replete) on decubitus ulcer healing in long-term tube-fed institutionalized patients. Investigators Final Report 1990. J Am Diet Assoc 1990;90:A–130.
18. Breslow RA, Hallfrisch J, Guy DG, et al. The importance of dietary protein in healing pressure ulcers. J Am Geriatr Soc 1993;41:357–362.
19. Gersovitz M, Motil K, Munro HN, et al. Human protein requirements: Assessment of the adequacy of the current Recommended Dietary Allowance for dietary protein in elderly men and women. Am J Clin Nutr 1982;35:6–14.
20. Long CL, Nelson KM, Akin JM Jr, et al. A physiologic bases for the provision of fuel mixtures in normal and stressed patients. J Trauma 1990;30:1077–1086.
21. McCauley R, Platell C, Hall J, McCulloch R. Effects of glutamine on colonic strength anastomosis in the rat. J Parenter Enter Nutr 1991;116:821.
22. Langkamp-Henken B, Herrlinger-Garcia KA, Stechmiller JK, et al. Arginine supplementation is well tolerated but does not enhance mitogen-induced lymphocyte proliferation in elderly nursing home residents with pressure ulcers. J Parenter Enteral Nutr 2000;24:280–289.
23. McCauley C, Platell C, Hall J, McCullock R. Influence of branched chain amino acid solutions on wound healing. Aust NZ J Surg 1990;60:471.
24. Choban PS, Burge JC, Flanobaum L. Nutrition support of obese hospitalized patients. Nutr Clin Prac 1997;12:149–154.
25. Ireton-Jones CS. Evaluation of energy expenditures in obese patients. Nutr Clin Prac 1989;4:127–129.
26. Crandon JH, Lind CC, Dill DB. Experimental human scurvy. N Eng J Med 1940;223:353.
27. Levenson SM, Upjohn HL, Preston JA, et al. Effect of thermal burns on wound healing. Ann Surg 1957;146:357–368.
28. Rackett SC, Rothe MJ, Grant-Kels JM. Diet and dermatology. The role of dietary manipulation in the prevention and treatment of cutaneous disorders. J Am Acad Dermatol 1993;29:447–461.
29. Vilter RW. Nutritional aspects of ascorbic acid: Uses and abuses. West J Med 1980;133:485.
30. ter Riet G, Kessels AG, Knipschild PG. Randomized clinical trial of ascorbic acid in the treatment of pressure ulcers. J Clin Epidemiol 1995;48:1453–1460.
31. Taylor TV, Rimmer S, Day B, et al. Ascorbic acid supplementation in the treatment of pressure sores. Lancet 1974;2:544–546.

32. Hunt TK. Vitamin A and wound healing. J Am Acad Dermatol 1986;15:817–821.

33. Ehrlich HP, Hunt TK. Effects of cortisone and vitamin A on wound healing. Ann Surg 1968;167:324.

34. Waldorf H, Fewkes J. Wound healing. Advances Dermatol 1995;10:77–96.

35. Pories WJ, Henzel WH, Rob CG, et al. Acceleration of healing with zinc sulfate. Ann Surg 1967; 165:423.

36. Hallbrook T, Lanner E. Serum zinc and healing of leg ulcers. Lancet 1972;2:780.

37. Sandstead SH, Henrikson LK, Greger JL, et al. Zinc nutriture in the elderly in relation to taste acuity, immune response, and wound healing. Am J Clin Nutr 1982;36(suppl):1046.

38. Goode HF, Burns E, Walker BE. Vitamin C depletion and pressure ulcers in elderly patients with femoral neck fracture. Brit Med J 1992:305:925–927.

39. Norris JR, Reynolds RE. The effect of oral zinc sulfate therapy on decubitus ulcers. JAGS 1971;19:793.

40. Goode P, Allman R. The prevention and management of pressure ulcers. Med Clin N Amer 1989;73: 1511–1524.

41. Thomas DR. The role of nutrition in prevention and healing of pressure ulcers. Clin Geriatr Med 1997; 13:497–511.

42. Reed BR, Clark RAF. Cutaneous tissue repair: Practical implications of current knowledge: II. J Am Acad Dermatol 1985;13:919–941.

43. Gregger JL. Potential for trace mineral deficiencies and toxicities in the elderly. In: Mineral Homeostasis in the Elderly. Bales CW, (ed.), Marcel Dekker, New York, 1989, pp. 171–200.

44. Albina JE. Nutrition and wound healing. JPEN 1994;18:367–376.

45. Thomas DR. Issues and Dilemmas in Managing Pressure Ulcers. J Gerontol Medical Sciences 2001;56: M238–M340.

46. Bergstrom N. Lack of nutrition in AHCPR prevention guideline. Decubitus 1993;6:4–6.

47. Thomas DR. Improving the outcome of pressure ulcers with nutritional intervention: A review of the evidence. Nutrition 2001;17:121–125.

48. Bourdel-Marchasson I, Barateau M, Sourgen C, et al. Prospective audits of quality of PEM recognition and nutritional support in critically ill elderly patients. Clin Nutr 1999;18:233–240.

49. Bourdel-Marchasson I, Barateau M, Rondeau V, et al. A multi-center trial of the effects of oral nutritional supplementation in critically ill older inpatients. GAGE Group. Groupe Aquitain Geriatrique d'Evaluation. Nutrition 2000;16:1–5.

50. Hartgrink HH, Wille J, Konig P, et al. Pressure sores and tube feeding in patients with a fracture of the hip: a randomized clinical trial. Clin Nutr 1998;17:287–292.

51. Henderson CT, Trumbore LS, Mobarhan S, et al. Prolonged tube feeding in long-term care: Nutritional status and clinical outcomes. J Am Coll Clin Nutr 1992;11:309.

52. Mitchell SL, Kiely DK, Lipsitz LA. The risk factors and impact on survival of feeding tube placement in nursing home residents with severe cognitive impairment. Arch Inter Med 1997;157:327–332

53. Thompson MP, Merria LK. Unexplained weight loss in ambulatory elderly. J Am Geriatr Soc 1991;39: 497–500.

54. Morley JE, Thomas DR. Anorexia and Aging: Pathophysiology. Nutrition 1999;15:499–503.

55. Shike M, Russell DM, Detsky AS, et al. Changes in body composition in patients with small-cell cancer. The effect of total parenteral nutrition as an adjunct to chemotherapy. Ann Inter Med 1984;101:303–309.

56. Toth MJ, Gottlieb SS, Goran MI, et al. Daily energy expenditure in free-living heart failure patients. Am J Physiol 1997;272:469–475.

57. Mitch WE. Mechanisms causing loss of lean body mass in kidney disease. Am J Clin Nutr 1998;67: 359–366.

58. Kotler DP, Wang J, Pierson RN. Body composition studies in patients with the acquired immunodeficiency syndrome. Am J Clin Nutr 1985;42:1255–1265.

59. Roubenoff R, Roubenoff RA, Cannon JG, et al. Rheumatoid cachexia: Cytokine-driven hypermetalboism accompanying reduced body cell mass in chronic inflammation. J Clin Invest 1994;93: 2379–2386.

60. Ikeda U, Yamamoto K, Akazawa H, et al. Plasma cytokine levels in cardiac chambers of patients with mitral stenssis with congestive heart failure. Cardiology 1996;87:476–478.

61. Pan W, Zadina JE, Harlan RE, et al. Tumor necrosis factor-α: a neuromodulator in the CNS. Neurosci Biobehav Rev 1997;21:603–613.

62. Liso Z, Tu JH, Small CB, et al. Increased urine IL-1 levels in aging. Gerontology 1993;39:19–27.

63. Cederholm T, Whetline B, Hollstrom K, et al. Enhanced generation of Interleukin 1β and 6 may contribute to the cachexia of chronic disease. Am J Clin Nutr 1997;65:876–882.
64. Chasse WT, Balasubramahiam A, Dayal R, et al. Hypothalamic concentration and release of neuropeptide Y into micordialyses is reduced in anorectic tumor bearing rates. Life Sci 1994;54:1869–1874.
65. Leibowitz SF. Neurochemical-neuroendocrine systems in the brain controlling macronutirent intake and metabolism. Trends Neurosci 1992;12:491–497.
66. Noguchi Y, Yoshikawa T, Marsumoto A, et al. Are cytokines possible mediators of cancer cachexia? Jpn J Surg 1996;26:467–475.
67. Keiler U. Pathophysiology of cancer cachexia. Support Care Cancer 1993;1:290–294.
68. Straton RJ, Dewit O, Crowe R, et al. Plasma leptin, energy intake and hunger following total hip replacement surgery. Clin Sci 1997;93:113–117.
69. Cederholm T, Arter P, Palmviad J. Low circulation leptin level in protein-energy malnourished chronically ill elderly patients. J Intern Med 1997;242:377–382.
70. Rosenthal AJ, Sanders KM, McMurtry CT, et al. Is malnutrition overdiagnosed in older hospitalized patients? Association between the soluble interleukin-2 receptor and serum markers of malnutrition. J Gerontol Series A, Biological Sciences Medical Sciences 1998;53:M81–M86.
71. Souba WW. Drug therapy: Nutritional support. N Eng J Med 1997;336:41–48.
72. Atkinson S, Sieffert E, Bihari D. A prospective, randomized, double-blind, controlled clinical trial of enteral immunonutrition in the critically ill. Crit Care Med 1998;26:1164–1172.
73. Matsuyama N, Takano K, Mashiko T, et al. Japanese J Clin Pathology 1999;47:1039–1145.
74. Barone EJ, Yager DR, Pozez AL, et al. Interleukin-1α and collagenase activity are elevated in chronic wounds. Plastic Reconstructive Surg 1998;102:1023–1027.
75. Segal JL, Gonzales E, Yousefi S, et al. Circulating levels of IL-2R, ICAM-1, and IL-6 in spinal cord injuries. Arch Physical Med Rehab 1997;78:44-47.
76. Bonnefoy M, Coulon L, Bienvenu J, et al. Implication of Cytokines in the aggravation of malnutrition and hypercatabolism in elderly patients with severe pressure sores. Age Ageing 1995;24:37–42.
77. Bruerra E, Macmillan K, Hanson J, et al. A controlled trial of megestrol acetate on appetite, caloric intake, nutritional status, and other symptoms in patients with advance cancer. Cancer 1990;66:1279–1282.
78. Allman RM, Goode PS, Patrick MM. Pressure ulcer risk factors among hospitalised patients with severe limitation. J Am Med Assoc 1995;273:865–870.
79. Schmoll E, Wilke H, Thole R. Megestrol acetate in cancer cachexia. Seminars Oncol 1991;12(suppl):32–34.
80. Heckmayr M, Gatzenneier U. Trreatment of cancer weight loss in patients with advance lung cancer. Oncology 1992;49(suppl)2:32–34.
81. Feliu J, Gonzalez-Baron M, Berrocal A. Usefulness of megestrol acetate in cancer cachexia and anorexia. Am J Clin Oncol 1992;15:436–440.
82. Azona C, Castro L, Crespo E, et al. Megestrol acetate therapy for anorexia and weight loss in childrren with malignant solid tumours. Aliment Pharmacol Ther 1996;10:577–586.
83. Mantovani G, Maccio A, Bianchi A, et al. Megestrol Acetate in Neoplastic Anorexia/Cachexia: Clinical Evaluation and Comparison with Cytokine Levels in Patients with Head and Neck Carcinoma Treated with Neoadjuvant Chemotherapy. Springer-Verlag, 1995. Int J Clin Lab Res 1995;25(3):135–141.
84. Christou NV, Meakins JL, Gordon J, et al. The delayed hypersensitivity response and host resistance in surgical patients: 20 years later. Ann Surg 1995;222:534–548.
85. Allman RM, Walker JM, Hart MK, et al. Air-fluidized beds or conventional therapy for pressure sores: A randomized trial. Ann Inter Med 1987;107:641–648.
86. Gorse GJ, Messner RL. Improved pressure sore healing with hydrocolloid dressings. Arch Dermatol 1987;123:766–771.
87. Inman KJ, Sibbald WJ, Rutledge FS. Clinical utility and cost-effectiveness of an air suspension bed in the prevention of pressure ulcers. JAMA 1993;269:1139–1143.
88. Anthony D, Reynolds T, Russell L. An investigation into the use of serum albumin in pressure sore prediction. J Adv Nurs 2000;32:359–365.
89. Moolten SE. Bedsores in the chronically ill patient. Arch Phys Med Rehab 1972;53:430–438.
90. Bennett RG, Bellantoni MF, Ouslander JG. Air-fluidized bed treatment of nursing home patients with pressure sores. J Am Geriatr Soc 1989;37:235–242.

91. Brandeis GH, Morris JN, Nash DJ, et al. Epidemiology and natural history of pressure ulcers in elderly nursing home residents. J Am Med Assoc 1990;264:2905–2909.
92. Trumbore LS, Miles TP, Henderson CT, et al. Hypocholesterolemia and pressure sore risk with chronic tube feeding. Clin Res 1990;38:760A.
93. Breslow RA, Hallfrisch J, Goldberg AP. Malnutrition in tubefed nursing home patients with pressure sores. J Parental Enteral Nutr 1991;15:663–668.
94. Ferrell BA, Osterweil D, Christenson P. A randomized trial of low-air-loss beds for treatment of pressure ulcers. JAMA 1993;269:494–497.
95. Guralnik JM, Harris TB, White LR, et al. Occurrence and predictors of pressure sores in the National Health and Nutrition Examination survey follow-up. J Am Geriatr Soc 1988;36:807–812.

13   Dementia

Heidi K. White

1. INTRODUCTION

Dementia is a progressive decline in memory and other cognitive functions that results in functional impairment. Alzheimer's disease (AD) is the most common, best-characterized, and most extensively studied cause of dementia. Although weight loss and malnutrition is possible regardless of the cause of dementia, research relating to the nutritional status of patients with dementia has been conducted almost exclusively in patients diagnosed with AD. This chapter focuses primarily on nutrition as it relates to AD. However, many of the principals regarding the evaluation and treatment of weight loss and malnutrition are applicable in vascular dementia and other causes of dementia.

The 20th century was marked by rapid growth in the US elderly population. The continued expansion of the older population expected during the first half of the 21st century will profoundly effect the prevalence of AD and other dementias. Because the incidence rate of AD increases with age *(1)*, expected growth in the oldest segment of the population will profoundly impact the prevalence of AD. Age-specific incidence rates, summarized from four major epidemiologic studies *(2)*, estimated the prevalence of AD in the United States to be 2.32 million, with a range of 1.09 to 4.58 million as of 1997. The prevalence is predicted to nearly quadruple in the next 50 yr, by which time approx 1 in 45 Americans will be afflicted with the disease *(1)*. Furthermore, the economic impact of caring for patients with AD will be substantial, with much of this cost a result of the need for formal services like institutional care *(3)*. Understanding the impact of AD on the nutritional status of these patients and finding effective means of meeting their nutritional needs is of fundamental importance as we attempt to provide appropriate medical care for this growing segment of older adults.

2. WEIGHT LOSS IN AD

Numerous studies have confirmed the tendency for patients with AD to lose weight *(4–10)*. For example, using data collected by the Consortium to Establish a Registry for Alzheimer's Disease (CERAD), which included weight measurement at yearly intervals, in comparison to control subjects, a general tendency toward weight loss in community-dwelling AD subjects was observed *(4,11)*. The overall tendency toward weight loss was

From: *Handbook of Clinical Nutrition and Aging*
Edited by: C. W. Bales and C. S. Ritchie © Humana Press Inc., Totowa, NJ

modest (estimated weight change per year of –0.7 lbs for AD subjects vs –0.1 lbs for controls; $p = 0.02$). Specific variables to assess the process of weight change indicated increased variability in weight over time and an episodic nature to weight loss in the disease process (*see* Fig. 1). More importantly, the proportion of AD subjects who lost 5% or more of their weight during study participation was significantly greater than that of controls (approx 35% compared to 18%). AD subjects were 2.30 times (odds ratio, 95% confidence interval [CI] 1.61–3.29) more likely to experience ≥5% weight loss when compared to controls. Surprisingly, a certain percentage of AD subjects were actually gaining weight, which points to the potential reversibility of this tendency toward weight loss (*see* Fig. 2).

Weight loss and subsequent malnutrition *(12)* in AD can lead to serious consequences. In the CERAD longitudinal data, weight loss was a predictor of mortality among subjects with AD; however, weight gain was associated with a reduced risk of mortality *(13)*. Furthermore, the risk of weight loss tended to increase with severity of disease. Unfortunately, this correlation does not address the question of whether malnutrition is simply the result of disease progression or whether malnutrition may contribute to the progression of AD. In general, malnutrition leads to reduced immune function, greater susceptibility to infection, impaired wound healing, and predisposition to pressure ulcers.

Weight loss and malnutrition are not simply a manifestation of severe or terminal AD. A study by Barrett-Connor and colleagues indicates that weight loss is an early manifestation of disease often occurring prior to diagnosis *(14)*. They followed community-dwelling subjects for 20 yr prior to diagnosis of AD and found weight loss significantly more common among those diagnosed with AD in a timeframe that was likely prior to the onset of symptoms. Further research is needed to understand the relationship between malnutrition and AD. Identifying risk factors may help to avoid weight loss and malnutrition. More aggressive nutritional interventions may improve the functional status and quality of life of persons with AD.

3. EATING BEHAVIORS

Abnormal eating behaviors appear to contribute to weight loss, especially as AD progresses. Aversive eating behaviors have been studied primarily in institutionalized patients, particularly as they relate to the need to be fed *(15–18)*. Typical behaviors include needing frequent verbal cues to complete the eating process, verbally refusing food, pocketing food in the cheeks without swallowing, clenching teeth, and spitting food. Little has been done to investigate the eating behaviors of noninstitutionalized subjects with AD *(19)*, even though weight loss is not restricted to the late stages of this disease. Earlier in the disease process, changes in eating behavior may be more subtle, such as a tendency to skip meals or experience fluctuations in appetite, delusions about food (e.g., believing food is poisoned), increased distractibility at meal time, and changes in food preferences. The few small studies that have reviewed swallowing in AD subjects suggest that aspiration is primarily a manifestation of late-stage AD *(20,21)*. However, an increased duration of the oral and pharyngeal components of swallowing have been observed in early-stage AD *(22)*. If inadequate caloric intake is the primary disturbance in AD, then measurement of caloric intake should confirm this hypothesis. However, studies regarding the adequacy of caloric intake in AD patients have arrived at differing conclusions *(23–30)* (*see* Table 1). This may be because of the imprecise methodology

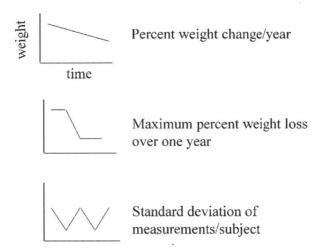

Fig. 1. Visual illustration of the dependent variables developed to model aspects of weight change in AD. Reprinted from the *Journal of the American Geriatric Society.*

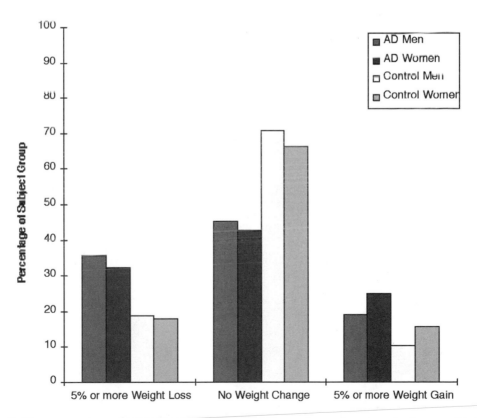

Fig. 2. The percentage of subjects by gender and AD case/control status who lost ≥ of initial weight, gained ≥5%, or stayed the same during the study period. Reprinted from the *Journal of the American Geriatric Society.*

Table 1
Estimated Caloric Intake in Patients with AD

Reference	Study population	Methods	Results	Conclusion
Spindler et al. (23)	17 Institutionalized AD patients 23 Nondemented community-dwelling controls	2-d Weighed dietary intake at 3 time points over 1 yr for AD and food diaries for controls	34 kcal/kg for AD 24 kcal/kg for controls Weight was maintained over the study period	Caloric intake for AD patients was sufficient to maintain current weight
Renvall et al. (24)	22 Community-dwelling AD 41 Nondemented community-dwelling controls	3-d Self-reported intake	29 kcal/kg for AD 26 kcal/kg for controls No difference in caloric or nutrient intake Biochemical values of nutrients revealed lower levels of B12 and folate for AD	Caloric and nutrient intake of community dwelling AD subjects is comparable to controls
Burns et al. (25)	28 Community-dwelling dementia patients 21 Institutionalized dementia patients 29 Community-dwelling controls	3-d Weighed dietary intake	38 kcal/kg com. dementia 32 kcal/kg inst. dementia 24 kcal/kg controls Institutionalized AD patients lost weight over a 6-mo study period Inst. dementia subjects had significantly lower BMI than com. dementia or controls	Despite higher caloric intake in institutionalized subjects compared to controls, their intake was less than community dementia subjects and their overall nutritional state was worse

Reference	Subjects	Method	Results	Conclusion
Niskanen et al. (26)	10 Institutionalized AD 10 Multi-infarct dementia (MID) 10 Nondemented community-dwelling controls	3-d Food intake recorded Indirect calorimetry	32 kcal/kg AD 27 kcal/kg MID 29 kcal/kg controls BMI similar in all groups AD had lower resting energy expenditure	Higher energy intake for AD compared to MID and controls, but no evidence for elevated resting energy expenditure
Franzoni et al. (27)	33 Institutionalized dementia patients 25 Institutionalized nondemented controls	3-d Weighed dietary intake	28 kcal/kg dementia 28 kcal/kg controls Equal survival over 28-mo of follow-up	Nutrient intake and nutritional status was similar in demented and nondemented, some evidence of general weight loss prior to measurement
Sandman et al. (6)	18 Institutionalized dementia No controls	5-d Weighed dietary intake on 2 occasions, 5 wk apart	38 kcal/kg dementia Low weight and mid-arm circumference indicated nutritional deficits for 50% of subjects and evidence of general weight loss prior to measurement	No difference in dietary intake between those with and without malnutrition
Litchford et al. (28)	15 Institutionalized AD 13 Inst. nondemented controls	Weighed dietary intake No reference to weight stability	1502 kcal/d AD 2034 kcal/d controls Lower nutrient intake for total calories, fat, carbohydrates, vitamin A, calcium, thiamine, riboflavin, and niacin in AD	Lower total calorie and specific nutrient intake in AD
Winograd et al. (30)	35 Community-dwelling AD 29 Nondemented community-dwelling controls	3-d Food diary	1899 kcal/d AD ♀ 1848 kcal/d controls ♀ 2012 kcal/d AD ♂ 2206 kcal/d control ♂ No evidence of caloric or nutrient deficits	Adequate caloric and nutrient intake for community-dwelling AD subjects

of caloric measurement and the inability to establish whether such measurements represent habitual energy intake *(31)*. Further description of changes in eating behavior, swallowing difficulties, and caloric intake in AD patients early in the disease process is necessary for understanding the clinical factors related to weight loss.

4. PATHOPHYSIOLOGY OF WEIGHT LOSS IN AD

Destruction of the hypocampus and surrounding cortical areas may explain certain behaviors that have the potential to influence both energy intake and expenditure, such as inability to prepare food, distraction from meals, agitation, and pacing. Additionally, plaques and tangles have been described in the hypothalamus in AD *(32–34)*. However, these explanations seem inadequate to explain weight loss early in the disease process when behavioral problems are less prominent and hypothalamic involvement is minimal. Anorexia or alterations in appetite perception would best explain early weight loss in AD. There are two primary physiologic mechanisms that might explain anorexia and, therefore, decreased caloric intake in AD: taste and smell dysfunction and the effect of inflammatory mediators (e.g., cytokines) on appetite.

4.1. Taste and Smell Dysfunction

Deficits in taste and smell function are likely to decrease appetite perception and food enjoyment. Taste and smell dysfunction occurs with normal aging and can be exacerbated by medications and disease (*see* Chapter 9) *(35–37)*. Although some changes in taste perception have been reported *(38)*, gustatory dysfunction has not been studied as thoroughly as olfactory dysfunction in AD. Multiple studies in subjects with mild-to-moderate AD have demonstrated deficits in odor identification *(39,40)*. Recent studies indicate that olfactory identification deficits are clearly present even prior to diagnosis of AD, particularly in individuals carrying the ApoE 4 allele *(41,42)*. Deficits in odor sensitivity have been reported by some investigators, but not others. It appears that odor threshold may become progressively more abnormal as the disease progresses *(43)*. Furthermore, Nordin et al. have found that both AD subjects and nondemented older adults are unaware of their decreased smell sensitivity *(44)*. In support of this interpretation, pathologic evaluations of autopsy specimens indicate that olfactory pathways are among the first areas of the brain to exhibit the typical pathology of amyloid plaques and neurofibrillary tangles *(45)*. Olfactory dysfunction may not be specific to AD; similar olfactory deficits have been noted in Parkinson's disease and vascular dementia *(46)*. Nevertheless, it seems likely that olfactory deficits and gustatory dysfunction impact the perception of flavor and potentially contribute to weight loss in AD.

4.2. Inflammatory Mediators

Cytokines like IL-6 are an integral part of anorexia-cachexia syndromes in other disease states, such as cancer and heart failure *(47,48)*. Additionally, IL-6 has been shown to correlate with functional disability and depression in older adults *(49,50)*. Cytokines, including IL-1, IL-6, and TNF-α, play an important role in the inflammatory process accompanying the hallmark changes of amyloid plaques and neurofibrillary tangles that occur with AD *(51–57)*. Some studies have shown elevation of serum levels of these cytokines *(58–64)* and even elevated levels in spontaneous or stimulated production from leukocytes *(65,66)*.Other studies have not demonstrated elevations in circulating cytokines *(67–70)*. Most studies have been small with little attention to potentially important variables other than disease severity. Factors including age of onset, behavioral symptoms, and systemic symptoms (e.g., weight loss) may produce variations in the overall inflammatory reaction experienced by AD subjects. Cytokines produced by the local inflammatory reaction in the brain may be sufficient to produce changes in neurotransmitters, neuropeptides, and hypothalamic neurons and thus cause anorexia. This leaves the relevance of peripheral cytokine levels in AD in question. However, weight loss may result from an overwhelming central inflammatory reaction that is mirrored by peripheral cytokine levels. As suggested in a recent study by Licastro et al., circulating cytokines may derive from cerebral inflammation rather than a peripheral inflammatory reaction *(58)*.

5. ENERGY EXPENDITURE

Weight loss results from a mismatch between energy intake and energy expenditure, yet the specific causes of this mismatch in AD remain unclear. Resting metabolic rate makes up the largest part of total energy expenditure. It has been suggested that resting metabolic rate may be elevated in AD. However, the results of several studies agree: there is no evidence that resting metabolic rate is elevated in AD subjects when compared to older adults without dementia *(71–74)*. The idea that physical activity in the form of behavioral disturbances (e.g., pacing) may contribute to increased energy expenditure has also not been supported by research evidence. The physical activity component of daily energy expenditure has been shown to be normal in AD subjects *(75)*. Unfortunately, there is no data on AD patients during the dynamic phase of weight loss. It is evident from our work and that of others that not all AD patients are losing weight all of the time *(4,76)*. There can be periods of acute weight loss, a slow gradual weight loss, and variations in weight, which may include substantial weight gain.

It is possible that only a subset of AD patients experience behavioral disturbances that would increase energy expenditure leading to weight loss. Furthermore, the possibility that this mismatch in energy intake vs expenditure may be episodic should be considered more fully in future research design. Preliminary data from institutionalized subjects with AD show that body mass index (BMI) is inversely correlated with a measure of behavioral symptoms, the Neuropsychological Inventory (Spearman Correlation Coefficient -0.52, $p < 0.01$), which indicates that as BMI decreased the frequency and severity of behavioral problems increased *(77)*. Individual behavior scores for agitation/aggression, irritability/lability, aberrant motor behavior (i.e., pacing; -0.42, $p < 0.05$), and eating disorders (-0.37, $p = 0.05$) were inversely correlated with baseline BMI. Behaviors that were not significantly correlated with BMI were delusions, hallucinations, elation, apathy, disinhibition, depression, and sleep. Although this was a small sample followed for a relatively short period of time (6 mo), change in behavior scores from baseline to month 6 were correlated with the change in weight over the 6-mo period. Both agitation/aggression and disinhibition showed significant inverse correlation with weight change, indicating that as these behaviors increased over time, weight tended to decrease. Social factors may also be of importance in explaining weight loss. A study by Gillette-Guyonnet et al. *(76)* focusing on clinical risk factors for weight loss in AD found only caregiver burden baseline measurements to be correlated with subsequent weight loss.

It seems possible that relatively subtle and perhaps intermittent changes in factors that influence both energy intake and energy expenditure may tip the balance toward weight loss for patients with AD. This imbalance may be multifactorial and intermittent. Rather than one particular cause or abnormality leading to weight loss, AD may lead to a condition in which changes in energy intake and expenditure are not easily compensated.

6. ROLE OF NUTRIENTS IN THE PATHOPHYSIOLOGY AND TREATMENT OF AD

In addition to AD pathology and various external factors contributing to weight loss and nutritional decline, the lack of certain nutrients may contribute to the development and progression of AD. Nutrient replacement may represent a means of prevention or treatment of AD.

Many studies suggest that oxidative stress and the accumulation of free radicals is involved in the pathology of AD leading to excessive lipid peroxidation and neuronal degeneration (78,79). Furthermore, the intake of flavinoids—antioxidant substances found in wine, tea, fruit, and vegetables—has been inversely related to the risk of developing dementia (80). Vitamin E is a lipid soluble vitamin that interacts with cell membranes, traps free radicals, and interrupts the oxidative reactions that damage cells (81). Vitamin E has been studied as a treatment for AD in one large 2-yr trial. Vitamin E significantly delayed clinical worsening, and fewer patients treated with vitamin E were institutionalized (82).

Vitamin B_{12} deficiency is known to not only cause anemia and peripheral neuropathy, but also psychiatric symptoms including memory loss (83). Resolution of cognitive symptoms have been reported with B_{12} treatment, especially when the memory symptoms are of recent onset (84,85). Low vitamin B_{12} levels and vitamin B_{12} deficiency have been reported in AD patients in comparison to control subjects and patients with other types of dementia. However, additional studies have not supported these results (86,87). In a population-based study, Basun et al. found no significant difference between vitamin B_{12} level/deficiency in AD vs nondemented subjects, but did find a tendency toward lower vitamin B_{12} levels in AD patients who were still living at home in comparison to those living in institutions (88). Furthermore, treatment of vitamin B_{12} deficiency in AD patients may reverse other symptoms of vitamin B_{12} deficiency, but the impact on cognitive symptoms has been disappointing (89,90).

Studies of the role of vitamin B_{12} in the development of AD have been mixed as well. In a longitudinal cohort of 410 volunteers with 5 yr of follow-up, a low serum B_{12} level—defined as <150 pg/mL—was not a significant risk factor for the development of AD (91). In another longitudinal cohort of 370 nondemented persons followed for 3 yr, a low level of B_{12} or folate resulted in a significantly higher risk of developing AD (92). This association was even stronger in participants with good baseline cognition. There is no convincing evidence that vitamin B_{12} deficiency can cause AD. However, some researchers have postulated that increased homocysteine concentrations associated with vitamin B_{12} and folate deficiency may contribute to neurologic degeneration. It appears that the recognition and treatment of vitamin B_{12} and folate deficiency may be most beneficial early in AD or prior to the diagnosis when cognitive symptoms are mild.

Apart from B_{12} and folate deficiency, plasma homocysteine levels may play an important role in the development of AD. Recently, Seshadri and colleagues provided strong epidemiolgic evidence that elevated homocysteine levels are associated with a significant increased risk of developing AD *(93)*. This risk increased with plasma homocysteine levels and was independent of vitamin B_{12} and folate levels. Homocysteine has also gained attention from its association with atherosclerotic disease. Epidemiologic evidence indicates an association between plasma homocysteine levels and the risk of vascular disease in the coronary, carotid, and peripheral circulation. The mechanisms by which homocysteine promotes AD or atherosclerosis are less clear. Possible mechanisms of promoting dementia may be through the development of cerebral microangiopathy, endothelial dysfunction, oxidative stress, as well as enhancement of β-amyloid peptide-dependent neurotoxicity and neural apoptosis *(94)*. The implication of this association between homocysteine levels and dementia (i.e., AD and vascular dementia) is that large doses of folate or vitamin B_{12} might substantially reduce homocysteine levels and prevent or delay the development of dementia. Clinical trials are needed to evaluate the effect of vitamin supplementation on the development and treatment of AD.

7. EVALUATING WEIGHT LOSS IN DEMENTIA

A physician should evaluate the patient with dementia who is losing weight (*see* Chapters 5 and 14), and medications should be reviewed. Drugs can cause many symptoms that potentially limit caloric intake like inattention (e.g., sedatives), movement disorders (e.g., antipsychotics), xerostomia (e.g., anticholinergics), esophagitis (e.g., alendronate), or anorexia (e.g., nonsteroidal anti-inflammatory drugs). Acetylcholinesterase inhibitors, which are the primary treatment for the cognitive symptoms of AD, have several potential adverse effects, including nausea, vomiting, and anorexia that may contribute to weight loss *(95–97)*. Additionally, galatamine has been associated with an increased incidence of weight loss *(98)*. Patients with dementia may not be able to voice symptoms attributable to these adverse effects.

A thorough medical history and physical examination should be done. The patient should be specifically evaluated for depression and aggressively treated when it is suspected to be present. Dental abnormalities like ill-fitting dentures, tooth decay, and abscess formation may contribute to weight loss as well. The possibility of a chronic pain syndrome or other chronic illness should be considered.

If the specific diagnosis of dementia has not been established, the possibility of nutritional deficiencies contributing to dementia should be considered. For example, patients with a history of gastrointestinal surgery or gastrointestinal disease should be evaluated for vitamin B_{12} deficiency, which can cause anemia, neuropathy, and cognitive impairment. Another less common cause of cognitive impairment is niacin deficiency (i.e., Pellagra).

There are many factors that may contribute to weight loss and nutritional deficits in AD, and they vary according to the stage of illness. The relationship of the most prominent factors to AD severity is illustrated in Fig. 3. Some of these factors can be related to the pathophysiology of AD, whereas others are related to external influences.

Weight, like blood pressure, is routinely monitored in the typical health care visit, thus, clinicians are often confronted with this issue. Presently, the extent of evaluation and appropriateness of intervention for clinically significant weight loss in the patient with AD remains unclear. Whether or not interventions for weight loss improve physical functioning or delay institutionalization has not been established. If nutritional interven-

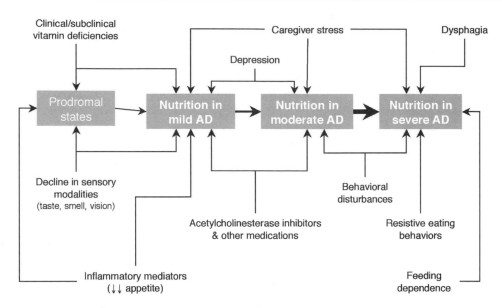

Fig. 3. Factors that influence nutrition in AD. Multiple factors can contribute to the occurrence of nutritional decline throughout the progression of AD. Weight loss is a common indicator of nutritional status in AD. The risk of weight loss increases with disease progression and severity (indicated by arrow size). Factors that are important early in the progression of disease may persist, but become less important as other factors exert greater influence. Factors intrinsic to AD pathology are bolded.

tions are proven beneficial, primary care physicians would be poised to recognize this problem and likely intervene more aggressively rather than remain fatalistic, as is often the case now.

The impact of nutritional deficits on symptoms in AD has not been vigorously explored. However, several studies indicate that even subtle deficits in nutritional status can impact cognitive performance in nondemented older adults (99–102). For example, Goodwin et al. (103) showed that healthy elderly subjects who had subclinically low blood concentrations or intakes of folate, vitamin B_{12}, vitamin C, and riboflavin scored more poorly on tests of memory and abstract thinking. Even if nutritional supplementation does not improve cognitive symptoms, nutritional interventions (e.g., multivitamin with minerals, calcium supplements, liquid calories and nutrient supplements, eliminating medications that inhibit intake) may help to maintain muscle and bone mass necessary for continued independent physical function and, in more disabled patients, prevent challenging complications like pressure ulcers.

8. INTERVENTIONS FOR WEIGHT LOSS IN AD

To date, only one intervention study, a combination of nutrition education and health promotion, has been undertaken to prevent weight loss and malnutrition in non-institutionalized subjects with AD (104). The intervention did result in a mean weight gain for the participants who received the intervention (0.7 ± 5.4 kg) over 12 mo whereas the comparison group experienced a mean weight loss (–0.7 ± 5.4 kg). However, when othr variables were considered in the analysis there was not a statistically significant difference between the two groups. Regardless of cognitive status, numerous large studies of older adults have indicated that weight loss and low body weight are markers for increased morbidity, mortality, and functional decline in older adults *(105–108)*. Nevertheless, the hypothesis that nutritional intervention can delay functional decline and morbidity is largely untested. However, observational data in institutionalized subjects with dementia show that weight gain in even small amounts can improve morbidity and mortality *(109)*, lending validity to the hypothesis that intervening to reverse weight loss and malnutrition in AD will improve the quality of life for AD patients.

Getting patients with dementia to eat is a process of trial and error. It is important to make sure that food is available. The inability to purchase and prepare food can go unrecognized early in the course of disease. Patients may forget to eat or skip meals. Take advantage of aromatous foods that stimulate the physiologic responses that prepare the individual for food intake and stimulate appetite. Serve foods that are flavorful and appealing. In most cases, dietary restrictions like low sodium and low cholesterol should be removed.

As the discase progresses, many patients need supervision, constant reminders, and simple directions to complete a meal. Providing finger foods can be helpful for patients who are challenged by the use of utensils *(110)*. Increasing the number of meals or providing between-meal snacks may be helpful. Appetite and alertness may be better early in the day so have breakfast and lunch become more substantial meals. Providing preferred foods can also increase intake *(111)*. Oral liquid supplements can be given between meals to boost calorie consumption. Simplifying the environment so that there are fewer distractions during mealtime may be helpful as well. Involving a nutritionist in the care of the patient will facilitate individualized interventions. Caregivers should realize that feeding a patient who can no longer feed himself or herself can be very time consuming. Patients entirely dependent in feeding should be encouraged to drink fluids because they will not be able to regulate fluid intake according to thirst on their own. If they refuse or have difficulty with liquids, then foods with a high-water content should be provided, such as ice cream, gelatin, and applesauce. In the institutional setting and even at home, some patients may respond better to a particular caregiver, special techniques that are particularly effective in feeding a patient should be shared and mimicked by other caregivers.

A routine vitamin/mineral supplement should be considered for all patients with moderate-to-advanced AD. Like all older adults, most patients with AD will require calcium and vitamin D supplementation. Weight should be monitored regularly so that weight loss can be recognized early. Family members and caregivers should be encouraged to report changes in eating behavior and signs of dysphagia, such as pocketing food in the cheeks and coughing during meals.

9. FEEDING TUBES IN PATIENTS WITH ADVANCED AD

Patients with advanced dementia often develop serious difficulties eating when they are no longer ambulatory and become dependent in all of their activities of daily living. They may resist food being placed in the mouth, fail to manage the food bolus once it is in the mouth (oral phase dysphagia), or aspirate when swallowing (pharyngeal phase dysphagia). The time and effort necessary to feed patients in this condition can be overwhelming. Feeding tubes are often considered as a possible intervention by families, physicians, or nurses.

There have not been randomized clinical trials that compare tube feeding with oral feeding in the severely demented. A review of existing literature by Finucane and colleagues found no evidence to support that tube feeding prevents aspiration pneumonia *(112)*. In fact, tube feeding does nothing to prevent the aspiration of oral secretions, nor can it prevent aspiration from regurgitated gastric contents. Jejunostomy, which places the feeding tube past the gastric outlet, is not associated with lower rates of pneumonia when compared to gastrostomy *(113,114)*. Furthermore, Finucane and colleagues did not find evidence to support prevention of other infections, the consequences of malnutrition, or pressure ulcers. They found no evidence to support a survival benefit, improved functional status, or greater patient comfort. Adverse events associated with feeding tubes include aspiration pneumonia, tube occlusion, leakage, and local infection. The mortality rate during percutaneous endoscopic gastrostomy tube placement is low (0–2%), but perioperative mortality ranges from 6–24%.

Coughing and gagging during eating are common signs of aspiration (*see* Chapter 24). A swallowing evaluation by a speech therapist that includes visualization of the swallow either in a barium study or by fiberoptic techniques can be helpful in determining the severity of the dysfunction. Altering food and liquid consistency can minimize the risk of aspiration. Semi-solid consistencies are generally tolerated better than liquids. Additional potentially helpful techniques to minimize the risk of aspiration are upright positioning of the patient during meals and for 30 min after meals, tucking the chin during swallowing, swallowing multiple times with each bolus, and keeping the bolus less than 1 teaspoon.

Careful attention to oral feeding may be quite effective in maintaining nutrition even in the most debilitated patients. However, in circumstances where careful hand feeding has not provided adequate nutrition, resulting in pneumonia or other complications of malnutrition, the possibility of providing food and liquid as tolerated, but allowing a natural death to occur should be considered. For the patient with severe dementia, the decision of whether or not to institute a feeding tube ultimately lies with the patient's family or guardian. However, families and physicians are often aided by advance directives that allow patients with dementia to convey their wishes relating to this issue either before or during the early stages of disease. It is important for health care providers to initiate these conversations with the patient regarding care at the end of life when cognitive abilities will still allow a meaningful discussion. The decision of whether or not to institute a feeding tube should be made with the knowledge that current research does not support the belief that a feeding tube will help the patient's condition.

10. RECOMMENDATIONS FOR CLINICIANS

Evaluation for patients who are losing weight:

1. A nutrition assessment should be conducted and evaluations for depression, dental status, and medication effects should also be considered. Medication review should target drugs that may cause inattention (e.g., sedatives), movement disorders (e.g., antipsychotics), xerostomia (e.g., anticholinergics), esophagitis (e.g., alendronate), or anorexia (e.g., nonsteroidal anti-inflammatory drugs, acetylcholinesterase inhibitors, NSAIDs, theophylline, digoxin).

2. Consider the possibility that nutritional deficiencies could contribute to the dementia. Patients with a history of gastrointestinal surgery/disease should be evaluated for vitamin B_{12} deficiency, which can cause cognitive impairment as well as anemia and neuropathy. Although less common, niacin deficiency (Pellagra) can also cause cognitive impairment.

Treatment for progressive weight loss:

1. Steps to halt or reverse the weight loss should be taken, including ensuring adequate access to food, as well as strategies for increasing food intake. These could include reminders about eating, verbal cues during meals, assistance with eating, removal of dietary restrictions (in most cases), provision of finger foods, flavorful preferred foods, and oral liquid supplements between meals or as a dessert. When dysphagia is suspected, a swallow evaluation by a speech language therapist should be conducted and food consistency/positioning altered as indicated.
2. Micronutrient (vitamin/mineral) deficiencies should also be corrected. Regardless of improvement in cognitive function, this will help maintain muscle and bone mass and avoid other complications such as pressure ulcers. A routine vitamin/mineral supplement should be considered for all patients with moderate to advanced dementia.
3. The use of tube feedings in dementia patients may be considered if hand feeding becomes extremely difficult or impossible. Although this will provide nutrition to the patient, it does not necessarily improve long-term outcomes or prevent the likelihood of aspiration. In addition to aspiration, associated adverse events may include tube occlusion, leakage, and local infection. The decision of whether or not to employ tube feeding should take into account previously expressed wishes of the person with dementia concerning this type of intervention and the knowledge that current research does not indicate that a feeding tube will help the patient's condition.

REFERENCES

1. Hebert LE, Scherr PA, Beckett LA, Albert MS, et al. Age-specific incidence of Alzheimer's disease in a community population. JAMA 1995;273:1354–1359.
2. Brookmeyer R, Gray S, Kawas C. Projections of Alzheimer's disease in the United States and the public health impact of delaying disease onset. Am J Public Health 1998;88:1337–1342.
3. Leon J, Cheng C, Neumann PJ. Alzheimer's disease care: costs and potential savings. Health Aff 1998;17:206–216.
4. White H, Pieper C, Schmader K, Fillenbaum G. Weight change in Alzheimer's disease. J Am Geriatr Soc 1996;44:265–272.
5. Cronnin-Stubbs D, Beckett L, Scherr P, Field T, et al. Weight loss in people with Alzheimer's disease: a prospective population based analysis. BMJ 1997;314:178–179.
6. Sandman O, Adolsson R, Nygren C, et al. Nutritional status and dietary in take in institutionalized patients with Alzheimer's disease and multiinfarct dementia. J Am Geriatr Soc 1987;35:31–38.
7. Singh S, Mullcy GP, Losowsky MS. Why are Alzheimer's disease patients thin? Age Aging 1988;17: 21–28.
8. Du W, DiLuca C, Growdon JH. Weight loss in Alzheimer's disease. J Geriatr Psychiatry Neurol 1993;6:34–38.
9. Wolf-Klein GP, Silerstone FA, Levy AP. Nutritional patterns and weight change in Alzheimer patients. Int Psychogeritr 1992;4:103–111.
10. Burns A, Marsh A, Bender DA. Dietary intake and clinical, anthropometric and biochemical indices of malnutrition in elderly demented patients and nondemented subjects. Psychol Med 1989;19: 383–391.
11. White H, Pieper C, Schmader K, Fillenbaum G. A longitudinal analysis of weight change in Alzheimer's disease. J Am Geriatr Soc 1997;45:531–532.
12. Renvall MJ, Spindler AA, Nichols JF, Ramsdell JW. Body composition of patients with Alzheimer's disease. J Am Diet Assoc 1993;93:47–52.

13. White H, Pieper C, Schmader K. The association of weight change in Alzheimer's disease with severity of disease and mortality: A longitudinal analysis. J Am Geriatr Soc 1998;46:1223–1227.
14. Barrett-Connor E, Edelstein S, Corey-Bloom J, Wiederholt W. Weight loss precedes dementia in community-dwelling older adults. J Am Geriatr Soc 1996;44:1147–1152.
15. Volicer L, Seltzer B, Rheume Y, et al. Eating difficulties in patients with probable dementia of the Alzheimer type. J Geriatr Psych Neurol 1989;2:188–195.
16. Blandford G, Watkins LB, Mulvihill M, Taylor B. Correlations of aversive feeding behaviors in dementia patients. J Am Geriatr Soc 1995;43:SA10:4.
17. Athlin E, Norberg A, Asplund K, Jansson L. Feeding problems in severely demented patients seen from task and relational aspects. Scand J Caring Sci 1989;3:113–121.
18. Norberg A, Athlin E. Eating problems in severely demented patients: Issues and dilemmas. Nurse Clin N Am 1989;24:781–788.
19. Morris CH, Hope RA, Fairburn CG. Eating habits in dementia. Br J Psych 1989;154:801–806.
20. Horner J, Alberts MJ, Dawson DV, Cook GM. Swallowing in Alzheimer's disease. Alzheimer's Dis Assoc Disorders 1994;8:177–189.
21. Chouinard J, Lavigne E, Villeneuve C. Weight loss, dysphagia, and outcome in advanced dementia. Dysphagia 1998;13:151–155.
22. Priefer BA, Robbins J. Eating changes in mild-stage Alzheimer's disease: a pilot study. Dysphagia 1997;12:212–221.
23. Spindler AA, Renvall MJ, Nichols JF, Ramsdell JW. Nutritional status of patients with Alzheimer's disease:a 1-year study. J Am Diet Assoc 1996;96:1013–1018.
24. Renvall MJ, Spindler AA, Ramsdell JW, Paskvan M. Nutritional status of free-living Alzheimer's patients. Am J Med Sci 1989;298:20–26.
25. Burns A, Marsh A, Bender DA. Dietary intake and clinical, anthropometric and biochemical indices of malnutrition in elderly demented patients and nondemented subjects. Psychol Med 1989;19:383–391.
26. Niskanen L, Piirainen M, Koljonen M, Uusitupa M. Resting energy expenditure in relation to energy intake in patients with Alzheimer's disease, multi-infarct dementia and in control women. Age Ageing 1993;22:132–137.
27. Franzoni S, Frisoni GB, Boffelli S, Rozzini R, Trabucchi M. Good nutritional oral intake is associated with equal survival in demented and nondemented very old patients. J Am Geriatr Soc 1996;44:1366–1370.
28. Litchford MD, Wakefield LM. Nutrient intakes and energy expenditures of residents with senile dementia of the Alzheimer's type. J Am Diet Assoc 1987;87:211.
29. Stahelin HB, Hofer HO, Vogel M, Held C, Seiler WO. Energy and protein consumption in patients with senile dementia. Gerontology 1983;29:145–148.
30. Winograd CH. Jacobson DH, Butterfield GE, Cragen E et al. Nutritional intake in patients with senile dementia of the Alzheimer's type. Alz Dis Assoc Disorders 1991;5:173–180.
31. Schoeller DA. How accurate is self reported energy intake? Nutr Rev 1990;48:373–379.
32. Goudsmit E, Hofman MA, Fliers E, Swaab DF. The supraoptic and paraventricular nuclei of the human hypothalamus in relation to sex, age, and Alzheimer's disease. Neurobiol Aging 1990;11:529–536.
33. van de Nes JAP, Kamphorst W, Ravid R, Swaab DF. The distribution of Alz-50 immunoreactivity in the hypothalamus and adjoining areas of Alzheimer's disease patients. Brain 1993;116:103–115.
34. Swaab DF, Grundke-Iqbal I, Iqbal K, et al. τ and ubiquitin in the human hypothalamus in aging and Alzheimer's disease. Brain Res 1992;590:239–249.
35. Schiffman SS, Pasternak M. Decreased discrimination of food odors in the elderly. J Gerontol 1979;34:73–79.
36. Doty RL, Reyes PF, Gregor T. Presence of both odor identification and detection deficits in Alzheimer's disease. Brain Res Bull 1987;18:597–600.
37. Schiffman S, Taste and smell losses in normal aging and disease. JAMA 1997;278:1357–1362.
38. Schiffman S, Clark C, Warwick Z. Gustatory and olfactory dysfunction in dementia: not specific to Alzheimer's disease. Neurobiol Aging 1990;11:597–600.
39. Serby M, Larson P, Kalkstein D. The nature and course of olfactory deficits in Alzheimer's disease. Am J Psychiat 1991;148:357–360.
40. Koss E, Weiffenbach J, Haxby J, Friedland R. Olfactory detection and identification performance are dissociated in early Alzheimer's diease. Neurology 1988;38:1228–1232.

41. Bacon A, Bondi M, Salmon D, Murphy C. Very early changes in olfactory function due to Alzheimer's disease and the role of apolipoprotein E in olfaction. Ann NY Acad Sci 1998;855:723–731.

42. Murphy C, Bacon A, Bondi M, Salmon D. Apolipoprotein E status is associated with odor identification deficits in nondemented older persons. Ann NY Acad Sci 1998;855:744–750.

43. Murphy C, Gilmore MM, Seery CS, Salmon DP, Lasker BR. Olfactory thresholds are associated with degree of dementia in Alzheimer's disease. Neurobiol Aging 1990;11:465–469.

44. Nordin S, Monsch AU, Murphy C. Unawareness of smell loss in normal aging and Alzheimer's disease: discrepancy between self-reported and diagnosed smell sensitivity. J Gerontol 1995;50B:P187–P192.

45. Price JL, Davis PB, Morris JC, White DL. The distribution of tangles, plaques and related immunohistochemical markers in healthy aging and Alzheimer's disease. Neurobiol Aging 1991;12:295–312.

46. Mesholam R, Moberg P, Mahr R, Doty R. Olfaction in neurodegenerative disease: a meta-analysis of olfactory function in Alzheimer's disease and Parkinson's disease. Arch Neurol 1998;55:84–90.

47. Inuii A. Cancer anorexia-cachexia syndrome: Are neuropeptides the key? Cancer Res 1999;59: 4493–4510.

48. Berry C. Clark AL. Catabolism in chronic heart failure. Eur Heart J 2000;21:521–532.

49. Cohen HJ, Pieper CF, Harris T, Rao MK, Currie MS. The association of plasma IL-6 levels with functional disability in community-dwelling elderly. J Gerontol: Med Sci 1997;52A:M201–M208.

50. Dentino AN, Pieper CF, Rao KMK, et al. Association of Interleukin-6 and other biologic variables with depression in older people living in the community. J Am Geriatr Soc 1999;47:6–11.

51. Griffin WS, Sheng JG, Roberts GW, Mrak RE. Interleukin-1 expression in different plaque types in Alzheimer's disease: significance in plaque evolution. J Neuropathol Exp Neurol 1995;54:276–281.

52. Griffin WS, Sheng JG, Royston MC, et al. Glial-neuronal interactions in Alzheimer's disease: the potential role of a 'cytokine cycle' in disease progression. Brain Pathol 1998;8:65–72.

53. Ringheim GE, Szczepanik AM, Petko W, et al. Enhancement of beta-amyloid precursor protein transcription and expression by the soluble interleukin-6 receptor/interleukin-6 complex, Mol Brain Res 1998;55:35–44.

54. Bauer J, Strauss S, Schreiter-Gasser U, et al. Interleukin-6 and alpha-2-macroglobulin indicate an acute-phase state in Alzheimer's disease cortices. FEBS Lett 1991;285:111–114.

55. Hull M, Berger M, Volk B, Bauer J. Occurrence of interleukin-6 in cortical plaques of Alzheimer's disease patients may precede transformation of diffuse into neuritic plaques. Ann NY Acad Sci 1996; 777:205–212.

56. Rogers I. Neuroinflammatory Mechanisms in Alzheimer's Disease. Birkhäuser, Basel, 2001.

57. Papassotiropoulos A, Bagli M, Jessen F, Bayer TA, et al. A genetic variation of the inflammatory cytokine interleukin-6 delays the intial onset and reduces the risk for sporadic Alzheimer's disease. Ann Neurol 1999;45:666–668.

58. Licastro F, Pedrini S, Caputo L, et al. Increased plasma levels of interleukin-1, interleukin-6 and alpha-1-antichymotrypsin in patients with Alzheimer's disease: peripheral inflammation or signals from the brain? J Neuroimmunol 2000;103:97–102.

59. Maes M, DeVos N, Wauters A, Demedts P, Maurits VW, Neels H, et al. Inflammatory markers in younger vs elderly normal volunteers and in patients with Alzheimer's disease. J Psychiatr Res 1999;33: 397–405.

60. Bonaccorso S, Lin A, Song C, et al. Serotonin-immune interactions in elderly volunteers and in patients with Alzheimer's disease (DAT): lower plasma tryptophan availability to the brain in the elderly and increased serum interleukin-6 in DAT. Aging (Milano) 1998;10:316–323.

61. Singh VK, Guthikonda P. Circulating cytokines in Alzheimer's disease. J Psychiatr Res 1997;31: 657–660.

62. Kalman J, Juhasz A, Laird G, et al. Serum interleukin-6 levels correlate with the severity of dementia in Down syndrome and in Alzheimer's disease. Acta Neurologica Scandinavica 1997;96:236–240.

63. Licastro F, Morini MC, Polazzi E, Davis LJ. Increased serum alpha 1-antichymotrypsin in patients with probable Alzheimer's disease: an acute phase reactant without the peripheral acute phase response. J Neuroimmunol 1995;57:71–75.

64. Fillit H, Ding WH, Buee L, et al. Elevated circulating tumor necrosis factor levels in Alzheimer's disease. Neurosci Lett 1991;129:318–320.

65. Shalit F, Sredni B, Stern L, Kott E, Huberman M. Elevated interleukin-6 secretion levels by mononuclear cells of Alzheimer's patients. Neurosci Lett 1994;174:130–132.

66. Lombardi VR, Garcia M, Rey L, Cacabelos R. Characterization of cytokine production, screening of lymphocyte subset patterns and in vitro apoptosis in healthy and Alzheimer's Disease (AD) individuals. J Neuroimmunol 1999;97:163–171.

67. Angelis P, Scharf S, Mander A, Vajda F, Christophidis N. Serum interleukin-6 and interleukin-6 soluble receptor in Alzheimer's disease. Neurosci Lett 1998;244:106–108.

68. Pirttila T, Mehta PD, Frey H, Wisniewski HM. Alpha 1-antichymotrypsin and IL-1 beta are not increased in CSF or serum in Alzheimer's disease. Neurobiol Aging 1994;15:313–317.

69. Esumi E, Araga S, Takahashi K. Serum interleukin-2 levels in patients with dementia of the Alzheimer type. Acta Neurologica Scandinavica 1991;84:65–67.

70. van Duijn CM, Hofman A, Nagelkerken L. Serum levels of interleukin-6 are not elevated in patients with Alzheimer's disease. Neurosci Lett 1990;108:350–354.

71. Poehlman ET. Regulation of energy expenditure in aging humans. J Am Geriatr Soc 1993;41:552–559.

72. Donaldson KE, Carpenter WH, Toth MJ, et al. No evidence for a higher resting metabolic rate in non-institutionalized Alzheimer's patients. J Am Geriatr Soc 1996;44:1232–1234.

73. Niskanen L, Piirainen M, Koljonen M, Uusitupa M. Resting energy expenditure in relation to energy intake in patients with Alzheimer's disease, multiinfarct dementia and in control women. Age Aging 1993;22:132–137.

74. Wolf-Klein GP, Silerstone FA, Lansey SC, et al. Energy requirements in Alzheimer's disease patients. Nutrition 1995;11:264–268.

75. Poehlman ET, Toth MJ, Goran MI, Carpenter WH, Newhouse P, Rosen CJ. Daily energy expenditure in free-living non-institutionalized Alzheimer's patients: a doubly labeled water study. Neurology 1997;48:997–1002.

76. Gillete-Guyonnet S, Nourhashemi F, Andrieu S, deGlisezinski I, Ousset PJ, Riviere D, et al. Weight Loss in Alzheimer's disease. Am J Clin Nutr 2000;71(suppl):637S–642S.

77. White HK, McConnell ES, Bales CW, Kuchibbahtia M. A 6-month observational study of the relationship between weight loss and behavioral symptoms in institutionalized AD subjects. J Am Geriatr Soc 2001;49:S44.

78. Smith MA, Perry G, Richey PL, et al. Oxidative damage in Alzheimer's. Nature 1996;382:120–121.

79. Jaendel C, Nicolas MB, Dubois F, et al. Lipid peroxidation and free radical scavengers in Alzheimer's disease. Gerontology 1989;35:275–282.

80. Commenges D, Scotet V, Renaud S, et al. Intake of flavinoids and risk of dementia. Eur J Epidem 2000;16:357–363.

81. Halliwell B, Gutteridge JMC. Oxygen radicals in the nervous system. Trends Neurosci 1985;8:22–26.

82. Sano M, Ernesto C, Thomas RG Klauber MR, et al. A controlled trial of selegiline, alpha-tocopheral, or both as treatment for Alzheimer's disease. N Eng J Med 1997;336:1216–1222.

83. Hector M, Burton JR, What are the psychiatric manifestations of B12 deficiency? J Am Geriatr Soc 1988;36:1105–1112.

84. Lindenbaum J, Healton EB, Savage DG et al. Neuropsychiatric disorders caused by cobalamin deficiency in the absence of anemia or macrocytosis. N Eng J Med 1988;318:1720–1728.

85. Martin DC, Francis j, Protechj et al. Time dependency of cogntive recovery with cobalamin replacement: report of a pilot study. J Am Geriatr Soc 1992;40:168–172.

86. Ikeda T, Furukawa Y, Nashimoto S, et al. Vitamin B12 levels in serum and cerobrospinal fluid of people with Alzheimer's disease. Acta Psychiatr Scand 1990;82:327–329.

87. Basun H, Forsell LG, Bendz R et al. Cobalamin in blood and cerebrospinal fluid in Alzheimer's disease and related disorders. Dementia 1991;2:324–332.

88. Basun H, Fratiglioni L, Winblad B. Cobalamin levels are not reduced in Alzheimer's disease: results from a population-based study. J Am Geriatr Soc 1994;42:132–136.

89. Carmel R, Gott PS, Waters CH et al. The frequently low cobalamin levels in dementia usually signify treatable metabolic, neurologic and electrophysiologic abnormalities. Eur J Haemat 1995;54:245–253.

90. Teunisse S, Bollen AE, van Gool WA, Walstra GJ. Dementia and subnormal levels of vitamin B12: effects of replacement therapy on dementia. J Neurol 1996;243:522–529.

91. Crystal HA, Ortof E, Frishman WH et al. Serum vitamin B12 levels and incidence of dementia in a healthy elderly population: a report from the Bronx longitudinal aging study. J Am Geriatr Soc 1994;42:933–936.

92. Clark R, Smith AD, Jobst KA et al. Folate, vitamin B12 and serum total homocysteine levels in confirmed Alzheimer's disease. Arch Neurol 1998;55:1407–1408.

93. Seshadri S, Beiser A, Selhub J, Jacques P et al. Plasma homocysteine as a risk factor for dementia and Alzheimer's disease. N Eng J Med 2002;346:476–483.

94. Loscalzo J. Homocysteine and dementias. N Eng J Med 2002;346:466–468.

95. Rogers SL, Farlow MR, Doody RS, et al. A 24-week, double-blind, placebo-controlled trial of donepezil in patients with Alzheimer's disease. Neurology 1998;50:136–145.

96. Rosler M, Anand R, Cicin-Sain A, Gauthier S, et al. Efficacy and safety of rivastigmine in patients with Alzheimer's disease: international randomized controlled trial. BMJ 1999;318:633–640.

97. Tariot PN, Solomon PR, Morris JC, Kershaw P, et al. A 5-month, randomized, placebo-controlled trial of galatamine in AD. Neurology 2000;54:2269–2276.

98. Rasking MA, Peskind ER, Wessel T, Yuan W et al. Galantamine in AD: a 6-month randomized, placebo-controlled trial with a 6-month extension. Neurology 2000;54:2261–2268.

99. Lauque S, Wegner A, Ousset PJ, et al. Comparative study on nutritional intake and cognitive functions (WAIS code). Age Nutr 1995;6:68–72 (in French).

100. LaRue A, Koehler KM, Wayne SJ, Chiulli SJ, Haaland KY, Garry PJ. Nutritional status and cognitive functioning in normally aging sample:a 6-year reassessment. Am J Clin Nutr 1997;65:20–29.

101. Perrig WJ, Perrig P, Stehclin B. The relation between antioxidants and memory performance in the old and very old. J Am Geriatr Soc 1997;45:718–724.

102. Ortega RM, Requejo AM, Andres P, et al. Dietary intake and cognitive function in a group of elderly people Am J Clin Nutr 1997;66:803–809.

103. Goodwin JS, Goodwin JM, Garry PJ. Association between nutritional status and cognitive functioning in a healthy elderly population. JAMA 1983;249:2917–2921.

104. Rivière S, Gillette-Guyonnet S, Voisin T, et al. A nutritional education program could prevent weight loss and slow cognitive decline in Alzheimer's Disease. J Nutr Health Aging 2001;5:295–299.

105. Tayback M, Kumanyika S, Chee E. Body weight as a risk factor in the elderly. Arch Intern Med 1990; 150:1065–1072.

106. Tully CL, Snowdon DA. Weight change and physical function in older women: findings from the nun study. J Am Geriatr Soc 1995;43:1394–1397.

107. Stevens J, Cai J, Pamuk E, Williamson D, Thun M, Wood J. The effect of age on the association between body-mass index and mortality. N Eng J Med 1998;338:1–7.

108. Payette H, Coulombe C, Boutier V, Gray-Donald K. Weight loss and mortality among free-living frail elders: a prospective study. J Gerontol 1999;54A:M440–M445.

109. Keller HH. Weight gain impacts morbidity and mortality in institutionalized oler persons. J Am Geriatr Soc 1995;43:165–169.

110. Soltesz KS, Dayton JH. Finger foods help those with Alzheimer's maintain weight. J Am Diet Assoc 1993;93:1106–1108.

111. Winograd CH, Brown EM. Aggressive oral refeeding in hosptitalized patients. Am J Clin Nutr 1990;52:967–968.

112. Finucane TE, Christmas C, Travis K. Tube feeding in patients with advanced dementia: a review of the evidence. JAMA 1999;282:1365–1370.

113. Lazarus BA, Murphy JB, Culpeper L. Aspiration associated with long-term gastric versus jejunal feeding: a critical analysis of the literature. Arch Phys Med Rehabil 1990;71:46–53

114. Fox KA, Mularski RA, Sarfati MR, et al. Aspiration pneumonia following surgically placed feeding tubes. Am J Surg 1995;170:564–566.

14 Nutrition and End-of-Life Care

*Christian Davis Furman
and Christine Seel Ritchie*

1. INTRODUCTION

Nutritional support during the last days of a dying patient is a critical issue that must be resolved by careful discussion between families, caregivers, and the health care team. Eating is such an integral part of life that when a loved one no longer wants to eat or cannot eat, some families and physicians feel they must do something to correct the situation. Food nourishes us, satisfies us when we are hungry, and comforts us in times of need. We celebrate everything with food and talk of food as "nourishing people back to health." We prepare and share meals as a way of expressing love and concern. In many instances, however, there is a natural decline in the desire and ability to eat by a family member with a terminal illness, which may be hard for caregivers to understand or accept. Health care providers need to be well-versed in issues regarding artificial nutrition and hydration in terminal illness in order to assist patients and their families in treatment decisions.

In this chapter, we review definitions regarding nutritional support, discuss legal and ethical issues surrounding nutrition, and review nutrition management challenges in patients with advanced malignancy and advanced dementia. Equipped with information regarding nutrition in terminal illnesses, health care professionals can help guide patients and assist families in respecting patient wishes.

2. DEFINITIONS

Non-oral feeding is the provision of food by a nasogastric tube, gastrostomy tube, gastrojejunostomy tube, or total parenteral nutrition (TPN). Artificial hydration is the provision of water or electrolyte solutions by any nonoral route. Artificial nutrition includes enteral nutrition by nasogastric tube, percutaneous endoscopic gastrostomy tube, percutaneous jejunostomy tube, gastrostomy tube, or gastrojejunostomy tube (*see* Chapter 26). Because TPN is rarely used in end-of-life care, it is not included in these definitions.

From: *Handbook of Clinical Nutrition and Aging*
Edited by: C. W. Bales and C. S. Ritchie © Humana Press Inc., Totowa, NJ

3. LEGAL AND ETHICAL ASPECTS

3.1. Legal Aspects

Multiple legal decisions provide guidance to physicians concerning the nutritional treatment of terminal patients. In the Karen Ann Quinlan Case in 1976, the court upheld the right to forgo life-sustaining care and clarified an important distinction between killing and allowing death *(1)*. The Barber Case in 1983 involved a patient in a deep coma after cardiopulmonary arrest following surgery to close an ileostomy. A California lower court indicted two doctors for murder who stopped intravenous fluids and feeding tubes. The spouse testified that the patient had stated "no Karen Quinlan." The appellate court disposed of the murder charges because the charge of murder requires proof of unlawful killing—an act of commission. Terminating artificial nutrition was considered an act of omission, not commission. For an omission to be unlawful, there must be a duty to act. There was no duty to act because of the patient's known prior wishes for no treatment *(2)*. In 1986, the appellate court in the Bouvia Case ruled that refusal of medical support by a competent patient is a fundamental right. The patient was a 29-yr-old female with severe cerebral palsy who was bedridden, immobile, in constant pain, and competent to make her own medical decisions. A feeding tube was placed against the patient's wishes. The patient then petitioned to remove the feeding tube. The lower court refused the petition, stating that it was a form of suicide. An appeals court later ruled in favor of the patient *(3)*. A more recent case involving nutrition in the terminally ill was the Cruzan Case in 1990. Parents of Nancy Cruzan, a woman in a persistent vegetative state, requested cessation of nutritional support. The US Supreme Court stated that patients have a right to die, and competent patients can refuse therapy, making it clear that artificial nutrition/ hydration was no different than any other medical treatment *(4)*.

In summary, enteral nutrition is considered medical treatment, not basic care. Patients have the right to refuse this form of medical treatment. Withdrawal of artificial nutritional support and allowing a patient to die is not equivalent to euthanasia. In the former instance, the goal of discontinuing therapy is to remove burdensome interventions; in the latter, the intended result is the death of the patient.

3.2. Ethical Aspects

In medicine, ethical principles guide how a patient should be treated or how a treatment dilemma should be handled. The ethical principle of autonomy states that a person should have the ability to govern oneself. This principle was applied in the court decisions of Barber in 1983, Bouvia in 1986, and Cruzan in 1990, which all stated that competent adults should be the final arbiters of decisions regarding their own health care. Benefi- cence is the ethical principle that states that physicians should always provide care that benefits the patient. In the case of artificial nutrition, the physician needs to ask if the artificial nutrition is actually "doing good" for their patient. The principle of nonmaleficence addresses the complimentary principle that one should not do harm— *primum non nocere*. In the case of artificial nutrition and hydration, physicians must ask if this medical treatment is harming their patient.

The argument for the discontinuation of nutritional support states that artificial nutri- tion and hydration are indistinguishable from other medical treatments. If this treatment is contributing to more harm than benefit, than the principle of nonmaleficence would

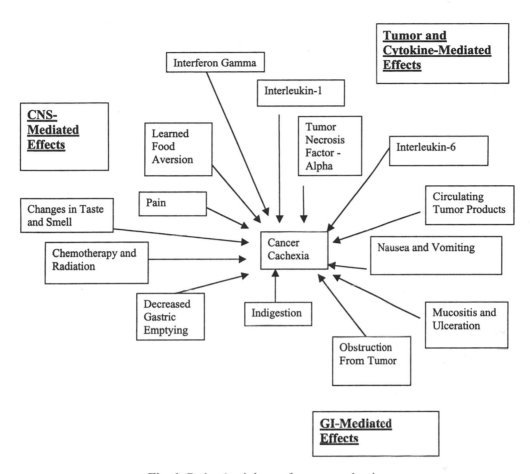

Fig. 1. Pathophysiology of cancer cachexia.

support its discontinuation. If the nutritional support is unwanted, then providing artificial nutrition does not adhere to the principle of autonomy and lessens patient dignity.

4. ARTIFICIAL NUTRITION AND HYDRATION IN TERMINAL CANCER

The primary signs of cancer cachexia include anorexia and weight loss. Cancer cachexia occurs in 50% of patients suffering from any form of cancer at any stage *(5)*. The degree of cachexia varies according to the pathology of the malignancy. It occurs in 30% of patients with lymphoma and 85% of patients with gastric or pancreatic cancer. It also varies according to the stage of the disease. Only 3% of patients receiving adjuvant therapy experience cachexia, but 75–80% of patients in the terminal stage experience it *(6)*.

The pathophysiology of cancer cachexia involves the interplay of the central nervous system (CNS) and psychological effects, tumor effects, treatment-induced effects, and endogenous mediators (Fig. 1). The CNS and psychological effects of pain, learned food aversion, and changes in taste and smell all lead to anorexia. Learned food aversion occurs when a certain food is given just before chemotherapy, then the person becomes averse to this food because of its association with chemotherapy. Changes in taste and smell occur from the chemotherapy and medications used to treat the side effects of chemotherapy. Chemotherapy and radiation can lead to anticipatory nausea, vomiting, and anorexia. These treatments can also lead to the development of mucositis and gastrointestinal ulceration. Food intake may be reduced in these cases as a result of extreme discomfort with eating. The direct effects of obstruction from the tumor and circulating tumor products lead to cancer cachexia. These tumor products are produced either directly by the tumor or by the body in response to the tumor. For example, tumor necrosis factor (TNF) and interleukin-1 are cytokines that cause cachexia. TNF, interleukin-1, and other endogenous mediators also cause nausea, vomiting, and decreased gastric emptying *(7)*.

The abnormal metabolism associated with cancer causes loss of cell mass with loss of weight. This abnormal metabolism is from numerous factors. Liver synthesis of protein and lipid increase, as does hepatic Cori cycle activity. Increased gluconeogenesis, increased PEP-CK activity, and increased amino acid release also occur. In the muscle, decreased protein synthesis and glucose uptake leads to increased skeletal muscle breakdown and an equal loss of muscle and fat mass *(8)*.

The impact of nutritional support in cancer cachexia remains in question. Nutritional support in cancer patients has not been shown to improve survival, improve tumor response, decrease toxicity, or decrease surgical complications *(9)*. In animal studies, nutritional support has actually been shown to increase rates of tumor growth. Also, nutritional support has not been shown to improve quality of life *(10)*.

In fact, the only exception to this lack of influence is the beneficial effect of nutritional support in head and neck cancer patients and esophageal cancer patients who are not able to swallow properly and still have an appetite *(14)*.

A number of treatment modalities have been used to address cancer cachexia. Corticosteroids, progestestational agents (e.g., Megace), cyproheptadine (Periactin), cannabinoids (marijuana), and pentoxifylline (Trental) are all medications that have been tried to treat cancer cachexia. Because of its positive effect on appetite, Megestrol acetate (Megace) is useful if profound anorexia is the main manifestation of cachexia and if expected survival is weeks to months. Megace has been shown to significantly increase appetite, but not survival *(10)*. In patients with a shorter predicted survival, a brief course of corticosteroids may be useful to stimulate appetite and have positive effects on nausea, pain, and asthenia. More data is needed before the other pharmacological treatments can be recommended as treatment for cancer cachexia.

A useful way to present to the family/caregiver the potential impact of withholding artificial nutrition might be to discuss a study that evaluated hunger and thirst in terminal patients. The authors completed a prospective study of patients in a comfort care unit—the majority had cancer or stroke as their terminal diagnosis. The patients were alert and competent. Food was offered and feeding was assisted, but not forced. The patients were followed for thirst, hunger, and dry mouth to see if food or fluid relieved the symptoms *(11)*. Hunger was not experienced by 63% of the patients studied; an additional 34% had hunger initially that subsequently resolved. Similarly, 62% had no thirst or thirst only initially. Most of the patients' symptoms were easily controlled with a small amount of food or water. The authors concluded by stating that hunger and thirst were uncommon in the terminal phase regardless of food and water intake inadequate to sustain basal energy requirements.

5. ARTIFICIAL NUTRITION AND HYDRATION IN TERMINAL DEMENTIA

5.1. Definitions and Prognosis of Advanced Dementia

Dementia is a progressive terminal condition possibly caused by one of a number of conditions including Alzheimer's disease (AD), cerebrovascular disease, congenital or acquired neurodegenerative diseases, brain tumors, AIDS, and Parkinson's disease. The features of dementia include loss of higher cognitive function, loss of intelligible speech, inability to maintain oral nutrition from loss of swallowing reflex, and inability to ambulate. In the United States, there are 4 million people with dementia *(12)*. In 1995, 30% of the 121,000 percutaneous endoscopic gastrostomy (PEG) tubes placed were in demented patients *(13)*.

Dementia is a progressive disease that worsens in recognizable stages. The functional assessment staging system (FAST) is one system used to follow the course of AD, thereby helping to decide how far the disease has progressed *(14)*. There are 7 stages with the first stage comprising of essentially no symptoms and the last stage describing advanced, end-stage dementia. At stage 6, the patient needs supervision in dressing, bathing, toileting, and eating, becoming dependent on the caregiver. Late deficits in this stage are incontinence and the inability to flush the toilet. Patients either die or are institutionalized after 3 yr in this stage. This is the stage when AD patients may stop eating spontaneously, but can be encouraged to eat. At stage 7, patients usually die within 1 yr. They lose the ability to speak, ambulate, eat, control their muscles, and smile. When patients reach this stage, it is very difficult to maintain nutrition because encouragement to eat becomes less successful. In this instance, difficulty eating is a marker for the terminal phase of AD. The same is not true in other forms of dementia. For example, patients with Parkinson's disease often lose the ability to maintain adequate caloric intake at an earlier stage of their disease; in this setting, a feeding tube may be required.

5.2. Addressing the Costs and Benefits of Artificial Nutrition and Hydration in Advanced Dementia

Physicians and families have difficulty discussing nutrition support in patients with advanced dementia. Nutrition may be a more emotional decision to some families than ventilator support or cardiac resuscitation. Families feel like they are "starving" their loved one, fearing the ill person will not survive as a direct result of not eating. These issues are so difficult that sometimes physicians and families do not ever initiate discussions of them. Also, the questions regarding the cost–benefit ratio of artificial nutrition in an advanced dementia patient have not been answered adequately to provide guidance to the general medical community.

Finucane attempted to address these difficult questions based on the limited clinical data available *(15)*. He reviewed primary concerns commonly cited as rationale for enteral nutrition, including aspiration pneumonia, skin breakdown, quality of life, and survival. His review of the literature does not indicate that enteral nutrition improves survival or quality of life. In addition, he reports 3 case-control studies that identified tube feeding as an independent risk factor for aspiration pneumonia. In fact, orally fed patients with dysphagia had significantly fewer major aspiration events than those fed by tube. Regarding skin breakdown, no prospective trial has been done, but 2 longitudinal studies showed that enteral nutrition did not improve healing of existing pressure ulcers *(16)* and provided no protection from new pressure ulcers *(17)*. Another concern about tube feedings is the issue of patient restraints. Bedfast patients with advanced dementia who receive artificial nutritional support are more likely to be restrained; the resulting immobility and incontinence may partially explain the lack of association between tube feeding and decreased skin breakdown.

Gillick addressed quality of life in her research and found that advanced dementia patients who were tube fed were often deprived of taste, touch, and social interaction *(18)*. Restraints were used 71% of the time in patients with dementia and feeding tubes, regardless of the type of tube. Restraints can lead to distress and agitation and sedating medications to control the behavior, all negatively impacting quality of life.

Sanders et al. address survival secondary to tube feeding *(19)*. They found that in a nursing home, the patients who were fed by a gastrostomy tube and those fed by hand had the same survival rates. Among gastrostomy patients, patients with dementia had a much worse prognosis (54% 1-mo mortality) when compared to those without dementia (28% 1-mo mortality). This study highlights that difficulty with eating may be a marker of the terminal phase of dementia; tube feeding is unlikely to prolong the patient's life at this stage.

5.3. Alternative Approaches to Artificial Nutrition and Hydration in Advanced Dementia

In AD patients, skillful feeding techniques need to be employed (*see* Chapters 11 and 13). The appropriate selection of food consistencies must take place, and adequate time for feeding and verbal cueing to chew the food and swallow must occur. Distractions must be kept to a minimum. The mid-day meal should be capitalized on because intake is often greatest at this time of day *(20)*.

6. ADDRESSING TREATMENT GOALS IN ADVANCED DEMENTIA AND ADVANCED CANCER

When treatment goals are discussed early in the diagnosis of a terminal condition, the patient can decide what their wishes are at the end of life. In this way, the goals will reflect the preferences and values of the patient. A discussion about feeding wishes should also take place. Unfortunately, patients' wishes are rarely known regarding tube feeding. Friedel and Ozick in 2000, exemplified the reality of how gastrostomy tubes become inserted. Of 18 patients in a New York municipal hospital scheduled for a gastrostomy tube, only one patient was deemed capable of giving informed consent. None of the other 17 patients had an Advanced Directive or Power of Attorney. The medical staff became the decision makers, and all 18 received a gastrostomy tube *(21)*.

The decision about feeding should be consistent with the overall goals of care. Treatment goals are not widely discussed because physicians feel pressed for time, feel uncomfortable discussing issues surrounding the end of life, and often were never taught how to discuss these sensitive topics. When discussing treatment goals, one must start by asking the patient what they already know. The next step is to review the patient's condition and prognosis. The physician should continue by discussing the patient's preferences and goals, then outlining appropriate treatment options—or goals as they relate to the patient's current condition: curative treatment, rehabilitative treatment, or palliative treatment *(22)*. Palliative treatment may include life-prolonging treatment or treatment solely aimed at comfort care. Finally, the physician should invite questions, allow time to reflect, and then decide if related issues of treatment withdrawal need to be discussed.

When a patient becomes terminal and is nondecisional, there are established guidelines as to how decisions are to be made. The advanced directive, if one exists, is the document that should be consulted first to know the patient's prior expressed wishes. If the advanced directive does not answer the specific question that needs to be addressed, then the legal guardian or the agent of the advanced directive makes the decision based on what they think the patient would have wanted or the wishes previously expressed by the patient. If there is no document and no designated decision maker, then the first-order relative makes decisions (usually the spouse, then adult children, then siblings, but this may vary by state). Finally, the opinion of other relatives can be considered. If none of the above exists, then the physician's judgment can be used to determine the best treatment for the patient.

7. PRACTICAL CONSIDERATIONS BEFORE PROVIDING ENTERAL/PARENTAL NUTRITION AND HYDRATION

The decision on whether to start tube feeding is never easy. There are some practical matters to consider before a decision is made. In a terminal patient, the usual goal of care should be aggressive palliative care. This means the goal is to provide comfort care by managing the symptoms of the disease or side effects of the treatment while maintaining optimal quality of life. The goal of nutrition support should be to maintain energy and strength while being attentive to potentially negative quality-of-life effects of coercive feeding or artificial nutrition and hydration.

During this time, the physician needs to understand the caregivers' feelings and needs to counsel the caregiver. The caregiver may feel frustrated over the inability to find and prepare foods that are tolerated by the patient. They may also sense that the food they are offering may not provide the comfort that the caregiver is trying to provide. The caregiver should realize that the loss of appetite and the inability to eat are common experiences in the terminally ill. Also, physical and emotional changes influence the ability to eat. For example, the disease itself, medications, fear, or depression may make it difficult to eat. Changes in the sense of smell, diarrhea, constipation, and nausea or vomiting also decrease the patient's appetite. Caregivers who push food on the patient with anorexia may be contributing to the patient's distress instead of comforting the patient. This was demonstrated by McCann et al. in a study of cancer patients *(23)*. Less information is known about dementia patients. It is hard to know if patients with dementia experience discomfort from not eating because they are noncommunicative at this stage.

A few practical suggestions are: eliminate most or all dietary restrictions if at all possible; give only amounts of food and beverages tolerated or accepted, because thirst and hunger are often diminished in the dying process; and have the patient assisted with meals; the patient should not be forced to eat.

Mild underhydration in the last days of life has a number of potential benefits. Without hydration, there are less oral and airway secretions, less congestion, and fewer symptoms associated with ascites and edema. Peripheral edema may increase pain and predispose the patient to pressure ulcers. In addition, the risk of aspiration is increased in terminal patients because they cannot always cough as a result of secondary weakness. However, the need to cough may decrease when oral secretions are reduced. Finally, increased gastrointestinal fluids can cause nausea and vomiting, especially for patients with intestinal strictures or obstruction from neoplasms. During the dying process, dehydration occurs from inadequate intake and losses from GI, renal, skin, and pulmonary secretions. Fluid deprivation at this stage rarely causes headache, nausea, cramps, or vomiting. Dehydration leads to mental changes, which may decrease the patient's awareness of their suffering. Families are sometimes concerned about the dry mouth that occurs as a person dies. Ice chips, sips of liquid, lip moisteners, salivary substitutes, mouth swabs, hard candy, and routine mouth care all help to relieve the xerostoma or dry mouth that occurs.

8. SUMMARY

Caring for patients with a terminal illness like cancer or advanced AD is difficult for the family and the physician. The issues surrounding feeding are some of the hardest to resolve. This chapter defines the problems and offers guidelines. To summarize, decisions regarding nutritional support in end-of-life care should be informed by treatment goals and patient preference. Case law regards enteral nutrition as medical treatment. With the exception of head and neck cancer and esophageal cancer, no studies have demonstrated improved survival in cancer or advanced dementia with enteral support. In advanced cancer patients, nausea and pain should be addressed, and corticosteroids and progestational agents considered. In advanced dementia, emphasis should be placed on oral food intake, allowing adequate time for feeding, avoiding distractions, and using verbal cueing. Every person, family, and physician must decide to what extent to nourish a person with a terminal illness based on available information on the risks and benefits.

9. RECOMMENDATIONS FOR CLINICIANS

1. Before deciding on a specific form of nutritional support, establish treatment goals.
2. With a few exceptions, artificial nutritional support in cancer patients does not improve survival, improve tumor response, decrease toxicity, or decrease surgical complications.
3. Artificial nutritional support may be appropriate in head and neck cancer patients and esophageal cancer patients that are unable to swallow properly and still have an appetite.
4. Megestrol acetate (Megace) may be useful in cancer patients if profound anorexia is the main manifestation of cachexia and if expected survival is weeks to months.
5. In advanced cancer patients with a shorter predicted survival, a brief course of corticosteroids may be useful to stimulate appetite and have positive effects on nausea, pain, and asthenia.
6. Current limited data do not demonstrate that artificial nutritional support improves survival or quality of life in advanced dementia patients.

REFERENCES

1. Bioethicists' statement on the US Supreme Court's Cruzan decision. NEJM 1990;323:686–687.
2. Burck R. Feeding, withdrawing, and withholding: ethical perspectives. Nutr Clin Prac 1996;11:243–253.
3. Bouvia v. Superior Court (Glenchur) 179 Cal. App. 3d 1127, 225 Cal. Rptr. 297 [Ct. App. 1986].
4. Bioethicists' statement on the US Supreme Court's Cruzan decision. NEJM 1990;323:686–687.

5. Dewys WD, Begg C, Lavin PT, et al. Prognostic effect of weight loss prior to chemotherapy in cancer patients. Am J Med 1980;69:491–497.

6. Nelson KA. The cancer anorexia-cachexia syndrome. Semin Oncol 2000;27:64–68.

7. Jaskowiak NT, Alexander HR. The pathophysiology of cancer cachexia. In: Oxford Textbook of Palliative Medicine, 2nd ed. Doyle D, Hanks GWC, MacDonald N (eds.), Oxford University Press, Oxford, 1998, pp. 534–547.

8. Tisdale MJ. Cancer cachexia: metabolic alterations and clinical manifestations. Nutrition 1997;13:1–7.

9. Maltoni M, Nanni O, Scarpi E, Rossi D, Serra P, Amadori D. High-dose progestins for the treatment of cancer anorexia-cachexia syndrome: a systematic review of randomized clinical trials. Ann Oncol 2001;12:289–300.

10. Bruera E, Fainsinger RL. Clinical management of cachexia and anorexia. In: Oxford Textbook of Palliative Medicine, 2nd ed. Doyle D, Hanks GWC, MacDonald N (eds.), Oxford University Press, Oxford, 1998, pp. 550–555.

11. McCann RM, Hall WJ, Groth-Juncker A. Comfort care for terminally ill patients: the appropriate use of nutrition and hydration. JAMA 1994;272:1263–1266.

12. Evans DA, et al. Prevalence of Alzheimer's Disease in a community population of older patients. JAMA 1989;262:2551–2556.

13. Gillick MR. Rethinking the value of tube feeding in patients with advanced dementia. NEJM 2000;342:206–210.

14. Primary Care Internal Medicine. In: Medical Knowledge Self-Assessment Program. American College of Physicians, Philadelphia, PA, 1998, p. 71.

15. Finucane TE, Christmas C, Travis K. Tube feeding in patients with advanced dementia: a review of the evidence. JAMA 1999;282:1365–1370.

16. Berlowitz DR, Brandeis GH, Anderson J, Brand HK. Predictors of pressure ulcer healing among long-term care residents. JAGS 1997;45:30–34.

17. Berlowitz DR, Ash AS, Brandeis GH, Brand HK, Halpern JL, Moskowitz MA. Rating long-term care facilities on pressure ulcer development: importance of case-mix adjustment. Ann Int Med 1996;124: 557–563.

18. Gillick MR. Rethinking the value of tube feeding in patients with advanced dementia. NEJM 2000;342:206–210.

19. Sanders DS, Carter MJ, D'Silva J, James G, Bolton RP, Bardham KD. Survival analysis in percutaneous endoscopic gastrostomy feeding: a worse outcome in patients with dementia. Am J Gastroenterol 2000; 95:1472–1475.

20. Suski NS, Nielsen CC. Factors affecting food intake of women with Alzheimer's type dementia in long-term care. JADA 1989;89:1770–1773.

21. Friedel DM, Ozick LA. Rethinking the role of tube feeding in patients with advanced dementia (letter; comment). NEJM 2000;342:1756.

22. Weissman DE. Establishing treatment goals, withdrawing treatments, DNR orders. In: Improving End-of-Life Care: A Resource Guide for Physician Education. Weissman DE (ed.), The Medical College of Wisconsin, Inc., Milwaukee, WI 1998, pp. 94–100.

23. McCann RM, Hall WJ, Groth-Juncker A. Comfort care for terminally ill patients: the appropriate use of nutrition and hydration. JAMA 1994;272:1263–1266.

IV

CLINICAL TOPICS
A. VASCULAR DISORDERS

15

Vascular Function, Aging, and the Impact of Diet

Daniel E. Forman, Paula A. Quatromoni, and Giulia L. Sheftel

1. INTRODUCTION

Although aging and disease are often regarded as independent processes, they are intertwined. Customary age-related changes in the walls and endothelium of blood vessels progressively increase susceptibility to cardiovascular disease. The growing awareness of these relationships leads to potential opportunities to modify aging patterns and thereby better preserve youthful physiology and natural resistance to disease. Lifestyle changes, including diet, are among the preventive measures that can bring about better maintenance of health. In this overview, we discuss some of the mechanisms underlying vascular senescence and the related rationale for dietary modification. Both general dietary recommendations and several specific diet-related categories, including cholesterol, salt, dietary antioxidants, and nutrients involved in homocysteine metabolism, are reviewed.

1.1. Customary Vascular Aging

Vascular senescence includes both predominant stiffening and diminished vasodilatory capacity (Fig. 1). Normal vascular histology in young adults includes a high proportion of elastin, a material tissue imparting elastic-type properties. Elastin-rich vessels distend to accommodate blood from the pumping heart, and then recoil to produce propagating pulsatility and its efficient transport into the periphery. However, with aging, elastin progressively fragments and pulsatility diminishes *(1)*. Deposits of calcium and crosslinked collagen accumulate in vessel walls, gradually transforming them into rigid, unyielding tubes. The hearts of older adults must therefore push blood into stiff, nonpulsating vessels *(2)*. As a result, blood is pumped against increased resistance without the benefit of intrinsic vascular pulsatility to ease and sustain distribution.

Biological changes in the endothelium lining the vessel lumen aggravate the impact of vascular stiffening. Endothelial synthesis of nitric oxide (NO), a key vasodilatory peptide, is reduced, diminishing maximal vasodilation particularly in the context of

From: *Handbook of Clinical Nutrition and Aging*
Edited by: C. W. Bales and C. S. Ritchie © Humana Press Inc., Totowa, NJ

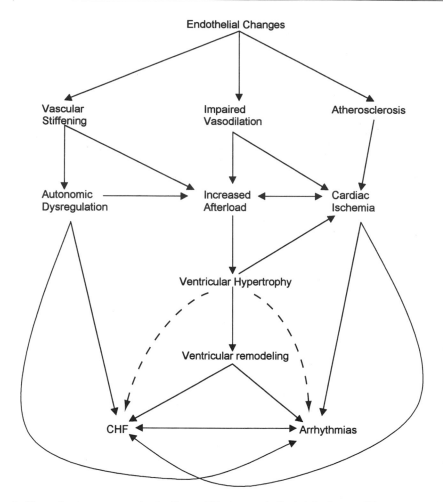

Fig. 1. Vascular senescence including stiffening and diminished vasodilatory capacity.

demand stresses that would normally stimulate dilation to facilitate augmented volume of blood *(3–5)*. Reduced vasodilation of the large central vessels compounds the workload on the heart, because dilation would normally ease the afterload stresses against which the heart must pump *(6,7)*. Further, reduced vasodilation of the coronary arteries also increases the likelihood of supply ischemia or inadequate supply of blood through the poorly dilating epicardial arteries *(8)*. Therefore, age-related proclivity to ischemia occurs at least in part independently of obstructive atherosclerotic lesions, because of impaired vasodilation. In addition, atherosclerosis is more likely to occur, compounding the likelihood of ischemia. Because endothelial NO is also an antioxidant, diminished NO leads to increasing concentrations of oxidized low-density lipoprotein (LDL) and an associated predisposition toward atherosclerosis. Animal studies have not only demonstrated that senescent coronary vessels are generally more susceptible to atherosclerosis *(9,10)*, but also to atheromatous lesions that are particularly abundant, complex, and unstable *(11)*.

The cumulative impact of vascular senescence is profound. In the heart, cardiac myocytes tend to hypertrophy, a natural response that modifies high-wall tensions, resulting from increased afterload pressures. Although this initially confers an advantageous reduction of wall tension and associated oxygen demands, the growth stimulation, especially in the context of oxidative stress (accumulates with age), also increases the likelihood of myocyte apoptosis and intrinsic cardiac weakening. Thus, vascular aging correlates with increased vulnerability to heart failure and arrhythmias (12).

Vascular senescence also leads to myocardial ischemia. This occurs in part as a result of the impaired coronary vasodilation, age-related atherosclerosis, and higher afterload work demands on the aging heart, which have already been discussed. Furthermore, ventricular hypertrophy itself adds to ischemic risk, particularly in the subendocardium, because of the added distance the myocardial blood must perfuse. Even the flow mechanics of blood through the coronary arteries change with age, compounding the risk of ischemia. Whereas intravascular pressure waves are normally dissipated into distensible elastin among younger adults, the intravascular pressure waves reflect off the stiffened peripheral walls of vessels in older adults and return toward the central vasculature (13). These reflected pressure waves consolidate as high-central impedance, even among adults who are normotensive. Not only does this add to the workload of the senescent heart (14), but because the reflected impedance peaks in late systole (when the heart is contracted and therefore resistant to perfusion), myocardial perfusion in diastole becomes unsynchronized from maximal perfusion pressure, and reduces intracardiac flow (15).

Age-related autonomic changes also stem from vascular stiffening. Autonomic regulation depends on vessel distension to trigger vagal outflow and associated modification of blood pressure and heart rate. As vessels stiffen, vagal responses progressively diminish, and sympathetic outflow becomes unopposed and excessive (16). Consequently, not only are tachyarrhytmias and hypertension more common among the elderly, but high norepinephrine confers direct toxic cellular effects (17,18), compounding the risks of myocyte apoptosis and heart failure. Furthermore, propensity to falls, exercise intolerance, and general frailty are among the many sequelae of autonomic impairment that typically stem from age-related vascular changes.

Despite the enormous toll of vascular aging, the research community has only recently recognized its implications. Therefore, only in the last decade have trials gradually re-oriented toward modification of vascular aging patterns and better preservation of cardiovascular health. One of the earliest manifestations of this shift in focus was the attention placed on systolic hypertension among the elderly. Although it had long been recognized that progressive stiffening of the peripheral blood vessels (i.e., smaller resistance vessels) led to high incidence of systolic blood pressure among the elderly, the clinical significance was unclear. However, in the last 10 yr, data have emerged that unequivocally demonstrate the impact of systolic hypertension on morbidity and mortality in older adults, including greater likelihood of strokes, ischemic heart disease, heart failure, cognitive decline, and even functional impairment (19,20). Moreover, benefits of diet and pharmacological therapy to modify hypertension and its associated risks have been observed. Yet, treatment of hypertension alone does not eliminate the vulnerabilities of aging. Atherosclerosis, hypercholesterolemia, and other potential sources of instability increase as functions of aging and predispose elders to increasing morbidity and mortality (7). Therefore, goals to improve vascular health have expanded beyond blood pressure management with a larger emphasis on prevention. Whereas specific pharmaceutical therapies are often under consideration, basic lifestyle choices remain critical, especially among age strata in which costs of medications, compliance with treatment regimens, and polypharmacology risks are common concerns.

Historically, blood pressure was the sole parameter by which vascular health was evaluated, new indices are now being employed with the assumption that they provide a more fundamental evaluation of vascular health. Novel indicators of vascular anatomy (e.g., vascular thickness) *(21)*, character (e.g., vascular stiffness, distensibility, compliance, and pulse pressure) *(22–24)*, and endothelial responsiveness (e.g., flow-mediated vasodilation) *(25,26)* are among those being evaluated in research and clinical settings. Nonetheless, it remains unclear which parameter is the most reliable and meaningful. When comparing different research studies, it is uncertain how or if these parameters correlate with one another *(27)*.

2. GENERAL DIETARY ISSUES FOR OLDER ADULTS

It has been demonstrated that the vulnerability of elders to many chronic health conditions is modifiable by lifestyle changes, including diet and exercise interventions. In fact, the role of diet in reducing cardiovascular disease (CVD) as well as diabetes mellitus and certain cancers has been well-established *(28)*. Studies show that older adults are capable of adopting lifestyle changes, particularly when they understand the benefits of behavior modification *(29)*. Research, at both national and community levels, has identified specific targets warranting dietary intervention, including inadequate intake of fruits, vegetables, whole grains, and dairy foods along with excessive dietary lipids *(30)* commonly observed among older populations. Inadequate intakes of protein and micronutrients and insufficient exercise are also problematic *(31–33)* and nearly two-thirds of the population over the age of 65 do not exercise regularly *(34)*.

The Dietary Guidelines for Americans form the foundation of the US federal nutrition policy *(35)*. Together with the Food Guide Pyramid *(36)*, they provide a basis for planning and promoting a healthy diet for children (aged 2 yr and older) and adults of any age. These guidelines promote three primary messages: aim for fitness; build a healthy base; and choose sensibly for good health. *Aim for fitness* urges adults to aim for a healthy weight and to be physically active every day. *Build a healthy base* recommends using the Food Guide Pyramid to guide food selections, eating a daily variety of grains (including whole grains), fruits and vegetables, and keeping foods safe to eat. *Choose sensibly* advocates selection of a diet that is low in saturated fat and cholesterol and moderate in total fat, beverages and foods with moderate sugar content, foods and food preparation methods that incorporate less salt, and moderation of alcohol consumption (if alcohol is consumed at all).

In addition to these general recommendations, a modified Food Guide Pyramid was developed by the Expert Committee of Nutrition and Health of Older Americans *(36a)*. This tool was designed specifically to assist older adults in making sensible food choices to achieve dietary variety and nutritional adequacy. It recommends daily consumption of 8 or more servings of water; 6 or more servings from the bread, fortified cereal, rice and pasta group (preferably whole-grain varieties); 2 or more servings of fruit; 3 or more servings of vegetables; 3 servings from the milk, yogurt and cheese group; and 2 or more servings from the meat, poultry, fish, dry beans, eggs, and nut group. Furthermore, the modified food pyramid for older adults advocates sparing ingestion of fats, oils, and sweets.

A third diet pyramid, the Traditional Healthy Mediterranean Diet Pyramid, is also widely promoted. This diet provides a set of guidelines applicable to foods and dietary patterns of diverse cultures and regions all over the world *(37)*. It evolved after it was observed in the 1960s that rates of chronic diseases were among the lowest in the world and adult life expectancy was among the highest among populations consuming the traditional Mediterranean diet *(38,39)*. In fact, reported reductions of chronic disease risk achieved with the Mediterranean diet exceed those achieved using the USDA Food Guide Pyramid.

The Mediterranean diet also incorporates daily physical activity at the base of the pyramid as an integral part of healthy weight, fitness, and well being. The basic nutrition message of the pyramid is emphasis on plant-based foods, low in saturated and *trans* fats. Other key dietary principles include: (1) an abundance of foods from plant sources, including fruits and vegetables, potatoes, bread and grains, beans, nuts, and seeds; (2) emphasis on a variety of minimally processed foods; (3) olive oil as the principal fat source; (4) total fat intake ranging from <25% to over 35% of total calories with saturated fat not to exceed 7–8% of calories; (5) daily consumption of low-to-moderate amounts of cheese and yogurt, preferably low-fat or nonfat versions; (6) weekly consumption of low-to-moderate amounts of fish and poultry with minimal use of eggs (0–4/wk); (7) fresh fruit used as the typical dessert to replace fat-dense sweets; and (8) red meat limited to a few times per month. Moderate consumption of wine is recommended to accompany meals, with the disclaimer that wine should be considered optional and avoided whenever consumption would put the individual or others "at risk."

The Mediterranean diet pyramid profiles a dietary pattern that is appropriate for most healthy adults, providing a model for a highly palatable, healthful framework to facilitate dietary behavior change. However, the nutritional needs of special populations require further consideration. In regard to older adults, the Mediterranean pyramid does not promote milk consumption since milk historically was a minor component of traditional Mediterranean diets *(37)*. Compromised calcium and vitamin D intake would be an undesirable consequence for the older population. For this reason, inclusion of calcium supplements and/or encouraged intake of nonfat milk would be appropriate recommendations for older persons using this diet.

In its most recent national health policy statement, Healthy People 2010, the US government similarly provides goals and guidelines for improving population health *(40)*, including 12 objectives related specifically to cardiovascular disease. These objectives emphasize the importance of maintaining a healthy weight, avoiding obesity, increasing physical activity, and providing nutrition education to patients with certain chronic diseases. Diet-related objectives promote increased consumption of fruits, vegetables and whole grains, reduced saturated fat intake, moderation in total fat, and reduced sodium intake. The similarity of these general dietary recommendations with those aimed at disease prevention is conspicuous. Age is a risk factor for CVD, and as a general rule, it is prudent to maintain a heart-healthy diet into older age.

Food is the best vehicle for nutrient consumption. Yet, many nutrition experts also believe that a daily multivitamin-mineral supplement for elders is a reasonable way to ensure adequacy of micronutrient intake *(41)*. A daily supplement that provides 100% of the US Recommended Dietary Allowances (RDA) with very low or no iron is often considered a prudent addition to an oral diet. The American Medical Association recommends this type of supplement particularly for seniors who have decreased food intake *(42)*. The American Dietetic Association encourages a vitamin supplement based on an individualized dietary assessment *(43)*.

In principle, dietary variety and nutrient adequacy are especially important for primary or secondary prevention of vascular disease. However, although older adults experience fundamental changes in their nutritional requirements, as well as changes in nutrient absorption, utilization, and excretion with aging *(44–46)*, standard dietary recommendations have typically not been tailored to address the unique needs of the elderly. While the RDAs are the levels of essential nutrients that the Food and Nutrition Board of the National Academy of Sciences judges to be adequate to meet the known needs of healthy people *(47)*, they do not provide separate recommendations for people in specific age categories above the age of 51 yr *(48)*. In contrast, the Dietary Reference Intakes (DRIs) *(49,50)* use newer reference values to guide nutrient adequacy. The DRIs provide guidelines for two segments of the older population: adults aged 51–70 yr and those over the age of 70. It is notable that DRIs for calcium, folate, and vitamin B_{12} are higher than the RDAs for these nutrients *(51,52)* Nonetheless, the RDAs are still considered by most experts to be the best guide for evaluating dietary intakes of most nutrients in the absence of DRI values *(53)*.

3. SPECIAL CHALLENGES OF DIET MODIFICATION IN A GERIATRIC POPULATION

Nutritional challenges in the older population encompass a range of issues, from undernutrition and cachexia to overnutrition and obesity *(54)*. Both ends of the spectrum are associated with high morbidity and mortality. Furthermore, the high prevalence of salt addiction, alcoholism, and multiple comorbidities (including diabetes mellitus) among the elderly adds to the complexity of the issue.

Multiple factors compound risks for malnutrition among elders. Poverty, social isolation, polypharmacy, frailty, dementia, depression, poor dentition and oral health, chewing and swallowing problems, sensory impairment, functional disability, presence of multiple acute or chronic comorbid conditions, and physiologic changes affecting digestion, absorption, and/or metabolism of nutrients *(55)* are among a long list of age-related barriers to adequate nutrition. In addition, many elderly cannot afford food, shop for groceries, prepare meals, or plan and obtain a balanced and varied diet. Research has demonstrated that those at greatest risk are the oldest-old, minorities, and those who either live alone or live in long-term care facilities *(43)*.

For elders who are particularly vulnerable to undernutrition, maintaining the desire to eat and the enjoyment of food is often the focus of supportive care *(56)*. In this circumstance, a fairly liberalized nutrition intervention is warranted to minimize the risk of weight loss and its associated mortality. A low-dose multivitamin-mineral supplement is also recommended *(43,57)*.

At the other end of the spectrum, weight management is the cornerstone of most therpeutic interventions since a high proportion of elders are overweight *(58)*. Approximately one quarter of the older US population is obese and only 36% of adults over age 60 are at a healthy body weight *(40)*. Obesity is a risk factor for multiple chronic health conditions, including CVD *(59,60)*. Diabetes and hypertension are also more common among obese adults, exacerbating the probability these adults will suffer from vascular stiffening, atherosclerosis, autonomic dysfunction, impaired vasodilation, and poor prognosis. The most appropriate range of body mass index (BMI) reflective of healthy body weight for older adults is controversial. The National Heart Lung and Blood Institute defines overweight as a BMI of 25–29.9 and obesity as a BMI of 30 *(61)*.

4. DIETARY MANAGEMENT OF LIPID DISORDERS IN OLDER ADULTS

Given the increasing prevalence of CVD with aging, and given that abnormal cholesterol levels unequivocally predict atherosclerosis and CVD in younger adults, interest in cholesterol as a disease predictor in the elderly has been extensively evaluated. National Health and Examination Survey III (NHANES III) demonstrated high total cholesterol (≥240 mg/dL) in 39% of adults aged 65–74 yr and 32% of those aged ≥75 *(62)*. However, multiple epidemiologic trials studying the predictive value of total cholesterol, LDL cholesterol, and low high-density lipoprotein (HDL)-cholesterol have led to divergent conclusions.

Several epidemiologic studies demonstrated positive correlations between cholesterol indices and CVD in older adults. In the Bronx Aging Study, a 10-yr prospective study of elders aged 75–85 yr, low HDL cholesterol predicted coronary events in men and elevated LDL cholesterol predicted coronary events in women *(63)*. Data from the Systolic Hypertension in the Elderly Program (SHEP) similarly demonstrated that total, non-HDL, and LDL cholesterol were predictive of coronary heart disease *(64)*. Corti et al. studied 4066 adults over 70 yr of age in the Established Populations for Epidemiologic Studies in Elderly and demonstrated that low HDL cholesterol predicted coronary heart disease events and mortality *(65)*.

In contrast, other epidemiologic studies indicated ambiguous and even inverse associations between cholesterol and both morbidity and mortality. Kronmal et al. demonstrated that although elevated total cholesterol and LDL cholesterol were predictive of cardiovascular mortality among adults aged 40 yr, their predictive significance attenuated with advancing age and became negative after age 80 *(66)*. Although high HDL cholesterol was predictive of cardiovascular survival, these benefits declined with age. The study also showed increased total mortality among those with lower LDL, presumably offsetting its cardiovascular benefits.

Similarly, Krumholz et al. demonstrated *(67)* that hypercholesterolemia and low HDL cholesterol did not predict coronary heart disease mortality or hospitalizations among a medicare population. In fact, higher total cholesterol (≥240 mg/dL) in women predicted relatively lower mortality when these women were compared to those with lower cholesterol values.

More recently, Schatz et al. published an analysis of 3572 Japanese American men, aged 71–93 yr, who were prospectively followed for 20 yr. In this population, low cholesterol had a significant association with mortality (risk ratio 1.64, 95% confidence interval [CI] 1.13–2.36), and long-term persistence of low cholesterol increased the risk of death *(68)*.

In the face of such disparate trial outcomes, conflicting hypotheses emerged. Some suggested that older adults most susceptible to the biological effects of cholesterol typically expired before they reached old age. According to this point of view, those surviving into old age were genetically constituted to endure, irrespective of lipid levels. Others suggested that certain ethnic or socioeconomic groups of patients studied in some investigations were relatively more at risk from cholesterol-related morbidity and mortality than those studied in other trials. Others hypothesized that low cholesterol was a marker of frailty and that frailty undermined overall survival, despite a marginal cardiac benefit (69).

Grundy, et al. suggested that a methodological nuance contributed to divergent conclusions concerning the role of cholesterol. Atherosclerosis is cumulative with aging, which implicitly narrows the quantification of the relative risk attributable to abnormal lipid indices, but not the absolute risk of disease (70). Manolio et al. (71) substantiated this point by demonstrating that total cholesterol and LDL cholesterol correlated with coronary heart disease mortality in men and women across a broad age range (including adults aged 65–100 yr), despite that the relative risk of hypercholesterolemia decreased with age.

In the midst of sometimes heated controversy about the implications and value of cholesterol indices, changes in the paradigms of CVD fundamentally impacted cholesterol management in all adults, including the elderly. Earlier conceptions of CVD envisage atherosclerosis with progressive accumulation of lipid deposits eventually clogging arteries. However, newer conceptions of CVD envisaged acute plaque rupture, platelet consolidation, and underlying endothelial function as key pathophysiological mechanisms, independent of lipid lesion size (72). Related notions of therapeutic cholesterol reduction shifted from an emphasis on reducing lesion size to goals of plaque stabilization and endothelial health. Moreover, atherosclerosis became recognized as a diffuse process, with an impact extending beyond the coronary vessels to include the cerebrovascular and peripheral arteries.

This evolution in the understanding and the implications of the disease itself changed the perception of cholesterol-lowering therapy. Study endpoints expanded beyond mortality to include broader effects, including reduced composite cardiovascular events, improved functional status, improved quality of life, and even improved cognition (i.e., reduced dementia). Likewise, indices of efficacy evolved from mere changes in lumen diameter to dynamic measurements of vascular performance (e.g., flow-mediated dilation of the brachial artery and/or acetylcholamine mediated vasoresponses of the coronary arteries). With these fundamental shifts in perspectives and therapeutic goals, the focus on lipids was catapulted from the realms of academic debates about epidemiologic data into the mainstream of clinical medicine with endpoints that often riveted the attention of physicians and patients, even before definitive data were available.

4.1. Cholesterol-Lowering Therapy with Statins

Coincident with the shifts in the paradigms of atherosclerotic disease, cholesterol reduction trials using statins and dietary therapy emerged. These trials demonstrated unequivocal therapeutic benefits of cholesterol lowering therapy. In the Scandinavian Simvastatin Survival Trial (4S trial) (73), patients with hypercholesterolemia and established coronary heart disease treated with simvastatin achieved 30% reduced mortality, 42% fewer cardiac endpoints, and 37% fewer cardiac procedures. Post hoc analyses demonstrated reduced secondary cardiovascular morbidity and mortality in adults aged 65 and 75 yr, with benefits comparable to those seen in younger age groups (74). In the Cholesterol and Recurrent Events (CARE) Trial, patients with average cholesterol levels treated with pravastatin achieved a 24% reduction in myocardial infarction and coronary events and a 27% reduction in coronary revascularization rates (75). Older patients in CARE derived benefits similar to those observed in younger adults (76). Similarly, in the Long-Term Intervention with Pravastatin in Ischemic Disease (LIPID) trial, results similar to the 4S and CARE trials were observed *(77)*. In LIPID, total mortality was reduced by 24% in those prescribed pravastatin, and the benefits of statin therapy extended to those older than 65 yr of age *(78)*. More recently, the Prospective Study of Pravastatin in the Elderly at Risk (PROSPER) trial was published *(78a)*. This trial focused specifically at elderly adults (70–82 yr) with a history or risk factors for vascular disease. Among the 2804 men and 3000 women enrolled, randomized treatment with 40 mg pravastatin yielded a 15% reduction in the primary composite endpoint of CHD-related death, nonfatal MI, and stroke (16.2% vs 14.1%; $p = 0.14$).

Even primary prevention trials with statins have demonstrated the efficacy of cholesterol reduction. In the West of Scotland Coronary Prevention Study (WOSCOPS), pravastatin reduced major coronary events by 31% with similar reductions in cardiac procedures and cardiac mortality *(79)*. Benefits extended to both younger and older adults. Likewise, in the Air Force/Texas Coronary Atherosclerosis Prevention Study (AFCAPS/TexCAPS study), lovastatin decreased major coronary events by 37% *(80)* in younger and older adults.

Not only does cholesterol reduction lower mortality and cardiac event rates related to hypercholesterolemia, but physiological studies demonstrate changes in artherosclerotic plaques consistent with stabilization *(81)* and improvement in endothelial function *(82,83)*. Therefore, even in older, frail adults with uncertain expectations of mortality benefit, the potential to change plaque constitution and reduce morbidity seems substantial. Cholesterol reduction has, for example, been demonstrated to reduce strokes *(84,85)*, to increase functional capacity among adults with peripheral arterial disease, and to possibly reduce dementia. All these benefits are logical with therapy that diffusely improves vascular function and related physiological manifestations. All are especially relevant to an older population *(86,87)* that is prone to these vascular limitations.

4.2. The National Cholesterol Education Program

The most recent recommendations from the expert panel that guides the National Cholesterol Education Program (NCEP) place strong emphasis on dietary intervention for both primary prevention and secondary management of coronary heart disease (CHD) *(88)*. The report specifically advocates for nutrition and lifestyle interventions among the older population. The panel urges the application of these recommendations to both men and women and across diverse racial and ethnic groups. It is noted that most new CHD events and most coronary deaths occur in older persons (65 yr and older), and that a high level of LDL cholesterol and low HDL cholesterol still carry predominant predictive power for the development of CHD in older adults *(88)*. For primary prevention, therapeutic lifestyle changes are the first line of therapy for older adults and replace Step 1 and Step 2 diets. In the case of secondary prevention, no firm age restrictions appear necessary when selecting persons with established CHD for LDL-lowering therapy.

Primary prevention of CHD requires a public health approach that emphasizes population-based behavioral lifestyle changes, including reduced intakes of saturated fat and dietary cholesterol, increased physical activity, and weight control *(88)*. For high-risk individuals, preventive strategies are intensified with clinical therapies and cholesterol-lowering drugs as appropriate. The goals of primary prevention are to lower population cholesterol levels (specifically LDL cholesterol) and to reduce CHD risk.

Secondary prevention also focuses on LDL cholesterol lowering. As discussed, recent clinical trials demonstrate that LDL-lowering therapy with statins reduces total mortality, coronary mortality, major coronary events, coronary artery procedures, and stroke in persons with established CHD *(88)*. For individuals requiring lipid-lowering drugs, adjunctive dietary therapy is indicated as a means of potentially reducing the dosage and/or the number of drugs required to reach NCEP targets for blood lipid levels *(89)*. Thus, lifestyle modifications and pharmacological interventions are appropriately targeted for candidates for secondary prevention. Medical and nutritional supervision is warranted for these individuals to monitor both the effectiveness of the therapy and the overall nutritional adequacy of the modified diet with respect to intake levels of micronutrients, essential fatty acids, and protein *(89)*.

NCEP's current dietary recommendations limit saturated fat intake to no more than 7% of total calories and dietary cholesterol to <200 mg/d *(88)*. NCEP's dietary advice is largely consistent with the Dietary Guidelines for Americans 2000 *(90)* calling for 50–60% of calories from carbohydrate and 20–30 g of fiber per day. One exception is that, in the NCEP diet, the total fat intake is allowed to range from 25–35% of total calories, as long as intake levels of saturated fats and *trans* fatty acids are kept low *(88)*. This is in contrast to the Dietary Guideline to keep total fat intake at or below 30% of calories. NCEP's flexibility on total fat intake is intended to encourage higher intakes of unsaturated fat, which can help reduce triglycerides and raise HDL cholesterol levels in persons with the metabolic syndrome.

Traits of abdominal obesity, atherogenic dyslipidemia, elevated blood pressure, insulin resistance, and prothrombic and proinflammatory states are recognized together as the metabolic syndrome mandating secondary risk-reduction therapeutic targets. Physiologic studies indicate that these traits correlate to increased likelihood of coronary heart disease as well as vascular stiffening *(91)*. In individuals with the metabolic syndrome, weight reduction and increased physical activity are emphasized in addition to the dietary modifications for saturated fat and cholesterol intake *(88)*. Weight reduction will enhance LDL lowering and will reduce all of the risk factors of the metabolic syndrome. Regular physical activity will reduce very low density lipoprotein (VLDL) cholesterol levels, increase HDL cholesterol, and in some individuals, lower LDL levels. Exercise offers other advantages because it can lower blood pressure, reduce insulin resistance, and improve cardiovascular function.

5. PREVENTION AND TREATMENT OF HYPERTENSION

Sodium intake, as well as obesity and alcohol consumption, influence blood pressure *(92)*. Despite proven benefits of antihypertensive medications to reduce strokes and CHD in middle-aged and older adults *(20,93)*, interest in lifestyle behavioral interventions for hypertension has grown. Observational and experimental evidence demonstrates a strong relationship between nutrition and blood pressure *(94)*.

Risks associated with salt ingestion have a strong physiological basis in older adults. A high-salt diet correlates to increased vessel stiffness *(95)*, particularly in relation to age *(96)*. Furthermore, among subsets of vulnerable adults, salt intake blunts production of nitrous oxide which diminishes normal vascular relaxation *(97,98)*. Such increased vascular stiffness and blunted vasodilation predispose elders to high intraluminal systolic stress because there is little compliance to modify volume-related pressures. Older adults are more likely to be "salt sensitive" with dietary indiscretion translating quickly into hypertension and fluid overload. The physiologic basis for this scenario is the intrinsically reduced vascular compliance in elders and reduced sodium clearance that occurs from natural senescent changes in the kidney.

National guidelines for the prevention and treatment of hypertension advocate a number of lifestyle and nutritional strategies, including reduced sodium intake, weight control, reduced alcohol consumption, and possibly increased dietary potassium *(99)*. Although alcohol and weight reduction strategies are widely embraced, concerns have been raised that sodium reduction might paradoxically worsen overall outcomes. An observational study by Alderman et al. suggested that consumption of a low-sodium diet was associated with increased coronary risk *(100)*. Likewise, Alderman et al. demonstrated an inverse relationship between dietary sodium and all-cause CVD mortality in a separate study *(101)*. Whereas these conclusions have been challenged on methodological grounds *(102)*, they do raise questions as to whether sodium restriction could inadvertently harm adults who, despite poor acute sodium excretion, are also more susceptible to impaired sodium homeostasis with natural vulnerability to hyponatremia. Therefore, there has been particular interest in clinical trial data to assess the safety and the clinical efficacy of sodium reduction, as well as the feasibility of sodium interventions in large, community-based populations.

Currently, average sodium intake in the United States is 150 mmol/d, which is equivalent to 3.5 g of sodium or 8.7 g of sodium chloride. National guidelines recommend limiting average daily salt consumption to 100 mmol/d (equivalent to 2.3 g of sodium or 5.8 g of sodium chloride) *(99)*. In practice, this may be difficult for many older adults. Taste sensation is often diminished as a function of age, producing a greater desire for salty foods, although there is evidence this might diminish with long-term dietary sodium reduction *(103)*. Elders also have reduced capacity to prepare fresh foods and rely more heavily on processed and convenience foods, accounting for a commonly observed increase in salt intake among older adults. Whereas several food manufacturers have created lines of low sodium products, their costs are often prohibitive and their distribution may be limited. These barriers have created much interest in trials testing the efficacy, safety, and durability of salt restriction among elderly adults.

5.1. Dietary Approaches to Stop Hypertension

The Dietary Approaches to Stop Hypertension (DASH) trial was a feeding study that enrolled 459 adults with systolic blood pressures of less than 160 mm Hg and diastolic blood pressures of 80–95 mm Hg *(92)*. A *fruits-and-vegetables diet* providing high amounts of fiber, potassium, and magnesium and a *combination diet* (rich in fruits and vegetables along with low-fat dairy foods, with reduced total fat, saturated fat and cholesterol content) were contrasted with a control diet (*see also* Chapter 16).

The combination diet lowered systolic blood pressure by 5.5 mm Hg and diastolic blood pressure by 3.0 mm Hg more than the control diet. The fruits-and-vegetables diet lowered blood pressure, but to a lesser extent (by 2.8 mm Hg for systolic and 1.1 mm Hg for diastolic). Furthermore, three different levels of daily salt consumption (142 mmol, 107 mmol, and 65 mmol) were analyzed for each group. At each level of decreased salt intake in each of the diets, there were significant stepwise reductions in blood pressures. The gradient of blood pressure reduction observed across the diets indicates that some aspects of the fruits-and-vegetables diet reduced blood pressure and that additional features of the combination diet reduced it even further. The reduction in blood pressure occurred within 2 wk and was sustained for the next 6 wk. Of additional importance, adherence to the modified diets was excellent *(92)*.

Among the study's implications, salt restriction seemed feasible and safe, and the dietary patterns tested in the DASH trial seem to be reasonable targets for the general US population. The fruits-and-vegetables diet provided 8–10 servings of fruits and vegetables per day. This level is higher than the 5–7 daily servings now recommended by the Dietary Guidelines for Americans. However, the combination diet provided 2.7 daily servings of low-fat dairy products, a level consistent with the 2–3 servings recommended by the Dietary Guidelines. Widespread adoption of the DASH combination diet could potentially shift the population distribution of blood pressure downward, reducing the occurrence of blood pressure-related CVD (104). A population-wide reduction in blood pressure of the magnitude observed in the DASH trial would reduce incident CHD by an estimated 15% and stroke by approx 27% (105).

5.2. Trial of Nonpharmacologic Interventions in the Elderly

The Trial of Nonpharmacologic Interventions in the Elderly (TONE) was conducted to determine the feasibility, efficacy, and safety of sodium reduction and weight loss specifically in older persons (aged 60–85 yr) with hypertension (94). In this study, 875 men and women aged 60–80 yr receiving antihypertensive medication were recruited. Those who were obese ($n = 585$) were randomized to reduced sodium intake, weight loss, both, or usual care. Those who were not obese ($n = 390$) were randomized to reduced sodium intake or usual care. Nutritionists and exercise counselors implemented the active interventions and monitored participants throughout intensive, extended, and maintenance phases of the program. Withdrawal of antihypertensive medication was a goal for all study participants and was attempted after 3 mo of intervention. Participants were followed for up to 36 mo (median 29 mo). Protocol completion was quite high, averaging approx 90% at follow-up and final evaluations (94).

The main outcome measure was diagnosis of high blood pressure at one or more follow-up visits, treatment with antihypertensive medication, or a cardiovascular event during follow-up. The combined hypertension outcome was less frequent among those assigned vs not assigned to reduced sodium intake (relative hazard ratio, 0.69; 95% CI, 0.59–0.81) and, in obese participants, among those assigned vs not assigned to weight loss (relative hazard ratio, 0.70; 95% CI, 0.57–0.87). Compared to usual care, reduced sodium intake and weight loss each contributed to lower risk among obese participants when tested individually (hazard ratios were 0.60 [95% CI, 0.45–0.80] and 0.64 [95% CI, 0.49–0.85], respectively). Combined sodium reduction and weight loss therapy resulted in a more dramatic lowering of risk among obese individuals (0.47 [95% CI, 0.35–0.64]). The frequency of cardiovascular events was similar in each of the six treatment groups.

The TONE trial provides compelling evidence in support of the feasibility, efficacy, and safety of a dietary lifestyle intervention for controlling blood pressure and lessening the need for antihypertensive medication in older patients with hypertension (94). Moderate decreases in sodium intake (40 mmol/d) and body weight (on average, 3.5 kg) were achieved among elders in this study. Because those receiving the combined intervention program were most successful in maintaining desirable blood pressure control after withdrawal of their antihypertensive medication, this strategy is considered the preferred management approach.

Elders in this study were highly motivated to change their lifestyle behaviors in order to reduce their dependence on medication. The interventions were well tolerated, and there was no suggestion that drug withdrawal contributed to any increase in morbidity or mortality. Nor was there any evidence that dietary interventions contributed to nutritional inadequacy or that exercise regimens resulted in any adverse physical effects *(94)*. Older patients with hypertension were capable of making and sustaining lifestyle modifications, demonstrating that specific behaviors are amenable to change with proper guidance and monitoring from trained health professionals. Such change translates directly into observable and measurable health benefits for older adults.

6. DIETARY ANTIOXIDANTS AND VASCULAR DISEASE

Observational epidemiologic studies, including descriptive, case-control, and cohort studies, have demonstrated that higher intakes of dietary antioxidants are associated with lower CVD risk *(89)*. Results from these studies have been most suggestive for an effect due to carotenoids and vitamin E, whereas results for other antioxidant nutrients have been inconsistent *(106,107)*. Because most of the studies have involved the consumption of antioxidant-rich foods including fruits, vegetables, and whole grains, AHA recommends achieving higher intakes of dietary antioxidants by increasing the consumption of these specific food groups *(89)*. The evidence necessary to recommend the use of antioxidant supplements, including vitamin E, for population-wide primary prevention of disease is considered insufficient *(108)*. Similarly, the balance of the evidence does not support the use of vitamin E supplements in individuals with established CVD or among those who are at high risk for CVD *(89)*.

7. B VITAMINS AND HOMOCYSTEINE

Homocysteine, a marker for the development of vascular disease *(109)*, requires an adequate supply of folate, vitamin B_6, vitamin B_{12}, and riboflavin for its metabolism. Levels of these vitamins correlate inversely with levels of circulating homocysteine, because they function as cofactors and substrates in the metabolism of methoinine and homocysteine. Normal levels of fasting plasma homocysteine are considered to be between 5 and 15 µmol/L, whereas moderate, intermediate, and severe hyperhomocysteinemia refer to concentrations between 16 and 30, between 31 and 100, and >100 µmol/L, respectively *(110)*.

Intake levels of folate and vitamin B_6 that exceed the current RDAs have been suggested to be important for the primary prevention of CHD. This suggestion is based on findings from a prospective study in more than 80,000 women followed for 14 yr, showing a significant reduction in CHD risk associated with higher intake levels of folate and vitamin B_6 *(111,112)*. Research has linked folate and vitamin B_6 nutritional status to the metabolism of homocysteine and CHD risk *(113,114)*. In a subset of participants of the Framingham Study, carotid artery atherosclerosis was inversely proportional to reported intakes of both folic acid and vitamin B_6 *(115)*.

In light of the apparent relationship of plasma homocysteine to CVD risk and the estimated influence of folic acid on homocysteine levels, it has been suggested that a 359 µg/d increase in folic acid intake in men and 280 µg/d increase in women could potentially prevent 30,500 and 19,000 vascular deaths annually in men and women, respectively *(116)*. However, the clinical benefits of such interventions remain unknown in the absence of any prospective, controlled intervention trials.

The most recent recommendations of the Food and Nutrition Board of the Academy of Sciences Institute of Medicine provides DRIs for folic acid, vitamin B_6 and vitmain B_{12} of 400 µg, 1.7 mg, and 2.4 µg, respectively (52). Because a large proportion of the population does not meet the current DRIs for folic acid, a prudent public health approach would recommend an increase in the intake of folate-rich foods, including ready-to-eat fortified cereals (preferably whole grain cereals), other whole grain foods, green leafy vegetables, fruits, and legumes. Promoting dietary adequacy for vitamin B_6 would emphasize the inclusion of ready-to-eat fortified cereals, non-citrus fruits, poultry, lean beef, and certain vegetables (artichokes, asparagus, beans, and cabbage). Vitamin B_{12} intake could be enhanced with the inclusion of lean beef, poultry, fish, dairy products, and ready-to-eat fortified cereals. Specifically, adults over the age of 50 are advised to consume foods fortified with vitamin B_{12} or a B_{12}-containing supplement since as many as 10–30% of older adults may malabsorb food-bound vitamin B_{12} (52). Dietary modifications such as these would result in improved vitamin nutritional status and may translate to lower homocysteine levels within the population (110).

Initial population studies have shown that fortification of food grains with folic acid, mandated by the FDA for the prevention of neural tube defects, has probably already lowered population homocysteine levels (89,117). Physiological studies add to the rationale to treat high homocysteine by demonstrating efficacy to improve indices of endothelial performance (118). Additional epidemiologic studies are needed to confirm preliminary observations and to assess the effects, if any, of increased folic acid intake on the prevalence of vascular disease.

8. VASCULAR INDICES TO GUIDE MANAGEMENT

Unfortunately, there is no gold standard by which vascular health can be definitively assessed. Thus, the precision of management will continue to be limited by the imprecision of the available diagnostic techniques. Whereas blood pressure was once the primary criteria of vascular health, even normotensive subsets of adults are prone to disease because of risk factors, including blood cholesterol, diabetes, and homocysteine, that contribute to persistent risk (7,119). Trying to ascertain an elemental measure of vascular health that incorporates all risk factors has remained elusive.

Even the utility of blood pressure as an index of vascular health has become complicated with greater consideration of pulse pressure to assess vascular performance. As adults age, vascular stiffening translates into higher systolic pressures, but lower diastolic pressures as a result of loss of intrinsic tone as the elastin tissue fragments. Multiple studies cite widened pulse pressure as a marker of these tissue changes and demonstrate the predictive power of pulse pressure on cardiovascular morbidity and mortality. However, the integration of blood pressure and pulse pressure in terms of clear therapeutic goals remains less clear (120,121). For example, treatment of mild hypertension pharmacologically is confounded if it also widens pulse pressure. Fortunately, diet and exercise have been demonstrated to produce a predominant clinical benefit.

Assessment of atherosclerotic burden and the benefits of vitamin therapy have also been complicated. Given that the sizes of atheromatous lesions do not predict their stability, a search for more sensitive and convenient indices of vascular health have been underway. Intimal-medial thickening is often used to assess the magnitude of atherosclerotic disease burden (122), but measures of vascular stiffness and flow-mediated vasodilation have also been used in different investigations (8,123). It becomes difficult to compare these studies and their conclusions, especially because there are growing insights that gender, age, and other population-specific variables probably confound these indices and their implications *(124)*.

9. THE AMERICAN HEART ASSOCIATION'S DIETARY GUIDELINES

As a convenient conclusion to this general overview of vascular aging and the therapeutic benefits of dietary intervention, the newly revised dietary guidelines from the American Heart Association (AHA) seem appropriate. These guidelines place a strong emphasis on foods (rather than nutrients) and an overall eating pattern that will promote dietary variety, balance, and nutritional adequacy *(89)*. Their focus is on population-wide recommendations for health maintenance and disease prevention among healthy individuals, yet they also identify strategies for medical nutrition therapy to treat those with specific risk factors or existing disease (i.e., further restricting saturated fat and cholesterol intakes among individuals with elevated LDL cholesterol levels or existing CVD).

The guidelines promote weight management, achieved through balanced energy intake and a regular pattern of physical exercise; moderate fat intake ($\leq$30% of calories); reduced saturated fat intake ($\leq$10% of calories); and restricted cholesterol intake (<300 mg/d). The AHA recommends an eating pattern that is rich in fruits, vegetables, and low-fat dairy products along with limited salt intake (<6 g/d; the equivalent of 2400 mg of sodium/d) and moderation of alcohol consumption (no more than 2 drinks/d for men and 1 for women). Vitamin, mineral, and fiber supplements should not be substituted for a balanced and nutritious diet that is designed to be rich in fruits, vegetables, and grains.

10. SUMMARY

The added dimension of this review is the understanding that dietary guidelines impact the vasculature of older adults. Vascular stiffening, vasomotor function, morphology, and vulnerability to atherosclerosis are all integrally related to food choices and related patterns of age-related change. There are multiple mechanisms of senescent vascular change that progressively predispose to disease in the vasculature itself, as well as the heart and bodily functions that depend on vascular flow. Although there is ever-present theoretical rationale to consider supplements or pharmaceutical products that might enhance vascular health, definitive indices to guide interventions are still controversial. In any case, basic dietary and lifestyle choices remain pivotal starting points for healthy living and prevention of otherwise likely vascular changes and clinical declines that typically occur with age.

11. RECOMMENDATIONS FOR CLINICIANS

1. General recommendations include maintaining a health weight, engaging regularly in physical activity, eating a variety of foods and selecting a diet low in saturated fat, salt, and processed foods; moderate in total fat and alcohol; and high in grains, fruits, and vegetables.
2. Treatment of lipid disorders should be carefully considered in older adults, given the potential benefit to reduce strokes, increase functional capacity in peripheral arterial disease and possibly reduce dementia. ATP guidelines for lipid disorders are to consume no more than 7% of total calories as saturated fat, avoid consumption of *trans*-saturated fats, and increase fiber in diet.

3. Salt restriction to 2.3 g of sodium per day for treatment of hypertension must be balanced against the risk of poor intake among some older adults because of decreased perceived flavor in a low-salt diet. Adoption of the DASH combination diet (rich in fruits, vegetables, and low-fat dairy foods) may be a more palatable alternative dietary intervention for older adults with hypertension.
4. Vitamin B_6, B_{12} and folate consumption should be encouraged in order to lower homocysteine levels and possibly cardiovascular risk.

REFERENCES

1. Hajdu MA , et al. Effects of aging on mechanics and composition of cerebral arterioles in rats. Circ Res 1990;66:1747–1754.
2. Safar M. Ageing and its effects on the cardiovascular system. Drugs 1990:39(suppl 1):1–8.
3. Gerhard M, et al. Aging progressively impairs endothelium-dependent vasodilation in forearm resistance vessels of humans. Hypertension 1996;27:849–853.
4. Jacob JM, Dorheim MA, Grammas P. The effect of age and injury on the expression of inducible nitric oxide synthase in facial motor neurons in F344 rats. Mech Ageing Dev 1999;107:205–218.
5. Taddei S, et al. Age-related reduction of NO availability and oxidative stress in humans. Hypertension 2001;38:274–279.
6. Pugh KG, Wei JY. Clinical implications of physiological changes in the aging heart. Drugs Aging 2001; 18:263–276.
7. Lakatta E. Aging effects on the vasculature in health: risk factors for cardiovascular disease. Am J Geriatr Cardiol 1994;3:11–17.
8. Zeiher AM, et al. Coronary atherosclerotic wall thickening and vascular reactivity in humans. Elevated high-density lipoprotein levels ameliorate abnormal vasoconstriction in early atherosclerosis. Circulation 1994;89:2525–2532.
9. Robert L. Aging of the vascular-wall and atherosclerosis. Exp Gerontol 1999;34:491–501.
10. Reaven PD, et al. Lipoprotein modification and atherosclerosis in aging. Exp Gerontol 1999;34:527–537.
11. Orlandi A, Marcellini M, Spagnoli LG. Aging influences development and progression of early aortic atherosclerotic lesions in cholesterol-fed rabbits. Arterioscler Thromb Vasc Biol 2000;20:1123–1136.
12. Wei JY. Age and the cardiovascular system. N Engl J Med 1992;327:1735–1739.
13. Karamanoglu M, et al. Functional origin of reflected pressure waves in a multibranched model of the human arterial system. Am J Physiol 1994;267:H1681–H1688.
14. Vaitkevicius PV, et al. Effects of age and aerobic capacity on arterial stiffness in healthy adults. Circulation 1993;88:1456–1462.
15. O'Rourke MF. Mechanical principles. Arterial stiffness and wave reflection. Pathol Biol (Paris) 1999; 47:623–633.
16. Lakatta EG. Catecholamines and cardiovascular function in aging. Endocrinol Metab Clin North Am 1987;16:877–891.
17. Colucci WS. The effects of norepinephrine on myocardial biology: implications for the therapy of heart failure. Clin Cardiol 1998;21(12 suppl 1):I20–I24.
18. Singh K, et al. Adrenergic regulation of myocardial apoptosis. Cardiovasc Res 2000;45:713–719.
19. Applegate WB. Systolic hypertension in older persons. Adv Intern Med 1992;37:37–54.
20. Staessen J, Fagard R, Amery A. Isolated systolic hypertension in the elderly: implications of Systolic Hypertension in the Elderly Program (SHEP) for clinical practice and for the ongoing trials. J Hum Hypertens 1991;5:469–474.
21. Nagai Y, et al. Increased carotid artery intimal-medial thickness in asymptomatic older subjects with exercise-induced myocardial ischemia. Circulation 1998;98:1504–1509.
22. Laurent S, et al. Arterial compliance is not diminished in hypertensive patients when compared at the same level of blood pressure. Arch Mal Coeur Vaiss 1994;87:1069–1072.
23. Laurent S, et al. Carotid artery distensibility and distending pressure in hypertensive humans. Hypertension 1994;23:878–883.
24. Laurent S. Arterial wall hypertrophy and stiffness in essential hypertensive patients. Hypertension 1995;26:355–362.

25. Celermajer DS, et al. Aging is associated with endothelial dysfunction in healthy men years before the age-related decline in women. J Am Coll Cardiol 1994;24:471–476.

26. Sorensen KE, et al. Impairment of endothelium-dependent dilation is an early event in children with familial hypercholesterolemia and is related to the lipoprotein(a) level. J Clin Invest 1994;93:50–55.

27. Muntinga JH, et al. Age-related differences in elastic properties of the upper arm vascular bed in healthy adults. J Vasc Res 1997;34:137–147.

28. Position of the American Dietetic Association: nutrition, aging, and the continuum of care. J Am Diet Assoc 2000;100:580–595.

29. Kumanyika S. Validating dietary guidance. J Am Coll Nutr 1995;14:215–216.

30. Marshall TA, et al. Inadequate nutrient intakes are common and are associated with low diet variety in rural, community-dwelling elderly. J Nutr 2001;131:2192–2196.

31. Lee J, Frongillo E. Nutritional and health consequences are asocated with food insecurity among US elderly persons. J Nutr 2001;131:1503–1509.

32. Cid-Ruzafa J, et al. Nutrition intakes and adequacy among an older population on the eastern shore of Maryland: the Salisbury eye evaluation. J Am Diet Assoc 1999;99:564–571.

33. Posner BM, et al. Nutritional risk in New England elders. J Gerontol 1994;49:M123–M132.

34. Grove NC, Spier BE. Motivating the well elderly to exercise. J Comm Health Nurs 1999;16:179–189.

35. Johnson RK, Kennedy E. The 2000 Dietary Guidelines for Americans: what are the changes and why were they made? The Dietary Guidelines Advisory Committee. J Am Diet Assoc 2000;100:769–774.

36. The Food Guide Pyramid, In: Home and Garden Bull. US Department of Agriculture, Washington, DC, 1992.

36a. Expert Committee of Nutrition and Health for Older Americans. The Nutrition and Health Campaign for Older Americans Toolkit. American Dietetic Association, Chicago, IL, 1998.

37. Nestle M. Mediterranean diets: science and policy implications. Am J Clin Nutrition 1995;61:6S.

38. Willet W. Diet and Health: What should we eat? Science 1994;264:532–537.

39. Lorgeril MD, et al. Mediterranean diet, traditional risk factors, and the rate of cardiovascular complications after myocardial infarction: final report of the Lyon Diet Heart Study. Circulation 1999;99: 779–785.

40. Healthy People 2010. US Department of Health and Human Services, Washington DC, 1999. http://web.health.gov//healthypeople.

41. Stampfer MJ, Willett WC. Homocysteine and marginal vitamin deficiency. The importance of adequate vitamin intake. JAMA 1993;270:2726–2727.

42. Vitamin preparations as dietary supplements and as therapeutic agents. Council on Scientific Affairs. JAMA 1987;257:1929–1936.

43. Nutrition recommendations and principles for people with diabetes mellitus. American Diabetes Association. Tenn Med 2000;93:430–433.

44. Das SK, et al. An underfeeding study in healthy men and women provides further evidence of impaired regulation of energy expenditure in old age. J Nutr 2001;131:1833–1838.

45. Wood RJ, Suter PM, Russell RM. Mineral requirements of elderly people. Am J Clin Nutr 1995;62: 493–505.

46. Blumberg, J., Nutritional needs of seniors. J Am Coll Nutr 1997;16:517–523.

47. Monsen ER. The 10th edition of the Recommended Dietary Allowances: what's new in the 1989 RDAs? J Am Diet Assoc 1989;89:1748–1752.

48. Food and nutrition board, National Academy of Sciences, Recommended Dietary Allowances, 10 ed. National Academy Press, Washington, DC, 1989.

49. Yates AA. Process and development of dietary reference intakes: basis, need, and application of recommended dietary allowances. Nutr Rev 1998;56:S5–S9.

50. Yates AA. Overview of key nutrients: energy and macronutrient aspects. Nutr Rev 1998;56:S29–S33.

51. Dietary reference intakes for calcium, phosphorus, magnesium, vitamin D, and fluoride, in Institute of Medicine, Food and Nutrition Board. National Academy Press, Washington, DC, 1997.

52. Dietary reference intakes for thiamin, riboflavin, niacin, vitamin B6, folate, vitamin B12, pantothenic acid, biotin, and choline, in Institute of Medicine, Food and Nutrition Board. National Academy Press, Washington, DC, 1998.

53. McCabe B, Dorey J. Health promotion and disease prevention in the elderly, In: Geriatric Nutrition. Chernoff R (ed.), Aspen Publishers, Gaithersburg, MD, 1999.

54. Millen B, Levine E. A continuum of nutrition services for older Americans, In: Geriatric Nutrition: A Health Professional's Handbook, Chernoff R (ed.), Aspen Publishers, Gaithersburg, MD, 1999, pp. 435–467.

55. Nutrition Screening Initiative. Report of Nutrition Screening 1. Toward a Common View. NSI, Washington, DC, 1991.

56. Liberalized diets for older adults in long-term care—Position of ADA. J Am Diet Assoc 1998;98: 201–204.

57. Tripp F. The use of dietary supplements in the elderly: current issues and recommendations. J Am Diet Assoc 1997;97(10 Suppl 2):S181–S183.

58. Mokdad AH, et al. The spread of the obesity epidemic in the United States, 1991–1998. JAMA 1999; 282:1519–1522.

59. Must A, Strauss RS. Risks and consequences of childhood and adolescent obesity. Int J Obes Relat Metab Disord 1999;23(Suppl)2:S2–S11.

60. Jensen GL, Rogers J. Obesity in older persons. J Am Diet Assoc 1998;98:1308–1311.

61. The National Heart, Lung, and Blood Institute Expert Panel on the identification, evaluation, and treatment of overweight and obesity in adults. Executive summary of the clinical guidelines of the identification, evaluation, and treatment of overweight and obesity in adults. J Am Diet Assoc 1998; 98:1178–1191.

62. Sundquist J, Winkleby MA, Pudaric S. Cardiovascular disease risk factors among older black, Mexican-American, and white women and men: an analysis of NHANES III, 1988-1994. Third National Health and Nutrition Examination Survey. J Am Geriatr Soc 2001;49:109–116.

63. Zimetbaum P, et al. Plasma lipids and lipoproteins and the incidence of cardiovascular disease in the very elderly. The Bronx Aging Study. Arterioscler Thromb 1992;12:416–423.

64. Frost PH, et al. Serum lipids and incidence of coronary heart disease. Findings from the Systolic Hypertension in the Elderly Program (SHEP). Circulation 1996;94:2381–2388.

65. Corti MC, et al. HDL cholesterol predicts coronary heart disease mortality in older persons. JAMA 1995;274:539–544.

66. Kronmal RA, et al. Total serum cholesterol levels and mortality risk as a function of age. A report based on the Framingham data. Arch Intern Med 1993;153:1065–1073.

67. Krumholz HM, et al. Lack of association between cholesterol and coronary heart disease mortality and morbidity and all-cause mortality in persons older than 70 years. JAMA 1994;272:1335–1340.

68. Schatz IJ, et al. Cholesterol and all-cause mortality in elderly people from the Honolulu Heart Program: a cohort study. Lancet 2001;358:351–355.

69. Corti MC, et al. Clarifying the direct relation between total cholesterol levels and death from coronary heart disease in older persons. Ann Intern Med 1997;126:753–760.

70. Grundy SM, et al. Cholesterol lowering in the elderly population. Coordinating Committee of the National Cholesterol Education Program. Arch Intern Med 1999;159:1670–1678.

71. Manolio TA, et al. Cholesterol and heart disease in older persons and women. Review of an NHLBI workshop. Ann Epidemiol 1992;2:161–176.

72. Brown BG, et al. Lipid lowering and plaque regression. New insights into prevention of plaque disruption and clinical events in coronary disease. Circulation 1993;87:1781–1791.

73. Randomised trial of cholesterol lowering in 4444 patients with coronary heart disease: the Scandinavian Simvastatin Survival Study (4S). Lancet 1994;344:1383–1389.

74. Miettinen TA, et al. Cholesterol-lowering therapy in women and elderly patients with myocardial infarction or angina pectoris: findings from the Scandinavian Simvastatin Survival Study (4S). Circulation 1997;96:4211–4218.

75. Sacks FM, et al. The effect of pravastatin on coronary events after myocardial infarction in patients with average cholesterol levels. Cholesterol and Recurrent Events Trial investigators. N Engl J Med 1996; 335:1001–1009.

76. Lewis SJ, et al. Effect of pravastatin on cardiovascular events in older patients with myocardial infarction and cholesterol levels in the average range. Results of the Cholesterol and Recurrent Events (CARE) trial. Ann Intern Med 1998;129:681–689.

77. Prevention of cardiovascular events and death with pravastatin in patients with coronary heart disease and a broad range of initial cholesterol levels. The Long-Term Intervention with Pravastatin in Ischaemic Disease (LIPID) Study Group. N Engl J Med 1998;339:1349–1357.

78. Hunt D, et al. Benefits of pravastatin on cardiovascular events and mortality in older patients with coronary heart disease are equal to or exceed those seen in younger patients: Results from the LIPID trial. Ann Intern Med 2001;134:931–940.

78a. Shepherd J, Blauw GJ, Murphy MB, et al. on behalf of the PROSPER study group. Pravastatin in elderly individuals at risk of vascular disease (PROSPER): a randomized controlled trial. Lancet 2002; 360:1623–1630.

79. Shepherd J, et al. Prevention of coronary heart disease with pravastatin in men with hypercholesterolemia. West of Scotland Coronary Prevention Study Group. N Engl J Med 1995;333:1301–1307.

80. Downs JR, et al. Primary prevention of acute coronary events with lovastatin in men and women with average cholesterol levels: results of AFCAPS/TexCAPS. Air Force/Texas Coronary Atherosclerosis Prevention Study. JAMA 1998;279:1615–1622.

81. Schartl M, et al. Use of intravascular ultrasound to compare effects of different strategies of lipid-lowering therapy on plaque volume and composition in patients with coronary artery disease. Circulation 2001;104:387–392.

82. Treasure CB, et al. Beneficial effects of cholesterol-lowering therapy on the coronary endothelium in patients with coronary artery disease. N Engl J Med 1995;332:481–487.

83. Anderson TJ, et al. The effect of cholesterol-lowering and antioxidant therapy on endothelium-dependent coronary vasomotion. N Engl J Med 1995;332:488–493.

84. Hebert PR, et al. Cholesterol lowering with statin drugs, risk of stroke, and total mortality. An overview of randomized trials. JAMA 1997;278:313–321.

85. Sacco RL, et al. High-density lipoprotein cholesterol and ischemic stroke in the elderly: the Northern Manhattan Stroke Study. JAMA 2001;285:2729–2735.

86. Simons M, et al. Cholesterol and Alzheimer's disease: is there a link? Neurology 2001;57:1089–1093.

87. Scott HD, Laake K. Statins for the reduction of risk of Alzheimer's disease (Cochrane Review). Cochrane Database Syst Rev 2001:3.

88. Executive Summary of The Third Report of The National Cholesterol Education Program (NCEP) Expert Panel on Detection, Evaluation, and Treatment of High Blood Cholesterol in Adults (Adult Treatment Panel III). JAMA 2001;285:2486–2497.

89. Krauss RM, et al. AHA Dietary Guidelines: revision 2000: A statement for healthcare professionals from the Nutrition Committee of the American Heart Association. Circulation 2000;102:2284–2299.

90. Service HNI. US Department of Health and Human Services, Nutrition and Your Health: Dietary Guidelines for Americans, US Department of Agriculture, Hyattsville, MD, 2000.

91. Sutton-Tyrrell K, et al. Aortic stiffness is associated with visceral adiposity in older adults enrolled in the study of health, aging, and body composition. Hypertension 2001;38:429–433.

92. Appel LJ, et al. A clinical trial of the effects of dietary patterns on blood pressure. DASH Collaborative Research Group. N Engl J Med 1997;336:1117–1124.

93. Hebert PR, et al. Recent evidence on drug therapy of mild to moderate hypertension and decreased risk of coronary heart disease. Arch Intern Med 1993;153:578–581.

94. Whelton PK, et al, Sodium reduction and weight loss in the treatment of hypertension in older persons: a randomized controlled trial of nonpharmacologic interventions in the elderly (TONE). TONE Collaborative Research Group. JAMA 1998;279:839–846.

95. Avolio AP, et al. Effects of aging on arterial distensibility in populations with high and low prevalence of hypertension: comparison between urban and rural communities in China. Circulation 1985;71: 202–210.

96. Khaw KT, Barrett-Connor E. Dietary potassium and blood pressure in a population. Am J Clin Nutr 1984;39:963–968.

97. Fujiwara N, et al. Study on the relationship between plasma nitrite and nitrate level and salt sensitivity in human hypertension: modulation of nitric oxide synthesis by salt intake. Circulation 2000;101:856–861.

98. Cubeddu LX, et al. Nitric oxide and salt sensitivity. Am J Hypertens 2000;13:973–979.

99. The sixth report of the Joint National Committee on prevention, detection, evaluation, and treatment of high blood pressure. Arch Intern Med 1997;157:2413–2446.

100. Alderman MH, et al., Association of the renin-sodium profile with the risk of myocardial infarction in patients with hypertension. N Engl J Med 1991;324:1098–1104.

101. Poulter NR. Dietary sodium intake and mortality: NHANES. The Faculty 31st International Society and Federation of Cardiology 10-day Teaching Seminar in Cardiovascular Disease, Epidemiology and Prevention. National Health and Nutrition Examination Survey. Lancet 1998;352:987–988.

102. He J, et al. Dietary sodium intake and subsequent risk of cardiovascular disease in overweight adults. JAMA 1999;282:2027–2034.

103. Bertino M, Beauchamp GK, Engelman K. Long-term reduction in dietary sodium alters the taste of salt. Am J Clin Nutr 1982;36:1134–1144.

104. Stamler J. Dietary salt and blood pressure. Ann NY Acad Sci 1993;676:122–156.

105. Cutler JA. Progress in life-style intervention for prevention and treatment of high blood pressure. Ann Epidemiol 1995;5:165–167.
106. Hennekens CH, et al. Antioxidant vitamin-cardiovascular disease hypothesis is still promising, but still unproven: the need for randomized trials. Am J Clin Nutr 1995;62(suppl 6):1377S–1380S.
107. Freedman JE. Antioxidant versus lipid-altering therapy—some answers, more questions. N Engl J Med 2001;345:1636–1637.
108. Tribble DL. AHA Science Advisory. Antioxidant consumption and risk of coronary heart disease: emphasison vitamin C, vitamin E, and beta-carotene: A statement for healthcare professionals from the American Heart Association. Circulation 1999;99:591–595.
109. Stampfer MJ, Malinow MR. Can lowering homocysteine levels reduce cardiovascular risk? N Engl J Med 1995;332:328–329.
110. Malinow M, Boston A, Krauss R. Homocyst(e)ine, diet, and cardiovascular disease: A statement for healthcare professionals from the nutrition committee, American Heart Association. Circulation 1999;99:178–182.
111. Koehler KM, et al. Association of folate intake and serum homocysteine in elderly persons according to vitamin supplementation and alcohol use. Am J Clin Nutr 2001;73:628–637.
112. Verhoef P, Stampfer MJ, Rimm EB. Folate and coronary heart disease. Curr Opin Lipidol 1998;9: 17–22.
113. Selhub J, et al. Vitamin status and intake as primary determinants of homocysteinemia in an elderly population. JAMA 1993;270:2693–2698.
114. Koehler KM, et al. Some vitamin sources relating to plasma homocysteine provide not only folate but also vitamins B-12 and B-6. J Nutr 1997;127:1534–1536.
115. Selhub J, et al. Assocation between homocysteine concentrations and extracranial carotid-artery stenosis. N Engl J Med 1995;332:286–291.
116. Boushey CJ, et al. A quantitative assessment of plasma homocysteine as a risk factor for vascular disease. Probable benefits of increasing folic acid intakes. JAMA 1995;274:1049–1057.
117. Jacques PF, et al. The effect of folic acid fortification on plasma folate and total homocysteine concentrations. N Engl J Med 1999;340:1449–1454.
118. Holven KB, et al. Effect of folic acid treatment on endothelium-dependent vasodilation and nitric oxide-derived end products in hyperhomocysteinemic subjects. Am J Med 2001;110:536–542.
119. Fraser GE. Diet and coronary heart disease: beyond dietary fats and low-density-lipoprotein cholesterol. Am J Clin Nutr 1994;59(suppl 5):1117S–1123S.
120. Weinberger MH, et al. Salt sensitivity, pulse pressure, and death in normal and hypertensive humans. Hypertension 2001;37:429–432.
121. Franklin SS. Cardiovascular risks related to increased diastolic, systolic and pulse pressure. An epidemiologist's point of view. Pathol Biol (Paris) 1999;47:594–603.
122. O'Leary DH, et al. Thickening of the carotid wall. A marker for atherosclerosis in the elderly? Cardiovascular Health Study Collaborative Research Group. Stroke 1996;27:224–231.
123. Ferrieres J, et al. Carotid intima-media thickness and coronary heart disease risk factors in a low-risk population. J Hypertens 1999;17:743–748.
124. Safar ME, et al. Stiffness of carotid artery wall material and blood pressure in humans: application to antihypertensive therapy and stroke prevention. Stroke 2000;31:782–790.

16 Nutritional Management of Hypertension in the Elderly

*Pao-Hwa Lin, Marji McCullough,
and Laura P. Svetkey*

1. INTRODUCTION

Hypertension, or high blood pressure, is prevalent in the United States and affects approx 50 million adults. It is a major risk factor for stroke and heart disease, which remain the first and third leading causes of death in the United States, and is therefore associated with a substantial financial and health care burden (*1*). Optimal blood pressure is defined as systolic blood pressure less than 120 mm Hg and diastolic blood pressure less than 80 mm Hg (or 120/80). Hypertension is defined as greater than or equal to 140/90 mm Hg. For most cases of hypertension (95%), also referred to as the essential hypertension, the causes are not clear. Although genetics may play a role, lifestyle factors like body weight, diet, and exercise are closely related.

1.1. Prevalence

Hypertension is common in US adults, particularly in the elderly. According to the phase I results of the National Health and Examination Survey (NHANES) III conducted between 1988 and 1991, the prevalence of hypertension was approx 25% among the overall population. This figure exceeded 50% in men and women aged 60 or older (Fig. 1) (*2*). Furthermore, among black women aged 60 and older, the prevalence of hypertension was nearly 80%. In some less industrialized nations, blood pressure does not rise with age (*3,4*), suggesting that the condition is not inevitable, but is somehow related to modernization. For the US population, NHANES III indicates that aging is not only associated with increasing prevalence of hypertension but also with an increasing severity. The shifting demographics in the United States, the growing segment of the elderly, and the high prevalence of hypertension all demand for more vigorous work in the areas of prevention, detection, and treatment of hypertension in this population.

From: *Handbook of Clinical Nutrition and Aging*
Edited by: C. W. Bales and C. S. Ritchie © Humana Press Inc., Totowa, NJ

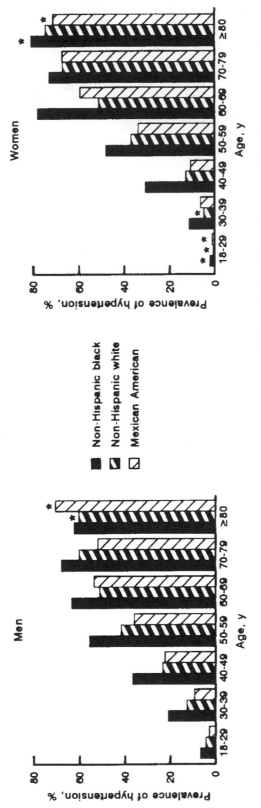

Fig. 1. Prevalence of hypertension by age and race/ethnicity for men and women, US population 18 yr of age and older. Hypertension defined as mean blood pressures greater or equal to 140/90 mm Hg or current treatment for hypertension with prescription medication. *Estimate based on sample size not meeting minimum requirements of the National Health and Nutrition Examination Survey III design or relative SEM greater than 30%. *Source:* ref. 2.

Table 1
Lifestyle Modifications for Hypertension Prevention and Management
as Recommended by the Sixth Report of the Joint National Committee
on Detection, Evaluation, and Treatment of High Blood Pressure (JNC VI)

1. Lose weight if overweight
2. Limit alcohol intake to less than 1 oz ethanol/d for men (2 drinks) or 0.5 oz ethanol/d for women
   and low-weight people (1 drink)
3. Increase aerobic physical activity, 30–45 min on most days
4. Reduce sodium intake to no more than 2300 mg/d
5. Maintain adequate intake of dietary potassium, about 3510 mg/d
6. Maintain adequate intake of dietary calcium and magnesium for general health
7. Stop smoking for overall cardiovascular health
8. Reduce intake of dietary saturated fat and cholesterol for overall cardiovascular health

1.2. Prevention and Treatment

Reducing blood pressure clearly decreases cardiovascular morbidity and mortality, and the benefit might even be more significant among older persons (5,6). Pharmacological treatment of hypertension has been shown to be very effective (7). Nonpharmacological strategies, also referred to as lifestyle modifications, have been efficient prevention and/or adjunct treatment strategy and are appropriate for adults of all ages (Table 1) (7).

Research has shown that the US population has made little progress in the JNC VI guidelines, including those directly related to diet. According to NHANES III, dietary intakes of potassium, calcium, and magnesium are all below the Recommended Daily Allowances (RDA) levels for those aged 50 and older, whereas, intakes of sodium, fat and saturated fat are greater than recommended in the same age group (8). These dietary patterns, either singularly or combined, may have contributed to the increasing prevalence of hypertension in the elderly.

This chapter presents an overview of the nutritional factors that have been associated with blood pressure control, their relevance to the elderly population, and a practical nutritional guideline for the prevention and management of hypertension in this population. It should be noted that keeping blood pressure within the optimal range (<120/80 mm Hg) is recommended for all adults, any reduction would confer health benefits on an individual level. In addition, small decreases in blood pressure across populations would result in a large decrease in the number of cardiovascular disease events (9).

2. INDIVIDUAL NUTRITIONAL FACTORS

Studies of individual nutrients and blood pressure are often subject to various design limitations, and thus results can be difficult to interpret. Whole food manipulation achieved under isocaloric conditions will inevitably change the intake of other nutrient(s) and dietary factors. As a result, it may be difficult to attribute the effect only to the change in any single nutrient. Nonetheless, there is evidence that certain nutrients play a role in blood pressure regulation.

2.1. Body Weight

Obesity is an important risk factor for both hypertension and cardiovascular diseases. Both observational and intervention trials have consistently shown the positive impact of weight loss on blood pressure control (10–18). Weight loss of approx 3–7 kg is associated with reduced blood pressure in individuals with high-normal blood pressure (16–18). In the Trials of Hypertension Prevention Phase I (TOHP) (19), weight loss was found to be the most successful factor in lowering blood pressure when compared to other nonpharmacological strategies. At the 6-mo follow-up, after rigorous counseling to reduce energy intake and increase exercise, men and women in the intervention group lost 6.5 and 3.7 kg, respectively. At study termination, blood pressure fell an average of 2.9/2.3 mm Hg overall after adjusting for the effect observed in the control group (18). After 7-yr follow-up in a subset of study participants, the odds of developing hypertension were reduced by 77% in the weight loss group (20), even though their long-term weight loss was nearly identical to that of the control group (4.9 kg and 4.5 kg, respectively). This addresses the potential effect of long-term weight loss and deserves further study. Additionally, significant weight loss (5%) is suggested to reduce the need for antihypertensive medication (21).

In the TOHP II (22), overweight adults received weight loss intervention during a 3-yr program. Blood pressure was significantly lower in the intervention group than in the control group at 6, 18, and 36 mo. In addition, the overall effect on blood pressure at 36 mo was a reduction of 0.35 mm Hg diastolic and 0.45 mm Hg systolic blood pressure per kg of weight loss. The trial of nonpharmacologic interventions in elderly (TONE) trial showed that obese older participants achieved a net reduction of 3.9 kg body weight at 30 mo. This weight loss reduced the hazard ratio, which indicates the rate of endpoints, including diagnosis of high blood pressure, treatment with antihypertensive medication, or a cardiovascular event, a measure describing how quickly subjects are dying, to 0.64 as compared to 1 for the usual care group. The hazard ratio for the sodium reduction and weight loss combined group was 0.47 as compared to the usual care. This study demonstrates that older individuals with hypertension were able to lose weight, sustain the weight lost, and improve their blood pressure control.

Energy needs decrease with advancing age, requiring a reduction in energy intake and contributing to the prevalence of obesity in the elderly. According to the NHANES III survey, the prevalence of overweight and obesity rises as the population ages (23). The subjects aged 70 and older had a combined prevalence of overweight and obesity greater than 50%. Table 2 shows the mean systolic blood pressure for different categories of BMI and different age groups among the US adult population. It is obvious that both age and body weight have a pronounced adverse impact on blood pressure.

It is not clear how weight loss reduces blood pressure, but it may involve mechanisms such as suppression of sympathetic nervous system activity, lowering insulin resistance, normalization of blood pressure regulating hormones (21), decreasing body sodium stores, decreasing blood volume and cardiac output, or increasing salt sensitivity (24–26).

2.2. Sodium

Sodium intake has been shown in observational studies to be associated with blood pressure (28,29). In the international study of salt and blood pressure (INTERSALT) study involving 10,079 men and women from 52 centers around the world (10), mean

Table 2
Mean Systolic Blood Pressure by Age and BMI from the NHANES III Survey

Mean ± SE	Total	BMI < 25	25 ≤ BMI < 27	27 ≤ BMI < 30	BMI > 30
Men					
20–39	118.7	116.3	118.8	120.2	125.2
40–59	125.6	122.2	123.9	125.9	130.7
60–79	137.1	135.7	137.5	136.4	139.4
80+	143.8	143.5	144.4	145.1	141.6
Women					
20–39	109.1	106.9	109.3	114.4	115.3
40–59	121.0	115.6	119.3	122.9	128.6
60–79	138.1	135.8	137.1	138.7	141.4
80+	149.5	148.3	150.5	151.9	149.1

From Brown et al. *(27)*.

urinary sodium excretion for each center was positively related to blood pressure. In a recent re-analysis of the original INTERSALT data, corrected for measurement error from use of single 24 h urine collections, 100 mmol/d (2300 mg sodium) increase in urinary sodium was associated with an increase of 3–6 mm Hg systolic and 0–3 mm Hg diastolic *(30)*. In a meta-analysis of observational studies, Law, et al. *(31)* reported somewhat stronger findings than INTERSALT, especially in the elderly and those with higher baseline blood pressures *(31)*, but diet and other confounders were not assessed in a standard manner across studies.

Intervention trials generally support the blood pressure lowering effect of sodium reduction, despite variability of study design, age, hypertension status, race and gender composition, amount and form of sodium provided, quantity and control of other nutrients in the diet, and degree of adherence to the diets *(32–35)*. Several meta-analyses of such trials have been conducted *(32,34,35)* and have found blood pressure reductions in both hypertensives and in nonhypertensives to varying degrees (range of systolic/diastolic blood pressure lowering in hypertensives: 3.7/0.9 to 5.8/2.5 mm Hg; range in nonhypertensives, 1.0/0.1 to 2.3/1.4 mm Hg). Graudal and colleagues also found that blood pressure regulating hormones, cholesterol, and LDL cholesterol levels increased on a low-salt diet in studies with extreme sodium reduction *(34)*. Many intervention trials have employed severe sodium restriction (e.g., 10 mEq, or 230 mg sodium per day), which is not practical to recommend outside a research setting, and most intervention studies of sodium reduction included younger subjects as research volunteers. In one study of 17 hypertensive participants with a mean age of 73, who were instructed to follow a 80–100 mEq sodium diet, only modest reductions and heterogeneous responses in blood pressure were observed. Using a crossover design, either a 80-mEq sodium supplementation or placebo was given to participants for 5 wk each. The placebo group had a significant reduction of 8 mm Hg in supine clinic systolic blood pressure only, but not standing or ambulatory blood pressures *(36)*. Perhaps the level of sodium in the diet was not low enough to produce important differences. This trial suggests that blood pressure readings in different settings (e.g., ambulatory monitoring) should be taken into consideration when evaluating the outcomes of intervention trials.

Although sodium reduction is recognized as an effective strategy in lowering blood pressure in the hypertensives, its effectiveness has been debated for individuals without hypertension *(37,38)*. However, some trials of sodium and blood pressure have found greater blood pressure responses among elderly nonhypertensives when compared to younger nonhypertensives *(39,40)*. Subjects over 50 yr of age changing from a 70 mEq to 200 mEq diet, the rise in supine systolic and diastolic blood pressure after 2 wk was 15/8 mm Hg, compared to 2.5/2.3 mm Hg observed in those under 50 yr of age *(40)*. The results of the dietary approach to stop hypertension (DASH)-Sodium multicenter trial *(41)* contributes to resolving this controversy. This study examined the effect of three sodium levels (resulting in urinary sodium excretion of 65, 107, and 142 mmol/d) on blood pressure in those with greater than optimal blood pressure or stage 1 hypertension. The sodium intervention was provided in conjunction with a typical American (control) diet or the DASH diet (*see* Section 3.) while keeping body weight stable. The lowest sodium intake (65 mmol/d), superimposed on the DASH diet, provided the most effective blood pressure lowering combination. Compared to the control diet with the highest sodium level, the DASH diet with the lowest sodium level reduced systolic blood pressure by 8.9 mm Hg in hypertensives and 7.1 mm Hg in nonhypertensives. Regardless of the diet, the lowering in systolic blood pressure because of sodium reduction was stronger in those over 45 yr of age than for those aged 45 and younger (Table 3) *(42)*. A similar trend was observed for diastolic blood pressure, but the difference was not statistically significant. Therefore, this study demonstrates that 65 mmol/d may be an optimal sodium guideline for prevention and treatment of hypertension in the general population and this strategy may be particularly effective for the elderly.

In the TONE clinical trial *(43)*, 681 hypertensive subjects aged 60–80 yr being treated with one medication were randomly assigned to a reduced sodium intervention or control group. After 3 mo of reduced sodium intake or usual care, medication was withdrawn. During the next 27 mo, as the intervention continued, mean urinary sodium excretion was 40 mmol/d less in the reduced sodium group than in the controls. This reduction in sodium was found in all subgroups and was associated with significant lowering of blood pressures by 4.3/2.0 mm Hg. In the TOHP II, overweight adults counseled to reduce sodium achieved a 2.9/1.6 mm Hg blood pressure reduction from sodium reaction alone and 4.0/2.8 mm Hg when coupled with weight loss after 6 mo. Although effects on average blood pressure declined over time with behavioral relapse, the incidence of hypertension was reduced by 20% and was still noted 48-mo follow-up in each intervention group *(44)*.

Salt-sensitivity, defined arbitrarily as a mean arterial pressure reduction of at least 10 mm Hg or 10% with salt restriction, is more common in the elderly and in African Americans *(45–48)*. The elderly may respond to a sodium load differently because of a decrease in ability of the vascular system to adjust to a change in circulating blood volume and because of blunted sodium excretion *(49)*. Decline in renal function with age will also reduce the ability of the kidney to handle a sodium load. Therefore, sodium reduction may be particularly effective in older individuals because they may retain sodium to a greater extent than younger persons. In addition, arterial compliance decreases with age. Therefore, any change in intravascular volume related to sodium intake should result in a greater blood pressure change in older than in younger persons. Weinberger and Fineberg

Table 3
Effects of Lower Minus Higher Sodium Intake on Blood Pressure (in mm Hg)
with the Control or DASH Diet *(42)*

Mean (95% CI)	Systolic blood pressure		Diastolic blood pressure	
	Control diet	DASH diet	Control diet	DASH diet
>45 yr	−7.5 (−8.9, −6.1)[a]	−4.5 (−6.0, −3.0)[b]	−3.8 (−4.8, −2.9)	−2.2 (−3.1, −1.2)
≤45 yr	−5.3 (−7.0, −3.5)	−1.4 (−2.9, 0.2)	−2.8 (−4.0, −1.7)	−1.1 (−2.1, 0.0)

[a]$p < 0.05$ comparing the two age groups.
[b]$p < 0.01$ comparing the two age groups.

(50) tested blood pressure responsiveness to a salt-sensitivity protocol of volume expansion and contraction in 28 individuals and found that hypertensive individuals had a progressive increase in sodium sensitivity with increasing age, but in nonhypertensive participants, sodium sensitivity was only seen among those 60 and older. Sodium reduction is not only an effective blood pressure-lowering strategy but also feasible in the elderly *(51,52)*. However, NHANES III indicates that average sodium intake in the US elderly (2500–3100 mg/d) continues to exceed the current recommendation for blood pressure control (2300 mg/d or less) *(8)* and is much higher than the sodium level proven to be effective in the DASH-Sodium trial (1500 mg/d/2100 kcal) *(41)*.

2.3. Potassium

Increased potassium intake has been associated with lower blood pressure in observational studies *(10,53)* and with decreased stroke-related mortality in a prospective study *(54)*. In intervention studies *(55,56)*, potassium provided as either a supplement (median 2925 mg) superimposed on a controlled research diet or added to participants' usual diets' lowered both systolic and diastolic blood pressure. In addition, greater blood pressure reductions occurred in those with progressively higher urinary sodium excretion during follow up and in studies that included >80% African Americans. This suggests that the effectiveness of potassium supplemention controlling blood pressure varies by race and level of sodium in the diet.

In the Nurses Health Study II, Sacks and colleagues *(57)* administered daily either supplemental potassium (1560 mg), calcium (1200 mg), magnesium (336 mg), all three minerals, or a placebo, to young women who habitually consume low levels of these nutrients for 6 mo. Potassium supplement alone was the only intervention that lowered blood pressure. In another study, 22 older (≥60 yr) participants with mild hypertension were given an isocaloric diet for 8 d with either 120 mmol (4680 mg) potassium or placebo using a crossover design *(58)*. Potassium supplementation decreased blood pressure significantly by 8.6/4.0 mm Hg. The authors postulated that this reduction in blood pressure may be a result in part to potassium-induced natriuresis.

Thus, the evidence for a role of potassium in lowering blood pressure is consistent across studies and is biologically plausible. Potassium may lower blood pressure through a direct vasodilatory role, alterations in the renin-angiotensin-aldosterone axis and renal sodium handling, and by natriuretic effects *(59)*. According to the NHANES III, the elderly consume similar amounts of potassium as other age groups (2800–3100 mg/d) and is less than that recommended by the JNCVI (3510 mg/d). There is a small risk that the high potassium intake (e.g., of the DASH diet) may lead to hyperkalemia in elderly individuals with reduced renal function and/or who are taking potassium-sparing diuretics. In the former case, dietary advice to increase potassium-rich fruit and vegetable intakes must be tempered by the risk in the onset of renal disease. In the latter case, the beneficial effect of increased fruit and vegetable intake may outweigh the benefit of the potassium-sparing diuretic, which can usually be replaced by thiazide or a loop diuretic. In either case, careful monitoring of serum potassium is essential while changes in diet or medication regimen are being made.

2.4. Calcium

Observational studies *(60–62)* have shown only modest and inconsistent associations between calcium and blood pressure. It should be noted that most studies used 24-h recall methods to assess dietary intake of calcium, and random day-to-day variation may have obscured any relationship with blood pressure *(61)*. Several meta-analyses of calcium-intervention trials *(63–66)* have shown a slight blood pressure reduction primarily of systolic blood pressure, with calcium supplementation of approx 1000 mg. Intervention studies using calcium from food sources have sometimes *(67,68)* been more effective, however, these studies involve simultaneous changes in other nutrients. Calcium supplementation also prevents a sodium-induced rise in blood pressure in salt-sensitive individuals *(69–72)*. Therefore, sodium intake should be controlled in any examination of the impact of calcium on blood pressure. Although calcium may play a role in blood pressure regulation, existing evidence does not warrant public health recommendations to increase calcium intake specifically for blood pressure control. However, the elderly in particular should be advised to consume adequate calcium for other health benefits, including bone health.

2.5. Alcohol

Observational studies have shown a link between excessive alcohol consumption and high blood pressure *(73)*. The mechanism for alcohol's impact on blood pressure is not clear, but it probably occurs via stimulation of the sympathetic nervous system, inhibition of vascular relaxing substances, calcium or magnesium depletion, and/or increased intracellular calcium in vascular smooth muscle *(73,74)*. In an observational study, men who reduced their alcohol consumption over a 20-yr period experienced less age-related increase in blood pressure than those who did not *(75)*. In 9 of 10 intervention studies reviewed by Cushman et al. *(76)*, reduction of 1–6 alcoholic beverages per day reduced systolic blood pressure significantly. Because of the limitation in existing evidence and variations in study design, it is difficult to arrive at a specific cut-off for blood pressure benefit. Men who consume ≥3–5 drinks/d *(77)*, and women who consume ≥2–3 drinks/d *(78)* may be at particularly higher risk. The relation of alcohol type to risk is inconsistent and chronic, habitual intake may be more related to blood pressure than recent intake *(77)*. Alcohol consumption has been shown to improve coronary heart disease risk *(79,80)*. To balance the positive with potentially adverse effects, the elderly should be advised to limit consumption to ≤2 drinks for men and ≤1 drink for women and low-weight people per day to improve blood pressure control.

2.6. Dietary Fat

Numerous studies have investigated the relationship between dietary fat and blood pressure. However, because of discrepancies in study design, lack of adequate sample size, and other design limitations, the issue is still controversial. Both the absolute total intake of dietary fat and the relative fatty acid composition may independently affect blood pressure control.

Most observational studies have not found an association between total fat intake and blood pressure (81–83). However, two large European studies (82,83) but not another (84) show a positive relationship between saturated fatty acids and blood pressure. In clinical intervention trials, lowering total fat intake from 38–40% to 20–25% of energy and/or increasing polyunsaturated to saturated fat ratio from 0.2 to 1.0 reduced blood pressure in several studies (85–88), but not all (89,90). Any change in total fat intake often introduces changes in other dietary factors as well, so the blood pressure responses may not be attributed solely to the change in fat intake. In addition, it is important to recognize that previous trials of dietary fat have had small sample sizes, and lacked sensitivity to detect 3–4 mm Hg effects.

Two large prospective studies have shown a significant positive relationship between dietary cholesterol intake and blood pressure (91–93). However, intakes of low-to-moderate levels of dietary cholesterol were found to have no significant effects on blood pressure in a short-term intervention study (94).

Both fish oil and corn oil supplements have been shown to reduce blood pressure among elderly hypertensives (95). However, pharmacological dosages of docosahexaenoic acid (DHA) were shown to lower blood pressure, although eicosapentaenoic acid (EPA) was not (96). It is suggested that the blood pressure-lowering effect of fish oil may be strongest in hypertensive individuals and in those with clinical atherosclerotic disease or hypercholesterolemia (97). Polyunsaturated fatty acids, particularly linoleic acid, have been suggested to lower blood pressure by increasing synthesis of prostaglandins (PG) (98). Animal studies have shown that n-6 fatty acids increase the tissue and circulating levels of PGs, prostaglandin-I (PGI), and PGE, which may affect blood pressure through control of vascular resistance, salt excretion, cardiac output or rennin secretion (98–100). Little research is available in humans examining how fat intake may affect blood pressure through this pathway. Thus, it is still unclear how fat intake and different fatty acids affect blood pressure and if an interaction exists among these factors.

2.7. Carbohydrates

Very few studies have been designed specifically to investigate the impact of the quantity of carbohydrate intake on blood pressure. However, studies examining the linkage between fat and blood pressure often change intake of carbohydrate and may indirectly provide data in this area, because a low fat diet usually corresponds with a high carbohydrate diet. A high carbohydrate diet has been suggested to adversely affect insulin metabolism and through that mechanism may be related to blood pressure regulation, however, research has not provided convincing evidence (101).

The impact of the type of carbohydrate ingested on blood pressure has been examined in a limited number of studies. For example, sucrose has been shown in some animal studies to have a hypertensive effect (102–104). Results regarding sucrose from human studies have not been consistent *(105,107)*. Fructose, nevertheless, has been shown to have a blood pressure lowering effect in humans *(106,108,109)* although glucose was found to be either hypertensive *(105,108)* or hypotensive *(110)*. Such inconsistencies in the study of various simple carbohydrates on blood pressure may be a result of the differences in study design or subject population, inadequate sample size, or length of feeding. More research is needed to clarify the effects of various carbohydrates on blood pressure using well-controlled designs in long-term situations.

2.8. Protein

A review of studies investigating the relationship between dietary protein and blood pressure from 1988 to 1994 has been published *(111)*, and very little new research has been conducted since this time period. In brief, many epidemiological studies have shown an inverse relationship between dietary protein and blood pressure *(91,112,113)*. Animal studies also demonstrated that low protein diets increase blood pressure and stroke, whereas high protein diets are protective *(114)*. Although most intervention trials in humans do not support findings from observational studies, most use protein supplements and many do not control for other nutrients. For example, studies using supplements ranging from 7 g of rice protein to 93 g of meat protein for 2 wk to 3 mo did not affect blood pressure *(115–122)*. However, in an 8-wk intervention study, skim milk supplementation significantly reduced blood pressure among nonhypertensive participants *(116)*. The skim milk supplements not only provided additional protein, but also other nutrients including calcium and magnesium and both may affect blood pressure. Thus, the blood pressure responses may be caused by multiple factors.

The underlying mechanism by which dietary protein may affect blood pressure is unclear. Specific amino acids, such as arginine, tyrosine, tryptophan, methionine, and glutamate, have been suggested to affect neurotransmitters or humoral factors that affect blood pressure *(111)*. More research is needed to understand the effects of various amino acids in humans, as well as the mechanisms underlying the relationship between dietary protein and blood pressure.

2.9. Magnesium

Several cross sectional *(123)* and prospective observational analyses *(124,125)* have found that high magnesium diets are associated with lower blood pressure. It should be noted that high magnesium diets tend to be high in other beneficial dietary factors as well. Adequate magnesium is required for the Na/K-ATPase pump, which regulates intracellular calcium—one of the critical determinants of vascular smooth muscle contraction *(126)*. Magnesium deficiency is recognized only rarely, being seen usually in the severely malnourished, chronic alcoholics, and in association with malabsorption syndromes *(126)*.

Some intervention studies have shown a blood pressure lowering effect of magnesium supplement *(127–131)*, although additional studies do not report these findings *(57,132–137)*. The blood pressure lowering was particularly effective in those who were magnesium-depleted (from diuretic treatment) *(127,128)*, in those with a low-baseline intake of dietary magnesium *(138)*, and in older men on antihypertensive medications *(131)*. Thus, evidence is not established to support a separate recommendation of magnesium supplementation for blood pressure control.

2.10. Fiber

Fiber has been shown to be inversely associated with blood pressure in both cross-sectional *(139–141)* and prospective analyses *(124)*. However, fiber has also been shown to be correlated with other nutrients and is difficult to separate from other dietary factors in studies using whole foods. In a prospective cohort analysis, Witteman and colleagues *(125)* found that the protective association with fiber was reduced when adjusting for magnesium and calcium in the statistical models. Conversely, in another study, dietary fiber was the only nutrient that remained significantly and inversely related to hypertension when adjusting for other nutrients *(124)*.

Several intervention studies have examined the effect of supplemental fiber on blood pressure, primarily by adding cereal fiber to the diet *(140)*. With an average supplementation of 14 g fiber, systolic and diastolic blood pressure are reduced by about 1.6/2.0 mm Hg *(140)*. In some studies, fiber has been provided as a mixture of soluble and insoluble fibers. Only soluble fiber influences gastrointestinal function and indirectly, insulin metabolism, possibly providing a mechanism by which fiber may lower blood pressure *(140)*. The weak effects of fiber in these studies may be the result of small-sample size, and the fact that many were conducted in young, nonhypertensive individuals in whom large changes in blood pressure are more difficult to detect. Further studies with adequate power to detect smaller differences in blood pressure are needed to clarify the role of fiber.

3. DIETARY PATTERNS

Other than potassium, sodium reduction, and weight loss, research examining single nutritional factors does not usually produce consistent findings, and there are several possible explanations. First, it is possible that the effect of individual nutrients may be too small to be detected, particularly when studies do not contain adequate sample size or statistical power. Second, most studies employed nutrient supplements that may function differently from nutrients naturally occurring in foods. Third, other factors existing in foods may also affect blood pressure. Lastly, nutrients occurring in foods simultaneously may exert synergistic effects on blood pressure. Thus, the DASH study was designed to test the impact of whole dietary patterns on blood pressure while controlling for multiple nutrients and dietary factors simultaneously *(142,143)*.

The main purpose of the DASH study was to examine the impact on blood pressure of three dietary patterns varying in the content of several nutrients and food groups *(144)*. The first dietary pattern was a control diet representing the typical American diet and containing relatively small amounts of fruits, vegetables, and dairy products. The typical American diet was high in total and saturated fats, cholesterol, and low in dietary fiber, calcium, potassium and magnesium. The second dietary pattern (the Fruits and Vegetables diet) had more fruits and vegetables and, thus, higher levels of dietary fiber, potassium and magnesium but was otherwise similar to the control diet. The DASH "combination" dietary pattern (also now referred to as the DASH diet) emphasized fruits, vegetables and low-fat dairy products, included whole grains, poultry, fish and nuts, and was reduced in fats, red meat, sweets, and sugar-containing beverages. The DASH diet had reduced amounts of total and saturated fat, and cholesterol, and increased amounts of potassium, calcium, magnesium, dietary fiber, and protein. Sodium intake, body weight, and alcohol consumption were kept constant throughout the study.

A total of 459 participants consumed the control diet for 3 wk first, then were randomly assigned to 1 of the 3 dietary patterns for an additional 8 wk. The DASH diet reduced systolic blood pressure by 5.5 mm Hg and diastolic by 3.0 mm Hg more than the control group (both SBP and DBP $p < 0.001$) *(145)*. The Fruits and Vegetables diet reduced blood pressures by 2.8 (systolic) and 1.1 (diastolic) mm Hg more than the control diet ($p < 0.001$ and $p = 0.07$). The reductions in blood pressures were significant after participants consumed the diets for 2 wk and were sustained for the following 6 wk (Fig. 2). In addition, blood pressure lowering was effective in men and women, younger and older persons alike, and particularly effective among minorities and those who had high blood pressure. These reductions occurred while body weight, sodium intake, alcohol consumption and exercise patterns remained stable. Among the 133 participants with hypertension (systolic blood pressure ≥140 mm Hg; diastolic blood pressure ≥90 mm Hg; or both), the combination diet lowered systolic and diastolic blood pressure by 11.4 and 5.5 mm Hg, respectively. These effects in hypertensives are similar to reductions seen with single drug therapy.

In a separate analysis, the impact of the DASH diet on blood pressure among those with isolated systolic hypertension (ISH) was examined *(146)*. The DASH diet significantly lowered systolic blood pressure by 11.2 mm Hg with a 95% confidence interval compared with the control diet [−6.1 to −16.2 mm Hg; $p < 0.001$]. Eighteen of the twenty three participants (78%) reduced their systolic blood pressure to <140 mm Hg compared to 24% in the control group. These results indicate that the DASH diet can be effective as first-line therapy in stage 1 ISH, which is particularly prevalent in the elderly.

The blood pressure-lowering effect of the DASH dietary pattern was recently reconfirmed in the DASH-Sodium trial (*see* Sodium section). This study supports the hypothesis that increasing foods rich in potassium, magnesium and dietary fiber reduces blood pressure. In addition, by further lowering total and saturated fat, cholesterol, and increasing low-fat dairy products in the DASH diet, blood pressure reduction was nearly doubled. However, it is also possible that other nutrients that were not controlled for in the study, and/or other beneficial factors as yet unrecognized, may have contributed to the overall blood pressure reduction.

4. PRACTICAL GUIDELINE: A WHOLE DIET APPROACH

In light of all the research evidence, elderly individuals should be advised to maintain a healthy body weight, reduce sodium, limit alcohol intake and follow the DASH dietary pattern (*see* Section 5.). The following section summarizes the guidelines that should be implemented to prevent or manage hypertension in the elderly. It is likely that one may gain benefit to blood pressure control following a combination of these strategies; therefore, individuals should be encouraged to implement as many as possible. Table 4 lists a sample DASH dietary pattern for individuals consuming approx 2000 kcal/d. This sample pattern provides the servings of various food groups recommended by the DASH study and can be modified to fit individual needs or for institutional menu planning. Individuals should be advised to make small and steady changes toward this dietary pattern. The benefit of following the DASH diet also extends to dyslipidemia *(147)* and osteoporosis *(148)*; both of which are common disease conditions in the elderly.

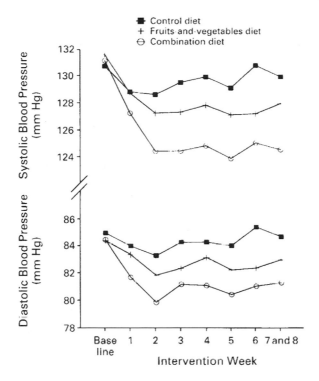

Fig. 2. Changes in blood pressures after consumption of the control diet, fruits-and-vegetables diet, or the combination (DASH) diet in the DASH study *(145)*.

Table 4
Sample DASH Dietary Pattern for a 2000 Kcal Level

Meals	Recommended pattern	Sample meal
Breakfast	Fruits (2 servings)	1/2 c Orange juice
	Grains (2 servings)	1 1/2 c Raisin bran with banana slices (1 small banana)
	Dairy (1 serving)	8 oz Skim milk
Lunch	Fruits (1 serving)	Med apple
	Vegetables (1 serving)	1 c Green salad (with fat-free dressing)
	Meat (1/2 serving)	1 1/2 oz Turkey on
	Grains (2 servings)	2 Slices whole wheat bread
	Dairy (1 serving)	1 Slice reduced fat cheese
Dinner	Fruits (1 serving)	Med peach
	Vegetables (3 servings)	1 1/2 c Steamed broccoli and carrots
	Grains (2 servings)	1 c Brown rice
	Dairy (1 serving)	8 oz Frozen yogurt
	Meat (1 serving)	3 oz Baked fish
Snack	Grains (1 serving)	1 c Unsalted light popcorn
	Nuts/seeds (1/2 serving)	1/2 oz Unsalted peanuts

5. SUMMARY

Although following the DASH dietary pattern, reducing sodium and losing weight offers the potential to lower blood pressure, the best approach to facilitate these lifestyle changes and to enhance long-term adherence remains a challenge for health professionals and patients alike. Changing lifestyle habits requires conscious effort on the part of the patient and support from various environmental avenues. Frequency of contact from health professionals and their counseling skills or styles may also affect patients' adherence (149). The impressive lifestyle changes observed in the TONE trial suggests that the elderly population may be particularly successful at implementing nonpharmacological strategies of prevention and treatment of hypertension (150). As the authors speculated, these hypertensive older patients may have been more motivated to reduce their dependence on medication, thus resulting in greater success in achieving and maintaining the lifestyle changes for blood pressure control.

6. RECOMMENDATIONS FOR CLINICIANS

1. Elderly patients should be advised to achieve or maintain ideal body weight, reduce sodium intake, limit alcohol intake (no more than 2 drinks for men, 1 drink for women and low-weight people), and follow the DASH dietary pattern (Table 4).
2. A goal for body weight should be a BMI < 25 unless there is an underlying health condition that compromises nutritional status (e.g., COPD).
3. Sodium intake should be initially limited to 2300–2400 mg/d and gradually reduced to 1500 mg/d.
4. In order to achieve the DASH dietary pattern, the patient should be taught the basics of planning the menu shown in Table 4. The patient should gradually adapt to a diet that emphasizes fruits, vegetables, and low-fat dairy products. The diet should also include whole grains, poultry, fish and nuts, and limit fats, red meats, sweets, and sugar-containing beverages.

REFERENCES

1. National Heart, Lung, and Blood Institute. Fact Book Fiscal Year 1996. US Department of Health and Human Services, National Institute of Health, Bethesda, MD, 1997.
2. Burt VL, Whelton P, Roccella EJ, Brown C, Cutler JA, Higgins M, et al. Prevalence of hypertension in the U.S. adult population. Results from the Third National Health and Nutrition Examination Survey, 1988–1991. Hypertension 1995;25:305–313.
3. James GD, Baker PT. Human population biology and hypertension. Evolutionary and ecological aspects of blood pressure. In Hypertension: Pathophysiology, diagnosis and management. Laragh JH, Brenner BM (eds.), Raven, New York, 1990, pp. 137–145.
4. Lowenstein FW. Blood-pressure in relation to age and sex in the tropics and subtropics. Lancet 1961;1:389–392.
5. Psaty BM, Smith NL, Siscovick DS, Koepsell TD, Weiss NS, Heckbert SR, et al. Health outcomes associated with antihypertensive therapies used as first-line agents. A systematic review and meta-analysis. JAMA 1997;277:739–745.
6. MacMahon S, Rodgers A. The effects of blood pressure reduction in older patients: an overview of five randomized controlled trials in elderly hypertensives. Clin Exp Hypertens 1993;15:967–978.
7. National Heart Lung and Blood Institute. The Sixth Report of the Joint National Committee on Prevention, Detection, Evaluation, and Treatment of High Blood Pressure. National Institutes of Health, 1997.
8. Alaimo K, McDowell M, Briefel R, Bischof A, Caughman C, Loria C, Johnson C. Dietary Intake of Vitamins, Minerals, and Fiber of Persons Ages 2 Months and Over in the United States: Third National Health and Nutrition Examination Survey, Phase 1, 1988–1991. Advance Data from Vital and Health Statistics, vol. 258, 1994.

9. Cutler J, Psaty B, MacMahon S, Furberg C. Public health issues in hypertension control: what has been learned from clinical trials. In Hypertension: Pathophysiology, Diagnosis, and Management. Laragh J, Brenner B (eds.) Raven, New York, 1995, pp. 253–270.

10. Intersalt Cooperative Research Group. Intersalt: An international study of electrolyte excretion and blood pressure: Results for 24-hour urinary sodium and potassium excretion. BMJ 1988;297:319–328.

11. Spiegelman D, Israel RG, Bouchard C, Willett WC. Absolute fat masss, percent body fat, and body-fat distribution: Which is the real determinant of blood pressure and serum glucose? Am J Clin Nutr 1992;55:1033–1044.

12. Stamler J. Epidemiologic findings on weight and blood pressure in adults. Ann Epidemiol 1991;1: 347–362.

13. Harlan WR, Hull AL, Schmouder RL, Landis JR, Thompson FE, Larkin FA. Blood pressure and nutrition in adults. The national health and nutrition examination survey. Am J Epidemiol 1984;120:17–28.

14. Ford ES, Cooper RS. Risk factors for hypertension in a national cohort study. Hypertension 1991; 18:598–606.

15. Okosun IS, Prewitt TE, Cooper RS. Abdominal obesity in the United States: Prevalence and attributable risk of hypertension. J Hum Hypertens 1999;13:425–430.

16. Stamler R, Stamler J, Gosch FC, Civinelli J, Fishman J, McKeever P, et al. Primary prevention of hypertension by nutritional-hygienic means. Final report of a randomized, controlled trial. JAMA 1989;262:1801–1807.

17. Hypertension Prevention Trial Research Group. The Hypertension Prevention Trial: Three-year effects of dietary changes on blood pressure. Arch Intern Med 1990;150:153–162.

18. Stevens VJ, Corrigan SA, Obarzanek E, Bernauer E, Cook NR, Hebert P, et al. Weight loss intervention in phase 1 of the Trials of Hypertension Prevention. The TOHP Collaborative Research Group. Arch Intern Med 1993;153:849–858.

19. The Trials of Hypertension Prevention Collaborative Research Group. The effects of nonpharmacologic interventions on blood pressure of persons with high normal levels. Results of the Trials of Hypertension, Phase I. JAMA 1992;267:1213–1220.

20. He J, Whelton PK, Appel LJ, Charleston J, Klag MJ. Long-term effects of weight loss and dietary sodium reduction on incidence of hypertension. Hypertension 2000;35:544–549.

21. Dustan HP, Weinsier RL. Treatment of obesity-associated hypertension. Ann Epidemiol 1991;1: 371–379.

22. Stevens VJ, Obarzanek E, Cook NR, Lee IM, Appel LJ, Smith West D, et al. Trials for the Hypertension Prevention Research. Long-term weight loss and changes in blood pressure: results of the Trials of Hypertension Prevention, phase II. Ann Intern Med 2001;134:1–11.

23. Flegal K, Carroll M, Kuczmarski R, Johnson C. Overweight and obesity in the United States: prevalence and trends. Intern J Obes 1998;22:39–47.

24. He J, Ogden LG, Vupputuri S, Bazzano LA, Loria C, Whelton PK. Dietary sodium intake and subsequent risk of cardiovascular disease in overweight adults. JAMA 1999;282:2027–2034.

25. Rocchini AP, Key J, Bondie D, Chico R, Moorehcad C, Katch V, et al. The effect of weight loss on the sensitivity of blood pressure to sodium in obese adolescents. N Engl J Med 1989;321:580–585.

26. McKnight JA, Moore TJ. The effects of dietary factors on blood pressure. Comp Ther 1994;20: 511–517.

27. Brown C, Higgins M, Donato K, Rohde F, Garrison R, Obarzanek E, et al. Body mass index and the prevalence of hypertension and dyslipidemia. Obes Res 2000;8:605–619.

28. Dahl L. Possible role of salt intake in the development of hypertension. In Essential hypertension: an international symposium. (Cottier P, Bock KD, eds.) Springer-Verlag, Berlin, 1960, pp. 53–65.

29. Elliott P. Observational studies of salt and blood pressure. Hypertension 1991;17(suppl):I–3-I–8.

30. Stamler J. The INTERSALT study: background, methods, findings and implications. Am J Clin Nutr 1997;65(suppl):626S–642S.

31. Law MR, Frost CD, Wald NJ. By how much does dietary salt reduction lower blood pressure? Analysis of observational data among populations. BMJ 1991;302:811–814.

32. Cutler JA, Follmann D, Allender PS. Randomized trials of sodium reduction: an overview. Am J Clin Nutr 1997;65:643S–651S.

33. Law MR, Frost CD, Wald III NJ. Analysis of data from trials of salt reduction. BMJ 1991;302: 819–824.

34. Graudal NA, Galloe AM, Garred P. Effects of sodium restriction on blood pressure, renin, aldosterone, catecholamines, cholesterols, and triglyceride. A Meta-analysis. JAMA 1998;279:1383–1391.

35. Midgley JP, Matthew AG, Greenwood CMT, Logan AG. Effect of reduced dietary sodium on blood pressure. JAMA 1996;275:1590–1597.

36. Fotherby M, Potter J. Effects of moderate sodium restriction on clinic and 24-hour ambulatory blood pressure in elderly hypertensive subjects. J Hypertens 1993;11:657–663.

37. McCarron DA. The dietary guideline for sodium: should we shake it up? Yes! Am J Clin Nutr 2000;71: 1013–1019.

38. Kaplan NM. The dietary guideline for sodium: should we shake it up? No. Am J Clin Nutr 2000;71: 1020–1026.

39. Nestel P, Clifton P, Noakes M, McArthur R, Howe P. Enhanced blood pressure response to dietary salt in elderly women, especially those with small waist:hip ratio. J Hypertens 1993;11:1387–3194.

40. Myers J, To M. Effect of alteration in sodium chloride intake on blood pressure of normotensive subjects. J Cardiovasc Pharmacol 1984;6:s204–s209.

41. Sacks F, Svetkey L, Vollmer W. Effects on blood pressure of reduced dietary sodium and the Dietary Approaches to Stop Hypertension (DASH) diet. DASH-Sodium Collaborative Research Group. N Engl J Med 2001;344:3–10.

42. Vollmer WMP, Sacks FMMD, Ard JMD, Appel LJMD, Bray GAMD, Simons-Morton DGMDP, et al. For the, Effects of Diet and Sodium Intake on Blood Pressure: Subgroup Analysis of the DASH-Sodium Trial. Ann Intern Med December, 2001;135:1019–1028.

43. Appel L, Espeland M, Easter L, Wilson A, Folmar S, Lacy C. Effects of reduced sodium intake on hypertension control in older individuals. Arch Intern Med 2001;161:685–693.

44. The Trials of Hypertension Prevention Collaborative Research Group. Effects of weight loss and sodium reduction intervention on BP and hypertension incidence in overweight people with high-normal blood pressure: the Trials of Hypertension Prevention, Phase II. Arch Intern Med 1997;157: 657–667.

45. Weinberger MH, Miller JZ, Luft FC, Grim CE, Fineberg NS. Definitions and characteristics of sodium sensitivity and blood pressure resistance. Hypertension 1986;8(Supp II):II–127-II–134.

46. Kawasaki T, Delea CS, Bartter FC, Smith H. The effect of high-sodium and low-sodium intakes on blood pressure and other related variables in human subjects with idiopathic hypertension. Am J Med 1978;4:193–198.

47. Fujita T, Henry WL, Bartter FC, Lake CR, Delea CS. Factors influencing blood pressure in salt-sensitive patients with hypertension. Am J Med 1980;69:334–344.

48. Luft FC, Weinberger MH. Heterogeneous responses to changes in dietary salt intake: the salt-sensitivity paradigm. Am J Clin Nutr 1997;65(Suppl):612S–617S.

49. Falkner B. Sodium sensitivity: a determinant of essential hypertension. J Am Coll Nutr 1988;7:35–41.

50. Weinberger MH, Fineberg NS. Sodium and volume sensitivity of blood pressure. Age and pressure change over time. Hypertension 1991;18:67–71.

51. Chobanian AV, Hill M. National Heart, Lung, and Blood Institute workshop on sodium and blood pressure. A critical review of current scientific evidence. Hypertension 2000;35:858–863.

52. Applegate W, Miller S, Elam J, et al. Nonpharmacologic intervention to reduce blood pressure in older patients with mild hypertension. Arch Intern Med 1992;152:1162–1166.

53. Ophir O, Peer G, Gilad J, Blum M, Aviram A. Low blood pressure in vegetarians: the possible role of potassium. Am J Clin Nutr 1983;37:755–762.

54. Khaw KT, Barrett-Connor E. Dietary potassium and stroke-associated mortality. A 12-year prospective population study. N Engl J Med 1987;316:235–240.

55. Whelton PK, He J, Cutler JA, Brancati FL, Appel LJ, Follmann D, et al. Effects of oral potassium on blood pressure. Meta-analysis of randomized controlled clinical trials. JAMA 1997;277:1624–1632.

56. Cappuccio FP, MacGregor GA. Does potassium supplementation lower blood pressure? A meta-analysis of published trials. J Hypertens 1991;9:465–473.

57. Sacks FM, Willett WC, Smith A, Brown LE, Rosner B, Moore TJ. Effect on blood pressure of potassium, calcium, and magnesium in women with low habitual intake. Hypertension 1998;31:131–138.

58. Smith S, Klotman P, Svetkey L. Potassium chloride lowers blood pressure and causes natriuresis in older patients with hypertension. J Am Soc Nephrol 1992;2:1302–1309.

59. Luft FC, Weinberger MH, Grim CE, Fineberg NS. Effects of volume expansion and contraction on potassium homeostasis in normal and hypertensive humans. J Am Coll Nutr 1986;5:357–369.

60. Birkett NJ. Comments on a meta-analysis of the relation between dietary calcium intake and blood pressure. Am J Epidemiol 1998;148:223–228.

61. Cutler JA, Brittain E. Calcium and blood pressure. An epidemiologic perspective. Am J Hypertens 1990;3:137S–146S.
62. Cappuccio FP, Elliott P, Allender PS, Pryer J, Follman DA, Cutler JA. Epidemiologic association between dietary calcium intake and blood pressure: A meta-analysis of published data. Am J Epidemiol 1995;142:935–945.
63. Cappuccio FP, Siani A, Strazzullo P. Oral calcium supplementation and blood pressure: An overview of randomized controlled trials. J Hypertens 1989;7:941–946.
64. Bucher HC, Cook RJ, Guyatt GH, Lang JD, Cook DJ, Hatala R, Hunt D. Effects of dietary calcium supplementation on blood pressure. JAMA 1986;275:1016–1022.
65. Allender PS, Cutler JA, Follmann D, Cappuccio FP, Pryer J, Elliott P. Dietary calcium and blood pressure: A meta-analysis of randomized clinical trials. Ann Intern Med 1996;124:825–831.
66. Griffith LE, Guyatt GH, Cook RJ, Bucher HC, Cook DJ. The influence of dietary and nondietary calcium supplementation on blood pressure. An updated meta-analysis of randomized controlled trials. Am J Hypertens 1999;12:84–92.
67. Cappuccio FP. The "calcium antihypertension theory." Am J Hypertens 1999;12:93–95.
68. Kynast-Gales SA, Massey LK. Effects of dietary calcium from dairy products on ambulatory blood pressure in hypertensive men. J Am Diet Assoc 1992;92:1497–1501.
69. Sowers JR, Zemel MB, Zemel PC, Standley PR. Calcium metabolism and dietary calcium in salt sensitive hypertension. Am J Hypertens 1991;4:557–563.
70. Zemel MB, Kraniak J, Standley PR, Sowers JR. Erythrocyte cation metabolism in salt-sensitive hypertensive blacks as affected by dietary sodium and calcium. Am J Hypertens 1988;1:386–392.
71. Saito K, Sano H, Furuta Y, Fukuzaki H. Effect of oral calcium on blood pressure response in salt-loaded borderline hypertensive patients. Hypertension 1989;13:219–226.
72. Rich GM, McCullough M, Olmedo A, Malarick C, Moore TJ. Blood pressure and renal blood flow responses to dietary calcium and sodium intake in humans. Am J Hypertens 1991;4:642S–645S.
73. MacMahon S. Alcohol consumption and hypertension. Hypertension 1987;9:111–121.
74. Cushman WC, Cutler JA, Hanna E, Bingham SF, Follmann D, Harford T, et al. Prevention and treatment of hypertension study (PATHS): Effects of an alcohol treatment program on blood pressure. Arch Intern Med 1998;158:1197–1207.
75. Gordon T, Doyle JT. Alcohol consumption and its relationship to smoking, weight, blood pressure, and blood lipids. Arch Intern Med 1986;146:262–265.
76. Cushman WC, Cutler JA, Bingham SF, Harford T, Hanna E, Dubbert P, et al. Prevention and treatment of hypertension study (PATHS). Rationale and design. Am J Hypertens 1994;7:814–823.
77. Klatsky AL, Friedman GD, Armstrong MA. The relationships between alcoholic beverage use and other traits to blood pressure: A new Kaiser-Permanente study. Circulation 1986;73:628–636.
78. Witteman JC, Willett WC, Stampfer MJ, Colditz GA, Kok FJ, Sacks FM, et al. Relation of moderate alcohol consumption and risk of systemic hypertension in women. Am J Cardiol 1990;65:633–637.
79. Beilin LJ. Alcohol, hypertension and cardiovascular disease. J Hypertens 1995;13:939–942.
80. Rimm EB, Giovannucci EL, Willett WC, Colditz GA, Ascherio A, Rosner B, Stampfer MJ. A prospective study of alcohol consumption and the risk of coronary disease in men. Lancet 1991;338:464–468.
81. Elliott P, Fehily A, Sweetnam P, Yarnell J. Diet, alcohol, body mass, and social factors in relation to blood pressure: the Caerphilly Heart Study. J Epidemiol Comm Health 1987;41:37–43.
82. Salonen J, Tuomilehto J, Tanskanen A. Relation of blood pressure to reported intake of salt, saturated fats, and alcohol in healthy middle-aged population. J Epidemiol Comm Health 1983;37:32–37.
83. Salonen J, Salonen R, Ihanainen M, Parviainen M, Seppanen R, Kantola M, et al. Blood pressure, dietary fats, and antioxidants. Am J Clin Nutr 1988;48:1226–1232.
84. Gruchow H, Sobocinski K, Barboriak J. Alcohol, nutrient intake and hypertension in U.S. adults. JAMA 1985;253:1567–1570.
85. Sandstrom B, Marckmann P, Bindslev N. An eight-month controlled study of a low-fat high-fiber diet: effects on blood lipids and blood pressure in healthy young subjects. Euro J Clin Nutr 1992;46:95–109.
86. Judd J, Marshal M, Dupont J. Relationship of dietary fat to plasma fatty acids, blood pressure, and urinary eicosanoids in adult men. J Am Coll Nutr 1989;8:386–399.
87. Mensink R, Janssen M, Katan M. Effect on blood pressure of two diets differing in total fat but not in saturated and polyunsaturated fatty acids in healthy volunteers. Am J Clin Nutr 1988;47:976–980.
88. Straznicky N, O'Callaghan C, Barrington V, Louis W. Hypotensive effect of low-fat, high carbohydrate diet can be independent of changes in plasma insulin concentrations. Hypertension 1999;34:580–585.

89. Aro A, Peitinen P, Valsta L, Salminen I, Turpeinen A, Virtanen M, et al. Lack of effect on blood pressure by low fat diets with different fatty acids compositions. J Hum Hypertens 1998;12:383–389.

90. National Diet Heart Study Research Group, The National Diet Heart Study Final Report. Circulation 1968;37,38:I-228–I-230.

91. Stamler J, Caggiula A, Grandits G, Kjelsberg M, Cutler J. Relationship to blood pressure of combinations of dietary macronutrients. Findings. Relationships of dietary variables to blood pressure (BP): findings of the Multiple Risk Factor Intervention Trial (MRFIT). Circulation 1996;94:2417–2423.

92. Liu K, Ruth K, Shekelle R, Stamler J. Macronutrients and long-term change in systolic blood pressure. Circulation 1993;87:679. Abstract 7.

93. Stamler J, Ruth KJ, Liu K, Shekelle RB. Dietary anti-oxidants and blood pressure change in the Western Electric Study 1958–1966. Circulation 1994;89:932. Abstract.

94. Sacks F, Marais G, Handysides G, Salazar J, Miller L, Foster J, et al. Lack of an effect of dietary saturated fat and cholesterol on blood pressure in normotensives. Hypertension 1984;6:193–198.

95. Margolin G, Huster G, Glueck C, Speirs J, Vandegrift J, Illig E, et al. Blood pressure lowering in elderly subjects: a double-blind crossover study of w-3 and w-6 fatty acids. Am J Clin Nutr 1991;53:562–572.

96. Mori T, Bao D, Burke V, Puddey I, Beilin L. Docosahexaenoic acid but not eicosapentaenoic acid lowers ambulatory blood pressure and heart rate in humans. Hypertension 1999;34:253–260.

97. Morris M, Sacks F, Rosner B. Does fish oil lower blood pressure? A meta-analysis of controlled trials. Circulation 1993;88:523–533.

98. Dunn M, Grone H. The relevance of prostaglandins in human hypertension. Advances in Prostaglandin, Thromboxane and Leukotriene Research 1985;13:179–187.

99. Adam O, Wolfram G. Effect of different linoleic acid intakes on prostagladin biosynthesis and kidney function in man. Am J Clin Nutr 1984;40:763–770.

100. Epstein M, Lifschitz M, Rappaport K. Augmentation of prostaglandin production by linoleic acid in man. Clin Sci 1982;63:565–571.

101. Affarah HB, Hall WD, Heymsfield SB, Kutner M, Wells JO, Tuttle Jr EP. High-carbohydrate diet: antinatriuretic and blood pressure response in normal men. Am J Clin Nutr 1986;44:341–348.

102. Ahrens, RA, Demula P, Lee MK, Majkowski JW. Moderate sucrose ingestion and blood pressure in the rat. J Nutr 1980;110:725–731.

103. Preuss H, Knapka J, MacArthy P, Yousufi A, Sabnis S, Antonovych T. High sucrose diets increase blood pressure of both salt-sensitive and salt-resistant rats. Am J Hypertens 1992;5:585–591.

104. Preuss H, Zein M, MacArthy P, Dipette D, Sabnis S, Knapka J. Sugar-induced blood pressure elevations over the lifespan of three substrains of Wistar rats. J Am Coll Nutr 1998;17:36–47.

105. Hodges R, Rebello T. Carbohydrates and blood pressure. Ann Intern Med 1983;98(Part 2):838–841.

106. Palumbo PJ, Briones ER, Nelson RA, Kottke BA. Sucrose sensitivity of patients with coronary-artery disease. Am J Clin Nutr 1977;30:394–401.

107. Surwit R, Feinglos M, McCaskill C, Clay S, Babyak R, Brownlow B, et al. Metabolic and behavioral effects of a high-sucrose diet during weight loss. Am J Clin Nutr 1997;65:908–915.

108. Koh E, Ard N, Mendoza F. Effects of fructose feeding on blood parameters and blood pressure in impaired glucose-tolerant subjects. J Am Diet Assoc 1988;88:932–938.

109. Hallfrisch J, Reiser S, Prather E. Blood lipid distribution of hyperinsulinemic men consuming three levels of fructose. Am J Clin Nutr 1983;37:740–748.

110. Jansen R, Penterman B, Van Lier H, Hoefnagels W. Blood pressure reduction after oral glucose loading and its relation to age, blood pressure and insulin. Am J Cardiol 1987;60:1087–1091.

111. Obarzanek E, Velletri P, Cutler J. Dietary protein and blood pressure. JAMA 1996;275:1598–1603.

112. Elliott P, Freeman J, Pryer J, Brunner E, Marmot M. Dietary protein and blood pressure: a report from the Dietary and Nutritional Survey of British Adults. J Hypertens 1992;10(suppl 4):S141. Abstract P105.

113. Stamler J, Elliott P, Kesteloot H, Nichols R, Claeys G, Dyer A, Stamler R. Inverse relation of dietary protein markers with blood pressure. Findings for 10,020 men and women in the INTERSALT Study. Circulation 1996;94:1629–1634.

114. Yamori Y, Horie R, Nara Y, Ikeda M, Ooshima A, Fukase M. Genetics of hypertensive diseases: Experimental studies on pathogenesis, detection of predisposition and prevention. Adv Nephrol 1981; 10:51–74.

115. Chapman C, Gibbons T, Henschel A. The effect of the rice-fruit diet on the composition of the body. N Engl J Med 1950;243:899–905.

116. Hatch F, Wertheim A, Eurman G, Watkin D, Froeb H, Epstein H. Effects of diet on essential hypertension, III: alterations in sodium chloride, protein, and fat intake. Am J Med 1954;17:499–513.

117. Brussaard J, van Raakj J, Strasse-Wolthuis M, Katan M, Hautvast J. Blood pressure and diet in normotensive volunteers: Absence of an effect of dietary fiber, protein, or fat. Am J Clin Nutr 1981; 34:2023–2029.

118. Sacks F, Donner A, Castelli W, Gronemeyer J, Pletka P, Margolius H, et al. Effect of ingestion of meat on plasma cholesterol of vegetarians. JAMA 1981;246:640–644.

119. Sacks F, Wood P, Kass E. Stability of blood pressure in vegetarians receiving dietary protein supplements. Hypertension 1984;6:199–201.

120. Prescott S, Jenner D, Beilin L, Margetts B, Vandongen R. Controlled study of the effects of dietary protein on blood pressure in normotensive humans. Clin Experim Pharmacol Physiol 1987;14:159–162.

121. Sacks F, Kass E. Low blood pressure in vegetarians: effects of specific foods and nutrients. Am J Clin Nutr 1988;48:795–800.

122. Kestin M, Rouse I, Correll R, Nestel, PJ. Cardiovascular disease risk factors in free-living men: comparison of two prudent diets, one based on lacto-ovovegetarianism and the other allowing lean meat. Am J Clin Nutr 1989;50:280–287.

123. Joffres MR, Reed DM, Yano K. Relationship of magnesium intake and other dietary factors to blood pressure: The Honolulu heart study. Am J Clin Nutr 1987;45:469–475.

124. Ascherio A, Rimm E, Giovannucci EL, Colditz GA, Rosner B, Willett WC, et al. A prospective study of nutritional factors and hypertension among U.S. men. Circulation 1992;86:1475–1484.

125. Witteman JCM, Willett WC, Stampfer MJ, Colditz GA, Sacks FM, Speizer FE, et al. A prospective study of nutritional factors and hypertension among U.S. women. Circulation 1989;80:1320–1327.

126. Moore TJ. The role of dietary electrolytes in hypertension. J Am Coll Nutr 1989;8(S):1–12.

127. Dyckner T, Wester PO. Effect of magnesium on blood pressure. BMJ 1983;286:1847–1849.

128. Reyes AJ, Leary WP, Acosta-Barrios TN, Davis WH. Magnesium supplementation in hypertension treated with hydrochlorothiazide. Curr Ther Res 1984;6:332 340.

129. Wirell MP, Wester PO, Stegmayr BG. Nutritional dose of magnesium in hypertensive patients on beta blockers lowers systolic blood pressure: a double-blind, cross-over study. J Int Med 1994;236:189 195.

130. Witteman JCM, Grobbee DE, Derkx FHM, Bouillon R, de Bruijn AM, Hofman A. Reduction of blood pressure with oral magnesium supplementation in women with mild to moderate hypertension. Am J Clin Nutr 1994;60:129–135.

131. Kawano Y, Matsuoka H, Takishita S, Omae T. Effects of magnesium supplementation in hypertensive patients. Assessment by office, home, and ambulatory blood pressures. Hypertension 1998;32:260–265.

132. Cappuccio FP, Markandu ND, Beynon GW, Shore AC, Sampson B, MacGregor GA. Lack of effect of oral magnesium on high blood pressure: A double blind study. BMJ 1985;291:235–238.

133. Henderson DG, Schierup J, Schodt T. Effect of magnesium supplementation on blood pressure and electrolyte concentrations in hypertensive patients receiving long term diuretic treatment. BMJ 1986; 293:664–665.

134. Nowson CA, Morgan TO. Magnesium supplementation in mild hypertensive patients on a moderately low sodium diet. Clin Exp Pharm Physiol 1989;16:299–302.

135. Zemel PC, Zemel MB, Urberg M, Douglas FL, Geiser R, Sowers JR. Metabolic and hemodynamic effects of magnesium supplementation in patients with essential hypertension. Am J Clin Nutr 1990; 51:665–669.

136. Yamamato ME, Applegate WB, Klag MJ, Borhani NO, Cohen JD, Kirchner KA, et al. Lack of blood pressure effect with calcium and magnesium supplementation in adults with high-normal blood pressure. Results from Phase I of the Trials of Hypertension Prevention (TOHP). Ann Epidemiol 1995;5:96–107.

137. Sacks FM, Brown LE, Appel L, Borhani NO, Evans D, Whelton P. Combinations of potassium, calcium, and magnesium supplements in hypertension. Hypertension 1995;26:950–956.

138. Lind L, Lithell H, Pollare T, Ljunghall S. Blood pressure response during long-term treatment with magnesium is dependent on magnesium status. A double-blind, placebo-controlled study in essential hypertension and in subjects with high-normal blood pressure. Am J Hypertens 1991;4:674–679.

139. Reed D, McGee D, Yano K, Hankin J. Diet, blood pressure, and multicollinearity. Hypertension 1985; 7:405–410.

140. He J, Whelton PK. Effect of dietary fiber and protein intake on blood pressure: A review of epidemiologic evidence. Clin Exp Hypertens 1999;21(5&6):785–796.

141. Ascerio A, Stampfer MJ, Colditz GA, Willett WC, McKinlay J. Nutrient intakes and blood pressure in normotensive males. Int J Epidemiol 1991;20:886–891.

142. Sacks F, Obarzanek E, Windhauser M, Svetkey L, Vollmer W, McCullough M, et al. Rationale and design of the dietary approaches to stop hypertension trial. Ann Epidemiol 1995;5:108–118.

143. Vogt TM, Appel LJ, Obarzanek E, Moore TJ, Vollmer WM, Svetkey LP, et al. Dietary approaches to stop hypertension: rationale, design, and methods. DASH collaborative research group. J Am Diet Assoc 1999;99(8 suppl):S12–S18.
144. Karanja N, Obarzanek E, Lin P-H, McCullough M, Phillips K, Swain J, et al. Descriptive characteristics of the dietary patterns used in the dietary approaches to stop hypertension trial. J Am Diet Assoc 1999; 99(suppl):S19–S27.
145. Appel LJ, Moore TJ, Obarzanek E, Vollmer WM, Svetkey LP, Sacks FM, et al. A clinical trial of the effects of dietary patterns on blood pressure. DASH Collaborative Research Group [see comments]. N Engl J Med 1997;336:1117–1124.
146. Moore TJ, Conlin PR, Ard J, Svetkey LP. DASH (Dietary Approaches to Stop Hypertension) diet is effective treatment for stage 1 isolated systolic hypertension. Hypertension 2001;38:155–158.
147. Obarzanek E, Sacks FM, Vollmer WM, Bray GA, Miller ER, et al. Effects on blood lipids of a blood pressure-lowering diet: the Dietary Approaches to Stop Hypertension (DASH) Trial. Am J Clin Nutr 2001;74:80–89.
148. Lin P-H, Ginty F, Appel L, Svetkey L, Bohannon A, Barclay D, et al. Impact of sodium intake and dietary patterns on biochemical markers of bone and calcium metabolism. American Society for Bone and Mineral Research Annual Meeting, October, 2001.
149. Smith D, Kratt P, Heckemeyer C, Mason D. Motivational interviewing to improve adherence to a behavioral weight-control program for older obese women with NIDDM. Diabetes Care 1997;20:52–54.
150. Whelton PK, Appel LJ, Espeland MA, Applegate WB, Ettingter WH, Kostis JB, et al. Sodium reduction and weight loss in the treatment of hypertension in older persons: A randomized controlled trial of nonpharmacologic interventions in the elderly (TONE). TONE Collaborative Research Group. JAMA 1998;279:839–846.

17 Cardiac Rehabilitation and Exercise

Kent J. Adams

1. INTRODUCTION

Despite the decrease in cardiovascular disease (CVD) related deaths *(1,2)* at the start of the new millenium, CVD is still the leading cause of death in the United States *(1–3)*. CVD accounts for over half of all deaths *(3)* and more than 900,000 deaths annually *(4)*. Over 12 million Americans have coronary heart disease (CHD) *(5)*, and CHD ranks first among CVD in actual causes of death *(1)*. Clinical manifestations of CHD include stable and unstable angina pectoris, acute myocardial infarction (MI), and sudden death *(3)*.

In the United States, CHD mortality has declined substantially over the last few decades, however, the social and economic burden of CHD remains high *(1,6)*. Approximately 1.5 million Americans experience a MI each year, with approx 0.5 million fatalities *(3)*. More than 50% of MIs occur in people over age 65 *(3)*, and CHD ranks number one as cause of death in older individuals *(2)*. The majority of physician visits in people over 75 are related to diagnosis or treatment of CHD *(2)*. Further, death as a result of CHD rises 7% (from 41% to 48%) as one moves from the >65- to 74 yr-old bracket to the >85-yr-old bracket *(2)*. Unfortunately, when one adds the demographic aging of America with the incidence of MI in those over 65, the picture does not look good. This is especially true among the oldest-old (85+ yr), the elderly population with the fastest growth *(2)*.

Adding the 1 million survivors of MI each year with over 7 million stable angina patients, over 300,000 coronary artery bypass graft surgery (CABG) patients (55% >65 yr), and over 350,000 percutaneous transluminal coronary angioplasty (PTCA) patients (46% >65 yr), brings the total number of candidates for cardiac rehabilitation services to about 10 million, with a significant portion over age 65 *(3,7)*. Additionally, with cardiac rehabilitation's documented benefits and safety, the approx 5 million patients experiencing heart failure and cardiac transplantation are increasingly referred to cardiac rehabilitation programs *(3)*. Unfortunately, the majority of these candidates (70–90%) never participate in cardiac rehabilitation programs *(1,3)*, with even fewer women (especially elderly women) participating *(7–11)*. Since the oldest-old are primarily women, lack of participation in secondary prevention programs, combined with high incidence of disease, are particularly troublesome *(2,7,12)*.

From: *Handbook of Clinical Nutrition and Aging*
Edited by: C. W. Bales and C. S. Ritchie © Humana Press Inc., Totowa, NJ

2. WHAT IS CARDIAC REHABILITATION?

According to the US Department of Health and Human Services Clinical Practice Guideline "Cardiac Rehabilitation" *(3)*:

Cardiac rehabilitation services are comprehensive, long-term programs involving medical evaluation, prescribed exercise, cardiac risk factor modification, education, and counseling. These programs are designed to limit the physiologic and psychological effects of cardiac illness, reduce the risk for sudden death or reinfarction, control cardiac symptoms, stabilize or reverse the atherosclerotic process, and enhance the psychosocial and vocational status of selected patients.

As opposed to primary prevention strategies (advice given to patients with no known CHD) *(7)* cardiac rehabilitation programs recognize their vital role in comprehensive secondary prevention (advice given to patients with diagnosed CHD) *(3)*. The American Heart Association (AHA) Consensus Panel Statement "Preventing Heart Attack and Death in Patients with Coronary Disease" *(13)* states that:

Compelling scientific evidence, including data from recent studies in patients with coronary artery disease, demonstrates that comprehensive risk factor interventions extend overall survival, improve quality of life, decrease need for interventional procedures such as angioplasty and bypass grafting, and, reduce the incidence of subsequent myocardial infarction.

This chapter focuses primarily on the role of exercise as a cornerstone in modern cardiac rehabilitation following hospitalization. However, specific core components of any comprehensive cardiac rehabilitation program are listed in Table 1 and are briefly discussed *(14)*. Overall, cardiac rehabilitation services focus on improving the physiological and psychosocial characteristics of the individual utilizing cardiac rehabilitation *(3)*. Key goals for the cardiac rehabilitation patient according to Thompson *(15)* are listed in Table 2. Additionally, the ability to resume and maintain functional independence is a specific goal for the elderly patient *(2,3,7,12)*. The principle benefits of comprehensive cardiac rehabilitation outlined by the Clinical Practice Guideline *(3)* are listed in Table 3.

2.1. Categorizations of Cardiac Rehabilitation Programs

Table 4 details the typical historic categorization of cardiac rehabilitation programs *(16)*. Recent guidelines however, have "de-emphasized the specifics of phases" *(7)* and have emphasized programs developed with a scientific basis, individualized in prescription and monitoring per specific patient risk characteristics and circumstance, and comprehensive in addressing the core components of comprehensive cardiac rehabilitation *(7,14,16–18)*.

2.2. Cost-Effectiveness of Cardiac Rehabilitation

Cardiovascular disease extracts a heavy toll on the citizens of the United States, costing greater than $135 billion *(2)*, with approx 75% ($100 billion) of this expenditure targeting the prevention and treatment of CHD *(2)*. Few studies document the cost of cardiac rehabilitation services, especially long-term services *(3,19)*. However, limited data does suggest that comprehensive cardiac rehabilitation is a cost-effective use of health care resources *(3,15,18–23)*, and compares favorably with other secondary prevention strategies *(15)*. The Clinical Practice Guideline *(3)*, however, emphasizes that

Table 1
Core Components of Cardiac Rehabilitation Programs

Baseline patient assessment
Nutritional counseling
Risk factor management (lipids, hypertension, weight, diabetes, and smoking)
Psychosocial management
Physical activity counseling
Exercise training

Source: Adapted from Balady et al. *(14)*.

Table 2
Key Goals of Cardiac Rehabilitation for the Patient

Maintenance or improvement of functional capacity
Improvement of quality of life
Prevention of future cardiac events

Source: Adapted from Thompson *(15)*.

Table 3
Principle Benefits of Comprehensive Cardiac Rehabilitation Programs

Improved exercise tolerance
Decreased symptoms and improved clinical measures
Improved blood lipids
Reduced cigarette smoking
Improved psychosocial well-being
Reduced stress
Reduced mortality

Source: Adapted from Wenger et al. *(3)*.

Table 4
Traditional Categories of Cardiac Rehabilitation Programs

Phase I—inpatient
Phase II—up to 12 wk of supervised exercise and/or education following
    hospital discharge
Phase III—variable length program of intermittent or no electrocardio-
    graphic (ECG) monitoring under supervision
Phase IV—no ECG monitoring, limited supervision

Source: Adapted from ref. *16*.

more comprehensive data from randomized controlled trials needs to be analyzed to determine cost effectiveness *(19)*. Additional studies are also necessary to determine cost effectiveness of nontraditional cardiac rehabilitation programs, especially with the continued evolution of comprehensive cardiac rehabilitation services *(19)*. There is no doubt, however, that long-term implementation of lifestyle changes related to healthy behaviors and physical activity in the elderly cardiac patient would significantly impact the economics of health care and the quality of life of the individual (24–29).

3. CARDIAC REHABILITATION AND THE ELDERLY

Unfortunately, comprehensive cardiac services are underutilized by the elderly (9,10). First, when faced with symptoms of MI and congestive heart failure, the elderly often make the fatal mistake of waiting longer to seek care (2). After treatment, cardiac rehabilitation is routinely underprescribed for the elderly by their primary caregivers (2,9–11). Lack of a referral to cardiac rehabilitation services is in direct contrast to the potential functional benefits comprehensive cardiac rehabilitation has the potential to provide (3,6–8,13–17), especially in the elderly (2,3,7,27,29–39).

In a 1992 study, Ades et al. (9) reported that hospital patients with a mean age of >70 yr had a 21% overall participation in cardiac rehabilitation. Importantly, the strongest predictor of entry into cardiac rehabilitation was the "primary physician's recommendation." This underscores the fact that health care providers stand at a crucial junction in providing incentives for their patients to implement positive lifestyle changes, such as participation in cardiac rehabilitation (1,9,10). Ades et al. (9) state:

> It is incumbent on the cardiac rehabilitation staff to ensure that community physicians do not have an inherent bias against referring their oldest patients for cardiac rehabilitation, as they are at greatest risk of cardiac disability.

Patient logistical and psychological factors impacted entry rate as well (9). Nonparticipation in cardiac rehabilitation decreases the likelihood of the patient receiving aggressive risk factor management (2,11). The American Association of Cardiovascular and Pulmonary Rehabilitation (AACVPR) (7) and Ades et al. (9) cite common barriers for lack of participation in cardiac rehabilitation in Table 5.

4. BENEFITS OF EXERCISE FOR THE ELDERLY CARDIAC PATIENT

Despite limited participation in cardiac rehabilitation by the elderly, cardiac rehabilitation is effective at increasing the positive outcomes related to health and function (3,6–8,31–39), a common goal regardless of the cardiac patient's age or background. Importantly, because of the typical lowered functional status of the elderly patient even before their cardiac event, the elderly cardiac patient can experience dramatic improvements in their functional ability through exercise. Clinicians must realize that including exercise in their overall prescription for health and quality of life is crucial in optimizing functional outcomes in their elderly patients. Properly prescribed and supervised exercise has proven to be safe and effective in prevention and treatment of diseases afflicting the elderly. The clinician "reluctant" to prescribe exercise to their elderly patient must realize that often it is more dangerous to the patient's health and functional abilities to remain sedentary. The Clinical Practice Guideline (3) and research by Ades et al. (9,10,31–36,38,39) suggests that elderly cardiac patients have similar potential when compared to younger cardiac patients to respond to exercise, despite limited clinical exercise studies of the older cardiac population (especially older females) (3,11,38). In addition, exercise is now an accepted therapeutic intervention for congestive heart failure patients, increas-

Table 5
Common Barriers to Participation in Cardiac Rehabilitation

Lack of physician referral
Transportation/logistical issues
Reimbursement issues
Lack of desire to alter lifestyle habits
Comorbidities
History of depression
Denial and social isolation

Table 6
Benefits of Aerobic Exercise for the Elderly Cardiac Patient

Increased functional capacity (maximal oxygen consumption)
Increased exercise tolerance
Increased exercise time to onset of angina and disease symptoms
Increased lactate threshold
Decreased heart rate and blood pressure at given submaximal workload
Decreased rate-pressure product at given submaximal workload
Decreased ventilation at given submaximal workload
Decreased respiratory exchange ratio at given submaximal workload
Decreased perceived exertion at given submaximal workload
Decreased resting heart rate and systolic blood pressure
Decreased body fat

ing physical capacity by improving both cardiopulmonary and musculoskeletal function *(40)*. Based on careful review of existing data, the Clinical Practice Guideline *(3)* states:

> *Elderly coronary patients have exercise trainability comparable to that of younger patients participating in similar exercise rehabilitation—no complications or adverse outcomes of exercise training at elderly age were described in any study. Elderly patients of both genders should be strongly encouraged to participate in exercise-based cardiac rehabilitation.*

Potential benefits of exercise to the elderly cardiac patient based on cardiac rehabilitation studies of younger and older patients and exercise studies of the elderly are presented in Tables 6, 7, and 8.

5. EXERCISE TRAINING

Detailed clinical guidelines and risk stratification for entry into inpatient and outpatient cardiac rehabilitation programs are published by the US Department of Health and Human Services *(3)*, the AACVPR *(7)*, and the ACSM *(16,17)*. Important baseline assessments for the older cardiac patient entering an exercise program include a medical evaluation which includes a detailed medical history, physical exam, resting electrocardiogram (ECG), and quality-of-life questionnaire (e.g., MOS SF-36) *(7,14,41)*. Table 9 lists contraindications to exercise training as set forth by the ACSM *(16)*. A graded

Table 7
Benefits of Resistance Exercise for the Elderly Cardiac Patient

Increased muscle strength, power, and endurance
Increased balance
Fall prevention
Increased function in activities of daily living
Increased time to exhaustion
Increased bone mineral density
Increased lean body mass (fights sarcopenia)
Maintenance of resting metabolism
Decreased body fat
Injury prevention
Decreased cardiovascular response to daily lifting tasks

Table 8
Benefits of Flexibility Exercise for the Elderly Cardiac Patient

Increased tendon flexibility
Increased joint function and range of motion
Increased muscular performance
Prevention and treatment of musculoskeletal injuries

Table 9
Contraindications for Exercise Training

Unstable angina
Severe arterial hypertension (SBP > 200 mm Hg or DBP > 110 mm Hg)
    or symptomatic orthostatic hypotension
Severe aortic stenosis
Tachy or bradyarrythmias
Uncontrolled sinus tachycardia at rest (>120 bpm)
Acute systemic illness or fever
Uncompensated congestive heart failure
Third-degree AV block without pacemaker
Active myocarditis or pericarditis
Recent embolism
Thrombophlebitis
>2 mm resting ST segment depression
Uncontrolled diabetes (blood glucose >400 mg/dL at rest)
Neuromuscular, musculoskeletal or rheumatoid disorders exacerbated
    by exercise
Additional metabolic conditions (e.g., acute thyroiditis, hypo- or hyper-
    kalemia, hypovolemia)

Source: Adapted from ref. *16*.

exercise test provides valuable information on normal and abnormal cardiovascular and musculoskeletal responses to increased activity and establishes thresholds for exertion-related abnormalities *(7)*, helping to set safe exercise levels *(27)*. The reader is referred to the AACVPR's *(7)* and ACSM's *(16,17)* guidelines for a more detailed look at clinical

Table 10
Key Conditions to Assess Prior to Initiating Exercise

Condition	Precaution
Hypertension	Patients with SBP > 180 mm Hg or DBP > 110 mm Hg should not start exercising until drug therapy is initiated. Endurance exercise (e.g., walking) at low intensities (i.e., 40–70% HRR) as effective at lowering BP as high intensity exercise. Add resistance training as secondary component of exercise regimen.
Pulmonary disease	Avoid early morning exercise when symptoms are worst. May benefit from interval training at higher intensities and resistance training. Maintain oxyhemoglobin saturation > 90%.
Diabetes mellitus	Delay exercise if blood glucose > 300 mg/dL or > 240 mg/dL with urinary ketone bodies. May need CHO snack before exercise if blood glucose <80–100 mg/dL, and during prolonged exercise (e.g., 20–30 g CHO/ 30 min of exercise). Measure blood glucose before, during, and after activity. Avoid insulin injections in areas of exercising muscle.
Frailty	Target balance and fall prevention. Emphasize resistance training. Be aware of medications. May benefit from exercise performed while sitting or using assistive devices.
Osteoporosis	Include strength, balance, and aerobic activities if possible. Avoid forward flexion of spine. Patients with kyphosis may need to exercise while sitting. Avoid quick trunk rotation and high spinal compressive forces. Emphasize fall prevention.
Arthritis	Avoid overstretching affected joints or high-impact, high-repetition, high-resistance exercise.

Source: Adapted from refs. *16,62*.

exercise testing. Additional key conditions to consider before initiating an exercise regimen are listed in Table 10. In order to optimize the exercise prescription for the elderly patient, a functional evaluation related to the physical requirements of activities of daily living (i.e., strength, power, endurance, balance, mobility, flexibility) should also be employed *(7,42)*. It is important for the clinician to remember that the impact of cardiac symptoms on the elderly patient exacerbate the combined effects of aging and a (typically) sedentary lifestyle, often leading to frailty and functional dependence. Therefore, therapeutic options must include exercise that combats frailty and functional dependence. General recommendations for exercise prescription apply to all ages *(16)*, however, because of their typically reduced functional status and presence of co-morbidities, special considerations specific to the individual elderly cardiac patient's limitations are recommended *(3,7,16,31–37,39)* (Table 11).

5.1. Fundamental Principles of Exercise Training

Whether designing an exercise prescription for the elderly cardiac patient or an elite athlete, certain fundamental principles of training need to be kept in mind.

5.1.1. INDIVIDUALITY

Individuals will respond and adapt differently to a given exercise prescription based on their physiological and perceptual responses to a stimulus *(16,43)*. The specific characteristics, needs and goals of the individual patient, including health status, medications,

Table 11
Considerations for Exercise with the Elderly Cardiac Patient

Exercise prescription

Be patient
Focus on fun
Start low, go slow—be conservative
Learn exercise preferences
Target functional independence (ability to perform ADLs)
Individualize the prescription
Use measured vs estimated peak heart rate to set workout
     intensities
Warm-up and cool-down
Emphasize a normal breathing pattern
Use complete range of motion within pain-free zone
Emphasize lifestyle changes in activity

Safety

Be aware of decreased functional ability (e.g., balance,
     comorbidities, cognitive function, memory)
Minimize orthopedic stress
Offer variety to prevent overuse injuries
Offer multi-joint exercises to minimize joint stress
Provide appropriate supervision and ECG monitoring
Know medications

Environment

Modify facilities and equipment
Emphasize fall prevention (e.g., floors, rugs, furniture)
Accommodate impaired senses such as vision (e.g., large
     type)
Understand transportation, weather, and darkness limitations
Involve family members and caregivers
Provide patient-familiar music

Source: Adapted from ref. 7.

risk factors, behaviors, goals, and preferences *(8,16,43–45)*, are always the cornerstone of any comprehensive exercise prescription. The "art and science" of an exercise prescription requires close monitoring of individual responses to the exercise program with such measures as heart rate, blood pressure, ECG monitoring, rate of perceived exertion, and verbal feedback on likes and dislikes of the program *(16)*. Recognizing the individuality of the elderly cardiac patient regarding comorbidities, functional limitations, preferences, and personality is crucial to optimizing outcomes and adherence to any exercise prescription *(2,12,16,17,37,43,45)*.

5.1.2. PROGRESSIVE OVERLOAD

In order for the patient's fitness level to improve, they must experience progressive and safe challenges to their physical capabilities *(16,43)*. With appropriate progression of the overload, variety of overload, and adequate rest (during and between workouts), positive adaptation will occur safely and progressively in response to the exercise stimulus *(43)*. One of the most common mistakes of exercise prescription, especially in the frail elderly, is application of excessive overload on the individual before they are prepared to tolerate and adapt to the stimulus *(2,12,16,37,43)*.

5.1.3. SPECIFICITY

Training effects are specific to muscle group recruitment patterns, modes of activity, speed of movement, range of motion, and energy systems involved *(16,43)*. For improved fitness to impact daily living and job-related tasks of the elderly patient, the exercise stimulus needs to be tailored to the specific needs of the individual *(7,12,16,37,43)*.

5.1.4. REVERSIBILITY

Without constant stimulus (maintenance or overload), gains in fitness and function will return to starting levels *(40)*. The principle of reversibility highlights the importance of making exercise part of a healthy lifestyle to be continued after formal cardiac rehabilitation is complete. Without long-term adherence, short-term gains in fitness achieved during cardiac rehabilitation (typically 8–12 wk) fail to give long-term benefit.

5.2. General Structure of an Exercise Training Session

5.2.1. WARM-UP

A proper warm-up in cardiac rehabilitation patients is always prudent *(16)*, especially for the elderly patient. Warm-up helps prepare the individual both physically and psychologically for the upcoming workout stress. Each exercise session should start with a 10–20 min warm-up period involving both low-intensity aerobic activities and mild calisthenics, along with stretching that elevate heart rate toward prescriptive exercise levels *(16,45)*.

5.2.2. WORKOUT

The workout period involves 20–60 min of exercise stress. Intensity and volume are inversely related (e.g., the higher the intensity, the lower the total volume of the workout) *(16)*. Aerobic training is emphasized in cardiac rehabilitation, but a variety of activities including resistance training and flexibility exercises are recommended additions to the aerobic exercise stress *(7,16)*. Games modified for low skill and intensity may also provide fun and effective alternatives to traditional exercise *(16)*. Individuality, progressive overload, specificity, and variety are keys to optimizing workout stress, enhancing outcomes, and minimizing boredom *(43)*.

5.2.3. COOL-DOWN

Proper cool-down is essential to the safety of the cardiac rehabilitation patient, helping to bring the body's physiology back to normal after the exercise stress *(16)*. As in warm-up, cool-down can involve low-intensity aerobics, calisthenics, and stretching activities. Relaxation skills can also be developed during the cool-down using modalities like meditation and mindful awareness techniques.

5.3. Characteristics of Aerobic Exercise

Aerobic exercise should be a cornerstone of the elderly patient's rehabilitation regimen. Aerobic exercise has positive benefits on many aspects of cardiovascular function, such as maximal oxygen consumption (VO_2 max), stroke volume, and increased capillary density and mitochondrial supply in muscle. These positive adaptations lower the physiological stress to a given workload, improve exercise tolerance, and delay the onset of angina during activities. Guidelines for basing the individualized aerobic exercise prescription of the elderly cardiac patient are based on the low end of the ACSM's recommendations for developing and maintaining cardiovascular fitness for the healthy adult *(44)*. Guidelines suggest performance of large muscle group, rhythmical activities that are easily maintained at a constant energy expenditure at an intensity of 55–90% of maximum heart rate (estimated HRmax = 220 – age), or 40–85% of maximum oxygen uptake reserve (VO$_2$R) or HR max reserve (HRR; Target HR range = [HRmax – HRrest] × target workout HR% + HRrest). A duration of 20–60 min of continuous or intermittent aerobic activity (minimum of 10-min bouts accumulated throughout the day) at a frequency of 3–5 d/wk is also recommended.

The elderly cardiac patient is typically more deconditioned than their younger counterpart *(16,35,36)*. Comorbidities that necessitate manipulation of the exercise prescription may also be present *(3,7,16,36,37)*. Therefore, the previous recommendations need a conservative, individualized approach when dealing with the elderly cardiac patient *(3,7,16,37,45)* such as mode, intensity, frequency, and duration.

Mode: Based on individual condition (balance, orthopedic problems, etc.) and preference, treadmill walking, stationary bicycling, arm ergometry, water aerobics, and rowing are examples of modalities useful in the rehabilitation process of the elderly adult *(7,16)*.

Intensity: The lower intensity values, i.e., 40–49% of VO$_2$R or HRR and 55%–64% of HRmax, are most applicable to individuals who are quite unfit *(16)*. The less fit the individual, the lower the intensity necessary to cause positive adaptations. The ACSM recommends a level high enough to convey a "training effect," but at least 10 bpm under the intensity that correlates with any of the signs of cardiovascular problems, angina, abnormal ECG, wall motion abnormalities, increased ventricular arrhythmias, or other signs of exercise intolerance *(16)*. It is recommended that measured peak heart rate be used when available because of the variability in peak heart rate in those older than 65 *(16,35,36)*. Ades et al. *(35,36)* also suggest that older patients work at a higher intensity than traditionally recommended during aerobic training, based on their observance that older coronary patients seldom achieve a true physiological maximum at baseline exercise testing for basing exercise intensity *(32)*. The presence of medications that affect peak heart rate should also be noted *(7,16)*. Conservative, progressive application of exercise stress is key to optimal outcome without complications.

Frequency: A minimum of 2–3 d/wk of exercise early in cardiac rehabilitation are recommended, with the goal of progressing to 3–5 d/wk for optimal benefit *(16)*. Caution must be exhibited so as not to orthopedically overstress the patient. Variety in mode of training can help change the stress on joints and alleviate boredom.

Duration: Many older cardiac patients will need to accumulate shorter bouts of exercise to achieve the recommended 20–60 min of activity each workout session. Duration should be increased before intensity to help ensure positive adaptation to the exercise stress *(16)*.

Focus, however, must also be on ensuring the elderly patient ability to perform activities of daily living, maintain functional independence, and achieve a high quality of life *(2,3,7,12,16,31–34,37)*. The lifestyle activity goal promoted by the Centers for Disease Control and Prevention (CDC) and ACSM *(46)* who recommend that every adult accumulate at least 30 min of moderate activity most days of the week should be emphasized. As appropriate to the individual patient, they should be counseled on how to incorporate activity into the daily routine *(14)*, such as walking, taking stairs, gardening, and other lifestyle-based activities. However, it is important to realize that for the older patient, performance of certain activities of daily living (e.g., stair climbing) may require a near maximal effort, and caution must be urged *(34–37)*.

5.4. Characteristics of Resistance Exercise Training

In general, the elderly benefit more from resistance training than other populations *(12,37,40,47–51)*. Becoming stronger and more powerful with greater endurance helps the older adult perform activities of daily living, improve bone mineral density, prevent falls, and remain functionally independent. Resistance training is the only exercise modality that has simultaneously impacted many factors that relate to the risk for falls and fractures, including muscle power, strength, mass, and dynamic balance *(49,50)*. Resistance training can help fight sarcopenia (age-related loss of muscle mass), which is related to many aspects of functional decline in the elderly. In the older cardiac patient, becoming stronger helps the person perform routine lifting tasks with a lower circulatory response, at a lower percent of their maximal strength level, and with greater efficiency of movement. For example, resistance training in older women has demonstrated a reduction in cardiovascular stress (e.g., heart rate, systolic blood pressure, and rate pressure product) while carrying the same absolute weight before and after training *(51)*. Greater walking endurance as a result of resistance training in the elderly has also been demonstrated *(31)*.

Traditionally, cardiac rehabilitation programs emphasized aerobic training and often omitted resistance training. However, the addition of resistance training to the aerobic exercise prescription has recently become the recommended course of action for most patients *(47)*. However, a recent review by McCartney *(52)*, found only two resistance training studies in cardiac patients over 60 (mean age 61 yr), demonstrating the need for research regarding resistance training in the older cardiac patient *(47)*. In 1999, Adams et al. *(53)* conducted a combined resistance training and aerobic training study using 61 cardiac rehabilitation patients with the majority (including high-risk patients) over 60 yr of age. High-intensity resistance training significantly improved the patient's strength with no complications. The same research group found similar results with combined resistance and aerobic training in 14 congestive heart failure patients who had a mean age of 60 yr *(40)*. In support, Fiatarone and colleagues *(2)* also found resistance training to be beneficial in 16 women with CHF averaging 77-yr-old. In response to the resistance training, subjects improved their musculoskeletal characteristics and metabolism, leading to improved functional performance.

Resulting from the lack of research studies using resistance training in the elderly patient (>65 yr) however, caution is urged in routine application of resistance training without careful consideration of the risk to benefit ratio for the individual elderly patient *(12,16,44,45,54,55)*. Contraindications to resistance training are similar to those for general exercise training (Table 9) and include uncontrolled hypertension (SBP >159 mm Hg or DBP > 99 mm Hg), uncontrolled dysrhythmias, unevaluated or untreated CHF, severe valvular disease, and hypertrophic cardiomyopathy *(7,16,47)*. Resistance training, however, may be a crucial addition to the exercise stress in order to return the elderly cardiac patient to functionally independent living. Resistance training has had dramatic and positive impact on frail and very old populations with no complications *(2,12,50,55)* and has become a highly recommended exercise therapy in even the oldest adults, often implemented before aerobic training *(2,12,30,37,49,50)*.

The AHA *(14,47)* and the ACSM *(16)* and the AACVPR *(7)* recommend the following guidelines on which to base the resistance training prescription for the elderly cardiac rehabilitation patient.

Mode: Weight machines, free weights (e.g., dumbbells and barbells, pulleys, rubber bands) are useful at providing resistance. Exercises chosen should involve large muscle groups of the body and mimic muscle action regularly encountered in daily living. Additionally, exercises involving movement around multiple joints will minimize the stress placed on any one structure, reducing the chance for injury.

Intensity: 10–15 repetitions at low resistance (i.e., 50–60% of one-repetition maximum) at first, with individualized, slow progression per the patient's condition, presence of comorbidities, and response to the resistance training program. As the patient adapts to the resistance training, individual adjustment in load keeps the patient in the 10–15 repetition range, similar to increasing a patient's workload on a treadmill to stay within a target heart range.

Volume: 1–2 sets each for major muscle groups (6–10 exercises total). Again, volume can be progressively increased per patient condition and tolerance.

Frequency: 2–3 d/wk for 20–30 min each day as an addition to the aerobic exercise training. With cautious application, studies suggest that adding resistance training to the aerobic exercise regimen can help the elderly cardiac patient's rehabilitation process and the return to functional independence *(2,3,12,16,47)*.

5.5. Characteristics of Flexibility Exercise Training

Limited data on outcomes of specific flexibility (range of motion) training are available, especially in the elderly *(37,44)*. However, poor flexibility is common in the elderly *(16,37,55)* and often contributes to functional decline and nursing home admission *(55)*. Flexibility exercise should be included in the individualized cardiac rehabilitation exercise prescription of the elderly participant and often can be incorporated in the overall workout (warm-up, between exercise sets and stations, and cool-down). Performing appropriate flexibility exercises (e.g., cat stretch, back-scratch stretch, seated toe-touch), individualized to the patient's joint health and physical condition, in a slow, controlled manner can help the elderly achieve and maintain functional range of motion *(16)*. The ACSM *(16)* recommends the following basic guidelines on which to base the flexibility exercise prescription for the elderly cardiac participant:

Mode: General static stretching.
Intensity: Light to mild discomfort.
Frequency: At least 2–3 d/wk.
Duration: Hold static stretch for 10–30 s.
Repetitions: 3–4 per stretch.

Effort should be made by the exercise technician to ensure the appropriate movement through the full range of motion in the variety of activities available to the participant (e.g., aerobics, resistance training, balance training) *(8,16,47)*. This will help optimize outcomes pertaining to joint range of motion *(12)*.

6. NUTRITIONAL COUNSELING

A comprehensive approach to combating the development and progression of cardiac disease in the elderly must include nutritional counseling *(56)*. In addition to senescence and disease, improper or inadequate nutritional intake contributes to disease progression, exercise capacity, and ultimately, frailty, functional dependence, and a poor quality of life in the elderly *(12,57,58)*. Additionally, it is crucial for the clinician to realize that sarcopenia (age-related loss of muscle mass) is directly related to functional disability in the older adult *(12,37,47,49,50,57)*. Inadequate calories and/or protein consumption, regardless of exercise stress, leads to sarcopenia, strongly contributing to low muscle strength and power, which increases risk for such things as falls, fractures, dependence, immune system impairment, and insulin insensitivity *(12,57)*.

Nutrition counseling for older adults in cardiac rehabilitation must recognize specific nutrient requirements related to age and presence of disease, plus additional demands related to increased physical activity and exercise *(56–59)*. Appropriate nutrition (Atherosclerosis chapter) can reduce the risk of a variety of chronic health problems, including heart disease, type 2 diabetes, and osteoporosis *(59)*. Additionally, obesity, a rapidly growing epidemic in all segments of our society, is strongly related to risk of CVD, improper lipoprotein metabolism, diabetes mellitus, and hypertension *(59,60)*. Patients may not always "look" obese, but the clinician must be aware that a high amount of intraabdominal fat may be present *(2,60)*. Also, sarcopenic obesity may be present where the patient's weight may be fairly stable, but there has been a consistent decline in lean body mass through the years and an accumulation of body fat *(57,61)*. Clinicians must recognize the complexity of treating obesity in the elderly because of an apparent decreased ability to regulate energy intake with energy expenditure *(56,58)*.

The AHA and AACVPR *(14)* recommend that the patient's diet be based on AHA guidelines *(59)* with consideration of the individual's age and disease status. Counseling should survey caloric and nutrient intake, dietary fat intake, eating habits, and preferences in order to optimally individualize the dietary plan *(14)*. Because the elderly have reduced energy needs with no change or increased nutrient requirements, counseling should include tools to select nutrient dense foods from each food group *(58,59)*. Dietary recommendations for elderly cardiac rehabilitation patients must also consider the impact of increased activity and exercise on dietary needs *(58)*. Table 12 outlines general recommendations considering both the AHA guidelines *(59)* and the needs related to exercise *(12,56–61)*.

7. RISK FACTOR MANAGEMENT

Risk factor management in cardiac rehabilitation encompasses lipid levels, hypertension, weight, diabetes, and smoking *(14)*. Once patient assessments have identified individual conditions, preferences, and needs, comprehensive risk factor intervention attempts to demonstrate improved clinical outcomes, improved quality of life, and an overall reduction in health care costs *(13)*. Unfortunately, approximately two-thirds of eligible patients fail to receive comprehensive treatment to modify risk factors *(7,13)*. Optimal risk factor reduction requires a team approach with doctors, nurses, nutritionists, behavioral counselors and exercise physiologists working together to develop the individualized treatment plan and to encourage adherence *(7,13)*. The importance of behavioral counseling to facilitate change cannot be overstated, since advice without action has

Table 12
General Dietary Recommendations for the Elderly Cardiac Rehabilitation Participant

1. Maintain appropriate body weight by balancing energy intake with energy expenditure. Gain or lose weight by combined manipulation of caloric intake and physical activity.

2. Drink plenty of fluids to avoid dehydration, especially before, during, and after the cardiac rehabilitation exercise session. Drink when thirsty and avoid exercise in hot, humid conditions. Limit alcohol intake to no more than 2 drinks per day for men and 1 for women.

3. Fat intake should be <30% of total caloric intake, with <7% coming from saturated fat and <200 mg of cholesterol per day. Limit intake of hydrogenated fat. Consume at least 2 servings of fish per week and consume additional unsaturated fats from vegetables, legumes, and nuts.

4. Protein intake should range from 1.0 to 1.2 g/kg/d, representing 12–15% of caloric intake. Emphasize lean sources, low in saturated fat, such as skim milk, low or nonfat dairy products, fish, soy, legumes and nuts.

5. Carbohydrates should represent approx 55–60% of caloric intake, and should primarily be complex carbohydrates, high in nutrients and fiber. Intake >5 servings per day of fruits and vegetables of many colors (i.e., dark green, orange, yellow), and >6 servings per day of various grain products (i.e, whole-grain cereals). Choose starches, such as cereal and potatoes, over refined, simple sugar products.

6. Vitamin and mineral intake (e.g., vitamin D and calcium, B vitamins) should meet RDA guidelines. Supplement with single or multivitamin as needed if dietary sources do not achieve appropriate levels.

no effect. Table 13 presents an overview of goals and recommendations of risk factor management in cardiac rehabilitation as recommended by the AHA and AACVPR (7,14).

8. RECOMMENDATIONS FOR CLINICIANS

Cardiovascular disease exacts a heavy toll, both socially and economically, on older adults. Unfortunately, the majority of older adults affected by CVD do not participate in comprehensive cardiac rehabilitation programs. Exercise is a cornerstone of modern cardiac rehabilitation and has the potential to dramatically alter the recovery and function of the older adult cardiac patient.

Recommendations for the clinician working with the elderly cardiac patient include:

1. Consider comprehensive cardiac rehabilitation for all older patients post-MI or diagnosed with CHF exacerbation and in cardiac patients interested in initiating an exercise program.
2. Perform a graded exercise test to identify thresholds for exertion-related abnormalities.
3. Make sure exercise regimens are individualized to the needs and goals of the patient.
4. Avoid overloading the physical capabilities of the patient when prescribing exercise (i.e., start slow, go slow).
5. Aerobic training intensity should be conservative (i.e., 55% HRmax), staying at least 10 bpm below the intensity that correlates with any signs of cardiovascular problems.
6. Frequency of exercise should begin at 2–3 d/wk and increase to 3–5 d/wk. Shorter bouts of exercise (e.g., 10 min at a time) may be necessary to achieve the recommended 20–60 min of activity per exercise session.

Table 13
Risk Factor Management in Cardiac Rehabilitation

Lipid management goals	*Recommendations*
LDL < 100 mg/dL; HDL > 35 mg/dL; Triglycerides < 200 mg/dL	Treatment strategies include: nutritional counseling per AHA guidelines; weight management; exercise; drug therapy; smoking cessation, achohol moderation.
Hypertension goals	*Recommendations*
BP < 130 mm Hg systolic and <85 mm Hg diastolic	Lifestyle modification (exercise, weight management, smoking cessation, alcohol moderation, moderate sodium restriction); drug therapy.
Weight goals	*Recommendations*
BMI < 25; waist < 40 inches (males), 35 inches (females), appropriate body weight	Combine diet, exercise, and behavior modification to reduce caloric intake, maintain adequate nutrition, and increase energy expenditure.
Diabetes goals	*Recommendations*
Fasting glucose normal (80–110 mg/dL or HbA₁C < 7.0); minimize diabetic complications; manage associated obesity, hypertension, and hyperlipidemia	Encourage dietary adherence and weight control. Use exercise, oral hypoglycemic agents, insulin therapy, and risk factor management as intervention strategies. Carefully monitor glucose before and after exercise.
Smoking goals	*Recommendations*
Abstinence from smoking and tobacco products at 12 mo from stop date	Provide formal smoking cessation program with group and/or individual counseling.

Source: Adapted from Balady et al. *(14)*.

7. Progressive resistance training should be performed 2–3 d/wk, targeting large muscle groups at a resistance that easily allows for 10–15 repetitions at a time with good technique.
8. Incorporate nutritional counseling into comprehensive cardiac rehabilitation efforts.

REFERENCES

1. Cooper R, Cutler J, Desvignes-Nickens P, Fortmann SP, Friedman L, Havlik R, et al. Trends and disparities in coronary heart disease, stroke, and other cardiovascular diseases in the United States. Findings of the National Conference on Cardiovascular Disease Prevention. Circulation 2000;102: 3137–3147.
2. Fiatarone Singh MA, Wei JY. Cardiovascular disease and hypertension. In: Exercise, Nutrition, and the Older Woman. Wellness for Women Over Fifty. Fiatarone Singh MA (ed.), CRC Press, Washington, DC, 2000, pp. 279–319.
3. Wenger NK, Froelicher ES, Smith LK, et al. Cardiac rehabilitation. Clinical practice guideline No. 17. U.S. Department of Health and Human Services, Rockville, MD, Public Health Service, Agency for Health Care Policy and Research and the National Heart, Lung, and Blood Institute. AHCPR Publication No. 96-0672, October 1995.

4. Hoyert DL, Kochanek KD, Murphy SL. Deaths: final data for 1997. In: National Vital Statistics Reports. DHHS Publication Number 99-1120, National Center for Health Statistics, Hyattsville, MD, 1999.

5. Morbidity and Mortality: 2000 Chart Book on Cardiovascular, Lung, and Blood Diseases. National Institutes of Health: National Heart, Lung, and Blood Institute; Bethesda, MD, 1998.

6. Balady GJ, Fletcher BJ, Froelicher ES, Hartley LH, Krauss RM, Oberman A, et al. Cardiac rehabilitation programs. A statement for healthcare professionals from the A H A. Circulation 1994;90:1602–1610.

7. American Association of Cardiovascular and Pulmonary Rehabilitation. Guidelines for Cardiac Rehabilitation and Secondary Prevention Programs. 3rd ed. Human Kinetics, Champaign, IL, 1999.

8. Leon AS. Exercise following myocardial infarction. Sports Med 2000;29:301–311.

9. Ades PA, Waldmann ML, McCann W, Weaver SO. Predictors of cardiac rehabilitation participation in older coronary patients. Arch Intern Med 1992;152:1033–1035.

10. Ades PA, Waldmann ML, Polk DM, Coflesky JT. Referral patterns and exercise response in the rehabilitation of female coronary patients aged ≥ 62 years. Am J Cardiol 1992;69:1422–1425.

11. Mosca L, Grundy SM, Judelson D, King K, Limacher M, Oparil S, et al. Guide to preventive cardiology in women. AHA/ACC Scientific Statement: Consensus Panel Statement. Circulation 1999;99: 2480–2484.

12. Fiatarone Singh MA. Exercise. In: Exercise, Nutrition, and the Older Woman. Wellness for Women Over Fifty. Fiatarone Singh MA (ed.), CRC Press, Washington, DC, 2000; pp. 3–128.

13. Smith SC Jr, Blair SN, Criqui MH, Fletcher GF, Fuster V, Gersh BJ, et al. Preventing heart attack and death in patients with coronary artery disease. Circulation 1995;92:2–4.

14. Balady GJ, Ades PA, Comoss P, Limacher M, Pina IL, Southard D, et al. Core components of cardiac rehabilitation/secondary prevention programs. A statement for healthcare professionals from the American Heart Association and the American Association of Cardiovascular and Pulmonary Rehabilitation. Circulation 2000;102:1069–1073.

15. Thompson PD. Exercise rehabilitation for cardiac patients. A beneficial but underused therapy. Physician Sports Med 2001;29:69–75.

16. American College of Sports Medicine. General principles of exercise prescription—exercise prescription for cardiac patients. In: ACSM's Guidelines for Exercise Testing and Prescription. 6th ed. Lippincott Williams & Wilkins, Baltimore, MD, 2000, pp. 135–199.

17. LaFontaine TP, Gordon NF. Comprehensive cardiovascular risk reduction in patients with coronary artery disease. In: American College of Sports Medicine. ACSM's Resource Manual for Guidelines for Exercise Testing and Prescription. 4th ed. Lippincott Williams & Wilkins, Baltimore, MD, 2001; pp. 263–273.

18. Froelicher VF, Herbert W, Myers J, Ribisl P. How cardiac rehabilitation is being influenced by changes in health-care delivery. J Cardiopulm Rehabil 1996;16:151–159.

19. Oldridge NB. Outcome assessment in cardiac rehabilitation. Health-related quality of life and economic evaluation. J Cardiopulm Rehabil 1997;17:179–194.

20. Oldridge NB, Furlong W, Feeny D, Torrance G, Guyatt G, Crowe J, Jones N. Economic evaluation of cardiac rehabilitation after acute myocardial infarction. Am J Cardiol 1993;72:154–161.

21. Ades PA, Huang G, Weaver SO. Cardiac rehabilitation participation predicts lower hospitalization costs. Am Heart J 1992;123:916–921.

22. Ades PA, Pashkow FJ, Nestor JR. Cost-effectiveness of cardiac rehabilitation after myocardial infarction. J Cardiopulm Rehabil 1997;17:222–231.

23. Bondestam E, Breikss A, Hartford M. Effects of early rehabilitation on consumption of medical care during the first year after acute myocardial infarction in patients ≥ 65 years of age. Am J Cardiol 1995; 75:767–771.

24. Fletcher GF, Balady G, Froelicher VF, Hartley LH, Haskell WL, Pollock ML. Exercise standards. A statement for healthcare professionals from the A H A. Circulation 1995;91:580–615.

25. Pearson T, Rapaport E, Criqui M, Furberg C, Fuster V, Hiratzka L, et al. Optimal risk factor management in the patient after coronary revascularization. A statement from the A H A for Healthcare Professionals. Circulation 1994;90:3125–3133.

26. Franklin BA, Balady GJ, Berra K, Gordon NF, Pollock ML. Exercise for persons with cardiovascular disease. American College of Sports Medicine. Current Comments, July, 1998.

27. Fletcher GF, Balady G, Blair SN, Blumenthal J, Casperson C, Chaitman B, et al. Statement on exercise: benefits and recommendations for health professionals by the Committee on Exercise and Cardiac Rehabilitation of the Council on Clinical Cardiology, A H A. Circulation 1996;94:857–862.

28. Fletcher GF. How to implement physical activity in primary and secondary prevention. A statement for healthcare professionals from the Task Force on Risk Reduction, A H A. Circulation 1997;96:355–377.

29. Perk J, Veress G. Cardiac rehabilitation: Applying exercise physiology in clinical practice. Eur J Appl Physiol 2000;83:457–462.
30. Adams KJ, Swank AM, Berning JM, Sevene-Adams PG, Barnard KL, Shimp-Bowerman J. Progressive strength training in sedentary older African American women. Med Sci Sports Exerc. 2001;33:1567–1576.
31. Ades PA, Ballor DL, Ashikaga T, Utton JL, Nair KS. Weight training improves walking endurance in healthy elderly persons. Ann Intern Med 1996;124:568–572.
32. Ades PA, Grunvald MH. Cardiopulmonary exercise testing before and after conditioning in older coronary patients. Am Heart J 1990;120:585–589.
33. Ades PA, Maloney A, Savage P, Carhart RL. Determinants of physical functioning in coronary patients. Response to cardiac rehabilitation. Arch Intern Med 1999;159:2357–2360.
34. Ades PA, Tischler MD, Savage PD, Dee J, Richman T, Henkin J. Determinants of disability in older coronary patients. Circulation 1996;94(suppl 1):I–497.
35. Ades PA, Waldmann ML, Gillespie C. A controlled trial of exercise training in older coronary patients. J Gerontol 1995;50A:M7–M11.
36. Ades PA, Waldmann ML, Poehlman ET, Gray P, Horton ED, Horton ES, et al. Exercise conditioning in older coronary patients. Submaximal lactate response and endurance capacity. Circulation 1993;88: 572–577.
37. American College of Sports Medicine position stand: exercise and physical activity for older adults. Med Sci Sports Exerc 1998;30:992–1008.
38. Ross SJ, Poehlman ET, Johnson RK, Ades PA. Body fat distribution predicts cardiac risk factors in older female coronary patients. J Cardiopulmonary Rehabil 1997;17:419–427.
39. Williams MA, Maresh CM, Esterbrooks DJ, Harbrecht JJ, Sketch MH. Early exercise training in patients older than age 65 years compared with that in younger patients after acute myocardial infarction or coronary artery bypass grafting. Am J Cardiol 1985;55:263–266.
40. Barnard KL, Adams KJ, Swank AM, Kaelin M, Kushnik MR, Denny DM. Combined high-intensity strength and aerobic training in patients with congestive heart failure. J Strength Cond Res 2000;14: 383–388.
41. Shephard RJ, Franklin B. Changes in quality of life: A major goal of cardiac rehabilitation. J Cardiopulm Rehabil 2001;21:189–200
42. Rikli RE, Jones CJ. Senior Fitness Test Manual. Human Kinetics, Champaign, IL, 2001.
43. Fleck SJ, Kraemer WJ. Designing Resistance Training Programs. 2nd ed. Human Kinetics, Champaign, IL, 1997.
44. American College of Sports Medicine position stand: the recommended quantity and quality of exercise for developing and maintaining cardiorespiratory and muscular fitness and flexibility in healthy adults. Med Sci Sports Exerc 1998;30:975–991.
45. American College of Sports Medicine position stand: exercise for patients with coronary artery disease. Med Sci Sports Exerc 1994;26:i–v.
46. Pate RR, Pratt M, Blair SN, Haskell WL, Macera CA, Bouchard C, et al. Physical activity and public health: A recommendation from the Centers for Disease Control and Prevention and the American College of Sports Medicine. JAMA 1995;273:402–407.
47. Pollock ML, Franklin BA, Balady GJ, Chaitman BL, Fleg JL, Fletcher B, et al. Resistance exercise in individuals with and without cardiovascular disease. Benefits, rationale, safety, and prescription. An advisory from the Committee on Exercise, Rehabilitation, and Prevention, Council on Clinical Cardiology, AHA. Circulation 2000;101:828–833.
48. Feigenbaum MS, Pollock ML. Strength training: Rationale for current guidelines for adult fitness programs. Physician Sports Med 1997;25:44–64.
49. Nelson ME, Fiatarone MA, Morganti CM, Trice I, Greenberg RA, Evans WJ. Effects of high-intensity strength training on multiple risk factors for osteoporotic fractures. JAMA 1994;272:1909–1914.
50. Fiatarone MA, O'Neil EF, Ryan ND, Meredith CN, Lipsitz LA, Evans WJ. Exercise training and nutritional supplementation for physical frailty in very elderly people. N Engl J Med 1994;330: 1769–1775.
51. Parker ND, Hunter GR, Treuth MS, Kekes-Szabo T, Kell SH, Weinser R, White M. Effects of strength training on cardiovascular responses during a submaximal walk and a weight-loaded walking test in older females. J Cardiopulm Rehabil 1996;16:56–62.
52. McCartney N. Role of resistance training in heart disease. Med Sci Sports Exerc 1998;30:S396–S402.
53. Adams KJ, Barnard KL, Swank AM, Mann E, Kushnik MR, Denny DM. Combined high-intensity strength and aerobic training in diverse phase II cardiac rehabilitation patients. J Cardiopulm Rehabil 1999;19:209–215.

54. Barnard KL, Adams KJ Swank AM, Mann E, Denny DM. Injuries and muscle soreness during the one repetition maximum assessment in a cardiac rehabilitation population. J Cardiopulm Rehabil 1999; 19:52–58.

55. Hurley BF, nd Hagberg JM. Optimizing health in older persons: aerobic or strength training? Exerc Sport Sci Rev 1998;26:61–89.

56. Deckelbaum RJ, Fisher EA, Winston M, Kumanyika S, Lauer RM, Pi-Sunyer FX, et al. Summary of a scientific conference on preventive nutrition: Pediatrics to geriatrics. Circulation 1999;100:450–456.

57. Evans WJ, Cyr-Campbell D. Nutrition, exercise, and healthy aging. J Am Diet Assoc 1997;97:632–638.

58. Sacheck JM, Roubenoff R. Nutrition in the exercising elderly. Clin Sports Med 1999;18:565–584.

59. Krauss RM, Eckel RH, Howard B, Appel LJ, Daniels SR, Deckelbaum RJ, et al. AHA Dietary Guidelines. Revision 2000: A statement for healthcare professionals from the Nutrition Committee for the A H A. Circulation 2000;102:2284–2299.

60. Krauss RM, Winston M, Fletcher BJ, Grundy SM. Obesity—Impact on cardiovascular disease. Circulation 1998;98:1472–1476.

61. Sceppa CC. Protein. In: Exercise, Nutrition, and the Older Woman. Wellness for Women Over Fifty. Fiatarone Singh MA (ed.), CRC Press, Washington, DC, 2000; pp. 145–154.

62. American College of Sports Medicine. ACSM's Exercise Management for Persons with Chronic Diseases and Disabilities. Human Kinetics, Champagne, IL, 1997.

18 Chronic Heart Failure

Michael W. Rich

*Dropsy [heart failure] is usually produced when a patient remains for
a long time with impurities of the body following a long illness. The flesh
is consumed and becomes water. The abdomen fills with fluid; the feet
and legs swell; the shoulders, clavicles, chest and thighs melt away.*

Hippocrates (1)

1. INTRODUCTION

Heart failure is a condition in which one or more abnormalities in cardiac function lead
to an inability of the heart to pump sufficient blood to meet the body's metabolic needs
while maintaining normal or near-normal intracardiac pressures and blood volumes.
Heart failure affects approx 5 million Americans, and more than 500,000 new cases are
diagnosed each year *(2)*. Importantly, both the incidence and prevalence of heart failure
increase with advancing age *(3)*, with approx 80% of hospital admissions for heart
failure occurring in persons over 65 yr of age *(4)*, and more than 50% occurring in persons
over the age of 75 *(5)*. As a result, heart failure is the leading cause of hospitalization in
the Medicare age group, and it is currently the most costly cardiovascular illness in the
United States *(6)*. Moreover, it is anticipated that the rapid growth in the older adult
population will result in a doubling in the number of older persons with heart failure
during the next two to three decades.

1.1. Etiology

In the United States, chronic hypertension and coronary heart disease account for
70–80% of heart failure cases *(7,8)*. Valvular heart disease (primarily aortic stenosis and
mitral regurgitation) and nonischemic cardiomyopathies (dilated, hypertrophic,
restrictive) are also common causes of heart failure in older adults. Less frequent causes
include infective endocarditis, pericardial disease, thyroid disorders, and drug toxicity
(e.g., anthracyclines). Of note is that with increasing age, the most common etiology of
heart failure shifts from coronary artery disease to hypertension, and this is particularly

From: *Handbook of Clinical Nutrition and Aging*
Edited by: C. W. Bales and C. S. Ritchie © Humana Press Inc., Totowa, NJ

evident in older women, among whom over 50% of heart failure cases may be attributed to hypertension *(8)*.

1.2. Pathophysiology

The cardiac cycle is divided into a filling phase (diastole) and an emptying or pumping phase (systole). Impaired cardiac filling from increased "stiffness" of the heart (e.g., from hypertension) results in increased intracardiac pressures and reduced cardiac output, leading to the syndrome of "diastolic heart failure." Conversely, damage to the heart muscle (e.g., from a myocardial infarction) results in impaired pumping action or "systolic heart failure." Although most patients with heart failure have evidence for both systolic and diastolic dysfunction, patients with significantly reduced systolic function (ejection fraction <40%) are often classified as having predominantly "systolic" heart failure, whereas patients with preserved systolic function at rest (ejection fraction ≥ 50%) are considered to have predominantly "diastolic" heart failure. Patients with heart failure and an ejection fraction of 40%–49% may be viewed as having "mixed" systolic and diastolic heart failure. Recent studies indicate that about half of heart failure cases are associated with impaired systolic function, whereas the remainder have normal or near-normal systolic function at rest *(7,9)*. Importantly, diastolic heart failure is more common in women than in men, in part because of the high prevalence of hypertension in women, and the proportion of patients with diastolic heart failure increases markedly with age. In the Cardiovascular Health Study, two-thirds of women over age 65 with heart failure had preserved systolic function, as compared with only 41% of men in this age group *(10)*.

Although treatment of systolic and diastolic heart failure is similar in many respects, it is important to evaluate ventricular function by echocardiography, radionuclide angiography, or cardiac catheterization in all patients with newly diagnosed heart failure because, as discussed below, there are important differences in pharmacotherapy depending on the degree of impairment in contractile function.

1.3. Clinical Features

The cardinal symptoms of heart failure include exertional shortness of breath and fatigue, reduced exercise tolerance, orthopnea, and lower extremity edema. Palpitations and orthostatic light-headedness are also common, but chest discomfort in the absence of ischemia is not usually present. Physical findings may include tachycardia, tachypnea, elevated jugular venous pressure, moist pulmonary rales, an S_3 or S_4 gallop, hepatomegaly, and dependent pitting edema. In patients with advanced or long-standing heart failure, there is loss of lean body mass, particularly muscle mass, which in severe cases leads to cardiac cachexia.

1.4. Prognosis

The prognosis for established heart failure in persons over age 65 is poor, with 5-yr survival rates of less than 50% in both men and women *(11)*. In addition, chronic heart failure is characterized by recurrent hospitalizations for acute exacerbations *(12,13)*, a marked increase in the risk of sudden death due to arrhythmia *(14)*, and substantially impaired quality of life as a result of diminished activity tolerance. Although the short-term prognosis (i.e., 3–6 mo) is somewhat more favorable in patients with diastolic compared to systolic heart failure, the long-term prognosis is similar *(15,16)*. In addition, hospitalization rates, symptom severity, and functional capacity do not differ significantly in patients with preserved vs impaired systolic function (17).

1.5. Treatment

Optimal treatment of chronic heart failure combines both nonpharmacological and pharmacological approaches (18). Nonpharmacological measures include patient education, dietary counseling, sodium, and in some cases, fluid restriction, attention to psychosocial and financial concerns, and close follow-up. Older patients with multiple comorbid conditions or complex environmental issues often benefit from a multidisciplinary approach to care delivery, involving nurses, social workers, dietitians, therapists, pharmacists, and physicians (19,20).

1.5.1. SYSTOLIC HEART FAILURE

The pharmacotherapy of systolic heart failure has been studied extensively over the last 20 yr. Angiotensin-converting enzyme (ACE) inhibitors are the cornerstone of treatment, and available evidence indicates that these agents are at least as effective in older as in younger heart failure patients (21). Angiotensin II receptor blockers (ARBs) and the combination of hydralazine and isosorbide dinitrate are suitable alternatives in patients who are unable to tolerate ACE inhibitors (22–25). Beta blockers have also been shown to reduce mortality and improve left ventricular function in stable heart failure patients at least up to the age of 80 (26,27). Digoxin improves symptoms and reduces hospitalizations for heart failure, but has no effect on survival; effects are similar in older and younger patients (28,29). Diuretics are important for maintaining normal volume status and for managing acute heart failure exacerbations, but with the exception of spironolactone, diuretics have no discernible effect on the natural history of heart failure. Spironolactone reduces mortality in patients with advanced heart failure and is indicated in patients who remain highly symptomatic despite the above therapeutic measures (30). Current pharmacotherapy of systolic heart failure is summarized in Fig. 1.

1.5.2. DIASTOLIC HEART FAILURE

In contrast to systolic heart failure, treatment of diastolic heart failure has been less well-studied and remains largely empiric (17). Hypertension should be treated aggressively and coronary artery disease should be managed with medications and/or revascularization as indicated. Diuretics are indicated for controlling volume overload, but overdiuresis should be avoided. Additional pharmacologic agents which have been shown to improve symptoms in selected patients with diastolic heart failure include nitrates, ACE inhibitors, ARBs, beta blockers, calcium channel blockers, and digoxin.

2. NUTRITIONAL ASPECTS OF HEART FAILURE

2.1. Heart Failure as a Metabolic Syndrome

Heart failure is a chronic progressive disorder characterized by a host of neurohormonal, immunologic, and metabolic derangements (Table 1) (31). In acute heart failure, activation of the sympathetic nervous system and renin-angiotensin-aldosterone axis serve to maintain cardiac output and preserve tissue perfusion. However, chronic activation of these systems is deleterious and perpetuates progression of the heart failure syndrome. Indeed, current therapy for heart failure focuses on antagonizing the harmful

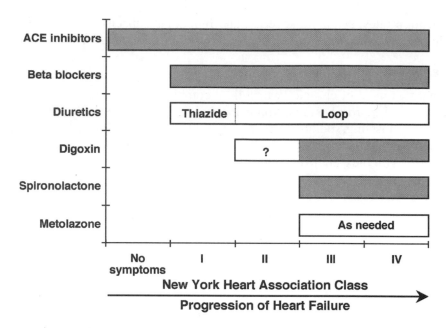

Fig. 1. Pharmacotherapy of left ventricular systolic dysfunction. Shaded regions denote conditions for which improved outcomes have been documented in prospective randomized clinical trials. ACE, angiotensin-converting enzyme.

Table 1
Neurohormonal and Metabolic Abnormalities in Chronic Heart Failure

Neurohormonal abnormalities

> Activation of sympathetic nervous system
>> Increased circulating norepinephrine and epinephrine
>> Sympathovagal imbalance with sympathetic dominance
> Activation of renin-angiotensin-aldosterone system
>> Increased angiotensin II levels
>> Increased aldosterone levels
> Increased atrial and brain natriuretic peptide levels
> Increased levels of endothelin-1
> Increased levels of vasopressin (anti-diuretic hormone)
> Increased cortisol levels
> Decreased levels of dehydroepiandrosterone (DHEA)*
> Increased insulin levels in noncachectic patients
> Increased growth hormone
> Normal or reduced insulin-like growth factor-1 (IGF-1)
> Thyroid dysfunction

Metabolic abnormalities

> Increased basal metabolic rate (BMR)
> Impaired peripheral blood flow (decreased nutrient delivery)
> Altered protein and fat metabolism
> Insulin resistance*

*Denotes antianabolic effect.

effects of these two neurohormonal pathways through the use of beta blockers and ACE inhibitors. Similarly, newer approaches to treating heart failure involve inhibiting the effects of other neurohormones (e.g., endothelin-1) or potentiating the effects of certain beneficial neurohormones (e.g., atrial natriuretic peptide).

In addition to activation of neurohormonal systems, chronic heart failure is associated with immunological dysregulation, as evidenced by increased levels of circulating tumor necrosis factor-α (TNF-α), interleukins 1, 2, 6, 8, and 10, soluble adhesion molecules, and certain leucocyte chemokines (32,33). Activation of these cytokines likely plays a pivotal role in the apoptosis (programmed cell death) and anorexia, which are features of chronic heart failure. In addition, some of these factors may exert direct cardiotoxic effects (e.g., through increased oxygen free radical activity), thereby contributing to heart failure progression.

Many of the neurohormonal and immulogic abnormalities in chronic heart failure are also associated with important effects on metabolism. Although the mechanisms underlying these effects are complex and not fully understood, the net effect is characterized by an imbalance between catabolic (tissue-wasting) and anabolic (tissue-building) factors (34). Cardinal features of advanced heart failure include an increase in basal metabolic rate (BMR) (35), altered protein and fat metabolism, and impaired peripheral blood flow with reduced nutrient delivery to bodily tissues. In the chronic setting, these effects lead to tissue wasting and loss of lean body mass (36).

2.2. Cardiac Cachexia

Hippocrates's early description of "dropsy" (i.e., heart failure) cited at the beginning of this chapter provides a remarkably apt characterization of cardiac cachexia. Although tissue wasting and loss of muscle mass occur early in chronic heart failure, marked tissue wasting and cachexia are hallmarks of advanced or end-stage heart failure.

Cardiac cachexia has been defined as a 7.5–10% or greater decline in lean body mass over a period of 6 mo or more (37). Estimates of the prevalence of cachexia in patients with heart failure vary widely, but typically range from 10% to 20%. Importantly, cachexia differs markedly from starvation (e.g., from anorexia nervosa). Although patients with heart failure may exhibit signs of malnutrition, in cachexia, there tends to be a greater loss of lean body mass, principally muscle mass but also bone mass, whereas in starvation there is preferential loss of adipose tissue in the early stages, with subsequent loss of muscle mass as malnutrition progresses (36). In addition, prolonged starvation is almost invariably associated with a very low body mass index (BMI), whereas patients with cardiac cachexia may experience only modest reductions in body weight, in part resulting from increased extracellular fluid accumulation (edema), as well as conversion of muscle tissue to fat.

As noted above, the complex cascade of metabolic disturbances leading to cardiac cachexia is incompletely understood. However, circulating levels of TNF-α are invariably elevated in patients with cardiac cachexia; indeed, the TNF-α level is the strongest predictor of weight loss in heart failure patients (34). Whether TNF-α plays a direct pathophysiological role in the development of cardiac cachexia, or merely serves as a marker for the cachectic state, and, concomitantly, the severity of heart failure, is currently unknown. In any case, circulating TNF-α levels have been shown to be a strong independent predictor of prognosis in heart failure patients. In contrast, plasma leptin levels, which correlate with BMI and percent body fat in healthy individuals, have not been shown to reliably predict nutritional status or prognosis in heart failure patients (38).

3. IMPACT ON SPECIFIC NUTRIENTS

3.1. Caloric Intake, Fat, and Protein

The occurrence of weight loss in patients with heart failure is somewhat paradoxical, because heart failure is often associated with reduced physical activity. In addition, loss of muscle mass is usually associated with a decline in resting energy expenditure (i.e., BMR). Furthermore, although some heart failure patients develop anorexia, due either to heart failure itself or as a result of medications (e.g., digoxin, captopril), in the absence of anorexia caloric intake is similar in heart failure patients (including those with cachexia) and persons without heart failure *(39)*. This combination of preserved caloric intake and apparently reduced energy expenditure both at rest and with activity would be expected to result in weight gain rather than weight loss. What, then, accounts for the net loss in nonedematous body mass so frequently encountered in heart failure patients?

First, as noted previously, most studies have shown that despite reduced muscle mass, there is an increase in BMR in most patients with heart failure, most likely as a result of increased energy requirements for respiration and the generalized catabolic state arising from neurohormonal dysregulation (especially increased circulating catecholamines) *(35,40)*, Second, although caloric intake is maintained, there is evidence that fat absorption is impaired in patients with heart failure, perhaps due to bowel edema *(41)*. In addition, although intestinal handling of protein appears to be preserved *(42)*, alterations in protein and carbohydrate metabolism result in impaired delivery of these nutrients to the body's tissues *(36)*. In summary, weight loss in heart failure is likely the result of both increased energy utilization and decreased availability of fat, protein (amino acids), and carbohydrates despite "normal" caloric intake.

To date, few studies have examined the role of nutritional support in heart failure patients. In one randomized trial involving 22 patients with advanced heart failure, a high caloric diet failed to result in significant changes in nutritional status or clinical outcomes *(43)*. However, only two subjects in this study were malnourished at the time of randomization. In another study, patients with moderate to severe heart failure and malnutrition received high-energy nasogastric tube feedings for 2 wk *(44)*. Total body weight and extracellular fluid weight declined, but lean body mass increased. There was, however, no change in oxygen consumption or cardiac function *(45)*. In a third study involving six patients undergoing mitral valve surgery, perioperative nutritional support was associated with improved clinical status and stable cardiac function. Finally, in a study of eight patients with cardiac cachexia, infusion of branched-chain amino acids had no discernible effect on protein metabolism *(46)*. In summary, there are insufficient data at present to assess the impact of various modes of nutritional support on metabolic parameters or clinical outcomes in patients with heart failure.

3.2. Water and Electrolytes

Activation of the renin-angiotensin-aldosterone system in patients with heart failure results in sodium and water retention. As a result, untreated heart failure is usually associated with increased total body water and total body sodium. Of note, total body sodium is generally increased even when serum sodium levels are reduced (i.e., hyponatremia). This situation occurs in patients with advanced heart failure because fluid retention is more pronounced than sodium retention, in part because of the action of vasopressin (antidiuretic hormone). Indeed, hyponatremia in patients with heart failure is associated with more severe hemodynamic and neurohormonal disturbances, and is a marker for poor prognosis *(47)*.

Diuretics are the mainstay of therapy for fluid overload in heart failure patients. Ideally, diuretic dosages are adjusted to maintain a normal state of hydration (i.e., "euvolemia"). However, over- and underdiuresis are both common, so that at any given time, a patient may be volume-overloaded, euvolemic, or relatively dehydrated, and careful assessment of volume status is thus essential in managing heart failure patients. From the practical standpoint, the simplest way to do this is by monitoring daily weights. Patients should be instructed to weigh themselves every morning without clothing, after voiding, and before eating, and weights should be recorded on a daily weight chart. An optimal or "dry" weight should be established, and variances of more than 2–3 lbs in either direction should lead to adjustments in diuretic dosage. The rationale behind this approach is that short-term variability in body weight primarily reflects changes in total body water. Note, however, that nonedematous weight may change over longer periods of time, usually decreasing but occasionally increasing if the overall nutritional status improves. Therefore, periodic reassessment of the patient's desirable weight is appropriate.

In addition to monitoring daily weights and adjusting diuretic dosages, dietary sodium restriction plays a pivotal role in maintaining normal volume status and avoiding acute heart failure exacerbations, as evidenced by the fact that several studies have shown that dietary sodium excess is a common precipitant of repetitive heart failure hospitalizations *(12,48)*. Dietary sodium excess contributes to fluid retention, and an acute dietary sodium load (e.g., potato chips, canned soup, "fast food") may result in a sudden increase in intravascular blood volume, triggering a rise in intracardiac pressures and precipitating acute heart failure. Older patients with diastolic heart failure are particularly sensitive to salt intake and changes in blood volume, and are thus less tolerant of a salt load. To minimize the risks of dietary sodium excess, heart failure patients, family members, and other caregivers should be educated about the importance of avoiding high sodium foods and limiting daily sodium intake to about 2 g *(18)*. Although some patients may find it difficult to adhere to a sodium-restricted diet, careful instruction and guidance from a dietitian is often effective in overcoming this barrier. It is also important to point out, in contrast to sodium restriction, fluid restriction is not usually required for most patients with mild to moderate heart failure unless significant renal impairment is also present. However, patients should be advised to avoid excess fluid intake: i.e., the oft-quoted dictum to "drink 8–10 glasses of water every day" does not apply to patients with heart failure. In addition, patients with advanced heart failure accompanied by hyponatremia may benefit from more stringent fluid restriction, 1.5 L/d total fluid intake.

Apart from the effect of diuretics on body water, these agents have important effects on key electrolytes, including sodium, potassium, chloride, magnesium, and calcium. Thiazides, "loop" diuretics (furosemide, bumetanide, torsemide), and metolazone promote natriuresis and kaliuresis, accompanied by increased urinary excretion of chloride and magnesium. As a result, all of these agents may be associated with hyponatremia, hypokalemia, hypochloremia, and hypomagnesemia. In addition, loop diuretics increase calcium excretion and may contribute to a negative calcium balance, although hypocalcemia from loop diuretics is uncommon. Conversely, the potassium-sparing diuretics spironolactone, triameterine, and amiloride, as well as the ACE inhibitors and angiotensin receptor blockers, are all associated with potassium retention and may occasionally induce significant hyperkalemia. For these reasons, serum electrolytes should be monitored periodically in patients receiving long-term diuretic therapy, especially during periods of dosage adjustment.

Diet and nutrition play an important role in managing body and serum electrolytes in heart failure patients. In general, patients with heart failure and preserved renal function should consume a diet rich in potassium, magnesium, and calcium, but low in sodium (as previously discussed). Most patients on chronic loop diuretic therapy will require potassium replacement, either through high-potassium foods (e.g., fresh fruits) or as potassium supplements (usually administered as potassium chloride, which also aids in chloride replacement). Diuretic-induced hyponatremia is potentially life-threatening and may require hospitalization, (e.g., if the serum Na^+ concentration falls to less than 120–125 meq/L). Treatment includes fluid restriction, reduction in diuretic dosage, and temporary liberalization of sodium intake. Hypomagnesemia is relatively common during long-term diuretic therapy, but may be overlooked unless serum magnesium levels are checked. Importantly, magnesium deficiency may contribute to muscle fatigue. Treatment consists of dietary therapy and magnesium supplements. Patients with chronic heart failure often suffer bone loss (osteopenia) because of low levels of vitamin D and secondary hyperparathyroidism *(33)*. However, the value of calcium supplements with or without vitamin D in heart failure patients is currently unknown.

3.3. Other Minerals

Zinc, manganese, copper, and selenium all have antioxidant effects, and deficiencies of these minerals may be associated with increased lipid peroxidation and oxidative stress *(49)*. In addition, severe copper and selenium deficiency have been associated with cardiomyopathies in humans *(50,51)*. Zinc and manganese deficiency have been associated with myocardial contractile dysfunction in laboratory animals *(52,53)*. Diuretics appear to increase urinary zinc excretion, and clinically significant zinc deficiency is common in older heart failure patients on chronic diuretic therapy *(54)*. Conversely, serious deficiencies of manganese, copper, and selenium occur infrequently in older adults consuming a normal diet. Based on currently available data, daily intake of each of these minerals should be sufficient to meet recommended dietary allowances (RDAs). Although some patients with diuretic-associated zinc deficiency may benefit from zinc supplements, there are currently no data to support routine use of such supplements in older heart failure patients.

Iron is essential for the production of hemoglobin, and iron deficiency is common in older adults. Although iron deficiency has no known direct cardiotoxic effects, chronic anemia leads to an increase in cardiac work in order to preserve tissue oxygen delivery, and in severe cases may lead to high-output cardiac failure. Conversely, iron overload from multiple blood transfusions or hemochromatosis has been associated with restrictive cardiomyopathy *(55)*. Therefore, iron intake should be sufficient to maintain tissue stores and prevent chronic iron-deficiency anemia, but excess iron intake should be avoided.

3.4. Vitamins

Vitamin B_1 (thiamine) deficiency impairs oxidative metabolism and has been unequivocally linked to high-output cardiac failure *(49,56)*. In addition, thiamine deficiency may contribute to "diuretic-resistance" in patients receiving moderate to high doses of loop diuretics over a prolonged period of time *(57,58)*. In the United States, clinically important thiamine deficiency is most commonly encountered in alcoholics and in older heart failure patients treated with loop diuretics. Of note, both digoxin and furosemide diminish uptake of thiamine by cardiac myocytes, and these drugs have potentiating effects *(59)*. Thiamine deficiency responds promptly to either oral or parenteral thiamine administration, which usually results in substantial improvement in cardiac function and symptoms. Although chronic thiamine supplementation may be considered in selected high-risk populations (e.g., alcoholics and poorly nourished older adults treated with high-dose loop diuretics), in most cases, maintaining a well-balanced diet will ensure adequate thiamine intake.

Vitamin C supplementation has been associated with improved endothelial function *(60–62)*, and some epidemiologic studies have suggested that increased intake of vitamin C correlates with reduced risk for cardiovascular disease *(63–65)*. However, there is no convincing evidence that vitamin C deficiency contributes to the development of heart failure or that vitamin C supplements are beneficial in heart failure patients *(49)*.

Vitamin E has antioxidant properties and reduces platelet adhesion *(66)*, and several epidemiologic studies have found that diets high in vitamin E, alone or in combination with vitamin C, are associated with a lower incidence of coronary heart disease *(67–70)*. However, two large prospective randomized trials of vitamin E therapy failed to show significant benefit *(71,72)*, and there is no evidence that vitamin E is of any value in the management of heart failure.

Deficiencies of folic acid, vitamin B_6, and vitamin B_{12} are common in older adults and contribute to age-associated increases in homocysteine levels *(73)*. However, although elevated homocysteine is an established marker for increased risk of coronary and cerebrovascular disease in both older and younger adults *(74–76)*, at present there is no evidence that folic acid or B vitamin supplements reduce the risk of clinical events. In addition, the importance of these vitamins in the development and treatment of heart failure is unknown.

Vitamin D is essential for maintaining normal calcium homeostasis, and marked vitamin D deficiency has been associated with decreased contractility in laboratory animals *(77)*. Vitamin D deficiency is common in older adults with or without heart failure *(78,79)*, and although vitamin D supplementation is appropriate in these individuals, there is no evidence that such treatment alters the clinical course of patients with heart failure.

Although high-dose niacin is an effective agent for the treatment of dyslipidemia, there is no evidence that niacin deficiency contributes to the development of cardiovascular disease *(49)*. Likewise, low beta-carotene intake has been associated with increased risk of myocardial infarction *(80)*, but there is no evidence that vitamin A levels correlate with heart failure risk or that vitamin A supplements are useful in the prevention of cardiovascular disease *(49)*. Similarly, there are no established links between vitamins B_2 (riboflavin) and B_{17} (pantothenic acid) and either the development or treatment of cardiac disorders *(49)*.

The role of ubiquinone (coenzyme Q_{10}) in the pathophysiology and treatment of heart failure remains controversial. Myocardial coenzyme Q_{10} levels are reduced in patients with heart failure, and low plasma coenzyme Q_{10} levels are associated with increased mortality *(49)*. In addition, the HMG-CoA reductase inhibitors ("statins"), which are commonly used to treat hyperlipidemia, have been associated with depletion of coenzyme Q_{10} (81). Observational studies indicate that coenzyme Q_{10} supplementation improves left ventricular (LV) function, symptoms, and exercise tolerance, but randomized controlled trials have failed to demonstrate significant benefit (82–84). At the present time, routine administration of coenzyme Q_{10} is not recommended.

3.5. Other Nutritional Supplements

Carnitine and creatine phosphate are nutritional supplements which may enhance skeletal muscle performance in some patients with heart failure (85–87), but there is little evidence that oral administration improves cardiac function. In addition, there is no evidence that these agents improve long-term clinical outcomes in heart failure patients, and there are also concerns about the safety of these agents during chronic use (49).

4. IMPACT OF HEART FAILURE MEDICATIONS ON NUTRITIONAL PARAMETERS

Many of the agents used in the treatment of chronic heart failure may have an effect on nutritional status. As noted above, diuretics directly impact fluid and electrolyte homeostasis, and diuretic-induced electrolyte abnormalities are very common. In addition, loop diuretics have been associated with thiamine deficiency and thiazide diuretics in particular may adversely affect carbohydrate and lipid metabolism. Digoxin may be associated with nausea and anorexia, and these symptoms may occur in older patients even at therapeutic dosages. The ACE-inhibitor captopril occasionally causes dysgeusia (altered taste), nausea, and anorexia, and other ACE inhibitors may be associated with similar side effects, although less frequently (Chapter 9). Beta blockers may also influence carbohydrate and lipid metabolism, and depressive symptoms, including reduced appetite, may occur in older patients treated with these agents. Finally, the calcium channel blockers diltiazem and especially verapamil are commonly associated with constipation in older individuals.

Because the heart failure syndrome is associated with progressive loss of muscle mass, culminating in the development of cardiac cachexia, several recent studies evaluating the impact of heart failure therapies on nutritional parameters are of interest. In one study involving eight patients with advanced heart failure and cardiac cachexia, 6 mo of treatment with the combination of digoxin, the ACE inhibitor enalapril, and the loop diuretic furosemide was associated with significant clinical improvement, as well as increased muscle bulk, subcutaneous fat, and serum albumin and hematocrit levels (88). In another study involving patients with advanced heart failure randomized to treatment with the beta-blocker carvedilol or placebo, carvedilol was associated with a small but significant increase in nonedematous body weight when compared to placebo (89). In contrast to these studies, two recent trials of etanercept, a tumor necrosis factor (TNF)-blocking agent, failed to demonstrate significant benefit and were discontinued (90). Because, as discussed previously, TNF-α has been thought to play an important role in the development of cardiac cachexia, the findings of the etanercept trials are particularly disappointing.

5. AGE-SPECIFIC NUTRITIONAL ISSUES

Older age is associated with increased risk for a broad range of nutritional deficiencies, and this risk is potentiated by the presence of cardiovascular disease in general, and by heart failure in particular. In addition, older adults are more susceptible to the adverse effects of pharmacological agents and dietary interventions on nutritional parameters, in part resulting from pre-existing nutritional deficiencies coupled with an increased prevalence of comorbid conditions. The latter issue may be particularly problematic, as the presence of several common comorbidities (e.g., coronary artery disease, diabetes mellitus, and renal insufficiency) may lead to serial dietary restrictions (low fat, low carbohydrate, low protein, low salt), culminating in a diet that is unpalatable and severely deficient in both calories and essential nutrients. Therefore, it is critically important that an appropriately detailed nutritional evaluation, including dietary history, body weight, selected laboratory tests (hemoglobin, albumin, cholesterol, electrolytes, creatinine, blood urea nitrogen), and in some cases, anthropometric assessments, be incorporated into the routine management of older patients with chronic illnesses, including heart failure.

6. RECOMMENDATIONS FOR CLINICIANS

Nutritional guidelines for managing chronic heart failure in older adults are summarized in Table 2. As noted previously, nutritional management of older patients begins with a nutritional assessment, ideally with the assistance of an experienced dietitian or nurse. As with other chronic illnesses, the guiding principal in making nutritional recommendations to older heart failure patients is the maintenance of a well-balanced diet with sufficient calories, nutrients, and fluids to meet daily requirements. In addition, the diet should be both palatable and "accessible," i.e., within the patient's financial means and physical capabilities. Few older patients with heart failure require a weight reduction diet; indeed, body weight correlates inversely with mortality in heart failure patients (91). In most cases it is appropriate to prescribe a diet that will either maintain current nonedematous weight or promote a modest increase in lean body mass. Although it has been suggested that the proportion of calories derived from protein and fat should be increased in older heart failure patients (36), there is little evidence to support this contention and current recommendations are that 15–20% of total calories be derived from protein, 25–30% from fat and the remaining 50–60% from complex carbohydrates.

Moderate dietary sodium restriction, such as a 2-g sodium diet, is appropriate for most patients with heart failure (18). Patients should be instructed to avoid high-sodium foods, such as canned soups and sauces, tomato juice, most prepared lunch meats and prepackaged frozen entrees, pickles, "fast foods," and certain ethnic foods that are high in sodium (e.g., Chinese cuisine). Moderate use of salt during cooking is acceptable, but use of salt at the table should be avoided. Dining out is potentially problematic, and patients should be advised to call ahead to see if low sodium options are available either on the menu or by request. Patients should also be instructed about the widespread availability of alternative seasonings that contain little or no salt.

Fluid intake should be adequate to maintain hydration while avoiding volume overload. In patients with preserved renal function, about 2 L of fluid per day is appropriate. Excess fluid intake (8–10 glasses of water a day) should be avoided, but fluid restriction is unnecessary in the absence of hyponatremia, severe renal failure, or advanced heart failure with diuretic resistance. In such cases, fluid intake should be limited to about 1.5 L per day.

Dietary potassium, calcium, and magnesium requirements vary considerably depending on medications, renal function, and comorbid conditions (e.g., osteoporosis). As a

Table 2
Nutritional Guidelines for Older Adults with Chronic Heart Failure

Component	Recommendation
Nutritional assessment	
Basic (all patients)	Obtain detailed dietary history
	Assess body weight and habitus
	Laboratory: hemoglobin, serum albumin, cholesterol, serum electrolytes (sodium, potassium, calcium, phosphorus, magnesium), creatinine, blood urea nitrogen
Supplemental (selected patients)	Anthropometric measures (e.g., skinfold thickness)
	Determination of lean body mass
	Folate, B_{12} levels
	Bone mineral density
General diet	Well-balanced, rich in fruits and vegetables, whole grains, dairy products, lean meats
Caloric intake	Sufficient to maintain lean body mass; 1600–2000 cal/d in most cases
Protein	15–20% of total calories
Fat	25–30% of total calories
Complex carbohydrates	50–60% of total calories
Fluids	~2 L/d
	1.5 L/d in setting of hyponatremia, severe renal failure, diuretic-resistance
	Avoid excess fluid intake
Electrolytes	
Sodium	2 g Na^+/d
Potassium, calcium, magnesium	Sufficient to maintain body stores and serum levels; supplement as indicated
Minerals	
Zinc, copper, manganese, selenium	Sufficient intake to meet RDAs; zinc supplements in selected patients
Iron	Sufficient to maintain body stores; avoid iron overload
Vitamins	
Thiamin (B_1)	Supplement in alcoholics, possibly patients on chronic high-dose loop diuretics
Folate, B_6, B_{12}	Supplement if deficient (common)
D	Supplement if deficient, especially if osteoporosis present (common)
A, riboflavin (B_2), niacin (B_3), Pantothenic acid (B_5), C, E	No known relation to heart failure; maintain RDAs
Dietary supplements	
Ubiquinone (coenzyme Q_{10})	Unproven benefit, not recommended
Carnitine	Unproven benefit, not recommended
Creatine phosphate	Unproven benefit, not recommended

RDA, recommended dietary allowance.

general principle, a well-balanced diet rich in fresh fruits and vegetables, whole-grain breads and cereals, and dairy products will provide sufficient amounts of potassium, calcium, and magnesium to meet normal needs. However, many older heart failure patients will require supplemental administration of one or more of these electrolytes to overcome losses through urinary excretion or as a result of other metabolic abnormalities. Because individual requirements cannot be easily predicted, periodic assessment of serum electrolyte levels is appropriate.

As discussed above, the importance of most vitamins and other micronutrients in the pathogenesis and treatment of chronic heart failure has not been well-characterized and it is therefore difficult to make specific nutritional recommendations. However, because older patients are at increased risk for multiple nutritional deficiencies, it is appropriate to maintain a high index of suspicion, particularly in frail, socially isolated, or institution-alized elders, as well as those with multiple comorbidities and those receiving multiple medications. In particular, deficiencies of folate, B_{12}, vitamin D, and zinc are common, and dietary or pharmacological supplementation is indicated when specific deficiencies are identified or suspected. Additionally, because long-term administration of loop diuretics may deplete thiamine stores, thiamine replacement should be considered in such cases, particularly in the setting of increasing diuretic-resistance. Finally, although there is no evidence to support the use of mega-dose vitamin or mineral supplements in older heart failure patients, routine daily use of an oral multivitamin and mineral supplement may ease concerns about deficiencies of these nutrients and is unlikely to be harmful. Conversely, the use of other dietary supplements, such as coenzyme Q_{10}, carnitine, or creatine phosphate, is not currently recommended.

7. SUMMARY

1. Nutritional management begins with a nutritional assessment. Obtain baseline body weight and monitor at regular intervals. Recognize that caloric needs may change as body weight changes and provide increased nutritional support if rapid unintentional weight loss occurs.
2. Patients should be encouraged to choose a well-balanced diet high in fruits and veg-etables as excellent sources of vitamins and electrolytes.
3. Sodium restriction to 2 g/d is usually sufficient; dietary counseling may be required to assist patients in achieving this goal.
4. Fluid restriction is not usually necessary except when hyponatremia, severe renal failure, or advanced heart failure is present; in these cases, fluid should be restricted to ~1.5 L/d. Excess fluid intake (8–10 glasses of water per day) should be avoided.
5. Magnesium, potassium, and calcium status should be monitored and supplemented as needed. Other nutrients of concern in high-risk patients include thiamine, folate, vitamin B_{12}, vitamin D, and zinc. Routine daily use of an oral vitamin/mineral supplement may be helpful in alleviating any deficits.

REFERENCES

1. Katz AM, Katz PB. Diseases of the heart in the works of Hippocrates. Br Heart J 1961;24:257–264.
2. American Heart Association. 2001 Heart and Stroke Statistical Update. A H A, Dallas, TX, 2000. http://www.americanheart.org/downloadable/heart/4838_HSSTATS2001_1.0.pdf
3. Kannel WB, Belanger AJ. Epidemiology of heart failure. Am Heart J 1991;121:951–957.

4. Popovic JR, Hall MJ. 1999 National Hospital Discharge Survey. Advance data from vital and health statistics; no. 319. National Center for Health Statistics, Hyattsville, MD, 2001.

5. Graves EJ. Detailed diagnoses and procedures. National Hospital Discharge Survey, 1990. Vital and health statistics, series 13, data from the National Health Survey. National Center for Health Statistics, Hyattsville, MD, 1992;113:1–225.

6. O'Connell JB, Bristow MR. Economic impact of heart failure in the United States: Time for a different approach. J Heart Lung Transplant 1994;13:S107–S112.

7. Gottdiener JS, Arnold AM, Aurigemma GP, et al. Predictors of congestive heart failure in the elderly: The Cardiovascular Health Study. J Am Coll Cardiol 2000;35:1628–1637.

8. Levy D, Larson MG, Vasan RS, Kannel WB, Ho KK. The progression from hypertension to congestive heart failure. JAMA 1996;275:1557–1562.

9. Vasan RS, Larson MG, Benjamin EJ, Evans JC, Reiss CK, Levy D. Congestive heart failure in subjects with normal versus reduced left ventricular ejection fraction: Prevalence and mortality in a population-based cohort. J Am Coll Cardiol 1999;33:1948–1955.

10. Kitzman DW, Gardin JM, Gottdiener JS, et al. Importance of heart failure with preserved systolic function in patients ≥ 65 yr of age. CHS Research Group. Cardiovascular Health Study. Am J Cardiol 2001;87:413–419.

11. Croft JB, Giles WH, Pollard RA, Keenan NL, Casper ML, Anda RF. Heart failure survival among older adults in the United States: A poor prognosis for an emerging epidemic in the Medicare population. Arch Intern Med 1999;159:505–510.

12. Vinson JM, Rich MW, Shah AS, Sperry JC. Early readmission of elderly patients with congestive heart failure. J Am Geriatr Soc 1990;38:1290–1295.

13. Krumholz HM, Parent EM, Tu N, et al. Readmission after hospitalization for congestive heart failure among Medicare beneficiaries. Arch Intern Med 1997;157:99–104.

14. Ho KK, Anderson KM, Kannel WB, Grossman W, Levy D. Survival after the onset of congestive heart failure in Framingham Heart Study subjects. Circulation 1993;88:107–115.

15. Pernenkil R, Vinson JM, Shah AS, Beckham V, Wittenberg C, Rich MW. Course and prognosis in patients ≥ 70 years of age with congestive heart failure and normal versus abnormal left ventricular ejection fraction. Am J Cardiol 1997;79:216–219.

16. Senni M, Tribouilloy CM, Rodeheffer RJ, et al. Congestive heart failure in the community: a study of all incident cases in Olmsted County, Minnesota, in 1991. Circulation 1998;98:2282–2289.

17. Kitzman DW. Heart failure with normal systolic function. Clin Geriatr Med 2000;16:489–512.

18. Hunt SA, Baker DW, Chin MH, et al. ACC/AHA Guidelines for the Evaluation and Management of Chronic Heart Failure in the Adult: Executive Summary. J Am Coll Cardiol 2001;38:2101–2113. www.acc.org/clinical/guidelines/failure/pdfs/hf_fulltext.pdf

19. Rich MW, Beckham V, Wittenberg C, Leven CL, Freedland KE, Carney RM. A multidisciplinary intervention to prevent the readmission of elderly patients with congestive heart failure. N Engl J Med 1995;333:1190–1195.

20. McAlister FA, Lawson FM, Teo KK, Armstrong PW. A systematic review of randomized trials of disease management programs in heart failure. Am J Med 2001;110:378–384.

21. Flather MD, Yusuf S, Køber L, et al. Long-term ACE-inhibitor therapy in patients with heart failure or left-ventricular dysfunction: a systematic overview of data from individual patients. Lancet 2000; 355:1575–1581.

22. Pitt B, Poole-Wilson PA, Segal R, et al. Effect of losartan compared with captopril on mortality in patients with symptomatic heart failure: randomized trial—the Losartan Heart Failure Survival Study ELITE II. Lancet 2000;355:1582–1587.

23. Cohn JN, Tognoni G, for the Valsartan Heart Failure Trial Investigators. A randomized trial of the angiotensin-receptor blocker valsartan in chronic heart failure. N Engl J Med 2001;345:1667–1675.

24. Cohn JN, Archibald DG, Ziesche S, et al. Effect of vasodilator therapy on mortality in chronic congestive heart failure. Results of a Veterans Administration Cooperative Study. N Engl J Med 1986;314: 1547–1552.

25. Cohn JN, Johnson G, Ziesche S, et al. A comparison of enalapril with hydralazine-isosorbide dinitrate in the treatment of chronic congestive heart failure. N Eng J Med 1991;325:303–310.

26. CIBIS-II Investigators and Committees. The Cardiac Insufficiency Bisoprolol Study II (CIBIS II): A randomized trial. Lancet 1999;353:9–13.

27. Effect of metoprolol CR/XL in chronic heart failure: Metoprolol CR/XL Randomized Intervention Trial in Congestive Heart Failure (MERIT-HF). Lancet 1999;353:2001–2007.

28. The Digitalis Investigation Group. The effect of digoxin on mortality and morbidity in patients with heart failure. N Engl J Med 1997;336:525–533.

29. Rich MW, McSherry F, Williford WO, Yusuf S, for the Digitalis Investigation Group. Effect of age on mortality, hospitalizations and response to digoxin in patients with heart failure: The DIG Study. J Am Coll Cardiol 2001;38:806–813.

30. Pitt B, Zannad F, Remme WJ, et al. The effect of spironolactone on morbidity and mortality in patients with severe heart failure. Randomized Aldactone Evaluation Study Investigators. N Engl J Med 1999; 341:709–717.

31. Anker SD, Rauchhaus M. Heart failure as a metabolic problem. Eur J Heart Failure 1999;1:127–131.

32. Anker SD, Rauchhaus M. Insights into the pathogenesis of chronic heart failure: Immune activation and cachexia. Curr Opin Cardiol 1999;14:211–216.

33. Berry C, Clark AL. Catabolism in chronic heart failure. Eur Heart J 2000;21:521–532.

34. Anker SD, Chua TP, Ponikowski P, et al. Hormonal changes and catabolic/anabolic imbalance in chronic heart failure and their importance for cardiac cachexia. Circulation 1997;96:526–534.

35. Poehlman ET, Scheffers J, Gottlieb SS, Fisher ML, Vaitkevicius P. Increased resting metabolic rates in patients with congestive heart failure. Ann Intern Med 1994;121:860–862.

36. Freeman LM, Roubenoff R. The nutrition implications of cardiac cachexia. Nutr Rev 1994;52:340–347.

37. Anker SD, Ponikowski P, Varney S, et al. Wasting as independent risk factor for mortality in chronic heart failure. Lancet 1997;349:1050–1053.

38. Murdoch DR, Rooney E, Dargie HJ, Shapiro D, Morton JJ, McMurray JJ. Inappropriately low plasma leptin concentration in the cachexia associated with chronic heart failure. Heart 1999;82:352–356.

39. Zhao SP, Zeng LH. Elevated plasma levels of tumor necrosis factor in chronic heart failure with cachexia. Int J Cardiol 1997;58:257–261.

40. Poehlman ET, Toth MJ, Fishman PS, et al. Sarcopenia in aging humans: The impact of menopause and disease. J Gerontol Biol Sci Med Sci 1995;50:73–77.

41. King D, Smith ML, Chapman TJ, Stockdale HR, Lye M. Fat malabsorption in elderly patients with cardiac cachexia Age Ageing 1996;25:144–149.

42. King D, Smith ML, Lye M. Gastro-intestinal protein loss in elderly patients with cardiac cachexia. Age Ageing 1996;25:221–223.

43. Broqvist M, Arnqvist H, Dahlstrom U, Larsson J, Nylander E, Permert J. Nutritional assessment and muscle energy metabolism in severe chronic congestive heart failure: Effects of long-term dietary supplementation. Eur Heart J 1994;15:1641–1650.

44. Heymsfield SB, Casper K. Congestive heart failure: Clinical management by use of continuous nasoenteric feeding. Am J Clin Nutr 1989;50:539–544.

45. Paccagnella A, Calo MA, Caenaro G, et al. Cardiac cachexia: Preoperative and postoperative nutritional management. J Parenteral Enteral Nutr 1994;18:409–416.

46. Morrison WL, Gibson JN, Rennie MJ. Skeletal muscle and whole body protein turnover in cardiac cachexia: Influence of branched chain amino acid administration. Eur J Clin Invest 1988;18:648–654.

47. Panciroli C, Galloni G, Oddone A, et al. Prognostic value of hyponatremia in patients with severe chronic heart failure. Angiology 1990;41:631–638.

48. Ghali JK, Kadakia S, Cooper R, Ferlinz J. Precipitating factors leading to decompensation of heart failure: Traits among urban blacks. Arch Intern Med 1988;148:2013–2016.

49. Witte KKA, Clark AL, Cleland JGF. Chronic heart failure and micronutrients. J Am Coll Cardiol 2001; 37:1765–174.

50. Kopp SJ, Klevay LM, Feliksik JM. Physiological and metabolic characterization of a cardiomyopathy induced by chronic copper deficiency. Am J Physiol 1983;245:H855–H866.

51. Lockitch G, Taylor GP, Wong LT, et al. Cardiomyopathy associated with nonendemic selenium deficiency in a Caucasian adolescent. Am J Clin Nutr 1990;52:572–527.

52. Coudray C, Boucher F, Richard MJ, et al. Zinc deficiency, ethanol and myocardial ischemia effect lipoperoxidation in rats. Biol Trace Elem Res 1991;30:103–118.

53. Li Y, Huang TT, Carlson EJ, et al. Dilated cardiomyopathy and neonatal lethality in mutant mice lacking manganese superoxide dismutase. Nat Genet 1995;11:376–381.

54. Golik A, Cohen N, Ramot Y, et al. Type II diabetes mellitus, congestive cardiac failure and zinc metabolism. Biol Trace Elem Res 1993;39:171–175.

55. Liu P, Olivieri N. Iron overload cardiomyopathies: new insights into an old disease. Cardiovasc Drugs Ther 1994;8:101–110.

56. Djoenaidi W, Notermans SL, Dunda G. Beriberi cardiomyopathy. Eur J Clin Nutr 1992;46:227–234.

57. Seligmann H, Halkin H, Rauchfleisch S, et al. Thiamine deficiency in patients with congestive heart failure receiving long-term furosemide therapy: A pilot study. Am J Med 1991;91:151–155.

58. Shimon I, Almog S, Vered Z, et al. Improved left ventricular function after thiamine supplementation in patients with congestive heart failure receiving long-term furosemide therapy. Am J Med 1995;98: 485–490.

59. Zangen A, Botzer D, Zangen R, Shainberg A. Furosemide and digoxin inhibit thiamine uptake in cardiac cells. Eur J Pharmacol 1998;13:151–155.

60. Ting HH, Timimi FK, Haley EA, et al. Vitamin C improves endothelium-dependent vasodilation in forearm resistance vessels of humans with hypercholesterolemia. Circulation 1997;95:2617–2622.

61. Gokce N, Keaney JF, Frei B, et al. Long-term ascorbic acid administration reverses endothelial vasomotor dysfunction in patients with coronary artery disease. Circulation 1999;99:3234–3240.

62. Hornig B, Arakawa N, Kohler C, Drexler H. Vitamin C improves endothelial function of conduit arteries in patients with chronic heart failure. Circulation 1998;97:363–368.

63. Khaw KT, Bingham S, Welch A, et al. Relation between plasma ascorbic acid and mortality in men and women in EPIC-Norfolk prospective study: A prospective population study. European Prospective Investigation into Cancer and Nutrition. Lancet 2001;357:657–663.

64. Gale CR, Martyn CN, Winter PD, Cooper C. Vitamin C and risk of death from stroke and coronary heart disease in cohort of elderly people. BMJ 1995;310:1563–1566.

65. Enstrom JE, Kanim LE, Klein MA. Vitamin C intake and mortality among a sample of the United States population. Epidemiology 1992;3:194–202.

66. Calzada C, Bruckdorfer KR, Rice-Evans CA. The influence of antioxidant nutrients on platelet function in healthy volunteers. Atherosclerosis 1997;128:97–105.

67. Rimm EB, Stampfer MJ, Ascherio A, et al. Vitamin E consumption and risk of coronary heart disease in men. N Engl J Med 1993;328:1450–1456.

68. Stampfer MJ, Hennekens CH, Manson JE, et al. Vitamin E consumption and the risk of coronary disease in women. N Engl J Med 1993;328:1444–1449.

69. Losonczy KG, Harris TB, Havlik RJ. Vitamin E and vitamin C supplement use and risk of all-cause and coronary heart disease mortality in older persons: The Established Populations for Epidemiologic Studies of the Elderly. Am J Clin Nutr 1996;64:190–196.

70. Kushi LH, Folsom AR, Prineas RJ, Mink PJ, Wu Y, Bostick RM. Dietary antioxidant vitamins and death from coronary heart disease in postmenopausal women. N Engl J Med 1996;334:1156–1162.

71. The Heart Outcomes Prevention Evaluation Study Investigators. Vitamin E supplementation and cardiovascular events in high-risk patients. N Engl J Med 2000;342:154–160.

72. Dietary supplementation with n-3 polyunsaturated fatty acids and vitamin E after myocardial infarction: Results of the GISSI-Prevenzione trial. Lancet 1999;354:447–455.

73. Selhub J, Jacques PF, Wilson PWF, et al. Vitamin status and intake as primary determinants of homocysteinemia in an elderly population. JAMA 1993;270:2693–2698.

74. Eikelboom JW, Lonn E, Genest J, Hankey G, Yusuf S. Homocyst(e)ine and cardiovascular disease: A critical review of the epidemiologic evidence. Ann Intern Med 1999;131:363–375.

75. Bots ML, Launer LJ, Lindemans J, et al. Homocysteine and short-term risk of myocardial infarction and stroke in the elderly: The Rotterdam Study. Arch Intern Med 1999;159:38–44.

76. Bostom AG, Rosenberg IH, Silbershatz H, et al. Nonfasting plasma total homocysteine levels and stroke incidence in elderly persons: The Framingham Study. Ann Intern Med 1999;131:352–355.

77. Weisshaar RE, Simpson RU. Involvement of vitamin D3 with cardiovascular function: direct and indirect effects. Am, J Physiol 1987;253:E675–E683.

78. MacLaughlin J, Holick MF. Aging decreases the capacity of human skin to produce vitamin D_3. J Clin Invest 1985;76:1536–1538.

79. Shane E, Mancini D, Aaronson K, et al. Bone mass, vitamin D deficiency and hypoparathyroidism in congestive heart failure. Am J Med 1997;103:197–207.

80. Tavani A, Negri E, D'Avanzo B, LaVecchia C. Beta-carotene intake and risk of nonfatal acute myocardial infarction in women. Eur J Epidemiol 1997;13:631–637.

81. DePinieux G, Chariot P, Ammi-Said M, et al. Lipid-lowering drugs and mitochondrial function: Effects of HMG-CoA reductase inhibitors on serum ubiquinone and blood lactate/pyruvate ratio. Br J Clin Pharmacol 1996;42:333–337.

82. Hofman-Bang C, Rehnqvist N, Swedberg K, Wiklund I, Astrom H. Coenzyme Q10 as an adjunctive in the treatment of chronic congestive heart failure. The Q10 Study Group. J Card Fail 1995;1:101–107.

83. Watson PS, Scalia GM, Galbraith A, Burstow DJ, Bett N, Aroney CN. Lack of effect of coenzyme Q on left ventricular function in patients with congestive heart failure. J Am Coll Cardiol 1999;33: 1549–1552.

84. Khatta M, Alexander BS, Krichten CM, et al. The effect of coenzyme Q10 in patients with congestive heart failure. Ann Intern Med 2000;132:636–640.

85. Anand I, Chandrashekhan Y, DeGiuli F, et al. Acute and chronic effects of propionyl-L-carnitine on the hemodynamics, exercise capacity and hormones in patients with congestive heart failure. Cardiovasc Drugs Ther 1998;12:291–299.

86. The Investigators of the Study on Propionyl-L-Carnitine in Chronic Heart Failure. Study on propionyl-l-carnitine in chronic heart failure. Eur Heart J 1999;20:70–76.

87. Gordon A, Hultman E, Kaijser L. Creatine supplementation in chronic heart failure increases skeletal muscle creatine phosphate and muscle performance. Cardiovasc Res 1995;30:413–418.

88. Adigun AQ, Ajayi AAL. The effects of enalapril-digoxin-diuretic combination therapy on nutritional and anthropometric indices in chronic congestive heart failure: Preliminary findings in cardiac cachexia. Eur J Heart Failure 2001;3:359–363.

89. Coats AJ, Anker SD, Roecker EB, et al. Prevention and reversal of cardiac cachexia in patients with severe heart failure by carvedilol: Results of the COPERNICUS study. Circulation 2001;104(suppl II): II-437 (abstract).

90. Louis A, Cleland JG, Crabbe S, et al. Clinical Trials Update: CAPRICORN, COPERNICUS, MIRACLE, STAF, RITZ-2, RECOVER and RENAISSANCE and cachexia and cholesterol in heart failure. Highlights of the Scientific Sessions of the American College of Cardiology, 2001. Eur J Heart Failure 2001; 3:381–387.

91. Horwich TB, Fonarow GC, Hamilton MA, MacLellan WR, Woo MA, Tillisch JH. The relationship between obesity and mortality in patients with heart failure. J Am Coll Cardiol 2001;38:789–795.

B. Pulmonary Diseases

19 Nutrition and Chronic Obstructive Pulmonary Disease

Katherine Gray-Donald
and Helga Saudny-Unterberger

1. INTRODUCTION

Chronic obstructive pulmonary disease (COPD) is an important cause of morbidity, hospitalization, and mortality worldwide. In the United States, COPD is the fourth leading cause of death and an estimated 119,340 deaths are attributable to COPD. Worldwide COPD ranks sixth among the 30 leading causes of death, accounting for 2,211,000 deaths. As the population ages, its is projected that by 2020, COPD will be the third leading cause of death worldwide *(1)*. COPD is still more common in men than women, however, the greatest increase in the COPD death rate between 1979 and 1989 occurred in females, reflecting the increased number of women who smoke cigarettes *(2)*. COPD interferes with the normal function of the respiratory system and depending on the severity of the disease can curtail activities of daily living. Weight loss is a common development in COPD and the clinical deterioration, diminished life expectancy, and decreased exercise capacity that are associated with weight loss have been acknowledged for many years *(3–5)*. Depending on the population studied and the indicator used to determine nutritional status, between 19% and 60% of COPD patients are classified as malnourished *(6)*. Evidence for the prevention or reversibility of this nutritional decline is accumulating and points to the importance of nutritional interventions in this area.

Patients with COPD have increased resting energy expenditure (REE) and total daily energy expenditure (TDEE) despite the apparent inactivity associated with the illness. This is presumably because of greater metabolic or mechanical demands for activities and the increased requirements for respiration. Insufficient energy intakes resulting from poor appetite and breathing difficulties, as well as elevated concentrations of tumor necrosis factor-α (TNF-α) and glucocorticosteroid-associated catabolism have also been implicated as possible reasons for weight loss.

From: *Handbook of Clinical Nutrition and Aging*
Edited by: C. W. Bales and C. S. Ritchie © Humana Press Inc., Totowa, NJ

2. PHYSIOLOGICAL BASIS OF THE DISORDER

Chronic obstructive pulmonary disease refers to a group of pathologic conditions affecting lung parenchyma, intrathoracic airways, or both, causing chronic airflow limitation *(7)*. The structural and functional abnormalities lead to the symptoms of cough, sputum production, dyspnea, and impaired gas exchange to varying degrees in different subjects. Chronic bronchitis is a clinical syndrome manifested by mucus hypersecretion, a daily productive cough, for at least 3 mo of the year for 2 consecutive years, and bronchial gland hypertrophy. Emphysema, on the other hand, is a chronic lung disorder characterized by the destruction of the gas-exchanging parenchyma distal to the terminal bronchioles, leading to the collapse of the abnormally enlarged air spaces and interfering with the transfer of O_2 and CO_2 between the blood and the alveolar air *(8)*.

Two prominent features of COPD are increased resistance to expiratory airflow and hyperinflation of the lungs. The expiratory airflow resistance causes air to be trapped in the lungs and is responsible for most of the hyperinflation. With increased airway resistance and hyperinflation, the work of breathing is noticeably elevated. The exchange of O_2 and CO_2 is impaired in COPD and as a consequence, the level of minute ventilation needed to maintain arterial carbon dioxide pressure at normal levels can be two to three times the normal rate *(9)*. Hyperinflation also affects the diaphragm, the primary muscle of inspiration, which normally assumes a dome shape that protrudes upward into the thoracic cavity. The negative pressure in a tightly curved diaphragm is necessary to move air into the lungs. With hyperinflation, the diaphragm is flattened, increasing the radius of the curvature and decreasing the pressure generated. A flattened diaphragm may not be able to produce any useful inspiratory pressure, thus adding to the work of breathing and often resulting in the recruitment of the muscles of the abdominal wall and other accessory muscles to increase ventilation *(10)*.

Although cigarette smoking is thought to be the most important environmental risk factor associated with COPD, long term exposure to pollution and occupational dust are also thought to be important risk factors for COPD. The disease can remain asymptomatic for many years and a diagnosis of COPD using spirometry is usually made at an advanced stage when dyspnea is severe enough to interfere with usual activities of daily living and a major loss in lung function has occurred. Carefully planned therapy that includes cessation of smoking, administration of bronchodilators and/or glucocorticosteroids, respiratory muscle training, and nutritional support will help alleviate some of the symptoms, but will not reverse the condition.

3. NUTRITIONAL CONCERNS

3.1. Weight Loss and Muscle Wasting in COPD Patients

There is no consensus regarding the definition of malnutrition for COPD patients (Table 1). Most studies in the 1990s included the use of the body mass index (BMI) (kg/height [m^2]) in their assessment. It has been clearly established that survival decreases significantly in both underweight (BMI < 20 kg/m^2) and even normal weight (BMI 20–25 kg/m^2) patients compared with overweight (BMI 25–29 kg/m^2) and obese patients (BMI > 29 kg/m^2) *(3)*. Total body weight used to determine BMI does not distinguish between fat tissue and lean body mass. Despite normal body weights, lean body mass is more depleted in COPD patients than in healthy controls *(11)*. Loss of

Table 1
Summary of Studies Determining the Nutritional Status of Patients with COPD

Criteria for malnutrition	Study sample	% Malnourished	Author(s)
<90% usual weight	38 Hospitalized patients	50	Hunter, 1981 (21)
<90% IBW	Retrospective assessment of nutritional status of 77 hospitalized patients	43	Openbrier, 1983 (62)
<90% IBW	135 Outpatients	24	Gray-Donald, 1989 (63)
<90% IBW	779 Outpatients	24	Wilson, 1989 (64)
Nutritional index comprising 4 parameters Alb, Palb, TLC, % IBW	153 Patients admitted to a rehabilitation center	19	Schols, 1989 (65)
BMI < 20 underweight and TSF <10th percentile MAC <5th percentile	126 Outpatients	23	Sahebjami, 1993 (66)
<90% IBW and <63% FFMPIBW	255 Patients admitted to a rehabilitation center	26	Schols, 1993 (67)
NI based on anthropometric and biochemical variables	50 Hospitalized patients	60	Laaban, 1993 (68)

TSF, triceps skinfold; MAC, midarm circumference; IBW, ideal body weight; NI, nutritional index; FFMPIBW, fat-free mass expressed as a percentage of ideal body weight; Alb, Albumin; Palb, prealbumin; TLC, total lymphocyte count.

459

weight, specifically loss of lean body mass, has deleterious effects on diaphragmatic and respiratory muscle functioning, resulting in decreased strength and endurance of the respiratory muscles which is evident in their impaired capacity for strenuous exercise *(11)*. Moreover, poor nutritional status will weaken the immune system and may interfere with the protection of the airways contributing to undesirable clinical outcomes. Recording body weight over time can be an informative measure of nutritional status, however, changes in body composition, particularly loss of lean body mass, may go unrecognized in COPD, and other methods of accurately determining loss of lean body mass in COPD patients need to be adopted *(16)* (*see* Section 4.4.).

3.2. Causes of Weight Loss and Muscle Mass Depletion

Weight loss is a common clinical feature in COPD and is related to decreased survival of patients, independent of the severity of the disease *(3,4)*. Weight loss is a complex interaction between the metabolic disturbances (increased total daily energy expenditure), a reduced food intake resulting from an increased sensation of dyspnea and a decreased appetite, changes in energy and protein requirements, frequent hospital admissions, the use of glucocorticosteroids, and the normal progression of the disease. The following sections discuss these factors.

3.2.1. HYPERMETABOLISM

Loss of weight occurs when energy expenditure is greater than energy intake. In most healthy sedentary adults, REE is the largest component (approx 60–70%) of daily TDEE with physical activity and metabolic responses to food intake being responsible for the balance of TDEE. It has long been recognized that the body's usual response to a decrease in food intake is to lower REE, an adaptive mechanism necessary to sustain life *(12)*. This adaptive mechanism fails in COPD and several studies over the years have pointed to an increased REE as one of the explanations for the observed weight loss in some patients with COPD. In a well-designed study by Schols and colleagues *(5)*, weight losing and weight stable COPD patients were compared. The weight losing patients exhibited higher REE (118 ± 17% predicted) than the weight stable patients (110 ± 11% predicted) and both groups of COPD patients had significantly higher REE than healthy controls (104 ± 6% predicted). The higher REE remained after adjusting for lean body mass and was significantly higher in the weight losing than in the weight stable COPD patients. In a subgroup of eight patients with moderate to severe COPD TDEE was also measured and was unexpectedly found to be higher when compared with healthy subjects. The investigators suggest that the physical activity component contributed to the significantly higher TDEE *(13)*. The energy needs of COPD patients are very high, despite their seemingly low level of physical activity, possibly because of the reduced efficiency of peripheral skeletal muscles leading to increased needs for the respiratory muscles to preserve an adequate level of ventilation.

It is well established that REE in many clinically stable patients with moderate to severe COPD is 10–20% higher than would normally be predicted from the Harris-Benedict equation *(14)*, and this higher need should be taken into account when dietary therapies are established.

3.2.2. CATABOLIC PROCESSES

COPD patients are frequently admitted to hospital with an acute exacerbation, triggered by an infection or some other environmental stimuli. Bacterial and viral infections are powerful catalysts for the body's immune system resulting in a complex and coordinated interaction to rid the body of these foreign substances. The production and release of stress hormones and cytokines contribute to the resulting changes in substrate metabolism and inappropriate mobilization of protein and fat. The prolonged or excess production of cytokines has been related to the unrestrained protein catabolism (cachexia) seen in patients with cancer and other critical illnesses (15). Tumor necrosis factor-alpha (TNF-α), a multipurpose cytokine has been implicated in the metabolic and nutritional disturbances seen in very ill patients (16). Elevated concentrations of serum TNF-α have also been found in weight losing COPD patients, whereas weight stable patients and healthy control subjects have much lower levels of TNF-α in their blood (17–19). TNF-α is but one of many cytokines involved in the inflammatory response process and more research is needed to clarify the relationship between the production of cytokines during the acute inflammatory process and their contribution to elevated REE, and weight loss seen in a subgroup of COPD patients.

3.2.3. Dyspnea/Fatigue/Depression

Some patients with COPD experience dyspnea during eating and may decrease their intake of food to avoid the unpleasant sensation. It has been suggested that the increased sense of breathlessness experienced during a meal by hypoxemic but not by normoxemic patients is due to decreased arterial oxygen saturation in the former, but not in the latter group of COPD patients (5). The entire process of preparing and eating a meal can be very tiring for some patients, and for that reason, can lead to a reduction in energy intake. In addition, the decline in functional status that often accompanies the progression of the disease can contribute to increased anxiety and depression and may lead to a decreased food intake (20).

3.2.4. Inadequate Food Intake

Weight maintenance relies on an energy intake that is balanced with energy expenditure, and when even a small but constant reduction in energy intake is not offset by a decrease in energy expenditure, weight loss will occur. Hypermetabolism can explain why some COPD patients lose weight despite seemingly normal or even above normal food intake.

Studies designed to investigate usual dietary intake in COPD are few, but one study in the early 1980s found that most subjects consumed seemingly adequate energy and protein intakes (21). However, Efthimiou, who conducted a feeding trial with COPD patients, found very low energy intakes at baseline (22). At present, we do not know the recommended energy or protein intake for COPD patients, but it is well documented that total energy needs are higher than those of healthy individuals.

3.2.5. Hospital-Associated Malnutrition

Patients with advanced COPD have frequent episodes of acute reversible airway obstruction, which in most instances, are likely triggered by viral infections. These episodes require hospitalization where the deterioration of nutritional status, (apart from the normal progression of the disease), is a likely consequence. It is well recognized that serious nutritional deficits can develop over the course of hospitalization in a variety of clinical problems (23–26). A recent prospective study of hospitalized patients may shed some light on the problem. Inadequate food intake (75% of calculated maintenance requirements) was common for prolonged periods. This may be explained by patients' dislike of the foods offered, lack of appetite, and diet prescriptions *(27)*. Failure to record patient's height and weight, lack of adequate nutritional support when problems were recognized, failure to observe and record patient's dietary intake, and prolonged use of glucose and saline IV fluids remain common *(28)*. Food delivery was cited as an additional cause of institutional malnutrition. Meals are delivered at times that suit the hospital routine, but not necessarily that of the patient. Patients also expressed dissatisfaction with portion size, the temperature of food, lack of availability of food between 6:00 and 8:00 PM, and meals that are frequently unpalatable or placed outside the reach of elderly or incapacitated patients *(29)*.

Adequate dietary intake is at the center of nutritional rehabilitation and weight gain, and the attending health care team is the patients' first line of defense against the protein and energy undernutrition during hospitalization. Some patients with COPD can maintain their weight and function reasonably well until an acute event leads to elevated energy requirements that cannot be met. Weight loss follows and the weight is not necessarily regained during the recovery period, leading to a stepped decline in body weight over time *(30)*.

3.2.6. Glucocorticosteroid Therapy

Oral or intravenous therapy with glucocorticosteroids is used in the treatment of an acute exacerbation of COPD. The anti-inflammatory and immunosuppressive properties of glucocorticosteroids are well established and are responsible for their widespread use in COPD and in other inflammatory diseases (asthma, rheumatoid arthritis). The catabolic effects of glucocorticosteroids on respiratory muscles are also well known. In a prospective examination of eight patients prescribed an average daily dose of 14.2 ± 8.2 mg of methylprednisolone or equivalent for the previous 6 mo, severe muscle weakness in both the respiratory and peripheral muscles developed *(31)*.

Glucose intolerance is a well-established side effect of systemic glucocorticosteroid use *(31a)*. The negative effect of glucocorticosteroids on protein metabolism is indicated by increased protein breakdown and possible reduced protein synthesis *(31b)*. Reduced muscle mass, thinning of skin, a reduction in the protein matrix of the bones followed by calcium loss, and a negative nitrogen balance are other well-known side effects of glucocorticosteroid treatment *(32)*.

The adverse effects of glucocorticosteroids on nitrogen balance have also been observed in other diseases. For example, patients with rheumatoid arthritis *(32)* who were in negative nitrogen balance during therapy with methylprednisolone, continued to be negative after therapy had stopped (4 d posttreatment) despite high energy (approx 47 kcal/kg) and protein (1.6 g/kg) intakes. The catabolic effects of glucocorticosteroids may override the positive effects of increased dietary intake.

4. NUTRITIONAL EVALUATION OF DEPLETION

4.1. Screening for Malnutrition

Given the poor prognosis for malnourished COPD patients and the possibility of frequent hospital admissions it is important that front-line health care workers in the community and in hospitals recognize malnutrition (weight loss and nutritional deterioration) early so that nutritional therapy can be initiated. A suggested screening process for COPD patients is provided in Fig. 1. Maintaining weight throughout the progression

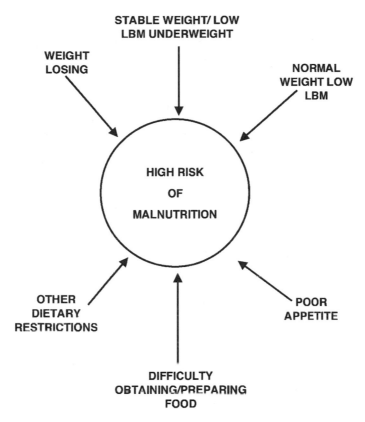

Fig. 1. Screening for high-risk individuals. The following factors may help identify individuals at high risk of becoming malnourished. LBM, lean body mass.

of the disease may be difficult to achieve, but weight maintenance in the early stages may be more beneficial than interventions to induce weight gain after depletion of lean body mass has occurred. Reports of recent weight loss can also be used to identify individuals at risk (>10% over the previous 6 mo or >5% during the previous month). Loss of lean body mass and other factors such as poor appetite, difficulty obtaining and/or preparing food, and other dietary restrictions may identify individuals at high risk of becoming malnourished. These individuals need to be brought to the attention of dietitians who can begin nutritional therapy as soon as possible.

4.2. Assessment of Nutritional Status of Patients with COPD

Nutritional assessment is defined as a comprehensive evaluation of nutritional status, including medical history, dietary history, physical examination, anthropometric measurements, and laboratory data (33). A summary of the studies determining the nutritional status of patients with COPD is shown in Table 1. Body weight alone may be misleading and will not identify all compromised individuals, in particular COPD patients where body water redistribution has masked malnutrition. However, weight loss is a distressing signal indicative of some catabolic event and should alert clinicians to investigate further. Simple measures of weight and height can be used to calculate BMI. In the elderly, a BMI in the range of 22–27 kg/m^2 is considered healthy and a BMI greater than 22 kg/m^2 has been shown to improve survival in COPD patients *(4,34,35)*. Bioelectrical impedance assay (BIA), a technique used to assess body composition, has been shown to be a safe, convenient, and feasible alternative in the evaluation and monitoring of nutritional status in normal and critically ill subjects *(36,37)*. The BIA has been used in COPD patients and has a high correlation ($r = 0.93$) with fat-free mass *(38)*. However, until BIA is readily available in a clinical setting, BMI is the most useful and inexpensive measure of nutritional status. BMI is easily calculated and only requires the measurement of body height and weight. If height cannot be measured, knee height *(39,40)* and arm-span measurements *(41,42)* can be used as substitutes.

4.3. Assessment of Visceral Protein Status

A more comprehensive review of the biochemical measures used in the assessment of nutritional status can be found elsewhere in this text (Chapters 5 and 6). Most patients with COPD have values within the normal range for serum albumin, transferrin and retinol-binding protein *(22,43–46)* and visceral proteins may not be objective markers of nutritional status in this population.

4.4. Assessment of Changes in Lean Body Mass

Depletion of lean body mass is a serious problem in a substantial portion of patients with COPD and affects their muscle strength, their ability to exercise, activities of daily living, and their survival. Short-term changes in body protein can be estimated using the nitrogen balance technique *(47)*, a noninvasive and useful measure available to clinicians, dietitians, and nurses in hospitals and in the community. This technique requires that nitrogen intake and 24-h urinary output are accurately determined. Agreement between urinary urea nitrogen and total urea nitrogen in critically ill patients with a variety of clinical conditions has been reported *(48,49)*. A negative nitrogen balance occurs when protein breakdown exceeds protein synthesis and can arise from infection, trauma, sepsis, burns, or surgery. In our study of COPD patients admitted to hospitals during an acute exacerbation of their disease, complete 24-h urine collections were available for 14 patients; 11 were in negative balance. As only one measure was available per patient we were left with the question of whether or not the state of negative nitrogen balance continued throughout the study period. To put our findings of the nitrogen balance studies in perspective, it is useful to underline that a nitrogen loss of approx 6 g/d will result in a loss of approx 37.5 g protein/d. Using the relationship that lean body tissue is 20% protein, an estimated loss of 187.5 g of lean tissue/d or 1.3 kg/wk can develop if the negative nitrogen balance is not corrected *(6)*.

5. NUTRITIONAL INTERVENTION IN STABLE, MALNOURISHED PATIENTS WITH COPD

The interest in using nutritional support to improve the outcome in stable, malnourished patients with COPD has grown over the last two decades and the refeeding trials among inpatients or outpatients have had mixed results (Table 2). Three studies have shown that under well controlled, experimental conditions, short-term (14–21 d) nutritional therapy will result in weight gain and improvements in respiratory muscle strength *(43,50,51)*. Mean weight gain in these studies have a range of 1.7–3 kg. The energy intake ranged between 1.4 × REE to 2.2 × REE. Of the 5 outpatient trials (Table 2), 4 did not

Table 2
Summary of Refeeding Trials Carried Out in Stable, Malnourished Patients with COPD

No. of subjects, type, duration	Total intake	Comments	Author(s)
6 Patients followed in a clinical research unit for 2 wk	$3 > 1.5 \times$ BMR $3 = 1.5 \times$ BMR	Gain of 3 kg, improvement in PI_{max}, no change in pulmonary function	Wilson et al., 1986 (43)
21 Patients, randomized and followed as outpatients for 8 wk	~2091 kcal $1.7 \times$ H.B.	No weight gain, no change in respiratory muscle or lung function	Lewis et al., 1987 (44)
25 Patients, randomized and crossover, followed as outpatients for 8 wk	~2350 kcal ~$1.8 \times$ REE	Small increase in weight, no effects on respiratory muscles or lung function	Knowles et al., 1988 (45)
21 Patients, randomized and followed as outpatients for 9 mo	~2118 kcal ~82 g protein ~$1.9 \times$ REE	Gain of 4 kg, improvement in respiratory muscles and grip, no change in lung function	Efthimiou et al., 1988 (22)
28 Patients, randomized, placebo-controlled, and followed for 13 wk	~2719 kcal $2.4 \times$ REE	Gain of 1.5 kg, no change in PI_{max}, PE_{max}	Otte et al., 1989 (69)
10 Patients, randomized, in hospital refeeding trial, 16 d	~2489 kcal $2.2 \times$ REE	Gain of 2.4 kg, improvement in PE_{max}, no change in FEV_1, FVC	Whittaker et al., 1990 (50)
27 Patients, randomized and followed in a clinical research unit for 3 wk followed by 3 mo as outpatients	$1.7 \times$ REE 1.5 g protein/kg/d	Gain of 1.7 kg, improvement in grip strength and PE_{max}	Rogers et al., 1992 (51)
12 Patients followed as outpatients for 4 mo	~1670 kcal	No change in weight, FEV_1 or respiratory muscles	Sridhar et al., 1994 (70)
217 Patients participating in an intensive inpatient rehabilitation program, randomized and followed for 8 wk	~2400 kcal	Weight gain in both depleted and nondepleted patients. Nutrition and steroids led to a greater increase in lean body mass in depleted patients	Schols et al., 1995 (61)

PI_{max}, maximal inspiratory pressure.
PE_{max}, maximal expiratory pressure.

observe any improvements in lung function or respiratory muscle strength over periods ranging from 8 wk to 4 mo. The one successful refeeding trial was a well-controlled study in which a mean weight gain of 4 kg over 3 mo was achieved in patients receiving a supplement. This weight gain was also associated with small improvements in respiratory muscle strength, hand grip strength, and distance walked. The energy intake of the treatment group was approx 43 kcal/kg body weight, and their protein intake was approx 1.7 g/kg body weight. However, this improvement was not sustained when patients were no longer part of the intervention *(22)*. The limited therapeutic effect of nutritional support in clinically stable outpatients is disappointing but may be related to the intensity of the intervention, complexity of the metabolic disturbances in COPD (presence of inflammation, shifts in body water compartments, relative anorexia) and the advanced age of the patients *(46)*. Additional therapy (anabolic agents) to reverse the weight loss has been successful but this is not yet a widely used strategy *(52)*.

5.1. Nutritional Intervention During an Acute Exacerbation

Although most feeding trials have focused on the rehabilitation of already malnourished patients, limited data are available evaluating the effect oral nutritional support has on functional status during an exacerbation of COPD. An acute exacerbation may result in a temporary low energy and protein intake, as well as an increased REE on admission to hospital. Food intake can be increased a few days after admission *(53)*. Our own data indicate that an increase in oral intake to approx 2370 kcal/d and 1.54 g protein/kg/d is possible during hospitalization *(6)*. This level of intake, although significantly better than among patients receiving usual care, did not result in improvements in muscle strength during the short period of hospitalization.

6. NUTRITION AND EXERCISE

While nutritional support alone in malnourished COPD patients has been met with limited success, the combination of nutritional support and an appropriate exercise program that helps improve respiratory muscle strength and increase fat-free mass, should be part of a comprehensive rehabilitation program in COPD patients. Adding a simple but effective weight training program may be as beneficial in COPD patients as it was found to be in healthy elderly whose walking capacity and respiratory and limb muscle strength improved after participating in an 18-mo nutritional supplementation and resistance training program *(54)*. In a group of frail elderly people, the combination of resistance training and supplementation was more beneficial in improving muscle strength and mobility than supplementation alone *(55)*.

7. WHAT ARE THE NUTRITIONAL REQUIREMENTS OF COPD PATIENTS?

Optimal amounts of carbohydrate, protein and fat have not been defined for individuals with COPD. Recommendations for energy and protein intake have mainly come from feeding trials in stable, malnourished patients and from hospitalized patients during an exacerbation of the disease.

7.1. Energy Intake

In malnourished, stable patients successful weight gain and nitrogen retention was achieved with energy intakes ranging from 1.4 to 2.2 × REE *(43,50,51)*. In patients hospitalized during an exacerbation, an energy intake of 1.9 × REE is achievable *(6)*. It is important that dequate energy intakes to cover the higher than expected energy expenditures needs be provided to COPD patients.

7.1.1. PROTEIN INTAKE

Protein intakes have been high in successful refeeding studies. While a protein intake of approx 1.4 g/kg/d was not associated with weight change *(44)* intakes of ≥1.7 g/kg/d lead to good weight gain and positive nitrogen balance *(22,56)*. To achieve such a level of protein intake from food requires a fairly high energy intake. In hospitalized COPD patients a protein intake of approx 1.5 g/kg/d resulted in a negative nitrogen balance *(6)*, thus it is not clear whether nitrogen balance can be achieved in the short term in this population.

7.1.2. THE MACRONUTRIENT COMPOSITION OF FOOD INTAKE

The macronutrient composition of the diet for patients with COPD has received attention because an increase in dyspnea resulting from diet-induced thermogenesis may be possible and could lead to changes in eating habits. A high intake of carbohydrate (≥74% of total energy) has been shown to increase carbon dioxide production and minute ventilation *(57)*, however, a more realistic intake of approx 53% energy from carbohydrate was shown to be well tolerated by normal-weight and underweight COPD patients. Some COPD patients require nutritional supplements between regular meals to reverse weight loss or maintain a stable weight. Recently, it was demonstrated that a carbohydrate-rich (60% of energy) supplement, while resulting in a higher respiratory quotient, led to faster gastric emptying and less shortness of breath than a fat-rich supplement (60% of energy) *(58)*. Although a very high intake of carbohydrate is not appropriate for this population, an intake of up to 60% of energy as carbohydrate is well tolerated. A high protein intake (≥1.7 g/kg) is needed to prevent lean body mass from being used as a source of energy. Fat intake is important as a source of energy but not at excessive levels as this may lead to slower gastric emptying and increase the feeling of bloating, abdominal discomfort and early satiety.

7.1.3. POLYUNSATURATED FATTY ACIDS AND FRUITS AND VEGETABLE INTAKE

Apart from determining which energy and protein requirements are needed to keep weight stable or reverse weight loss seen in COPD patients, attention has started to focus on other dietary constituents. Antioxidants and omega-3-fatty acids and how they are potentially protective factors in lung function have been of recent interest. The beneficial effect of increased fruits and vegetable intake and lung function in COPD has not been clearly demonstrated. A high intake of omega-3-fatty acids, which are abundantly present in mackerel, lake trout, tuna, herring, salmon and anchovy as well as in seeds and nuts, (particularly flaxseeds and walnuts), may have beneficial effects on lung function in the general population *(58a)* but no clear evidence is available for COPD. Clear benefits of a high intake of omega-3-fatty acids have been shown for coronary heart disease and stroke *(59)*, but the evidence for other diseases is only speculative at this time. Nonetheless, omega-3-fatty acids are important components of the phospholipid membrane of all cells and membrane elasticity is necessary for cells and tissues, (including the lungs), to function properly. Omega-3-fatty acids may confer their health benefits through anti-inflammatory properties and their inhibitory effects in the synthesis of cytokines and mitogens, and may be beneficial in COPD *(59)*.

High-risk individuals (Fig. 1) should also undergo a dietary evaluation assessing the adequacy of energy and protein intake, and acceptable foods that are nutrient-dense should be offered to enhance intakes. Micronutrient requirements are likely met by using the food guide pyramid as a resource. Patients in hospitals need close monitoring to ensure that meals are not missed due to procedures, snacks and meals are consumed and missed foods are replaced.

8. RECOMMENDATIONS

Weight loss is a common clinical feature of COPD and because the adverse effects of weight loss are well understood, adequate nutritional support and an appropriate exercise program should be part of an inclusive rehabilitation program in COPD patients. Weight gain, positive nitrogen balance and improvements in muscle strength, hand-grip strength and walking distance are possible with energy intakes ranging from 1.4 to 2.2 × REE and protein intakes of ≥1.7 g/kg/d. For overweight patients, appropriate nutritious food choices are important and weight loss, if necessary, should be very gradual. Other food constituents, particularly antioxidants and omega-3-fatty acids, may be beneficial in lung function. Every effort should be made to identify patients with poor nutritional status as soon as possible so that appropriate therapy can be delivered as *secondary prevention* rather than as *treatment* once serious losses have occurred.

8.1. Maintaining or Improving Nutritional and Respiratory Function

8.1.1. ROLE OF THE DIETITIAN

Because of the existing problems of undernutrition in this patient group, the dietitian should focus on the obviously malnourished patient or the patient who is starting to lose or has lost lean body mass. COPD patients often have a poor appetite, may suffer from fatigue and breathlessness, and dietary advice should include enjoyable, energy- and nutrient-dense foods as eating can tire some COPD patients. The patient's usual food habits, tastes, and preferences need to be considered. It is important for the patient to try to eat what he/she enjoys. Sustaining an adequate intake at all times is a challenge. Extra food may be needed and could come in the form of energy-dense supplements spread out over the day to avoid feelings of bloating and breathlessness.

Many concurrent health problems may be evident but nutritional interventions in hospitals need to assure the adequate intake of protein and energy. This can be achieved through tempting food choices (having family members bring in favorite foods), offering snacks on a very regular basis, having food available at frequent intervals without disruptions, and helping the patient and family understand the importance of nutritional therapy (despite their major preoccupation with breathing problems). At home, family support or such services as meal delivery (Meals on Wheels), home care or community meals can help assure adequate nutritional support. Nutritious snacks, such as cheese, puddings or commercial supplements, are very important for COPD patients, as many find it difficult to eat a lot during one meal. Simple foods with a minimum of preparation time are important so as to not tire or discourage the patient. Patients should eat frequent meals of the foods they enjoy (*see* Tables 3 and 4). Income can also be a problem as many COPD patients may be on disability or early retirement from work, and affordable food suggestions are important.

8.1.2. MAINTAINING OR IMPROVING RESPIRATORY FUNCTION

Whenever possible, patients should participate in an endurance and strength exercise program to preserve and/or improve respiratory muscle strength and build peripheral muscles. Severely depleted patients may need an exercise program adapted to their special situation. The benefits of exercise are well known *(54,55)*, and in COPD patients, they can enhance the nutritional therapy, owing to improved appetite and well being. If weight gain has been successful and respiratory muscle function has been restored or improved, patients can move on to a maintenance regimen.

It is possible that despite adherence to an exercise program and aggressive therapy some individuals cannot arrive at the desired outcome, and in such instances anabolic agents may be considered. Treatment with recombinant human growth hormone (rhGH) has been investigated in nutritionally depleted patients with COPD, but failed to show any improvements in muscle function *(60)*. A treatment combining nutritional supplementation with the injection of the anabolic steroid nandrolone decanoate resulted in an increase in fat-free mass and improved respiratory muscle function *(61)*. Clearly, more work needs to be done to unravel the factors that make some patients more able to maintain nutritional adequacy, whereas others have great difficulty in this area.

In conclusion, COPD patients need to be screened to detect those who are starting to lose weight, as well as those already undernourished. Dietary interventions are thought to be more useful early on in the disease process to stop the loss of lean body mass, rather than refeed to rebuild. Waiting until patients show clear signs of undernutrition is not in their best interest. Offering appealing foods with high energy and protein density is important and needs to be institutionalized. Disruptions in food intake from testing should be minimized. Support at home is crucial. Appealing meals need to be provided with a minimum of effort on the patient's part. Fatigue, discomfort, depression, anxiety, and reduced income from leaving a job can all lead to poor intakes. It is clear that a treatment plan for discharged patients is very important to their well being, as breathlessness and exercise intolerance are their most distressing symptoms.

9. RECOMMENDATIONS FOR CLINICIANS

1. Routine nutritional assessment (weight and height measurements, recent weight loss) for elderly patients with COPD will help identify patients with poor status so that intervention can be initiated as early as possible.
2. Patients found to be at risk should receive nutritional surveillance, be provided adequate protein ($\geq$1.7 g/kg/d) and energy (1.4–2.2 × REE), supplements as needed, be given an appropriate exercise program and be encouraged to include food sources rich in antioxidants and omega-3-fatty acids.
3. Interventions should emphasize weight gain (Recommendation 5), positive nitrogen balance, and improvements in muscle strength, handgrip strength, and distance walked.

Table 3
Suggestions for a Menu Plan a for Female COPD Patient

Day 1

Breakfast:	1 soft-boil egg, 1 slice of whole-wheat toast with 3 slices of cheese, coffee, or tea with 3.7% milk and sugar
Snack:	~200 g rice pudding with raisins
Lunch:	1 bowl of chunky vegetable soup homemade or canned and 1 turkey sandwich (2 slices of whole-wheat bread, mustard, ~90 g sliced turkey, tomatoes, and lettuce)
Dinner:	~100 g fried salmon, 100 g boiled carrots, 40 g boiled peas, 1 small scoop (~16 g) of ice cream and ~240 (1 cup) of applesauce
Snack:	~200 g rice pudding with raisins

This menu supplies approx 2190 kcal or ≥1.7 × REE for a 75-yr-old female COPD patient weighing 64 kg. Her protein intake is ~1.7 g/kg body weight. The caloric beakdown is follows: 19% protein, 50% carbohydrates, and 31% fat.

Table 4
Suggestions for a Menu Plan for a Male COPD Patient

Day 2

Breakfast:	60 g raisin bran cereal with 2% milk, coffee or tea with milk and sugar
Snack:	1 5-oz can of chocolate pudding
Lunch:	~490 g (2 cups) of beef and vegetable stew—homemade or canned, 2 slices of bread with 2 teaspoons of butter, a few slices of tomatoes, and 3 thin slices of cheese, 1 small scoop (16 g) of ice cream, and ~244 g (1 cup) of applesauce
Snack:	Tea or coffee with 2% milk
Dinner:	~150 g fried, skinless chicken, 200 g (1 cup) of rice, ~70 g (1/2 cup) boiled carrots fresh or frozen, ~184 (1 cup) boiled broccoli, fresh or frozen
Snack:	1 5-oz can of chocolate pudding

This menu supplies approx 2470 kcal or ≥1.7 × REE for a 73-yr-old male COPD patient weighing 70 kg. The protein intake is ~1.8 g/kg body weigh. The caloric breakdown is as follows: 20% protein, 50% carbohydrates, and 30% fat.

4. For undernourished patients at home, family support is crucial so that the patient can receive appealing meals with a minimum of effort in a supportive social environment. Social support is also important in the hospital setting, as is the need to minimize disruptions of food intake for medical tests.
5. Patients who are overweight should lose weight very gradually and a weight reduction diet should emphasize overall dietary adequacy (protein and micronutrients).

REFERENCES

1. Hirsh RS, Dasbach EJ. An economic overview of chronic obstructive pulmonary disease. Pharmaco-economics 2001;19:623–642.
2. Monthly vital statistics report, vol. 48, no. 11, www.cdc.gov/nchs/fastats/copd.htm
3. Schols AMWJ, Slangen, JOS, Volovics Lex, Wouters FM. Weight loss is a reversible factor in the prognosis of chronic obstructive pulmonary disease. Am J Respir Crit Care Med 1998;157:1791–1797.
4. Gray-Donald K, Gibbons S, Shapiro H, Macklem PT, Martin JG. Nutritional status and mortality in chronic obstructive pulmonary disease. Am J Respir Crit Care Med 1996;153:961–966.
5. Schols AMWJ, Mostert R, Soeter PB, Wouters EFM. Body composition and exercise performance in chronic obstructive pulmonary disease. Thorax 1991;46:695–699.
6. Saudny-Unterberger H, Martin G, Gray-Donald K. Impact of nutritional support on functional status during an acute exacerbation of chronic obstructive pulmonary disease. Am J Respir Crit Care Med 1997;156:794–799.
7. Cherniack NS. Chronic Obstructive Pulmonary Disease. W.B. Saunders Company, 1991.
8. Hubmayr RD, Rodarte JR. Cellular effects and physiologic responses: Lung mechanics. In: Chronic Obstructive Pulmonary Disease Cherniack NS (ed.), 1991;9:79–90.
9. Rochester DF. Effects of COPD on the respiratory muscles. In: Chronic Obstructive Pulmonary Disease Cherniack NS (ed.), 1991, pp. 134–152.
10. Tobin MJ. Respiratory muscles in disease. Clin Chest Med 1988;9:2.
11. Wouters EFM. Nutrition and metabolism in COPD. Chest 2000;117:274S–280S.
12. Benedict F, Miles W, Roth P, et al. Human Vitality and Efficiency Under Prolonged Restricted Diet. Carnegie Institute, Washington, DC, publication no. 280, 1919.
13. Baarends EM, Schols AMWJ, Pannemans DLE, Westerterp KR, Wouters EFM. Total free living energy expenditure in patients with severe chronic obstructive pulmonary disease. Am J Respir Crit Care Med 1997;155:549–554.
14. Harris JA, Benedict EG. A Biometric Study of Basal Metabolism. Carnegie Institution of Washington, Washington, DC, 1919.
15. Tracey KJ, Cerami A. Tumor necrosis factor: a pleiotropic cytokine and therapeutic target. Annu Rev Med 1994;45:491–503.
16. Van Der Poll T, Sauerwein HP. Tumor necrosis factor-α: its role in the metabolic response to sepsis. Clin Sci 1993;84:247–256.
17. Di Francia M, Barbier D, Mege Jean L, Orehek J. Tumor necrosis factor-alpha. Levels and weight loss in chronic obstructive pulmonary disease. Am J Respir Crit Care Med 1994;150:1453–1455.
18. De Godoy I, Calhoun WJ, Donahoe M, Mancino J, Rogers RM. Elevated TNF-α production by peripheral blood monocytes of weight losing COPD patients. Am J Respir Crit Care Med 1996;153:633–637.
19. Takabatake N, Nakamura H, Abe S, et al. The relationship between chronic hypoxemia and activation of the tumor necrosis factor-α system in patients with chronic obstructive pulmonary disease. Am J Respir Crit Care Med 2000;1161:1179–1184.
20. Braun SR, Keim NL, Dixon RM, et al. The prevalence and determinants of nutritional changes in chronic obsturctive pulmonary disease. Chest 1984;4:558–563.
21. Hunter AM, Carey MA, Larsh HW. The nutritional status of patients with chronic obstructive pulmonary disease. Am Rev Respir Dis 1981;124:376–381.
22. Efthimiou J, Fleming J, Gomes C, Spiro SG. The effect of supplementary oral nutrition in poorly nourished patients with chronic obstructive pulmonary disease. Am Rev Respir Dis 1988;137:1075–1082.
23. Weinsier RL, Hunker EM, Krumdieck CL, Butterworth CE. Hospital malnutrition: A prospective evaluation of general medical patients during the course of hospitalization. Am Clin Nutr 1979;32:418–426.
24. Coats KG, Morgan SL, Bartolucci AA, Weinsier RL. Hospital-associated malnutrition: a reevaluation 12 years later. Am Diet Assoc 1993;93:27–33.
25. McWhirter JP, Pennington CR. Incidence and recognition of malnutrition in hospital. BMJ 1994;308:945–948.
26. Corish C, Flood P, Mulligan S, Kennedy NP. Prevalence of undernutrition and weight loss changes during the course of hospitalization among patients admitted to two Dublin hospitals. Proc Nutr Soc 1998;57:10A.

27. Sullivan DH, Sun S, Walls RC. Protein-energy undernutrition among elderly hospitalized patients. A Prospective Study. JAMA 1999;281:2013–2019.

28. Corish CA, Kennedy NP. Protein-energy undernutrition in hospital in-patients. Br Nutr 2000;83: 575–591.

29. Rushe F, Moloney M. Patient satisfaction, nutrient content and actual intake of food served in two Dublin teaching hospitals. Proc Nutr Soc 1998;57:166A.

30. Wilson DO, Rogers RM, Hoffman RM. Nutrition and chronic lung disease. State of the art. Am Rev Respir Dis 1985;132:1347–1365.

31. Decramer M, De Bock V, Dom R. Functional and histologic picture of steroid-induced myopathy in chronic obstructive pulmonary disease. Am J Respir Crit Care Med 1996;153:1958–1964.

31a. McEvoy CE, Niewoehner DE. Corticosteroids in chronic obstructive pulmonary disease. Clinical benefits and risks. Clin Chest Med 2000; 21:739–752.

31b. Löfberg E, Gutierrez A, Wernerman J, et al. Effects of high doses of glucocorticoids on free amino acids, ribosomes, and protein turnover in human muscle. Eur J Clin Invest 2002;32:345–353.

32. Roubenoff R, Roubenoff RA, Ward LM, Stevens MB. Catabolic effects of high-dose corticosteroids persist despite therapeutic benefit in rheumatoid arthritis. Am J Clin Nutr 1990;52:1113–1117.

33. American Society for Parenteral and Enteral Nutrition. Standards for nutrition support: hospitalized patients. Nutr Clin Prac 1995;10:208–219.

34. Cornoni-Huntley JC, Harris TB, Everett DF, et al. An Overview of body weight of older persons, including the impact on mortality. The National Health and Nutrition Examination survey 1-epidemiologic follow-up study. J Clin Epidemiol 1991;44:743–753.

35. Conners AF, Dawson NV, Thomas C, et al. Outcomes following an acute exacerbation of severe chronic obstructive lung disease. Am J Respir Crit Care Med 1996;154:959–967.

36. Lukaski HC, Johnson PE, Bolonchuk W, Lykken GI. Assessment of fat free mass using bioelectrical measurements of the body. Am J Clin Nutr 1985;41:810–817.

37. Robert S, Zarowitz BJ, Hyzy R, Eichenhorn M, Peterson EL, Popovich J. Bioelectric impedance assessment of nutritional status in critically ill patients. Am J Clin Nutr 1993;57:840–844.

38. Schols AMWJ, Wouters EFM, Soeters PB, Westerterp KR. Body composition by bioelectrical-impedance analysis compared with deuterium dilution and skinfold anthropometry in patients with chronic obstructive pulmonary disease. Am J Clin Nutr 1991;53:421–424.

39. Chumlea WC, Roche AF, Steinbaugh ML. Estimating stature from knee height for persons 60–90 years of age. J Am Geriatr Soc 1985;33:116–120.

40. Han TS, Lean ME. Lower leg length as an index of stature in adults. Int J Obes Relat Metab Dis 1996;20:21–27.

41. Kwok T, Whitelaw MN. The use of armspan in nutritional assessment of the elderly. J Am Geriatr Soc 1991;39:492–496.

42. Reeves SL, Varakamin C, Henry CJK. The relationship between arm-span measurement and height with special reference to gender and ethnicity. Eur J Clin Nutr 1996;50:398–400.

43. Wilson DO, Rogers RM, Sanders MH, et al. Nutritional intervention in malnourished patients with emphysema. Am Rev Respir Dis 1986;134:672–677.

44. Lewis MI, Belman MJ, Dorr-Uyemura L. Nutritional supplementation in ambulatory patients with chronic obstructive pulmonary disease. Am Rev Respir Dis 1987;135:1062–1068.

45. Knowles JB, Fairbarn MS, Wiggs BJ, et al. Dietary supplementation and respiratory muscle performance in patients with COPD. Chest 1988;93:977–983.

46. Creutzberg Eva C, Schols AMWJ, Weling-Scheepers CAPM, Buurman WA, Wouters EFM. Characterization of nonresponse to high caloric oral nutritional therapy in depleted patients with chronic obstructive pulmonary disease. Am J Respir Crit Care Med 2000;161:745–752.

47. Mackenzie Th, Clark N, Bistrian BR, et al. A simple method for estimating nitrogen balance in hospitalized patients: A Review and Supporting Data for a Previously Proposed Technique. J Am Coll Nutr 1985;4:575–581.

48. Blackburn GL, Bistrian BR, Maini BS, et al. Nutritional and metabolic assessment of the hospitalized patient. J Parent Enteral Nutr 1977;1:11–22.

49. Milner A. Accuracy of urinary nitrogen for predicting total urinary nitrogen in thermally injured patients. J Parent Enteral Nutr 1993;17:414–416.

50. Whitaker JS, Ryan CG, Buckley PA. The effects of refeeding on peripheral and respiratory muscle function in malnourished chronic obstructive pulmonary disease patients. Am Rev Respir Dis 1990; 142:283–288.

51. Rogers RM, Donahoe M, Costantino J. Physiologic effects of oral supplemental feeding in malnourished patients with chronic obstructive pulmonary disease. Am Rev Respir Dis 1992;146:1511–1517.

52. Schols AMWJ, Slangen J, Volovics L, Wouters EFM. Weight loss is a reversible factor in the prognosis of chronic obstructive pulmonary disease. Am J Respir Crit Car Med 1998;157:1791–1797.

53. Vermeeren MAP, Schols AMWJ, Wouters EFM. Effects of an acute exacerbation on nutritional and metabolic profile of patients with COPD. Eur Respir J 1997;10:2264–2269.

54. Bunout D, Barrera G, De la Maza P, et al. The impact of nutritional supplementation and resistance training on the health functioning of free-living chilean elders: Results of 18 months of follow-up. J Nutr 2001;131:2441S–2446S.

55. Fiatarone MA, O'Neill EF, Ryan ND, Clements KM, Solares GR, et al. Exercise training and nutritional supplementation for physical frailty in very elderly people. N Eng J Med 1994;330:1769–1775.

56. Goldstein SA, Thomashow BM, Kvetan V, et al. Nitrogen and energy relationships in malnourished patients with emphysema. Am Rev Respir Dis 1988;138:636–644.

57. Angelillo VA, Bedi S, Durfee D, et al. Effects of low and high carbohydrate feedings in ambulatory patients with chronic obstructive pulmonary disease and chronic hypercapnia. Ann Intern Med 1985; 103:883–885.

58. Vermeeren MAP, Wouters EF, Nelissen LH, et al. Acute effects of different nutritional supplements on symptoms and functional capacity in patients with chronic obstructive pulmonary disease. Am J Clin Nutr 2001;73:295–301.

58a. Smit HA, Grievink L, Tabak C. Dietary influences on chronic obstructive lung disease and asthma: a review of the epidemiological evidence. Proc Nutr Soc 1999;58:309–319.

59. Connor WE. Importance of n-3 fatty acds in health and disease. Am J Clin Nutr 2000;71(suppl): 171S–175S.

60. Schols AM, Wouters EFM. Nutritional abnormalities and supplementation in chronic obstructive pulmonary disease. Clin Chest Med 2000;214:753–762.

61. Schols AM, Soeters PB, Mostert R, et al. Physiologic effects of nutritional support and anabolic steroids in patients with chronic obstructive pulmonary disease. A placebo-controlled randomized trial. Am J Respir Crit Care Med 1995;152:1268–1274.

62. Openbrier DR, Irwin MM, Rogers RM, et al. Nutritional status and lung function in patients with emphysema and chronic bronchitis. Chest 1983;1:17–22.

63. Gray-Donald K, Gibbons L, Shapiro SH, et al. Effect of nutritional status on exercise performance in patients with chronic obstructive pulmonary disease. Am Rev Respir Dis 1989;140:1544–1548.

64. Wilson DO, Rogers RM, Wright EC, et al. Body weight in chronic obstructive pulmonary disease. Am Rev Respir Dis 1989;139:1435–1438.

65. Schols MWJ, Mostert R, Soeters P, et al. Inventory of nutritional status in patients with COPD. Chest 1989;96:247–249.

66. Sahebjami H, Doers JT, Render ML, et al. Anthropometric and pulmonary function test profiles outpatients with stable chronic obstructive pulmonary disease. Am J Med 1993;94:469–474.

67. Schols MWJ, Soeters PB, Dingemans AM, et al. Prevalence and characteristics of nutritional depletion in patients with stable COPD eligible for pulmonary rehabilitation. Am Rev Respir Dis 1993;147: 1151–1156.

68. Laaban JP, Kouchakji B, Dore MF, et al. Nutritional status of patients with chronic obstructive pulmonary disease and acute respiratory failure. Chest 1993;103:1362–1368.

69. Otte KE, Ahlburg P, D'Amore F, et al. Nutritional repletion in malnourished patients with emphysema. J Parent Enteral Nutr 1989;13:152–156.

70. Sridhar MK, Galloway A, Lean MEJ. Study of an outpatient nutritional supplementation programme in malnourished patients with emphysematous COPD. Eur Respir J 1994;7:720–724.

C. Cancer

20 Nutritional Requirements Following Cancer Treatment/Surgery

Selwyn M. Vickers and Peter A. Nagi

1. INTRODUCTION

Malnutrition represents one of the most common causes of morbidity and mortality in the cancer patient. Over 50% of patients diagnosed with cancer report significant weight loss and related symptoms of malnutrition (1). Gastrointestinal malignancies have some of the highest incidence of nutritional problems, with pancreatic and gastric cancers each reporting more than an 80% incidence of malnutrition (2). Breast, prostate, and lung cancers also have significant incidences, from 35% to 60% according to recent studies (2,3). In addition to the symptoms caused by malnutrition, the response to treatment and overall survival of cancer patients has been shown to correlate inversely with their degree of malnutrition (4). Thus, any prognostic determination in a patient diagnosed with cancer must ultimately consider their nutritional status and any interventions must be considered in parallel.

Malnutrition in the cancer patient, often referred to as the "cancer cachexia syndrome," is a multifactoral disorder involving physical, metabolic, and psychosocial factors. Initially, patients present with symptoms of fatigue, malaise, and anorexia. Without intervention, these can progress to more serious signs of skeletal muscle atrophy, tissue wasting, and subsequent immune dysfunction (4). Appropriate nutritional support, along with other treatment modalities, can aid in the effectiveness of antineoplastic therapy and reduce complications of treatment (5). However, nutritional intervention is not indicated in all patients and initiation requires a careful consideration of an individual's overall health condition. A detailed assessment of nutritional parameters and an understanding of the physiology of cancer cachexia are essential to proper nutritional management. Selected treatment options should be based on the evidence of clinical trials designed to improve the longevity and quality of life of patients with cancer.

2. CANCER CACHEXIA

Cancer cachexia is a complex phenomenon that results from several interrelated processes. Specifically, a decrease in nutrient intake combined with an inefficient utilization

From: *Handbook of Clinical Nutrition and Aging*
Edited by: C. W. Bales and C. S. Ritchie © Humana Press Inc., Totowa, NJ

of these nutrients results in a large net loss of energy. The underlying reasons for these concomitant processes is not yet completely understood, but they are likely related to the direct and indirect effects of tumor burden.

2.1. Tumor Effects

Directly, tumor burden can cause dysphagia, early satiety, malabsorption, abdominal pain, and intestinal obstruction *(5)*. The location and size of the tumor dictate the extent of direct tumor effects. For example, a large oropharyngeal tumor can cause dysphagia and odynophagia from encroachment into the lumen and ulceration of the upper gastrointestinal tract. Pancreatic and bile duct tumors can obstruct the normal flow of bile and lead to fat malabsorption and deficiencies of fat-soluble vitamins *(6)*. Disseminated tumors of the peritoneal cavity can cause intestinal obstruction and electrolyte imbalances by infiltration of lymphatic vessels. Indirectly, tumor presence can cause anorexia, nausea, vomiting, and alterations in taste and smell *(7)*. Typically resulting from the body's immune response, these symptoms can be further exacerbated by learned food aversions, anxiety, depression, and even physical weaknesses further detracting from adequate nutritional intake. The ultimate causes of the indirect effects of tumor presence are the subject of ongoing research, however, early studies indicate that the host response to tumor is a complex process.

2.2. Host Response

Many of the indirect effects of tumor burden can be related to host cytokine production (Fig. 1) Several studies in cancer patients have documented elevated levels of circulating cytokines (e.g., IL-1, IL-6, λ-interferon, and TNF-α) that have detrimental effects on many host metabolic processes *(8–10)*. In animal models, exogenous administration of these cytokines can produce a condition identical to cancer anorexia and cachexia *(11,12)*. These cytokines are related not only to the symptomatic decrease in nutrient intake of cancer patients, but they can also alter the utilization of these nutrients.

Tumor-related abnormalities have been studied in carbohydrate, fat and protein metabolism. In fact, abnormal carbohydrate metabolism is a hallmark of cancer cachexia *(13)*. Glucose intolerance and peripheral insulin resistance are common findings in malnourished cancer patients, in contrast to the euglycemic or hypoglycemic state of nonstressed, starved patients *(14)*. This results in a net wasting of energy through inefficient utilization of these carbohydrates. Additionally, energy wasting may further result from increased tumor glycolysis resulting in lactate production that must then be converted to glucose by the liver *(15)*. Energy-inefficient processes are also demonstrated in the lipid metabolism of cachetic cancer patients. To further sequester energy stores, cancer patients have increased hydrolysis of lipid stores, despite abnormally high levels of plasma triglycerides *(16,17)*. Perhaps the most significant metabolic alteration noted in cancer patients pertains to protein synthesis and degradation. In contrast to the protein sparing to conserve organ function that occurs during normal starvation, cancer patients exhibit excessive protein turnover and wasting, leading to excessive muscle atrophy and organ dysfunction *(18)*. These changes often occur early in tumor growth and can be only partly explained by tumor gluconeogenesis, in which the tumor uses amino acids to produce energy *(19)*. Clearly, these metabolic derangements are very different from the adaptations seen during starvation, and reversal of these processes is difficult even with adequate nutritional support.

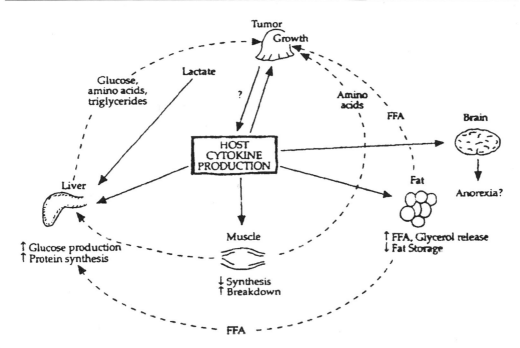

Fig. 1. Proposed mechanism of the cancer cachexia syndrome. Reprinted from ref. *1* with permission from JPEN.

3. NUTRITIONAL ASSESSMENT

The first step in determining whether a patient with cancer would benefit from nutritional support involves a detailed analysis of the patient's nutritional status.

3.1. History and Physical

A history and physical exam by the treating clinician should focus on recent weight changes and relative preillness body weight, appetite, eating habits, gastrointestinal tract symptoms, and preexisting medical conditions, as well as current medications or treatments the patient is receiving. Several standardized patient evaluation forms have been developed to aid clinicians in this capacity (e.g., Patient-Generated Subjective Global Assessment). In general, an unintended weight loss of greater than 5% of usual body weight in 1 mo or 10% in 6 mo is considered high risk for nutrition-related complications *(20)*. The physical exam should focus on evidence of muscle wasting, decreased strength, or depleted fat stores. Anthropometic measurements involving body mass index and mid-arm muscle area can be helpful references when performed by a trained professional.

3.2. Laboratory Tests

In conjunction with a history and physical, biochemical parameters can be used to objectively assess nutritional status. However, the accuracy of laboratory values hinges on the absence of multiple confounding factors and should never be evaluated in isolation. Among the most commonly used laboratory indicators of malnutrition are retinol-binding protein, transferrin and serum albumin. Synthesized in the liver, these markers can reflect the degree of visceral protein depletion at various time intervals. With half-lives of 2, 8, and 20 d respectively, these proteins have been used to estimate recent and prolonged periods of malnutrition *(14)*. Specifically, serum albumin levels less than 3.5 g/dL are most consistently associated with severe malnutrition and subsequent nutritional complications *(21)*. Current controversy exists regarding the reliability of serum albumin levels in chronic disease states, as biological factors, such as dehydration, renal dysfunction, liver failure, or recent blood transfusions can dramatically alter laboratory results. Until better objective indices are developed, these laboratory values should be evaluated only in the context of the underlying disease process.

3.3. Other Tests

Other tools for patient evaluation include functional assessments of the immune system as evidenced by delayed hypersensitivity testing of the skin. Allergies to common antigens (mumps, *Candida*, or dermatophytes) has been associated with malnutrition and a subsequent increase in related morbidity *(22)*.

Several comprehensive indexes have been devised to incorporate assessment data into a stratified scale of patient risk. Buzby and collegues devised the Prognostic Nutritional Index based on serum albumin, transferrin, triceps skin-fold thickness, and delayed cutaneous hypersensitivity that has been shown to correlate with clinical outcome in cancer patients *(23,24)*. These parameters can be useful to the clinician in conjunction with a complete history and physical exam to determine the severity of malnutrition and subsequent indications for intervention.

4. NUTRITIONAL SUPPORT

Nutritional support in cancer patients is primarily intended to prevent or reverse the effects of cachexia. Long-term treatment is only indicated when the patient is unable to meet basic nutritional requirements without assistance.

4.1. Oral Nutrition

The preferred route of nutrient administration is through oral supplementation. Oral supplementation should first be attempted through the use of natural, high-energy foods. If this proves unsuccessful, high-calorie liquid shakes are a cheap and easily attainable form of nutrition that can augment the inadequate dietary intake of many cancer patients. Most commercially available products contain sufficient amounts of protein, carbohydrate, and fat to sustain good health, and their composition can be catered to each patient's specific needs. Their main drawback is taste fatigue, which often limits patient compliance.

4.2. Enteral Nutrition

Enteral feeding involves the provision of nutrients directly into the gastrointestinal tract by means of a tube or catheter. A small, pliable nasogastic tube can be useful for short-term nutrient supplementation and has the advantage of easy placement and continuous or bolus feeding schedules. This method is preferred over parenteral nutrition when the gastrointestinal tract is functional, as it is less expensive and has fewer complications. Some disadvantages include patient discomfort and an increased risk of sinusitis and aspiration *(16)*. In some cancer patients, enteral feeding can be utilized to deliver nutrients distal to areas of partial obstruction, such as from oropharyngeal or esophageal tumors. For intervals of support expected to last longer than 4 wk, a surgically or endo-scopically placed gastrostomy or jejunostomy tube is recommended *(14)*.

Nutritional supplements such as arginine, omega-3 fatty acids, and ribonucleic acids can be added to enteral feedings to attain further immunologic and metabolic benefits *(25,26)*. A recent prospective study in cancer patients by Daly et al. demonstrated fewer complications and a shorter length of stay for patients receiving nutrient-enriched post-operative tube feedings when compared to a standard formula *(27)*.

4.3. Total Parenteral Nutrition

Total parenteral nutrition (TPN) involves the central venous cannulation of a patient's circulatory system in order to provide nutrients directly into the bloodstream. The com-position of TPN can be altered to specific needs of cancer patients and additives or immune-enhancing substances can be added for additional benefit. Glutamine, for example, has been shown to protect the mucosal integrity of the gastrointestinal tract and decrease the incidence of bacterial translocation *(28)*. However, parenteral nutrition has many associated risks and should only be considered in patients unsuitable for oral or enteral nutrition. Long-term access is typically gained by means of Hickman or Broviac catheters inserted into the subclavian or internal jugular vein or by peripherally inserted central catheters *(1)*. Placement complications include pneumothorax, venous thrombo-sis and arterial injury. Also, these catheters must be aseptically placed and maintained and used solely for nutrient administration to prevent the complications of catheter infection and sepsis *(29)*.

The use of TPN in cancer patients has been extensively studied, however, as a result of the heterogeneity of these studies, the results are often difficult to interpret. Overall, the routine use of TPN in cancer patients without severe malnutrition should be discour-aged, as it offers little to no benefit and can often lead to higher morbidity from infectious complications *(30)*. In certain situations, however, clinical studies have demonstrated the benefits of TPN. For example, Weisdorf et al. compared TPN to intravenous fluids administered 6 d prior to cytoreductive therapy in bone marrow transplant recipients. His results showed that TPN administration decreased malignant relapse and increased long-term survival in these patients *(31)*. In another study by Muller et al. severely malnour-ished patients undergoing celiotomy for a variety of gastrointestinal malignancies demonstrated a decrease in mortality and major postoperative complications in patients that received 10 d of preoperative TPN *(32)*.

5. ADJUVANT THERAPY

In addition to the deleterious effects of the cancer itself, the treatment of cancer can have significant impact on the nutritional status of a patient. Both surgical and medical approaches to therapy for cancer often incur physiologic consequences that can com-pound the adverse affects of cancer. To understand these ramifications, analysis of the effects of treatment modalities is warranted.

5.1. Surgery

Cancer patients are particularly sensitive to the catabolic stresses of surgery. In patients who are already deemed protein-calorie deficient, the stress of surgery can result in increased complications of infection, poor wound healing, and protracted recovery *(33)*.

Yamanda et al. demonstrated a strong correlation between nutritional status and postoperative complications *(34)*. In these cases, delaying elective surgery until nutritional status is improved becomes an important consideration. Preoperative nutritional support in patients with severe malnutrition is supported by several studies and has been shown to improve clinical outcomes *(32,35,36)*. However, Klein and Koretz demonstrate that there is little evidence to support this approach in patients without severe malnutrition *(30)*.

In general, the type of surgery planned will dictate the necessity for nutritional support. Oropharyngeal or gastric resections often have complications of anastomic stenosis, malabsorbtion, delayed gastric emptying, dumping syndrome, or fistula development and warrant pre-emptive consideration for feeding tube placement *(37)*. Intestinal resections also have a high instance of associated complications that are compounded by the effects of cancer. Impaired nutrient utilization from cancer cachexia can be compounded by B_{12} deficiency from ileal resection, water and electrolyte imbalances from ileostomy or colostomy, or decreased nutrient absorption from short gut syndrome *(23)*. Other abnormalities, such as exocrine and endocrine insufficiencies from pancreatic resections, can further complicate recovery if they are not recognized and treated. In all cases of surgery where postoperative nutrient intake might be suboptimal for a period of 7–10 d, postoperative nutritional support should be considered *(38,39)*.

5.2. Radiation

Radiation therapy presents problems of acute and late consequence that can have a significant nutritional impact. The severity of these complications depends largely on the site, intensity and duration of radiation *(40)*. Radiation to the head and neck region often results in acute nausea, alterations in taste, and decreased salivation that hamper adequate nutritional intake *(41)*. In addition to altering nutritional intake, decreased salivation or xerostomia can cause dental caries, especially if sugar-containing beverages or candy are used to combat it. Sugar free mints and gums, artificial saliva, increased intake of water, or medical inducement by pilocarpine hydrochloride may minimize symptoms. Secondary infections, such as candidiasis (thrush), often cause ulcerations of the oral cavity and throat and can further decrease food intake. This can be partly alleviated by the frequent intake of small meals and the use of anesthetic sprays (e.g., lidocaine) or mouthwashes *(6)*.

Radiation to the abdomen can cause intestinal dysfunction from tissue edema and congestion with resultant decreased peristalsis and endarteritis of small vessels *(6)*. In addition to acute pain, nausea, vomiting, and diarrhea, these effects can lead to long term sequellae, such as gastrointestinal tract fibrosis, stenosis, ulceration, or necrosis *(42)*. Radiation-induced hepatitis and pancreatitis, though usually self-limiting, are also complications that can severely impair adequate nutrition *(43)*. There is no proven benefit for the routine use of enteral or parenteral nutritional support in radiation-treated patients without severe malnutrition *(30,44,45)*.

5.3. Chemotherapy

Almost every major class of chemotherapeutic agent can cause some degree of nausea, vomiting, and anorexia *(46)*. These side effects, combined with the direct toxicity of most chemotherapy agents to rapidly dividing cells, can result in significant nutritional consequences in cancer patients. Gastrointestinal mucosal cells are among the most frequently affected by chemotherapy. Stomatitis, oral ulcerations and pharyngitis can lead to odynophagia and anorexia that exacerbates cancer cachexia (47). Some commonly used agents, such as actinomycin D, cytarabine, 5-flurouracil, hydroxyurea and methotrexate can induce ulceration of the entire gastrointestinal tract (48,49). Other effects include bone marrow toxicity with resultant anemia, hepatotoxicity, that further aggravates hypoalbuminemia, and renal toxicity that can complicate preexisting metabolic derangements (49). These effects of chemotherapy can have a profound impact on the nutritional status of a patient and their subsequent response to treatment.

However, treatment of these toxicities can be difficult some pharmacological interventions have shown clinical benefits. Prophylactic administration of antiemetics such as prochlorperazine (Compazine) 10 mg q6 (po, iv, im) or 25 mg suppository per rectum every 12 h prior to the start of chemotherapy can reduce the associated nausea and vomiting. Ondansetron hydrochloride (Zofran) 10 mg IV q8 or 4–8 mg per oral every 8 h, given alone or in combination with dexamethasone, can also be used to treat episodic nausea and vomiting associated with chemotherapy (6). Other pharmacological treatments, such as corticosteroids and the marijuana derivative dronabinol, continue to be studied for clinical applicability and side effect profiles (50). In the absence of severe malnutrition, the routine institution of enteral or parenteral nutrition does not provide additional benefits to chemotherapy patients in terms of improved survival, tumor response, or chemotherapy toxicity (30,51,52).

6. NUTRITIONAL INTERVENTION

Numerous studies have been done to evaluate the effectiveness of nutritional support in the cancer patient. This heterogeneous collection of studies compares many variables in treatment options, such as timing of nutritional intervention, types of intervention, and duration of nutritional support. As such, specific recommendations for nutritional intervention depend on individual circumstances. Generally, however, recommendations exist for intervention in certain situations.

6.1. Cancer Cachexia

Mild and moderately malnourished patients can benefit from protein-calorie rich diets in the form of natural or commercially available food supplements scheduled 3–4 times daily. If lack of appetite continues to be a problem, megestrol acetate (Megace) has shown promise in treating nausea as well as anorexia in cancer patients (53). In doses of 160–800 mg/d, megestrol acetate can increase appetite with a resultant increase in true body mass (53,54). These results, however, have not translated to an increase in overall survival of cancer patients (60).

When oral intake is inadequate or not feasible, enteral or parenteral supplementation may be indicated. These situations include the presence of malignant gastrointestinal obstruction and the presence of severe malnutrition as evidenced by serum albumin less than 3.5 g/dL and weight loss greater than 10% of usual body weight (1,55).

Nutritional support should not be instituted in patients who have evidence of terminal disease and are not candidates for further antitumor therapy unless the natural history of the disease is of a protracted nature and survival can be expected to be greater than 6 mo (1).

6.2. Perioperative

Nutritional support should be utilized in patients undergoing major oncologic surgery in whom no oral intake is anticipated for 7–10 d postoperatively or in patients with severe preoperative malnutrition, again defined by serum albumin less than 3.5 g/dL and weight loss greater than 10% of usual body weight *(38)*. The preferred route of delivery is enteral, with TPN reserved for patients without enteral access. In these patients, nutritional support should begin prior to or in conjunction with surgical intervention.

6.3. Radiation and Chemotherapy

The routine use of enteral or parenteral nutrition in patients receiving chemotherapy or radiation therapy has not demonstrated therapeutic benefit in terms of increased survival, tumor response, or reduced toxicity *(23,56)*. However, in patients whom severe gastrointestinal dysfunction or treatment toxicities preclude adequate enteral intake for a period anticipated to be 5 d or longer, nutritional intervention is indicated *(1)*. Patients who are severely malnourished and have rapidly progressive tumors that have not responded to chemotherapy or radiation, will not likely benefit from nutritional support *(57)*.

7. CONCLUSION

The treatment of malnutrition in cancer patients is a complex and evolving process that requires an integrated approach. Physicians, nurses, dieticians, and pharmacists should all be involved in providing the appropriate nutritional support for cancer patients. In the future, nutritional support in cancer patients may be directed toward attenuating the host response to malignancy and targeting cytokine production and its downstream effects *(23)*. Currently, however, the goal of nutritional care in the cancer patient should always be considered supportive whether the aim of primary therapy is cure or palliation *(14)*.

8. RECOMMENDATIONS FOR CLINICIANS

1. Clinicians should evaluate all cancer patients for changes in weight, appetite, eating habits, and gastrointestinal symptoms that may affect nutritional status.
2. Appetite stimulants such as megastrol acetate, raging in doses from 240 to 1600 mg/d, can be useful to improve caloric intake and increase weight gain.
3. If a patient is unable to obtain adequate energy intake with oral intake, enteral feeding is preferred over parenteral nutrition.
4. In patients with a malignant gastrointestinal obstruction or severe malnutrition, enteral or parenteral support may be required.
5. For intervals of support expected to last longer than 4 wk, a surgically or endoscopically placed gastrostomy or jejunostomy tube is recommended.
6. In patients who are severely malnourished, delaying elective surgery until nutritional status is improved is desirable. Perioperative nutritional supplementation is beneficial to these patients.
7. Nutritional support should be utilized in patients undergoing major surgery in whom no oral intake is anticipated for 7–10 d postoperatively.

REFERENCES

1. Laviano A, Meguid MM. Nutritional issues in cancer management. Nutrition 1996;12:358–371.
2. DeWys WD, Begg C, Lavin PT, et al. Prognostic effect of weight loss prior to chemotherapy in cancer patients. Am J Med 1980;69:491.

3. American Society for Parenteral and Enteral Nutrition Board of Directors: Guidelines for use of parenteral and enteral nutrition in adults and pediatric patients: Nutritional support for adults with specific diseases and conditions. JPEN J Parenter Enteral Nutr 1993;17:7A–12A.
4. Kern K, Norton J. Cancer cachexia. J Parenter Enter Nutr 198;12:286–298.
5. Donaldson SS, Lenon RA. Alterations of nutritional status: impact of chemotherapy and radiation. Cancer 1979;43:2036–2052.
6. Howard RB, Herbold NH. Nutrition and cancer. In: Nutrition in Clinical Care, 2nd ed. Howard R (ed.), McGraw-Hill, New York, 1982, pp. 672–681.
7. Carson JA. Gormican A. Taste accuity and food attitudes of selected patients with cancer. J Am Diet Assoc 1977;70:361–365
8. Moldawer LL, Gelin J, Schersten T, et al. Circulating interleukin 1 and tumor necrosis factor during inflammation. Am J Physiol 1987;253:922–928.
9. Moldawer LL, Rogy MA, Lowry SF. The role of cytokines in cancer cachexia 1992;16:34S–49S.
10. Strassmann G, Jacob CO, Evans R, et al. Evidence for the involvement of interleukin-6 in experimental cancer cachexia. J Clin Invest 1992;89:1681–1684.
11. Langstein HN, Doberty GM, Fraker DL, et al. The role of gamma interferon and tumor necrosis factor-alpha in an experimental rat model of cancer cachexia. Cancer Res 1991;51:415–421.
12. Gelin J, Moldawer LL, Lonnroth C, et al. Role of endogenous tumor necrosis factor and interleukin-1 for experimental tumor growth and development of cancer cachexia. Cancer Res 1991;51:415–421.
13. Kokal WA, McCulloch A, Wright PD, et al. Glucose turnover and recycling in colorectal cancer. Ann Surg 1983;198:601–604.
14. Rivadeneira DE, Evoy D, Fahey TJ, et al. Nutritional support of the cancer patient. CA Cancer J Clin 1998;48:69–80.
15. Hers HG, Hue L. Gluconeogenesis and related aspects of glycolysis. Ann Rev Biochem 1983;53:617.
16. Gentilini Q, Fahey TJ, Daly JM. Nutrition and the cancer patient. In: Cancer Surgery for the General Surgeon. Winchester DP, Jones RS, Murphy GP (eds.) Lippincott-Raven, Philadelphia, PA, 1998.
17. Masuno H, Yoshimura H, Ogawa N, et al. Isolation of lipolytic factor from ascites fluid of patients with hepatoma and its effect on feeding behavior. Eur J Cancer Clin Oncol 1984;20:1177.
18. Shaw JH, Humberstone DM, Douglas RG, et al. Leucine kinetics in patients with benign disease, non-weight losing cancer, and cancer cachexia: Studies at the whole body and tissue level and the response to nutritional support. Surgery 1991;109:37–50.
19. Norton JA, Burt ME, Brennan MF. In vivo utilization of substrate by human sarcoma-bearing limbs. Cancer 1980;45:2934.
20. Blackburn GL, Bistrian BR, Maini BS, et al. Nutrition and metabolic assessment of the hospitalized patient. J Parenter Enteral Nutr 1977;1:11.
21. Rich MW, Keller AJ, Schechtman KB. Increased complications and prolonged hospital stay in elderly cardiac surgical patients with low serum albumin. Am J Cardiol 1989;63:714–718.
22. Pietsch JB, Meakins JL, MacLean LD. The delayed hypersensitivity response: Application in clinical surgery. Surgery 1977;82:349–355.
23. Apovian CM, Still CD, Blackburn GL. In. Principles and Practice of Supportive Oncology. Berger A (ed.), Lippencott-Raven, Philadelphia, PA, 1998, pp. 571–587.
24. Busby GP, Mullen JL, Mathews DC, et al. Prognostic nutritional index in gastrointestinal surgery. Am J Surg 1980;139:160–167.
25. Daly JM, Reynolds J, Thom A, et al. Immune and metabolic effects of arginine in the surgical patient. Ann Surg 1988;208:512–523.
26. Daly JM, Weintraub FN, Shou J, et al. Enteral nutrition during multimodality therapy in upper GI cancer patients. Ann Surg 1995;221:327–338.
27. Daly JM, Lieberman MD, Goldfine J, et al. Enteral nutrition with supplemental arginine, RNA, and omega-3 fatty acids in patients after operation: Immunologic, metabolic and clinical outcome. Surgery 1982;112:56–67.
28. Souba WW. Glutamine and cancer. Ann Surg 1993;218:715.
29. MacKersie, Campbell AR, Cammarano WB. Principles of critical care. In: Trauma Mattox KL (ed.) McGraw-Hill, New York, 2000, pp. 1231–1266.
30. Klein S, Koretz RL. Nutrition support in cancer patients: What do the data really show? Nutr Clin Pract 1994;9:91–100.
31. Weisdorf SA, Lysne J, Wind D, et al. Positive effect of prophylactic total parenteral nutrition on long-term outcome of bone marrow transplantation. Transplantation 1987;43:833–838.

32. Muller JM, Brenner U, Dienst C, et al. Pre-operative parenteral feeding in patients with gastrointestinal cancer. Lancet 1982;1:68–71.
33. Blackburn GL, Harvey KB. Nutrition in surgical patients. In: Surgery: Basic Priciples and Practice, 2nd ed. Hardy JD (ed.), JB Lippincott, Philadelphia, PA, 1988.
34. Yamanda N, Koyama H, Hioki K, et al. Effect of postoperative total parenteral nutrition as an adjunct to gastrectomy for advanced gastric carcinoma. Br J Surg 1993;70:267.
35. Smith RC, Hartemink RJ, Hollinshead JW, et al. Fine bore jejunostomy feeding following major abdominal surgery: a controlled randomized clinical trial. Br J Surg 1986;201:1–8.
36. Fletcher JP, Little JM. A comparison of parenteral nutrition and early postoperative enteral feeding on the nitrogen balance after major surgery. Surgery 1986;100:21–24.
37. Bray GA. Intestinal bypass operation and the treatment for obesity. Ann Intern Med 1976;85:97.
38. Heslin MJ, Brennan MF. Advances in perioperative nutrition: cancer. World J Surg 2000;24:1477–1485.
39. Guidelines for use of total parenteral nutrition in the hospitalized adult patient. A.S.P.E.N. Board of Directors. J Parenter Enteral Nutr 1986;10:441–445.
40. Donaldson SS. Nutritional consequences of radiotherapy. Cancer Res 1977;37:2407.
41. Donaldson SS. Nutritional problems associated with radiotherapy. In: Nutrition and Cancer: Etiology and Treatment. Newell GR (ed.), Raven Press, New York, 1981.
42. Theil HJ, Feitkau R, Sauer R. Malnutrition and the role of nutritional support for radiation therapy patients. Recent Results Cancer Res 1988;108:205–226.
43. Darbinian JA, Coulston AM. Impact of radiation therapy on the nutrition status of the cancer patient: acute and chronic complications. In: Nutrition Management of the Cancer Patient. Bloch AS (ed.), Aspen, Rockville, MD, 1990, pp. 181–198.
44. Valerio D, Overett L, Malcolm A, et al. Nutritional support for cancer patients receiving abdominal and pelvic radiotherapy: A randomized prospective clinical experiment of intravenous versus oral feeding. Surgical Forum 1978;29:145–148.
45. Daly JM, Hearne B, Dunaj J et al. Nutritional rehabilitation in patients with advanced head and neck cancer receiving radiation therapy. Am Surg 1984;148:514–520.
46. Ohnuma T, Holland JS. Nutritional consequences of cancer therapy and immunotherapy. Cancer Res 1977;37:2395.
47. Kokal WA. The impact of anti-tumor therapy on nutrition. Cancer 1985;55:273–278.
48. Mitchell EP, Schein PS. Gastrointestinal toxicity of chemotherapeutic agents. Semin Oncol 1982;9:52.
49. Darbinian JA, Coulston AM. Impact of chemotherapy on the nutrition status of the cancer patient: acute and chronic complications. In: Nutrition Management of the Cancer Patient. Bloch AS (ed.), Aspen, Rockville, MD, 1990, pp. 161–172.
50. Loprinzi CL, Goldberg RM, Peethambaram, Cancer anorexia/cachexia. In: Principles and Practice of Supportive Oncology. Berger A (ed.), Lippincott-Raven, Philadelphia, PA, 1998, pp. 133–139.
51. Elkort RJ, Baker FL, Vitale JJ, et al. Long-term nutritional support as an adjunct to chemotherapy for breast cancer. J Parenter Enter Nutr 1981;5:385–390.
52. Popp MB, Fisher RI, Wesley R, et al. A prospective randomized study of adjunctive parenteral nutrition in the treatment of advanced diffuse lymphoma: Influence on survival. Surgery 1981;90:195–203.
53. Gregory EJ, Cohen SC, Oines DW, et al. Megesterol acetate therapy for advanced breast cancer. J Clin Oncol 1985;3:155–160.
54. Bruera E, Macmillan K, Kuehn N, et al. A controlled trial of megesterol acetate on appetite, caloric intake, nutritional status, and other symptoms in patients with advanced cancer. Cancer 1990;66:1279–1282.
55. Copeland EM, Souchon EA, MacFayden BV, et al. Intravenous hyperalimentation as an adjunct to radiation therapy. Cancer 1977;36:609.
56. Tandon SP, Gupta SC, Sinha SN et al. Nutritional support as an adjunct therapy of advanced cancer patients. Indian J Med Res 1984;80:180–188.
57. Solassol C, Joyeux J, Dubois JB. TPN with complete nutritive mixtures: An artificial gut in cancer patients. Nutr Cancer 1979;1:13–18.

D. Endocrine Disorders

21

Nutrition and Lifestyle Change in Older Adults with Diabetes Mellitus

*Barbara Stetson
and Sri Prakash Mokshagundam*

1. INTRODUCTION

Diabetes mellitus (diabetes) is a major health problem in the United States, affecting an estimated 16 million individuals, of whom 5 million are undiagnosed. Type 2 diabetes disproportionately affects minority populations, including African Americans, Hispanics, Native Americans, Asian Americans, and Pacific Islanders. The Pima Indians of Arizona have one of the highest rates of diabetes in the world. Risk factors for diabetes that are specific to these populations include genetic, behavioral, and lifestyle factors *(1)*.

The prevalence of obesity is rising so rapidly that the World Health Organization has declared that there is now a global epidemic of obesity. Obesity is common in Western market economies (Europe, United States, Canada, Australia, etc.) and in Latin America, and rates are increasing in sub-Saharan Africa and Asia, where rates have traditionally been low. Internationally, emergence of new cases of diabetes parallels the increases seen in Western countries and the prevalence is increasing even more quickly in Asia. The risks of type 2 diabetes in these countries tend to increase at levels of body mass index generally classified as nonobese in Caucasian westerners *(2)*. These worldwide changes are the result of an accelerated prevalence of obesity, today's predominance of sedentary lifestyle and the rapidly growing population of older adults *(3)*.

2. DIABETES IN OLDER US ADULTS

The graying of America also contributes to the increasing cases of diabetes, as diabetes prevalence increases with age. In developing countries, the majority of people with diabetes are between 45–64 yr of age. In developed countries, the majority of people with diabetes are age 65 or older. In the United States, the oldest of the large baby boom cohort are now approaching age 60, and increasing numbers will soon join these ranks. The Third National Health and Nutrition Examination Survey (NHANES III) included information on type 2 diabetes and included persons age 75 and older. Extrapolation from this

From: *Handbook of Clinical Nutrition and Aging*
Edited by: C. W. Bales and C. S. Ritchie © Humana Press Inc., Totowa, NJ

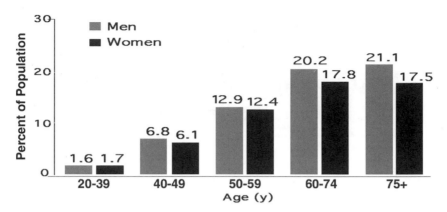

Fig. 1. Prevalence of diabetes in the United States by age group. *Source*: Harris et al. Diabetes Care 1998;21:518–524.

nationally representative sample indicates that in the United States, 44% of persons with self-reported diagnosed diabetes are age 65 or older and 18% are over age 75 (Fig. 1) *(4)*.

3. HEALTH CONSEQUENCES OF DIABETES

Diabetes is a chronic disease that leads to a variety of micro- and macrovascular complications that affect almost all systems in the body. Although the primary abnormality in diabetes, elevated blood glucose level, remains largely asymptomatic, the consequences of sustained elevation in blood glucose are potentially devastating. Diabetes is the leading cause of blindness, chronic renal insufficiency, peripheral neuropathy, and nontraumatic limb amputations.

Type 2 diabetes exerts a tremendous economic burden, accounting for over $100 billion in annual health care expenditures in the United States and 28% of the Medicare budget for older Americans *(5)*. In NHANES III, among persons with type 2 diabetes over age 65, 21% reported being in poor health, and 35% reported having at least one hospitalization in the preceding year *(6)*.

Cardiovascular disease (CVD) is the most frequent and costly complication of type 2 diabetes. A recent review indicates that when cardiovascular events are stratified by diabetes status, relative risk for men and women is twofold and threefold, respectively, of gender-matched nondiabetics. Among all CVD events, diabetes accounted for 56% of events in men and 78% of events in women. A number of diabetes-related risk factors have been associated with CVD. Diabetics with albuminuria have been shown to have a CVD risk that is 4–5 times that of diabetics without albuminuria. This highlights the importance of identifying such persons in order to provide more aggressive preventive strategies *(7)*.

4. GENERAL AIMS OF DIABETES TREATMENT

The management of diabetes requires a combination of lifestyle interventions and medications. Diabetes is often a progressive disease, requiring changing therapeutic strategies. The interaction between lifestyle changes and medications must be carefully

Table 1
ADA Criteria for Diagnosis of Diabetes

	Normal	Impaired fasting glucose	Diabetes mellitus
Fasting blood glucose	<110 mg/dL	111–125 mg/dL	>125 mg/dL

considered. Dietary intervention to maintain optimal glycemic indices is a key component of management. The aims of diabetes treatment are to: decrease or prevent the development of long-term complications of high blood glucose and related metabolic abnormalities; improve the quality of life of individuals with diabetes, and treat or prevent the development of symptoms of high or low blood glucose.

5. DIAGNOSIS AND CLASSIFICATION

The American Diabetes Association (ADA) and the World Health Organization revised the criteria for the diagnosis of diabetes in 1997 (8,9) (Table 1). The new diagnostic criteria are based mainly on fasting blood glucose levels (8). In addition to the occurrence of chronically elevated blood glucose levels, isolated postchallenge hyperglycemia is a particularly common problem among older adults who have abnormal glucose tolerance, however, this is not incorporated into current diagnostic criteria (10). The ADA diagnostic criteria were developed for general use and apply broadly to all age groups. No specific ADA guidelines exist for older adults.

5.1. Typologies of Diabetes in Older Adults

The proper classification of diabetes is important in setting goals for nutritional management of individuals with diabetes. Diabetes mellitus is broadly classified into type 1 and type 2 diabetes.

5.1.1. TYPE 1 DIABETES

Type 1 diabetes is an autoimmune disorder resulting from cell-mediated and antibody-mediated destruction of beta cells of the islets (11). Insulin is required for the management of type 1 diabetes. Failure to treat with insulin results in development of acute metabolic complication—diabetic ketoacidosis. Although type 1 diabetes most commonly occurs in the first three decades of life, it can develop at any age, even in older adults. The basic underlying mechanism of disease is autoimmune destruction of the pancreatic islets. Circulating islet cell antibodies can be demonstrated in the majority of individuals, especially in the first few years after diagnosis. Alternatively, to new onset type 1 diabetes, older adults may have preexisting type 1 diabetes. Type 1 diabetes, particularly of long duration, is often very "brittle" with wide fluctuations in blood glucose levels and episodes of recurrent and severe hypoglycemia.

5.1.2. TYPE 2 DIABETES

The majority of older adults with diabetes have type 2 diabetes. Type 2 diabetes is characterized by two defects—insulin resistance and defective insulin secretion (12). The majority of individuals with type 2 diabetes are obese. However, in the older population the proportion of subjects with type 2 diabetes who are underweight increases and could be as high as 20%. This is particularly true in the nursing home population. In addition to elevated blood glucose levels, individuals with type 2 diabetes typically have one or more components of the insulin resistance syndrome (also called Syndrome X, cardiovascular dysmetabolic syndrome, or Reaven's syndrome) *(13)*. These include hypertension, obesity (particularly abdominal obesity), dyslipidemia (elevated serum triglyceride and low HDL-cholesterol levels), hyperinsulinemia, hyperuricemia, and high levels of plasminogen activator inhibitor 1 (PAI-1). Insulin resistance appears to be a central defect in individuals with the insulin resistance syndrome. The mechanisms that lead to the development of insulin resistance and the evolution of diabetes in these individuals remain unclear. Persons with type 2 diabetes may be treated with either diet and lifestyle change alone or by a variety of oral medications and insulin.

Type 2 diabetes results from a combination of insulin resistance, increased hepatic glucose production, and defective insulin secretion *(14)*. Insulin resistance is generally considered the early defect in type 2 diabetes. Insulin resistance is often present in nondiabetic relatives of individuals with type 2 diabetes and in persons with impaired glucose tolerance. Several studies have also demonstrated defective insulin secretion in these at-risk individuals. Studies of Pima Indians have demonstrated that the progression form normal glucose tolerance to diabetes mellitus is associated with a progressive decline in acute insulin response to glucose *(15)*.

The exact mechanism of insulin resistance in type 2 diabetes is unclear. A variety of genetic and environmental factors lead to decreased insulin sensitivity. Obesity and decreased physical activity have been known to decrease insulin sensitivity. Aging is associated with a change in body composition with increase in fat mass and decrease in muscle mass *(16,17)*. This could be partly responsible for the increase in insulin resistance with aging. Aging is also associated with a decline in insulin secretion, particularly a blunting of the first-phase insulin secretion *(18)*. First-phase insulin secretion is an important determinant of postchallenge blood glucose levels. Age-related changes in health behaviors, such as increased sedentary lifestyle, may also further compound these changes. Type 2 diabetes is a progressive disorder. The progression of the clinical picture with increasing blood glucose levels, requiring increasing doses of medications, results from a progressive decline in beta-cell function. When beta-cell function is markedly reduced, exogenous insulin will be necessary to regulate blood glucose levels.

The diagnosis of type 1 and type 2 diabetes can usually be made without difficulty based on clinical criteria alone. However, some individuals may require additional testing. Latent autoimmune diabetes of adults (LADA) is an autoimmune disorder with destruction of islets similar to type 1 diabetes *(19)*. However, the destruction of islets is very gradual, along with a gradual, rather than dramatic, decline in islet function. Thus, individuals present with features similar to type 2 diabetes mellitus, but eventually develop complete loss of islet function. The proportion of subjects with this type of diabetes is not known, but up to 10% of individuals with type 2 diabetes might have LADA. LADA should be suspected in lean individuals with adult onset diabetes who do not respond well to oral agents, and those individuals who only require small amounts of insulin and develop marked hyperglycemia or hypoglycemia with small changes in insulin doses (indicating high sensitivity to insulin). The diagnosis can be confirmed by measurement of islet cell antibodies. Measurement of c-peptide level might be helpful but is not confirmatory, because low c-peptide levels can be seen in type 2 diabetes after severe reduction in beta-cell function. Diabetes might also occur as a result of drugs, such as corticosteroids, or because of pancreatitis or following pancreatectomy.

An additional diabetes-related syndrome is postchallenge hyperglycemia, in which high blood glucose levels are present in the fasting state and after an oral glucose challenge. Postchallenge hyperglycemia has been recognized as a risk factor for diabetes-related complications. In recent years, the absolute level of blood glucose level after a meal and the increment in blood glucose after a meal (glycemic spikes) have been shown to be independent risk factors for the development of CVD *(20)*.

6. ESTABLISHING MEDICATION AND NUTRITIONAL MANAGEMENT GOALS

Once the type of diabetes is established, medication and nutritional management goals should be developed. In addition to tailoring the nutritional recommendations to assist glycemic control, consideration of other important risk factors is critical. Obesity, dyslipidemia, hypertension, and insulin resistance are important and often overlapping factors warranting consideration when planning dietary interventions for older adults with type 2 diabetes. Avoidance of hypoglycemia, particularly recurrent and/or severe hypoglycemia, is a major consideration in type 1 diabetes. Lifestyle interventions recommended for the management of diabetes have positive effects on both insulin secretion and insulin resistance. Aggressive lifestyle intervention can prevent the progression of impaired glucose tolerance to diabetes and could decrease the dose and number of medications for the management of type 2 diabetes.

6.1. Medication Use and Glycemic Control in Older Adults with Diabetes

Two landmark trials have served as the basis for current recommendations for the management of blood glucose levels in diabetes mellitus. The Diabetes Control and Complications Trial (DCCT) was conducted in adults with type 1 diabetes and compared intensive insulin treatment using multiple insulin injections or an insulin pump to conventional treatment using twice-daily injections of intermediate and short-acting insulin *(21,22)*. The results showed significant reduction in risk of all microvascular disease endpoints in the intensively treated group. However, the DCCT did not include older adults and did not have the statistical power to analyze benefits on macrovascular risk reduction. The clear demonstration of a relationship between glycemic control, measured by reduction in hemoglobin A1c, and improved outcomes indicate that similar outcomes would be expected in older adults.

The United Kingdom Prospective Diabetes Study (UKPDS) was a long-term study of a variety of treatment options in adults with type 2 diabetes *(22)*. The important findings of the UKPDS can be summarized as follows: (1) A reduction of 1% in Hemoglobin A1c results in approx 22% reduction in microvascular complications. (2) Reduction in microvascular complications with reduction in Hemoglobin A1c is observed irrespective of type of intervention. (3) Glycemic control in type 2 diabetes mellitus worsens over time and necessitates changes in medication, irrespective of initial management approach. (4) In a subgroup of subjects treated with metformin, there was a significant reduction in macrovascular disease. There was a trend toward lower cardiovascular disease in the intensively treated group, irrespective of initial therapy of choice. Although the UKPDS included an older population, subgroup analysis of the older age group is not available.

The results of the DCCT and UKPDS played a major role in the selection of the glycemic targets recommended by the ADA.

Results of the UKPDS have guided the medical management approach to type 2 diabetes. A wide variety of therapeutic options are now available for the management of type 2 diabetes. These include use of dietary interventions alone to a variety of oral medications, alone, and in combination, and insulins, with or without oral agents.

Data from NHANES III indicate that use of anti-hyperglycemic medications by adults with type 2 diabetes varies across the continuum of ages, with greater use of oral agents in younger age groups (54% age 20–54, 52% age 55–64, 43% age 65–74, 44% age ≥75) and greater use of insulin in the older groups (19% age 20–54, 28% age 55–64, 35% age 65–74, 31% age ≥ 75). When ethnicity, gender, education and duration of diabetes were controlled, age was not significantly associated with glycemic control. When compared with younger persons, older adults were actually less likely to have glycemic control at a level at which ADA guidelines would recommend further intervention (HbA1c > 8; 42% for the age group 20–54, 38% age 55–64, 37% age 65–74, 27% age ≥ 75). Most older adults not achieving optimal glycemic control were already using drug therapy. Of course, persons with suboptimal control or severe health problems persons may have declined participation in NHANES, and adults residing in long-term care were excluded. If these rates of glycemic control are generalized to the US population, more than 2 million community-dwelling adults over age 65 with diagnosed type 2 diabetes would not be meeting ADA goals for HbA1c, and over 1 million would require further actions to promote acceptable metabolic control (6).

6.1.1. BALANCING DIET AND MEDICATION

The interaction of diet and medication is of particular importance in the management of diabetes. Insulin and drugs that increase insulin secretion are likely to induce hypoglycemia if meals are not taken at appropriate times. Erratic eating habits might require readjustment of medications, either dose, timing, or both. Poor eating habits might also necessitate change to medications that are less likely to cause hypoglycemia when used alone. Metformin (Glucophage) and the thiazolidenediones (Pioglitazone and Rosiglitazone) are least likely to cause hypoglycemia when used alone. The problem of unwanted weight gain is another issue for consideration for many overweight individuals. Insulin and the thiazolidenediones, particularly when used in combination are most likely to result in weight gain. The deleterious effect of weight gain in overweight older adults must be evaluated in tandem with the potential benefits of improved glycemic control. Loss of appetite may occur with Metformin and would be of concern in the undernourished person with diabetes.

7. GOALS OF DIABETES TREATMENT IN OLDER ADULTS

The major goal of treating diabetes is to decrease the rate of micro- and macrovascular disease associated with elevated blood glucose. Convincing evidence of the benefits of tight blood glucose control in type 1 (from the DCCT) and type 2 (from the UKPDS) diabetes has been presented in the last decade (21,22). The ADA goals for glycemic control are for maintenance of a HbA1c level of 7.0% or less. ADA dietary guidelines include a diet relatively high in carbohydrates, low in fat, and moderate in protein (23) (see also Table 2). More recent recommendations by the American Association of Clinical Endocrinologists (AACE)/American College of Endocrinology (ACE) have advo-

Table 2
Macronutrient Content of General Diabetic Diet

Carbohydrates	55–60% of total caloric intake
Protein	12–20% of caloric intake
Fat	<30% of total caloric intake
	<300 mg/d of cholesterol
	Saturated and polyunsaturated fat
	<10% of total caloric intake
	(2–40 g/d)

Table 3
Veterans Health Administration
Clinical Guidelines for Metabolic Control in Diabetes

Clinical assessment	Glycemic goal
Life expectancy ≥ 5–10 yr and microvascular disease absent	HbA1c < 8.0%
Life expectancy < 5 yr or microvascular disease present	HbA1c < 9.0%

cated lower Hemoglobin A1c targets (<6.5%) and attention to postprandial blood glucose levels (2 h postmeal glucose level <140 mg/dL).

8. GENERAL DIABETES DIETARY RECOMMENDATIONS

The general goals of nutritional recommendations for the management of diabetes mellitus include:

1. Achieve and maintain blood glucose levels as outlined previously.
2. Achieve and maintain optimum lipid levels.
3. Achieve and maintain reasonable body weight. This would include weight loss if overweight and weight gain if undernourished.
4. Prevent acute complications.
5. Maintain overall health.

The ADA goals listed above are general and written to apply to all persons with diabetes. However, older adults persons with diabetes require special consideration and require reassessment of goals. The Department of Veterans Affairs Clinical Guidelines for the Management of Diabetes Mellitus has also written specific guidelines for metabolic control (HbA1c), which attempt to incorporate years and quality of life and the presence of chronic disease in the consideration of more liberal goals for metabolic control (23). An example of these guidelines applied to goals for metabolic control is in Table 3.

In addition to glycemic goals, several metabolic and cardiovascular risk factors must also be considered because of the higher rates of CVD and its substantial impact on morbidity and mortality in persons with diabetes. The high risk of cardiovascular morbidity and mortality in diabetes is the result of a variety of factors. These include overall blood glucose control, glycemic fluctuation, postprandial blood glucose levels, high

Table 4
Lifestyle and Pharmacological Approaches to Risk Factor Management

Risk factor	Lifestyle intervention	Pharmacological intervention
Hba1c	Diet and exercise	Insulin sensitizing agents, insulin secretagogues, insulin
Postprandial glucose/glycemic	Carbohydrate content of meals excursion	Repaglinide (prandin), nateglinide (starlix), short-acting insulins (insulin lispro, insulin aspart, regular insulin)
LDL cholesterol	Low-cholesterol diet Exercise	Statins Bile acid-binding agents Niacin
Triglyceride	Low-fat diet Exercise/weight loss	Gemfibrozil/fenofibrate Niacin (long acting) Omega-3 fatty acids
Low HDL cholesterol	Exercise Smoking cessation	Niacin Gemfibrozil/fenofibrate
High blood pressure	Low-sodium diet Exercise Weight loss	Variety of antihypertensive agents (ACE inhibitors preferred)
Procoagulant state	Exercise/weight loss	Aspirin
Proinflammatory state		Aspirin

LDL cholesterol, low HDL cholesterol, elevated serum triglycerides, blood pressure, and altered coagulation profile. In addition inflammation, pro-oxidant state, and endothelial dysfunction play a significant role. Recommendations to focus on maintaining optimal control of blood pressure in persons with diabetes are based on the positive results of such control as demonstrated in the UKPDS, Hypertension Optimal Treatment trial (HOT), and Arterial Blood Pressure Control in Diabetes (ABCD) studies (25–27). Additionally, the benefits of lowering total and LDL cholesterol have also been demonstrated in intervention studies (4S, CARE studies) (28,29). Any nutritional approach to the management of diabetes mellitus must specifically address the issues related to cardiovascular risk. Cardiovascular risk reduction in diabetes mellitus is achieved through a combination of lifestyle changes and pharmacological interventions that address the multiple risk factors. A general outline of lifestyle and pharmacological approaches is shown in Table 4.

Taken together, these lifestyle and pharmacological interventions can play a major role in the management of cardiovascular risk reduction in persons with diabetes. The recommended goals for management of weight, blood pressure, and lipids are outlined in Table 5.

The carbohydrate composition of the diet has been a focus of many recommendations. The amount and type of carbohydrate in the diet has been a subject of controversy. There are no well-designed studies that have compared different dietary approaches. In a study

Table 5
Recommended Assessment and Management Goals for CVD Risk Factors in Diabetes

Parameter	Frequency	Goal
HbA1c	3–4 mo	<7% (<6.5%)[a]
Fasting blood glucose	2–7 times a week[b]	80–120 mg/dL
Postprandial blood glucose	2–7 times a week[b]	<140 mg/dL[a]
LDL cholesterol	Annual 3–4 mo, if abnormal	<100 mg/dL
HDL cholesterol	Annual 3–4 mo, if abnormal	>45 mg/dL
Triglyceride	Annual 3–4 mo, if abnormal	<200 mg/dL
Systolic blood pressure	Each visit	<130 mm Hg
Diastolic blood pressure	Each visit	<85 mm Hg
Microalbuminuria	Annual	Normal or no progression
Eye examination	Annual	Normal or no progression
Neurological examination	Annual	Normal or no progression

[a]Recommended by AACE/ACE.
[b]No clear recommendation (need to individualize).

of a high-carbohydrate (60%) low-fat (25%) diet when compared to a low-carbohydrate (35%) high monounsaturated fat (50%) diet (30), plasma glucose, triglyceride, and very low-density lipoprotein (VLDL) cholesterol were lower in subjects in the high-fat diet group. Use of complex carbohydrates is preferred. The use of lower fat content in the diet is based on the need to restrict caloric intake, improve lipid levels, and assist weight loss. Use of high-fat/low-carbohydrate diets could lead to more hypoglycemic episodes and ketosis. Higher protein diets have been recommended and have been popular for weight loss. However, the efficacies of these diets in persons with diabetes have not been well tested. Higher protein content has been shown to increase risk of development and progression of diabetic nephropathy, contraindicating this type of diet for persons with poorly controlled diabetes or complications.

9. BODY WEIGHT AND FUNCTIONAL STATUS IN OLDER ADULTS WITH DIABETES

9.1. Overweight and Obesity

Being overweight is not only an important risk factor for the development of diabetes; it also has a significant impact on diabetes progression and the development of complications (31). Obesity is known to be a critical problem in children and young and middle-aged adults with type 2 diabetes. Only recently has the problem of obesity been systematically examined in older adults. Obesity appears to be common in older adults until the eighth decade of life and then declines in the oldest old. Data from NHANES III indicate that type 2 diabetes strongly increases in prevalence with increasing bodyweight in older as well as younger adults. Personal risks for diabetes were observed to be stronger for obese younger adults, but still substantially elevated in older adults with risks of 3.4 (95% CI, 1.1–8.3) for the most obese men over age 55 and 5.8 (95% CI, 4.2–7.4) for the most obese women over age 55.

Recent findings from NHANES III illustrate the current trends in weight classification for community-dwelling older adults, for the age group of 55 yr and older (Table 6). It is notable that nearly two-thirds of these older adults were overweight or obese.

Table 6
Nationally Representative Trends in Weight Classification for Older Adults

	Under weight	Normal weight	Over weight	Obesity I	Obesity II	Obesity III
BMI	<18.5	18.5–24.9	25.0–29.9	30.0–34.9	35.0–39.9	≥40
%Men ≥55	1.44%	31.56%	43.72%	18.29	4.17%	0.82%
%Women ≥55	3.00%	36.36%	33.02%	17.19%	6.99%	3.43%

9.2. Underweight and Malnutrition

Although obesity is clearly a problem that greatly impacts diabetes in older adults, for many individuals, malnutrition may be the more pressing nutritional concern. Even with the problem of increasingly prevalent overweight, obesity and diabetes, the prevalence of obesity in older persons with diabetes is still less than that in younger persons with type 2 diabetes. This may be particularly true for the oldest old, and those who have impaired functional status. One study found that at least 21% of nursing home patients with type 2 diabetes were underweight *(32)*.

10. SPECIAL NUTRITION INTERVENTION SITUATIONS FOR PERSONS WITH DIABETES

10.1. Acute Illness, Hospitalization, Enteral and Parenteral Nutrition

Acute illness and hospitalization occur more frequently in older adults. Older adults with diabetes are more likely to be hospitalized than nonelderly and nondiabetics. Nutrition concerns in older adults with acute illness, in addition to meeting short-term nutritional needs common to all acutely ill individuals, must also include avoidance of hypoglycemia and wide fluctuations in blood glucose. Older persons residing in the community who are ill, as well as those who are in nursing home facilities, should follow standard sick-day rules. Sick-day rules are usually a part of all diabetes self-management education programs and include instructions on blood glucose monitoring, maintaining adequate fluid intake, and also consuming carbohydrate to meet minimal nutritional needs and avoid hypoglycemia. The goals of management of diabetes are also different during acute illness. The primary aim is to avoid severe hypo and hyperglycemic episodes. Blood glucose levels should be maintained at 100–200 mg/dL. This level of glycemic control is recommended based on studies that revealed impaired granulocyte function and wound healing when blood glucose levels were over 200 mg/dL. A recent study showed that intensive blood glucose control, even in the severely ill, reduces mortality in individuals with type 2 diabetes hospitalized in an intensive care unit. It is particularly important for individuals with type 1 diabetes to maintain adequate hydration, check blood glucose and urine ketones, and when appropriate, to administer insulin to avoid ketoacidosis. When using intravenous fluids, dextrose should be used along with insulin. Failure to use dextrose in intravenous fluids leads to inadequate use of insulin and could lead to development of ketosis and ketoacidosis. The general recommendations for insulin use with intravenous nutritional fluids are outlined in Table 7.

Enteral and parenteral nutrition might present additional challenges in the management of patients with diabetes. Although the glycemic goals for individuals receiving

Table 7
Insulin Use with IV Nutritional Fluids

Use IV dextrose 5% at ~100 cc/h unless blood glucose > 250 mg/dL
Start insulin infusion at ~1–2 U/h
Check blood glucose q1 h
Increase insulin infusion by 1 U/h if blood glucose is > 200 mg/dL
Decrease insulin by 1 U/h if blood glucose less than 100 mg/dL

enteral and parenteral nutrition are the same as glycemic goals for the general population of diabetics, achievement of normoglycemia may be more difficult in patients who are acutely ill. It is estimated that up to 30% of patients who receive parenteral nutrition have diabetes. Many of these patients have no previous history of diagnosed diabetes and develop diabetes as a result of stress-induced increases in counter-regulatory hormones and cytokines.

The relative value of high-carbohydrate vs high-fat enteral feeds for persons with diabetes has been debated *(33)*. The most widely used commercial enteral preparations for individuals with diabetes provide approx 1 cal/mL, 40 % (Choice DM TF) to 34% (Glucerna) carbohydrate, and 43% (Choice DM TF) to 49% (Glucerna) fat. They also have high Monounsaturated fatty acids (35% MUFA in Glucerna). MUFA has been shown to be beneficial in improving lipid profile, glycemic control, and lower insulin level *(34)*. Choice DM TF has a higher content of medium chain triglycerides and has no fructose. The use of insulin or oral agents in persons receiving enteral nutrition should be tailored to match the timing of feeds. Parenteral nutrition fluids are high in carbohydrate and derive few calories from fat. In persons with diabetes, particularly in less severely stressed individuals, the proportion of carbohydrate may be decreased, but is still very high. The usual rate of glucose infusion is 4–5 g/kg body weight and lipid infusion of 1–1/5 g/kg body weight. This requires adequate use of insulin to maintain normoglycemia *(35)*. Insulin infusion not only maintains glycemic control, but prevents protein breakdown and promotes protein synthesis.

10.2. Hypoglycemia in Older Adults

Hypoglycemia is a major limiting factor in the management of diabetes. The incidence of hypoglycemia is relatively high in older compared to younger adults. A variety of factors may play a role in the increased risk of hypoglycemia in older adults. These include poor nutritional status, cognitive dysfunction, polypharmacy, and comorbid illnesses. Except in the severely malnourished, poor dietary intake by itself does not lead to hypoglycemia. The most common cause of hypoglycemia remains the use of blood glucose-lowering agents. Drugs that increase insulin secretion and insulin itself can cause hypoglycemia. A major finding of the DCCT, which was conducted with young, healthy adults, was that the major deleterious health consequence of tight blood glucose control in persons with type 1 diabetes is hypoglycemia. Drugs that enhance insulin sensitivity (thiazolidenediones) decrease hepatic glucose production (metformin), or decrease carbohydrate absorption (alpha-glucosidase inhibitors) have very low risk of hypoglycemia, except when used in combination with insulin or an insulin secretagogue. When medication use creates problems of consistent hypoglycemia, patients must learn how to avoid and manage hypoglycemic episodes. Older adults taking insulin who have high variability in blood glucose levels, exhibit very low average blood glucose concentrations, have had diabetes for a long duration, have a low body mass index, or have high levels of vigorous physical activity, may be at particular risk of severe hypoglycemia (36).

10.2.1. SELF-MONITORING AND DIETARY TREATMENT OF HYPOGLYCEMIA

Frequent self-monitoring of blood glucose levels provides specific information that may serve as feedback for guiding decisions about moment-to-moment treatment needs, thus helping patients to anticipate or prevent severely low glucose levels. Frequent blood glucose testing may be perceived as too expensive, too inconvenient or painful by many persons with diabetes, and unfortunately, rather than performing frequent blood glucose testing, many individuals simply rely on their symptoms or estimates about their blood glucose levels when deciding what to eat or how vigorously to exercise or whether to operate a motor vehicle (37). By increasing the frequency of blood glucose testing (at least four times per day for persons taking insulin) and making informed decisions about when to eat additional carbohydrate (e.g., eat 15 g of carbohydrate to raise blood glucose levels about 45 mg/dL) or identify personal sources of vigorous physical activity contributing to low blood glucose levels, patients may learn to prevent severe hypoglycemia. Educating patients about the importance of always carrying glucose tabs, gel or fast-acting carbohydrate snacks, placing them in various locations, such as the car or relative's homes, may also aid in the treatment of mild-to-moderate hypoglycemic episodes. Recommendations for management of hypoglycemia in adults are presented in Table 8.

10.2.2. HYPOGLYCEMIA UNAWARENESS AND TREATMENT OF HYPOGLYCEMIA

As previously described, older adults with type 1 diabetes and those with type 2 diabetes who are on exogenous insulin regimens are at risk for hypoglycemia. Many individuals develop the syndrome of hypoglycemia unawareness, in which the warning symptoms that indicate that hypoglycemia is developing (e.g., tremulousness, tachycardia) are decreased or not detected. Without these warning symptoms, individuals are not able to take actions, such as eating to prevent continued reductions in blood glucose levels and severe hypoglycemic episodes, may result. Following episodes of hypoglycemia, counterregulatory hormone stores may not be available, and thresholds for symptoms of hypoglycemia may shift to lower glucose concentrations. Therefore, patients with recurrent hypoglycemia may be particularly at risk for unawareness and for severely low hypoglycemic episodes. Failure to test blood glucose levels regularly can contribute to the problem of hypoglycemia unawareness. This cycle is particularly problematic for older adults who are highly physically active or who skip meals, do not eat sufficient quantities of food to match their insulin doses or consume a high-fat diet, which delays carbohydrate absorption and is not accounted for in the timing of insulin administration.

Alcohol consumption, although not typically problematic when consumed in moderation, can pose risks for hypoglycemia in older adults taking insulin. In particular, the major risk of alcohol-related hypoglycemia relates to persons in a fasting state and those who are alcohol dependent. The disinhibiting effect of alcohol poses the risk of hypoglycemia unawareness, making blood glucose monitoring essential. The potential for a delayed risk of hypoglycemia the morning after evening alcohol intake should also be emphasized (38). The problem of patient hypoglycemia unawareness should be considered if the patient's HbA1c is low (e.g., <6.0), and he/she describes inability to detect counterregulatory autonomic symptoms (e.g., tremulousness, pounding heart, anxiety, queasy stomach, sweating, flushed face) when blood glucose levels are low (39). Poten-

Table 8
Dietary Management of Hypoglycemia

Check blood glucose level by glucose monitor:

1. If blood glucose less than 60 mg/dL or symptomatic—treat with 15 g of carbohydrate (1/2 cup juice, 1 cup regular soft drink, glucose gel).
2. Repeat blood sugar reading in 15 min after treatment.
3. Repeat step 1 until blood glucose is >60 mg/dL.
4. If meals are due within 60 min—eat meal now.
5. If meals are not due within 60 min, follow the glucose treatment with a snack containing carbohydrates and one protein (cheese and crackers, peanut butter and crackers, skim milk and crackers, or a small sandwich).
6. If blood glucose <40 mg/dL and/or subject is stuporous, confused, or unresponsive—give 1 amp of D50W as IV push and start D10W at 60 cc/h. Check blood glucose every 5 min and repeat until blood glucose > 60 mg/dL or until awake. Give oral carbohydrate once awake.

tial barriers to blood glucose testing or adequate food consumption, such as financial constraints, fear of pain, depression, or feelings of being overwhelmed by diabetes should be assessed.

Structured psychoeducational intervention and print materials to reduce hypoglycemia unawareness have been developed and systematically evaluated for nearly 20 yr in the Blood Glucose Awareness Training (BGAT) program developed by Cox and colleagues (37). The BGAT program focuses on improving the accuracy of patients' detection and interpretation of relevant blood glucose symptoms and other internal and external cues. Prospective, controlled studies including long-term follow-up indicate that training in BGAT results in improved accuracy of recognition of current blood glucose levels, improved detection of hypoglycemia in individuals with hypoglycemia unawareness, improved judgment regarding when to treat low blood glucose levels, reduced occurrence of severe hypoglycemia, improved judgment about not driving while hypoglycemic, reduction in rate of motor vehicle violations, and better-preserved counterregulatory hormonal response during intensive insulin treatment (37). Overall, intensive training to promote blood glucose awareness can have significant and sustained benefits and aid in more consistent dietary management of older adults who take insulin.

11. DIABETES LIFESTYLE CHANGE AND PHYSICAL LIMITATIONS

Physical disabilities, such as diabetic retinopathy, CVD, peripheral vascular disease, and congestive heart failure, may result in decreased activity, including limited transportation options, limited ability to shop for food or ability to read restaurant menus. These limitations may, in turn, lead to dietary intake that is less than optimal as well as sedentary lifestyles, placing individuals at risk for weight gain and enhanced cardiovascular risk.

12. CONSIDERING DIABETES DIETARY GUIDELINES WITHIN THE CONTEXT OF OLDER ADULT LIVES

The reader will note that while published guidelines are available to assist the health provider in setting general goals for metabolic control and diet and medication diabetes self-care regimens, these recommendations must of course, be considered in the context of what older adults are actually doing in terms of their diabetes diet care and in the context of the demands of their day to day lives. The ADA guidelines, developed to be practical for the general population, recommend consideration of comorbid health problems and the specific needs of older adults, in developing dietary interventions. However, the domains of these diet-related needs are not specified and strategies for adapting the recommendations to fit the special needs of older adults with diabetes are not presented. It follows that few systematic diabetes nutrition and lifestyle change studies have included older persons *(40)*. Lifestyle issues influencing dietary behavior in older adults and shaping the adaptation of dietary goals and interventions to best meet the needs of older adults with diabetes will be discussed in the subsequent section.

13. DIETARY HABITS OF OLDER ADULTS WITH DIABETES

A number of studies have examined the actual dietary practices of children and young to mid-life adults with diabetes, however few studies have evaluated dietary intake in older adults with diabetes. Of the few systematic studies available, both the type of food consumed and the pattern of eating behaviors emerge as important influences on nutritional intake. An Australian study of adults over age 65 found that both diabetic and nondiabetic age-matched subjects' typical dietary habits exceeded recommended levels of dietary fat and provided inadequate fiber. Only 6% of the diabetic subjects consumed a diet with at least 50% carbohydrate and less than 30% fat *(41)*. This suggests that recommendations to increase fiber and decrease fat may be beneficial for the majority of older adults with diabetes.

Persons with diabetes must follow a diet that incorporates healthy food choices and spacing of meals to be consistent with exogenous insulin use and physical activity, with the goal of maintaining euglycemia. Unhealthful snacking is one area that threatens optimal nutrition in older adults. A random telephone survey of 335 community-dwelling adults age 55 and older residing in the continental United States found that 98% of older adults reported snacking at least once each day, with evening the most common time for snacking and nearly all snacking occurring at home *(42)*. Taste outranked nutrition as a snack selection criteria. Fruits were popular but were chosen less often than other less healthful snacks. This suggests that the context of snacking is an important consideration influencing choices made when snacking and should be addressed when providing nutritional guidance to older patients with diabetes. Concrete suggestions for replacing highly processed, high-fat snack foods with fruits and vegetables and other nutritious snacks may assist older adults in selection of healthier snacks. This may be accomplished by asking patients to generate a list of problematic meal and snack foods along with a list healthy items that they personally deem to be healthy and tasty alternatives. Patients may be encouraged to incorporate these alternatives into their shopping lists and keep them in the home as replacements for preferred but unhealthy items. Evening activities that are alternatives to snacking (e.g., walking, crafts) may also be encouraged.

14. PSYCHOSOCIAL AND BEHAVIORAL ISSUES RELATED TO DIETARY INTAKE IN OLDER ADULTS WITH DIABETES

14.1. Depression

Depression is a significant cause of suffering in many older adults and may play an important role in the course of their treatment. Data from the Epidemiological Catchment

Area study of more than 18,000 adults conducted in five sites found depressive symptoms in 15% of adults over age 65 and lifetime rate of depression in 2% of women and 3% of men *(43)*. Estimates of the prevalence of depression in primary care geriatric clinic populations are 5%. In nursing homes, estimates have ranged from 15% to 25% at any given point, with an incidence of 13% per year *(44,45)*.

In older adults with diabetes, rates of depression are likely even higher. Estimates of the prevalence of depression in the general adult population with diabetes indicate a rate of 2–3 times that of the general population *(46)*. A systematic review of the published literature on depression in diabetes indicates a mean prevalence rate of depression in 23.4% of persons with diabetes (vs 14.5% in controls), with rates for both type 1 and type 2 diabetes.

Depression has been linked to elevated death rates in older persons with diabetes. Data from the Hispanic Established Population for the Epidemiologic Study of the Elderly (EPESE) were used to examine the prevalence of comorbid depressive symptomology and chronic medical conditions and their influence on death rates in older Mexican Americans *(47)*. Death rates were substantially higher when a high level of depressive symptoms was comorbid with diabetes, cardiovascular disease, hypertension, stroke and cancer. The odds of having died among persons with diabetes with high levels of depressive symptoms were three times that of diabetics without high levels of depressive symptoms. Hence, an interaction between depression and diabetes and the prevalence of other risk factors greatly increased absolute risk of mortality. Recidivism of depression in persons with diabetes may be relatively higher than in the general population *(48)*. Following treatment for depression, nonremission appears to be associated with lower adherence to blood glucose monitoring, higher HbA1c levels and higher body weight in adults with type 2 diabetes *(49)*.

14.2. Depression and Dietary Intake in Older Adults

In depressed older adults, indirect self-destructive behavior, such as not eating and medication nonadherence, may be more common than overt self-harming gestures such as suicide attempts, and are associated with decreased survival. Many older adults might consider depression to be a normal part of aging and may not report their symptoms to a health care provider. Health providers may also attribute some depressive symptoms to old age or other physical ailments or mood disturbance may be less prominent than multiple somatic complaints. Some older patients with depression may present with "failure to thrive" rather than specific complaints *(50)*.

For the older adult who suffers from dysphoric mood, a new diagnosis of diabetes may be perceived as catastrophic and overwhelming. For both newly diagnosed and those with ongoing diabetes, the demands of the regimen, particularly the often complicated dietary issues may be perceived as "one more thing" to do in what may be seen as an already stressful existence. A study of older adults with type 2 diabetes (median age 64 yr) found that depressive symptoms were associated with poor outcomes and poor adherence to diabetes diet *(51)*. Subjects with greater depressive symptomology had greater consumption of high fat foods and desserts, exercised less, and tested their blood glucose levels less frequently. Depression was not significantly associated with HbA1c or blood pressure but was positively associated with microalbumin level, total cholesterol, and LDL cholesterol. Given the high rates of depression in this population, careful assessment of depressive symptomology and its impact on dietary intake, related aspects of diabetes self-care and health outcomes are critical.

14.3. Social Support

Social isolation is an established risk factor for morbidity and mortality in numerous disease states, with the largest body of literature linking it to CVD, a common outcome of diabetes (52). One avenue in which social support may impact outcomes in chronic diseases such as diabetes is through its impact on self-care behaviors. Recently widowed persons may have limited cooking skills or access to shopping. Such persons may also be depressed and withdraw from usual daily activities, including social, food-related activities such as dining out or even preparing regular meals.

Interestingly, studies of the impact of social support and health behavior in persons with diabetes indicate substantial gender differences. Higher levels of social support have been associated with improved glycemic control in women with type 2 diabetes. However, several studies have found that a high level of perceived support is associated with less diabetes control in men, and it may be that forms of support that are satisfactory to men may reinforce patterns of eating, drinking, and exercise that are inconsistent with optimal diabetes self-care (53). In older adults who continue to live with a spouse, husband's food preference, regardless of nutritional content, is often the best predictor of family meals that are eaten (54). This indicates that not only is social isolation an important influence on dietary intake, but day-to-day social support and interactions among family and friends may both positively and negatively impact dietary intake in older persons with diabetes. Thus, it is imperative to evaluate the social context of patients' food purchases and dietary intake patterns.

Diabetes education programs that include the older adult's spouse may help to promote optimal social support for healthful dietary and lifestyle changes. Substantial improvements were found for diabetes knowledge, psychosocial functioning and metabolic control in a 6-wk diabetes education program for male diabetes patients (and their spouses) aged 65–82 years of age (55).

14.4. Cognitive Dysfunction

A number of studies have indicated that older adults with both type 1 and type 2 diabetes have impaired cognitive function compared with age matched groups, and the level of impairment worsens with increases in hyperglycemia. Tightened blood glucose control, even in the absence of normoglycemia, can result in cognitive improvements in older persons with diabetes (56,57). If frequent self-monitoring and adherence to specific dietary guidelines is within the abilities of the older patient with diabetes, then attainment of tight blood glucose control may be a reasonable goal. However, intensive self-management may not always be realistic for many cognitively impaired older adults. Unfortunately, despite the potential physical benefits, intensive management and tight control may require so many day-to-day demands, that this may be difficult to achieve. Cognitive dysfunction can make adherence to dietary recommendations particularly difficult. For example, older adults who are cognitively impaired may not remember structured mealtimes that are coordinated with their insulin regimen. Difficulty following a complicated meal plan, such as carbohydrate counting or using a sliding scale to match insulin units to intake, may make such treatment regimens too overwhelming to be practical. For some older individuals, a concrete, structured meal plan can help minimize ambiguity regarding their diabetes diet. Such plans may be made in conjunction with a diabetes educator or dietitian.

In addition, provision of home-based caretakers or meal services may also assist the older person with cognitive impairment or significant physical disability or other barriers to obtain access to optimal nutrition that is consistent with diabetes goals.

14.5. Attitudes and Dietary Intake in Older Adults with Diabetes

Older patients' personal views of diabetes appear to impact their levels of diabetes self-care. A study of adults over age 60 with type 2 diabetes found that perceptions regarding cause of diabetes, treatment effectiveness and seriousness of one's diabetes were significantly associated with quality of life and negative affect. Beliefs regarding treatment effectiveness were particularly predictive of dietary intake and physical activity *(58)*. Studies of women reflecting heterogeneous ethnic groups and socioeconomic status indicate that they conceptualize diabetes in terms of their own cognitive explanatory models, which are not necessarily congruent with the way in which health providers conceptualize diabetes *(59)*. A study of first national adults in Canada who had type 2 diabetes *(60)* found that women tended to emphasize the importance of the impact of diabetes on their lives and the psychosocial difficulties encountered, while their healthcare providers focused instead on the pathophysiology and physical impact of diabetes. This suggests that diabetes diet intervention strategies must take patient perspectives into account or they may be perceived as irrelevant by patients and be destined for failure.

14.6. Ethnic/Cultural Issues Influencing Dietary Intake

Research also suggests that ethnic minority, older adults, and traditionally "hard to reach" persons may have culturally unique health-related perspectives that are not effectively targeted by traditionally delivered health promotion interventions *(61)*. Although being healthy appears to be important and a general awareness of what to do to stay healthy is evident, operational definitions of health in these populations are often somewhat different than that typically used in health promotion efforts. For example, focus group studies with underserved ethnic minorities found that a prevailing belief was that better health behaviors could build resistance to acute illnesses and keep them healthy, but that chronic diseases such as diabetes, were the result of fate and heredity and beyond their individual control. In general, participants did not appear to make the cognitive "link" between chronic disease prevention and the importance of diet, physical activity, and weight control. Most participants expressed an interest in "doing better" but were not able to specify how such healthful changes might be made.

Qualitative evaluations of cultural influences on diabetes reveal the complexity of psychosocial influences on diabetes lifestyle change and why traditional health provider perspective based dietary interventions with minority persons often fail. An interview-based study of 20 middle-aged Mexican-American women with type 2 diabetes revealed that their personal understanding and interpretation of their diabetes was most heavily based on their family's experiences and on community influences *(59)*. From the participants' perspectives, the severity of their diabetes was indicated by being treated with insulin injections and the provider being vigilant, although treatment with oral medications and the perception that providers had a lax attitude was taken to mean that the diabetes was not severe. Having diabetes was also viewed as a confusing, silent illness and provider provision of information was often viewed as insufficient. Participants' actual comments may be eye opening for the health care provider striving to understand patients' perspectives. For example, respondent comments included, "The doctor always says I'm not doing what I'm supposed to, writes his note and leaves, what's he talking about?" "The doctor tells you one thing, like I'm borderline, then he puts me on pills and doesn't say anything, and I guess I figured diabetes was like an infection or something like that they would take care of it, a pill"; "My doctor told me if I wasn't so obese I wouldn't have diabetes. No one has ever called me obese. Obese, what is that? Why was he so petty? That hurt, after he said that, I didn't remember a word he said."

The strong influence of family and culture on adherence to a diabetes diet and lifestyle change is also evident in focus group-based qualitative research of African-American women with type 2 diabetes. Factors influencing optimal diabetes diet and physical activity behaviors were evaluated in a study of 70 Southern, predominantly rural African-American women, of whom 65% were age 55 and older (62). These women described the psychological impact of diabetes as being stronger than the physical impact. The psychological issues reported included feelings of nervousness, fatigue, worrying and having feelings of dietary deprivation, including craving for sweets. Rather than attributing fatigue to poor diabetes control and linking this to self-care patterns, participants tended to associate feeling tired to stress-related factors. Women in the focus groups reported considerable life stress other than diabetes, particularly having a multicaregiver role. Care was generally provided to homebound parents and adult children and grandchildren living in their home or spending large amounts of time there and was seen as a barrier to personal diabetes management, particularly for diet and physical activity. Family members complaining about and resistant toward healthy food preparation methods was an example of such a barrier. Positive family support for diabetes was evident in the form of instrumental support from adult daughters or other female family members or friends to older, single, or widowed women. In addition, spirituality and religion emerged as a main theme in all groups. Spirituality was largely viewed as a primary source of emotional support, a positive influence on diabetes and a contributor to quality of life. Church was described as an important source of social and emotional support and resource for coping. This study exemplifies the importance of incorporating family and the church in self-care behaviors of many Southern African-American women.

Cultural and social influences on diabetes self-care have also been examined in Pacific Islander Americans in a low-income community in Hawaii (63). As in Hispanic and African-American groups, family and cultural factors play a prominent role in their diabetes diet and lifestyle behavior patterns. Barriers to diet and exercise identified from focus groups include a cultural expectation combined with direct social pressure to over eat at community or family events; cultural values that associate being overweight with wealth or happiness and ideal body weight; limited financial resources to purchase healthy foods; lack of knowledge about how to prepare healthful foods and disinterest; lack of motivation to engage in structured exercise; feelings of anxiety, anger and depressed mood.

This rich, qualitative work with minority ethnic groups with diabetes demonstrates why consideration of the social and cultural context of older adult's lives is critical for the development of interventions to promote diet and lifestyle change. Family-centered and church based approaches may offer appropriate avenues for efforts to promote optimal diabetes care and maximize the effective delivery of dietary interventions for many older adults with diabetes, who are over represented in ethnic minority populations.

14.7. Quality of Life and Diabetes Diet in Older Adults

In considering prescribing a diabetes diet or when addressing issues related to dietary adherence, it is important to consider the impact of dietary change on the individual's quality of life. Diabetes itself poses numerous challenges, and the many lifestyle demands are among the most difficult for patients. Both type 1 and type 2 diabetes appear to have an impact on health-related quality of life (64). Persons with type 2 diabetes treated with insulin injections appear to experience poorer health-related quality of life than those taking oral agents only or who are treated with lifestyle change alone. This treatment-related difference in quality of life is also apparent in older and inner-city populations and controlling for age, gender, BMI, and diabetes duration (65). Diabetes-specific quality of life issues are associated with overall well-being, and dietary restrictions and daily hassles related to diabetes care are associated with treatment satisfaction, as well as with general well-being. A liberalized diet and flexible insulin therapy are among the diabetes-related factors most associated with favorable quality of life in persons with type 1 diabetes (66).

A Japanese study of diabetic adults over age 60 examined the burden related to having to make changes related to caloric restriction, dietary balance, regular dietary habits, restriction of favorite foods, and the amount of snacks and restrictions when eating out (67). Women, relatively younger subjects, those with lower family support, chronic hyperglycemia and taking oral diabogenic agents reported a higher level of burden from lifestyle changes required by the diabetes diet.

From the previous information, it is apparent that psychosocial influences play a substantial role in the dietary and lifestyle behaviors of older adults with diabetes. Such influences are summarized in Table 9.

15. THEORETICAL CONCEPTUALIZATIONS OF LIFESTYLE CHANGE IN OLDER ADULTS WITH TYPE 2 DIABETES

Lifestyle modification involves a complex series of behavior changes that consider the social and physical environment as well as cognitive and dispositional factors. Theories of changes in health behavior provide a framework for understanding such behaviors as well as providing a framework for interventions to enhance lifestyle change. Two theories efficacious in promoting nutrition and lifestyle change in type 2 diabetes are briefly presented here.

15.1. Social Cognitive Theory

Social cognitive theory (SCT) is one of the most influential and well-documented models of behavior change (68,69). The goal of SCT based interventions is acquisition of knowledge and skills. In this model, behavior, cognition, other personal factors, and the environment are seen as reciprocally influencing one another. The relative influence of each factor varies from one activity to another and from one individual to another, but each must be considered in developing a behavior change intervention. Important in the development and maintenance of behavior change are self-efficacy, belief in personal ability or competence to perform the desired behaviors, and social support. Interventions involve setting small goals, teaching cognitive and behavioral skills, and enhancing environmental factors to enhance their change. In order to maximize the individuals'

Table 9
Psychosocial Influences on Diet and Lifestyle Change in Older Adults

Psychosocial influences on diabetes dietary intake

    Dietary changes and quality of life
    Social isolation/impact of social support
    Depression
    Hypoglycemia unawareness
    Dementia/cognitive dysfunction
    Competing priorities
    Dislike of healthful foods or structured physical activity
    Financial difficulty
    Limited access to healthy foods or safe activity resources
    Cultural norms that are not supportive of optimal diabetes self-care

ability to perform needed behaviors, obstacles are evaluated and their self-efficacy for overcoming obstacles addressed. Strategies involve monitoring progress and address the importance of long-term maintenance of behavior changes.

15.2. Transtheoretical Model

The Transtheoretical Model, or Stages of Change Model (SCM) was developed to describe and explain changes that people appear to go through in initiating and maintaining behavior change. This can help both providers and patients develop more realistic expectations of the potential for making changes by identifying where a patient is on a continuum of stages for change *(70)*. The SCM has been widely used in studying health behaviors, including exercise *(71)* and weight control *(72)*. This model postulates that people move through an orderly sequence of change, although some may stay at one stage for a long period of time, some may move forward more rapidly than others, and some may move back and forth between stages. The SCM also considers a number of processes of change that can be used in altering a variety of behaviors, which may be more or less appropriate at different stages. These processes are consistent with behavior change strategies utilized in SCT-based interventions and may be the focus of counseling strategies. Greatest success in implementing stage-matched behavior change counseling is likely to be attained by targeting one area of behavior change at a time. The individual behaviors to be targeted for change in persons with diabetes might include specific dietary behaviors (e.g., increasing fruit and vegetable intake, reducing high fat snacks), increasing physical activity (or decreasing sedentary activity such as watching television), or increasing blood glucose monitoring. The stages of change of the SCM and examples of stage-matched counseling approaches are depicted in Table 10.

16. BEHAVIOR CHANGE INTERVENTIONS TO PROMOTE DIETARY CHANGE IN OLDER ADULTS WITH DIABETES

The two models described may be used to guide development of dietary and lifestyle interventions to increase the likelihood that older adults with diabetes actually adopt and maintain the recommended behaviors. An example of one of the few theoretically based lifestyle change intervention programs developed specifically for older adults with diabetes is the Sixty-something study *(73)*. Principles of SCT were used to develop a

Table 10
Stage-Based Counseling Strategies

Stages in behavior* change process	Patient needs	Counseling messages
Not interested in adopting the behavior (*Precontemplation*)	Motivation to engage in behavior	Ask what patient likes, dislikes about the health behavior in question Discuss pros and cons of the behavior* Reinforce and build on patient's personal reasons for doing the behavior Discuss effects of the behavior on diabetes, lifestyle, and wellness Let patient know you want to help and you'll bring it up at the next visit
Interested in adopting the behavior* in next 6 mo, but not in next 30 d (*Contemplation*)	Motivation to engage in behavior sooner rather than later	Need to strengthen benefits for the behavior and weaken cons for doing it– tipping the balance in favor of healthy diabetes behaviors
Interested in adopting the behavior* in next 30 d (*Preparation*)	Skill-building Support Specific planning strategies	Encourage patient to make a specific plan to fit in the behavior using small steps; Tell others about plans to gain social support for changes to be made Make specific plans to address expected obstacles (e.g., time demands, feelings of discouragement)
In process of doing the behavior consistently within past 6 mo (*Action*)	Relapse prevention	Congratulate on success Review concerns Reinforce plans to avoid temptation to skip behavior of focus and drift to previous lifestyle If patient relapses, encourage to cycle back to the behavior of focus right away; use the experience as an opportunity for learning to help manage difficulties the next time around
Have engaged in the behavior* regularly for more than 6 mo (*Maintenance*)	Relapse prevention or nothing	Support Encourage Review concerns and plans for relapse prevention, if appropriate

*Individual behaviors targeted for change in persons with diabetes might include specific dietary changes, such as fruit and vegetable intake, high-fat snack foods, episodes of unplanned snacking, sessions of physical activity, time engaged in sedentary activity, such as watching television or videos, and frequency of self-monitoring of blood glucose or rates of appropriately taking medications.

10-session self-management training program with 102 adults over 60 yr of age with type 2 diabetes. Subjects were randomly assigned to immediate or delayed intervention conditions. The intervention conditions taught problem solving skills and strategies for enhancing self-efficacy from overcoming personal barriers to adhering to their diabetes diet and other aspects of the diabetes regimen. The immediate intervention produced greater reductions in caloric intake and percent of calories from fat, greater weight loss, and increases in the frequency of blood glucose testing compared to delayed controls. Improvements were generally maintained at 6-mo follow-up. Results from subjects receiving the delayed intervention closely approximated those for the immediate intervention subjects.

Theoretical and practical approaches to diet and lifestyle change may address the physiological and psychosocial needs of older and minority persons with diabetes. A primary care clinic and community-based diabetes intervention was conducted with an older group of 200 African-American women with type 2 diabetes to improve dietary behaviors, physical activity and other aspects of diabetes self-care. A useful description of the practical cognitive and behavioral strategies used in the program has been presented in the literature (74). In order to aquaint the reader with these practical strategies, which may be used in their own clinical nutrition encounters, they will be briefly presented here.

Concrete behavioral counseling strategies utilized in intervention study included using a single illustrated page of recommendations in the form of a tip sheet for diet and physical activity. Suggestions for behavior change were broken down into small, achievable steps in an efforts to promote self-efficacy. Group sessions were conducted to promote progress in readiness to change diet and physical activity behaviors and to provide helpful social support. Both health professionals and peer counselors assisted with groups. The content areas included not only diabetes knowledge deficits and skills but also strategies for managing the situational and psychological barriers to appropriate eating habits and activity. Peer counselors provided social support and feedback, reinforced diet, and activity goals using monthly telephone contacts and addressed issues related to cultural translation. These types of practical, theoretically based strategies may be useful for the busy practitioner, because they may increase the likelihood of dietary change, and be incorporated into individual patient contacts.

17. WEIGHT LOSS INTERVENTION IN OLDER ADULTS WITH DIABETES

Weight loss issues that must be considered for older adults with diabetes include the impact of restrictions on quality of life and potential loss of lean muscle mass from decreased protein intake.

In research undertaken with diabetic younger adults, weight loss programs that combine diet, physical activity, and behavior modification techniques have been shown to be the most effective over the short term (1,75). Hypocaloric diets, which can improve glucose tolerance and lipid levels, may also be appropriate for older, obese persons with diabetes. There are a large number of studies in younger adults that have shown weight loss and exercise are a key aspect of the treatment of diabetes. Weight loss and exercise have both been shown to decrease insulin resistance and to improve glycemic control (1). Behavioral weight control interventions with persons with type 2 diabetes have found that even reductions of approx 10% of weight loss can decrease hypertension and lipid abnormalities and improve glycemic control, with improvements related to the magnitude of weight loss *(1)*. A study of 15 obese patients over age 65 with type 2 diabetes found that participation in a diet-based weight loss program resulted in moderate weight loss, and improved glycemic control despite the fact that patients did not achieve ideal body weight *(76)*.

The major difficulty in weight control and obesity intervention is the problem of long-term maintenance of behavior change and weight loss. There is some evidence to suggest that weight regain is more common for persons with diabetes *(77)*. The most efficacious strategies for persons with diabetes and older adults are as yet, unknown. Structured behavioral weight loss programs based on SCT and SCM have been published for use by individuals or groups, a good example of such published a self-paced program is the LEARN Program for Weight Control, which is referenced in the Section 21.

17.1. Role of Physical Activity in Diabetes Lifestyle Change

Most state of the art weight loss programs now incorporate physical activity intervention. Lifestyle changes including diet and physical activity, are often recommended for young adults with diabetes, independent of weight management efforts, and interventions have been conducted in several studies. A major benefit of physical activity in diabetes is its beneficial role in the management of hyperglycemia and in cardiovascular risk factor reduction. Regular physical activity is recommended for the general population of older adults with diabetes. In the case of underweight, malnourished older adults, regular physical activity can help to promote appetite. Inactivity can lead to frailty and limited mobility, which in turn, may limit access to shopping and other food-related activities like meal preparation. Training to increase strength, flexibility, and endurance can promote increased functioning and independence in older adults, including the oldest old. Unfortunately, in today's culture, prevalence of inactivity is high, particularly in older adults and minorities and even when activity is initiated, maintenance over time remains a challenge.

Data from adults age 60 and over who participated in NHANES III indicates high prevalence of disability in older adults with diabetes, with 32% of women and 15% of men reporting inability to walk one-fourth of a mile, climb stairs, or do housework when compared with 14% of women and 8% of men without diabetes. Diabetes was associated with 2–3-fold increased odds of not being able to do all three tasks. Among women, diabetes was also associated with slower walking speed, inferior lower extremity function, decreased balance, and an increased risk of falling. Thus, physical disability in older adults with diabetes is sufficiently prevalent to play a major role in basic activities of daily living and may substantially impact diabetes self-care abilities and impair their quality of life *(78)*.

Few physical activity interventions have been specifically conducted with older adults with diabetes, so the efficacy of physical activity intervention approaches for older adults with diabetes is unclear. A review of physical activity efficacy studies with younger adults with type 2 diabetes indicates that moderate intensity physical activity is associated with 15% to 20% lower HbA1c over 3 to 4 mo *(79)*.

A randomized study evaluated the impact of exercise in Caucasian adults who were over age 65, with type 2 diabetes who were not taking exogenous insulin. The intervention was a supervised, 16-wk aerobic exercise program that did not include dietary intervention *(80)*. The intervention group showed improved fitness and improved glucose tolerance on oral glucose tolerance test, with the absence of weight loss. Exercise participation did not decrease reported diabetes quality of life and resulted in an improvement in positive attitudes toward diabetes.

A small randomized study conducted in Australia compared usual care to a 6-mo structured education and physical activity program with 26 middle-aged and older men and women (median age 61 yr) *(81)*. Activity levels were increased and metabolic control improved in the intervention group at the end of the program but these gains were not maintained at 1-yr follow-up. An increase in activity over 6 mo was associated with significant weight loss, decreased body fat and fasting insulin over 6 mo and predicted a reduction in fasting glucose over 12 mo. Changes in caloric intake and diet composition did not explain these associations.

A randomized weight loss and exercise program conducted with older African-Americans aged 55–79 found that lifestyle intervention resulted in greater weight loss, activity, reduced intake of fat and saturated fat, lower HbA1c and cholesterol levels and improved nutrition knowledge relative to a usual care group at a three month follow-up and maintenance of improved weight and HbA1c at a 6-mo follow-up. Decreases in HbA1c were generally independent of the changes in diet, weight and physical activity. Blood pressure increases in persons in the usual care condition resulted in group differences at 3- and 6-mo follow-ups as well *(82)*.

Overall, research with older adults with type 2 diabetes suggests that combining dietary changes with physical activity is more likely to result in long-term maintenance of weight loss and improved physiological outcomes than either approach on its own *(83)*.

17.2. Addressing Concerns Regarding Activity in Older Adults with Diabetes

Once concern in recommending physical exercise to older adults with diabetes is the possible impact of comorbid health problems on their ability to safely exercise. Among people over age 60 with type 2 diabetes, the prevalence of peripheral neuropathy is greater than 50% *(84)*. A randomized study of 20 older adults (median age 64 yr) with type 2 diabetes and confirmed peripheral neuropathy compared a 3-wk exercise intervention designed to increase available distal strength and balance to a control exercise program *(85)*. Intervention subjects but not controls had significant improvements in all clinical measures of balance. This suggests that incorporation of strength and balance training may increase the safety of activity interventions in older adults with diabetes. It is unclear if such exercise intervention translates to reduced frequency of falls.

Another area of concern regarding exercise recommendations for older adults with diabetes is the prevalence of silent coronary artery disease in this population. Screening via an exercise tolerance test may be prudent before at-risk individuals begin any exercise program. Other comorbid conditions potentially influencing physical activity interventions in older persons with diabetes not systematically studied in this population are osteoporosis, arthritis, and low muscle mass and related frailty.

18. FUTURE TRENDS AND CONTROVERSIES IN DIABETES INTERVENTION APPROACHES

In addition to conventional dietary approaches, several vitamin and mineral supplements have been proposed as resources to optimize nutritional intervention in individuals with diabetes. These include the use of vitamin E, omega-3 fatty acids, alpha-lipoic acid, and chromium supplements. Oxidative stress has been implicated in many of the complications of diabetes *(85)*. Vitamin E is the major chain-breaking antioxidant and has been shown to inhibit lipid peroxidation. It has also been postulated to have beneficial effects on platelet function. However, the optimal dose for persons with diabetes is unclear. At doses of 400 IU daily, there were no significant benefits on cardiovascular disease in the HOPE study *(86)*. Higher dose (800 IU or more) have been suggested by some investigators. In addition, prevention of diabetic microvascular disease has also been reported in one study *(87)*.

Omega-3 fatty acids have also been associated with reductions in CVD. Dietary omega-3 fatty acids can be obtained through fish oil. The two-long-chain fatty acids—eicosapentanoic acid (EPA) and docosahesanoic acid (DHA)—have been the most widely used. At doses of 750–1000 mg daily, antioxidant effects may be seen. However, triglyceride-lowering effects are only seen at doses of 5–15 g daily *(88)*. This might require the use of daily multiple tablets, and efficacy trials are needed for persons with diabetes, since higher doses do carry a small risk of worsening glycemic control, bleeding, and elevation in LDL cholesterol level.

Supplemental use of chromium has also been investigated. It has been shown to improve insulin sensitivity and hence blood glucose levels in type 2 diabetes *(89)*. Alpha-lipoic acid has also been shown to improve insulin sensitivity, especially when given intravenously. However, its benefits when used orally need to be established *(90)*. None of these supplements have been evaluated in large clinical trials.

19. RECOMMENDATIONS FOR IMPARTING DIETARY INFORMATION

In order to impart diabetes diet information in a fashion that will lead to actual changes in behavior and maintenance of these changes, it is critical to consider the psychosocial and cultural influences that are present for each individual patient. Simple and concrete statements such as "eat less fat" or "eat less food" or "get more walking in each day" may promote learning and minimize failure. Nutrition information is best presented in sequenced manageable steps that can then be individualized to the patient's setting *(91)*. Simple tip sheets and problem solving approaches discussed in earlier sections may also be helpful. It is also important to be mindful of the range of functioning in older adults. Older adults of the World War II generation, and tended to be characterized as somewhat reverential toward physicians and the health care system. However, baby boomers, who are now entering the realm of older adulthood, tend to differ from previous generations and have high expectations of their health providers *(92)*. This generation of "new" older adults tend to want a collaborative relationship with their health care provider, desire additional information including resources such as self-help publications, Internet, video and audiotapes, demand convenience, expect hard evidence of quality and expertise, be skeptical of advice at face value, and to be willing to explore alternative therapies *(91)*. In order to meet the needs of the range of older adults with diabetes, it is clear that a "one size fits all" approach will not be effective. Rather, issues related to culture and ethnicity and generational cohort must be considered.

20. RECOMMENDATIONS FOR CLINICIANS

1. Establish the type of diabetes and medication regimen in order to appropriately integrate dietary goals.

2. Consider the importance of cardiovascular risk, ncluding obesity and lipids, in developing diabetes dietary goals and routine assessment (*see* Table 5).
3. Work with the patient to set a goal of achieving and maintaining reasonable body weight. For obese older adults, moderate weight loss may achieve dramatic results and exercise may greatly enhance dietary intervention. Maintenance of behavior change and weight loss is critical. For underweight adults, focus on promotion of optimal nutritional intake and functional status.
4. Educate older adults with diabetes about the rationale for diet and lifestyle change and link to health outcomes; promote self-efficacy for change.
5. Consider the risk of hypoglycemia for older adults taking insulin—particularly those with poor nutritional status, cognitive dysfunction, polypharmacy, suspected or confirmed heavy alcohol use, and comorbid illness. Encourage frequent self-monitoring and dietary self-treatment and preventive strategies.
6. Assess older adults' specific dietary patterns, such as food choices, quantity eaten, and unplanned snacking as well as the lifestyle contexts in which they occur.
7. Address psychosocial issues that may influence dietary intake, including depression, social support, cognitive status, attitudes and perceptions, and the impact of the diabetes regimen on quality of life.
8. Address and intervene within individuals' cultural context, including family influences and church, when appropriate.
9. Provide a collaborative relationship with each patient, offer resources, and provide concrete, behavioral strategies to promote behavior change.
10. When appropriate, provide self-help materials including Internet and ADA resources (*see* Section 21.).

21. NUTRITION AND LIFESTYLE CHANGE IN OLDER ADULTS WITH DIABETES MELLITUS

21.1. Internet Resources

American Diabetes Association: www.ada.org
American Association of Diabetes Educators (includes "find an educator" service locator): www.aadenet.org
Joslin Diabetes Center: www.joslin.harvard.edu

21.2. Books

(Books from the American Diabetes Association may be ordered at: 1-800-ADA-ORDER)
Franz MJ, Battle JP (eds.) American Diabetes Association Guide to Medical Nutrition Therapy. American Diabetes Association, Alexandria, VA, 2000.
Anderson RM, Barr PA, Funnell MM, Arnold MS, Edwards GJ, Fitzgerald JT. Living with Diabetes: Challenges in the African American Community. American Diabetes Association, Alexandria, VA, 2000.
Warshaw HS, Bolderman KM. Practical Carbohydrate Counting: A How to Teach Guide for Health Professionals. American Diabetes Association, Alexandria, VA, 2001.
American Diabetes Association. The Health Professional's Guide to Diabetes and Exercise. American Diabetes Association, Alexandria, VA, 1995.
American Council on Exercise. Exercise for Older Adults. ACE's Guide for Fitness Professionals. American Council on Exercise, San Diego, CA, 1998.
Warshaw HS, Webb R. The Diabetes Food and Nutrition Bible. American Diabetes Association, Alexandria, VA, 2001.

Brownell KD. The LEARN Program for Weight Management 2000 (10th ed.) American Health Publishing Company, Dallas, TX, 2000.

Demps-Gaines F, Weaver R. The New Soul Food Cookbook for People with Diabetes. American Diabetes Association, Alexandria, VA, 1999.

Anderson BJ, Rubin RR (eds.) Practical Psychology for Diabetes Clinicians. How to Deal with the Key Behavioral Issues Faced by Patients and Health Care Teams. American Diabetes Association, Alexandria, VA, 1996.

Polonsky WH. Diabetes Burnout: What to Do When You Can't Take It Anymore. American Diabetes Association, Alexandria, VA, 1999.

Lincoln TA, Eaddy JA. Beating the Blood Sugar Blues: Proven Methods and Wisdom for Controlling Hypoglycemia. American Diabetes Association, Alexandria, VA, 2001.

REFERENCES

1. Wing RR, Goldstein MG, Acton KJ, Birch LL, Jakicic JM, Sallis JF Jr, et al. Behavioral science research in diabetes: Lifestyle changes related to obesity, eating behavior, and physical activity. Diabetes Care 2001;24:1–2.
2. Seidell JC. Obesity, insulin resistance and diabetes a worldwide epidemic. Br J Nutr 2000;83(suppl 1): S5–S8.
3. Visscher TL, Seidell JC. The public health impact of obesity. Annu Rev Public Health 2001;22:355–375.
4. King H, Aubert RE, Herman WH. Global burden of diabetes 1995–2025: Prevalence, numerical estimates, and projections. Diabetes Care 1998;21:1414–1431.
5. Ratner RE. Type 2 diabetes mellitus: The grand overview. Diabet Med 1998;15(suppl 4):S4–S7
6. Shorr RI, Franse LV, Resnick HE, DiBari M, Johnson KC, Pahor M. Glycemic control of older adults with type 2 diabetes: Findings from the Third National Health and Nutrition Examination Survey, 1988–1994. J Am Geriatr Soc 2000;48:264–267.
7. Howard BV, Magee MF. Diabetes and cardiovascular disease. Curr Atheroscler Rep 2000;2:476–481.
8. The Expert Committee on the Diagnosis and Classification of Diabetes Mellitus: Diabetes Care 1997; 20:1183–1197.
9. World Health Organization: Definition, diagnosis and classification of diabetes mellitus and its complications: Report of a WHO consultation. Part 1, Diagnosis and Classification of Diabetes Mellitus (WHO/NCD/NCS/99.2) Geneva, World Health Organization, 1999.
10. Barzilay JI, Spiekerman CF, Wahl PW, Kuller LH, Cushman M, Furberg CD, et al. Cardiovascular disease in older adults with glucose disorders: Comparison of American Diabetes Association criteria for diabetes mellitus with WHO criteria. Lancet 1999;354:622–625.
11. Falorni A, Kockum I, Sanjeevi CB, Lernmark A. Pathogenesis of insulin-dependent diabetes mellitus. Baillieres Clin Endocrinol Metab 1995;9:25–46.
12. Morley JE. An overview of diabetes mellitus in older persons. Clin Geriatr Med 1999;15:211–224.
13. Hansen BC. The metabolic syndrome X. Ann NY Acad Sci 1999;892:1–24.
14. Dagogo-Jack S, Santiago J. Pathophysiology of Type 2 diabetes and modes of action of therapeutic interventions. Arch Intern Med 1997;157:1802–1817.
15. Weyer C, Bogardus C, Mott DM, Pratley RE. The natural history of insulin secretory dysfunction and insulin resistance in the pathogenesis of type 2 diabetes mellitus. J Clin Invest 1999;104:787–794.
16. Elahi D, Muller DC. Carbohydrate metabolism in the elderly. Eur J Clin Nutr 2000;54(suppl 3): S112–S120.
17. Beaufrere B, Morio B. Fat and protein redistribution with aging: Metabolic considerations. Eur J Clin Nutr 2000;54(suppl 3):S48–S53.
18. Chiu KC, Lee NP, Cohan P, Chuang LM. Beta cell function declines with age in glucose tolerant Caucasians. Clin Endocrinol (Oxf) 2000;53:569–575.
19. Pozzilli P, Di Mario U. Autoimmune diabetes not requiring insulin at diagnosis (latent autoimmune diabetes of the adult): Definition, characterization, and potential prevention. Diabetes Care 2001;24: 1460–1467.
20. Resnick HE, Shorr RI, Kuller L, Franse L, Harris TB. Prevalence and clinical implications of American Diabetes Association-defined diabetes and other categories of glucose dysregulation in older adults: The health, aging and body composition study. J Clin Epidemiol 2001;54:869–876.

21. The Diabetes Control and Complications Trial Research Group. N Engl J Med 1993;30:977–8623. Turner RC, Holman RR. Lessons from UK prospective diabetes study. Diabet Res Clin Pract 1995; 28(suppl):S151–S157.

22. Turner RC, Holman RR. Lessons from UK prospective diabetes study. Diabet Res Clin Pract 1995; 28(suppl):S151–S157.

23. American Diabetes Association. Evidence-based nutrition principles and recommendations for the treatment and prevention of diabetes and related complications. Diabet Care 2002;25:202–212.

24. Clark MJ, Sterrett JJ, Carson DS. Diabetes guidelines: A summary and comparison of the recommendations of the American Diabetes Association, Veterans Health Administration, and American Association of Clinical Endocrinologists. Clin Ther 2000;22:899–910.

25. Adler AI, Stratton IM, Neil HA, Yudkin JS, Matthews DR, Cull CA, et al. Association of systolic blood pressure with macrovascular and microvascular complications of type 2 diabetes (UKPDS 36): Prospective observational study. BMJ 2000;12;321:412–419.

26. Hansson L, Zanchetti A, Carruthers SG, Dahlof B, Elmfeldt D, Julius S, Menard J, et al. Effects of intensive blood-pressure lowering and low-dose aspirin in patients with hypertension: Principal results of the Hypertension Optimal Treatment (HOT) randomised trial. HOT Study Group. Lancet 1998;351: 1755–1762.

27. Villarosa IP, Bakris GL. The appropriate blood pressure control in diabetes (ABCD) Trial. J Hum Hypertens 1998;12:653–655.

28. Goldberg RB, Mellies MJ, Sacks FM, Moye LA, Howard BV, Howard WJ, et al. Cardiovascular events and their reduction with pravastatin in diabetic and glucose-intolerant myocardial infarction survivors with average cholesterol levels: Subgroup analyses in the cholesterol and recurrent events (CARE) trial. The Care Investigators. Circulation 1998;98:2513–2519.

29. Haffner SM. The Scandinavian Simvastatin Survival Study (4S) subgroup analysis of diabetic subjects: implications for the prevention of coronary heart disease. Diabet Care 1997;20:469–471.

30. Garg A, Bonanome A, Grundy SM, Zhang ZJ, Unger RH. Comparison of a high-carbohydrate diet with a high-monosaturated fat diet in patients with non-insulin-dependent diabetes mellitus. N Engl J Med 1988;319:829–834.

31. Jovanovic L, Gondos B. Type 2 diabetes: The epidemic of the new millennium. Ann Clin Lab Sci 1999; 29:33–42.

32. Mooradian AD, Osterwil D, Petrawek D, Morley JE. Diabetes mellitus in elderly nursing home patients. J Am Geriatr Soc 1988;36:391–396.

33. Wright J. Total parenteral nutrition and enteral nutrition in diabetes. Curr Opin Clin Nutr Metab Care 2000;3:5–10.

34. Garg A. High-MUFA diets for patients with DM: a meta-analysis. Am J Clin Nutr 1998;67(suppl 3): 577S–582S.

35. Hongsermeier T, Bistrian BR. Evaluation of a practical technique of determining insulin requirements in diabetic patients receiving total parenteral nutrition. J Parenter Enter Nutr 1993;17:16–19.

36. Janssen MM, Snoek FJ, de Jongh RT, Casteleijn S, Deville W, Heine RJ. Biological and behavioural determinants of the frequency of mild, biochemical hypoglycaemia in patients with type 1 diabetes on multiple injection therapy. Diabetes Metab Res Rev 2000;16:157–163.

37. Cox DJ, Gonder-Frederick L, Polonsky W, Schlundt D, Kovatchev B, Clarke W. Blood glucose awareness training (BGAT-2): long-term benefits. Diabetes Care 2001;24:637–642.

38. Meeking DR, Cavan DA. Alcohol ingestion and glycemic control in patients with insulin-dependent diabetes mellitus. Diabet Med 1997;14:279–283.

39. Bolli GB. How to ameliorate the problem of hypoglycemia in intensive as well as nonintensive treatment of type 1 diabetes. Diabetes Care 1999;22(suppl 2):B43–B52.

40. Strano-Paul L, Phanumas D. Diabetes management. Analysis of the American Diabetes Association's clinical practice recommendations. Geriatrics 2000;55:57–62.

41. Horwatch CC, Worsley A. Dietary habits of elderly persons with diabetes. J Am Diet Assoc 91:553–557.

42. Cross AT, Babicz D, Cushman LF. Snacking habits of senior Americans. J Nutr Elder 1995;14:27–38.

43. Fombonne E. Increased rates of depression: Update of epidemiological findings and analytic problems. Acta Psychiatr Scand 1994;90:145–156.

44. Consensus Panel, Diagnosis and treatment of depression in late life. JAMA 1992;268:1018–1024.

45. Slater SL, Katz IR. Prevalence of depression in the aged: Formal calculations versus clinical facts. J Am Geriatr Soc 1995;43:778–779.

46. Lustman P, Griffith L, Freedland K, Kissel S, Clouse R. Prevalence of depression in adults with diabetes. An epidemiological evaluation. Diabetes Care 1993;16:1167–1178.

47. Black SA, Markides KS. Depressive symptoms and mortality in older Mexican Americans. Ann Epidemiol 1999;9:45–52.

48. Lustman P, Griffith L, Freedland K, Clouse R. The course of major depression in diabetes; Gen Hosp Psychiatry 1997;19:138–143.

49. Lustman PJ, Freedland KE, Griffity LS, Clouse RE. Predicting response to cognitive behavior therapy of depression in type 2 diabetes. Gen Hosp Psychiatry 1998;20:302–306.

50. Sarkisian CA, Lachs MS. "Failure to thrive" in older adults. Ann Intern Med 1996;124:1072–1078.

51. Polonsky WH, Dudl RJ, Peterson M, Steffian G, Lees J, Hokai H. Depression in type 2 diabetes: Links to health care utilization, self-care and medical markers. Diabetes 2000;49(suppl):A64.

52. Orth-Gomer K. International epidemiological evidence for a relationship between social support and cardiovascular disease, 97–117. In: Social Support and Cardiovascular Disease. Shumaker SA, Czajkowski SM (eds.), Plenum, New York, 1994.

53. Kaplan RM, Hartwell SL. Differential effects of social support and social network on physiological and social outcomes in men and women with type II diabetes mellitus. Health Psychology 1987;6:387–398.

54. Weidner G, Healy AB, Matarazzo JD. Family consumption of low fat foods: Stated preference versus actual consumption. J App Soc Psychol 1985;15:773–779.

55. Gilden JL, Hendryx M, Casia C, Singh SP. The effectiveness of diabetes education programs for older patients and their spouses. J Am Geriatric Soc 1989;37:1023–1030.

56. Bent N, Rabitt P, Metcalfe D. Diabetes mellitus and the rate of cognitive aging. Br J Clin Psychol 2000; 39:349–362.

57. Meneilly GS, Cheung E, Tessier D, Yakura C, Tuokko H. The effect of improved glycemic control on cognitive functions in the elderly patient with diabetes. II Gerontol 1993;48:M117–M121.

58. Hampson SE, Glasgow RE, Foster LS. Personal models of diabetes among older adults: Relationship to self-management and other variables. Diabetes Educ 1995;21:300–307.

59. Alcozer F. Secondary analysis of perceptions and meanings of type 2 diabetes among Mexican American women. Diabetes Educ 2000;2:785–795.

60. Hernandez CA, Antone I, Cornelius I. A grounded theory study of the experience of type 2 diabetes in first national adults in Canada. J Transcultural Nurs 1999;10:220–228.

61. White SL, Maloney SK. Promoting healthy diets and active lives to hard-to-reach groups: market research study. Public Health Rep 1990;105:224–231.

62. Samuel-Hodge CD, Headen SW, Skelly AH, Ingram AF, Keyserling TC, Jackson EJ, et al. Influences on day-to-day self-management of type 2 diabetes among African-American women: Spirituality, the multi-caregiver role, and other social context factors. Diabetes Care 2000;23:928–933.

63. Wang CY, Abbott L, Goodbody AK, Hui WTY, Rausch C. Development of a community-based diabetes management program for Pacific Islanders. Diabetes Educ 1999;25:738–746.

64. Jacobson AM. Quality of life in patients with diabetes mellitus. Semin Clin Neuropsychiatry 1997;2: 82–93.

65. Petterson T, Lee P, Hollis S, Young B, Newton P, Dornan T. Well being and treatment satisfaction in older people with diabetes. Diabetes Care 1998;21:930–935.

66. Bott U, Muhlhauser I, Overmann H, Berger M. Validation of a diabetes-specific quality-of-life scale for patients with type 1 diabetes. Diabetes Care 1998;21:757–769.

67. Araki A, Izumo Y, Inoue J, Hattori A, Nakamura T, Takahashi R, et al. Burden of dietary therapy on elderly patients with diabetes mellitus. Nippon Ronen Igakkai Zasshi 1995;32:904–909.

68. Bandura, A. Self-efficacy: Toward a unifying theory of behavioral change. Psychol Rev 1977;84:191–215.

69. Bandura, A. Social Foundations of Thought and Action. Prentice-Hall, Englewood Cliffs, NJ, 1986.

70. Prochaska JO, DiClemente CC. The Transtheoretical Approach: Crossing Traditional Boundaries of Therapy. Dow Jones Irwin, Homewood, IL, 1984.

71. Marcus BH, Selby VC, Niaura RS, Rossi JS. Self-efficacy and the stages of exercise behavior change. Res Q Exer Sport 1992;63:60–66.

72. O'Connell DO, Velicer WF. A decisional balance measure and the stages of change model for weight loss. Intern J Addictions 1988;23:729–750.

73. Glasgow RE, Toobert DJ, Hampson SE, Brown JE, Lewinsohn PM, Donnelly J. Improving self-care among older patients with type II diabetes: The sixty something study. Patient Education Counseling 1992;19:61–74.

74. Keyserling TC, Ammerman AS, Samuel-Hodge CD, Ingram AF, Skelly AH, Elasy TA, et al. A diabetes management program for African American women with type 2 diabetes. Diabetes Educ 2000;26: 796–805.

75. NHLBI obesity education initiative expert panel on the identification, evaluation, and treatment of overweight and obesity in adults: Clinical guidelines on the identification, evaluation, and treatment of overweight and obesity in adults: the evidence report. Obes Res 1998;6(suppl 2):51S–210S.

76. Reaven GM. Beneficial effect of moderate weight loss in older patients with no-insulin-dependent diabetes mellitus poorly controlled with insulin. J Am Geriatr Soc 1985;33:93–95.

77. Guare JC, Wing RR, Grant A. Comparison of obese NIDDM and nondiabetic women: Short- and long-term weight loss. Obes Res 1995;3:329–335.

78. Gregg EW, Beckles GL, Williamson DF, Leveille SG, Langlois JA, Engelgau MM, Narayan KM. Diabetes and physical disability among older U.S. adults. Diabetes Care 2000;23:1272–1277.

79. Clark DO. Physical activity efficacy and effectiveness among older adults and minorities. Diabetes Care 1997;20:1176–1182.

80. Tessier D, Menard J, Fulop T, Ardilouze J, Roey MA, Dubuc N, et al. Effects of aerobic physical exercise in the elderly with type 2 diabetes mellitus. Arch Gerontol Geriatr 2000;31:121–132.

81. Samaras K, Ashwell S, Mackintosh AM, Fleury AC ,Campbell LV, Chisholm DJ. Will older sedentary people with non-insulin-dependent diabetes start exercising? A health promotion model. Diabetes Res Clin Pract 1997;37:121–128.

82. Agurs-Collins TD, Kumanyika SK, Ten Have TR, Adams-Campbell LL. A randomized controlled trial of weight reduction and exercise for diabetes management in older African American subjects. Diabetes Care 1997;20:1503–1511.

83. Young M, Boultin A, Maclead A, Williams D, Sonksen P. A multicentre study of the prevalence of diabetic peripheral neuropathy in the United Kingdom hospital clinic population. Diabetologia 1993; 36:150–154.

84. Richardson JK, Sandman D, Vela S. A focused exercise regimen improves clinical measures of balance in patients with peripheral neuropathy. Arch Phys Med Rehabil 2001;82:205–209.

85. Mann JI. The role of nutritional modifications in the prevention of macrovascular complications of diabetes. Diabetes 1997;46(suppl 2):S125–S130.

86. Ruhe RC, McDonald RB. Use of antioxidant nutrients in the prevention and treatment of type 2 diabetes. J Am Coll Nutr 2001;20:363S–369S.

87. Gaede P, Poulsen HE, Parving HH, Pederson O. Double-blind, randomized study of the effect of combined treatment with vitamin C and E on albuminuria in Type 2 diabetic patients. Diabet Med 2001; 18:756–760.

88. Harris WS, Connor WE, Alam N, Illingworth DR. Reduction of postprandial triglyceridemia in humans by dietary n-3 fatty aids. J Lipid Res 1988;29:1451–1460.

89. Anderson RA. Chromium and diabetes. Nutrition 1999;15:720–722.

90. Evans JL, Goldfine ID. Alpha-lipoic acid: A multifunctional antioxidant that improves insulin sensitivity in patients with type 2 diabetes. Diabetes Technol Ther 2000;2:401–413.

91. Gohdes D. Diet therapy for minority patients with diabetes. Diabetes Care 1988;11:189–191.

92. Clark B. Older, sicker, smarter, and redefining quality: The older consumer's quest for service. In: Healthy Aging. Challenges and Solutions. K Dychtwald (ed.), Aspen, Inc., Gaithersburg, MD, 1999.

22 Obesity in Middle and Older Age

Gordon L. Jensen and Melanie Berg

1. INTRODUCTION

Obesity is a growing concern among middle- and older-aged adults as a result of its increasing prevalence and profound impact on health and quality of life. Obesity is associated with functional decline and increased risk for chronic medical conditions including hypertension, type II diabetes, hyperlipidemia, coronary artery disease, and osteoarthritis. Obesity is a complex multifactorial disease that is chronic in nature. The successful management of obesity involves comprehensive medical, lifestyle, and nutritional interventions. The most effective treatments of this disease are medically supervised and require a skilled multidisciplinary approach. A combination of prudent diet, exercise, and behavior modification are the mainstay of treatment. This chapter addresses each of these topics as it examines the growing problem of obesity in middle and older age.

2. THE PREVALENCE OF OBESITY

Obesity continues to grow in prevalence in the United States (1). Data from the National Health and Nutrition Examination Surveys (NHANES) reveals that the percentage of obese persons increased from 14.5% from 1976 to 1980 to 22.9% from 1988 to 1994. The most recent data from NHANES 1999 to 2000 shows further increases in obesity prevalence for men and women of all ages. The age-adjusted prevalence of obesity has increased from 22.9% in NHANES III (1994–1998) to 30.5% in 1999 to 2000. The prevalence of overweight has increased during this time period from 55.9% to 64.5% (1a). Trends were similar for all genders, age, and racial/ethnic groups (2) and detailed subanalysis shows that African American and Hispanic women are particularly susceptible. There is a greater prevalence of obesity among older women compared to older men (2,3). Obesity is common up to age 80 yr with prevalence then declining precipitously, likely reflecting both weight loss and mortality. Many obese older persons were obese as middle-aged adults.

3. THE CAUSES OF OBESITY

Environmental factors that may contribute to obesity include lifestyle as well as behavioral issues. Obesity is highly prevalent in the Arizona Pima Indian population (4).

From: *Handbook of Clinical Nutrition and Aging*
Edited by: C. W. Bales and C. S. Ritchie © Humana Press Inc., Totowa, NJ

Arizona Pima Indians have been compared to both Mexican Pima Indians and groups of unrelated Non-Pima individuals living in the same environment as the Mexican Pima Indians to evaluate the effect of environmental factors on the incidence of obesity. It was observed that Arizona Pimas consumed a more energy-rich diet and were less active than the other groups. Obesity was present in only 13% of Mexican Pimas when compared to 69% of Arizona Pimas with a 30-kg average difference in body weight *(4)*.

Weight gain often occurs in middle age. Women typically manifest additional gain in body fat during the perimenopausal period. Peak body fat tends to occur somewhat later in women than in men and may occur as late as ages 50–60 yr *(5)*. Lifestyles of middle- and older-aged adults are often sedentary, likely being a major contributor to obesity. Unfortunately, many middle- and older-aged adults view weight gain and sedentary lifestyle as inevitable parts of the aging process. Increased dietary energy intake also promotes positive energy balance with resulting weight gain. Mean daily energy intakes for adults are 100–300 cal higher in NHANES III (1988–1991) when compared with NHANES II (1976–1980) *(6)*.

Certain medications including antidepressants (e.g., fluoxetine, mirtazapine, phenelzine sulfate), antipsychotics (e.g., piperazine phenothiazine, risperidone, olanza- pine), anticonvulsants (e.g., carbamazepine, valproic acid), corticosteroids (e.g., corti- sone, prednisone), and oral contraceptives (e.g., combination, biphasic, and triphasic preparations) contribute to weight gain by promoting increased energy intake and increased body fat. Neuroendocrine abnormalities including polycystic ovarian syn- drome and hypothyroidism are sometimes associated with obesity, but these conditions contribute to less than 1% of obesity cases and rarely cause severe obesity.

It also appears that there may be susceptible genes that contribute to obesity. This susceptible gene hypothesis is supported by findings from twin studies in which pairs of twins were exposed to periods of positive and negative energy balance *(7)*. The differ- ences in the rate of weight gain, the proportion of weight gain, and the site of fat depo- sition showed greater similarities within pairs rather than between pairs. Obesity related syndromes such as Prader Willi are rare and usually detected in early childhood, resulting from overt clinical manifestations including hypogonadism, mental retardation, and short stature.

Recent research interest has focused on the molecular level of appetite modulation with factors like *leptin (8)* and *melanocortin (9)*. Genetic defects have been identified in animal models that are now being correlated with human obesity phenotypes.

4. DEFINING OBESITY

4.1. Body Mass Index

In clinical practice, it is practical to indirectly assess body fat by using an empirical formula that combines weight and height. Although there are exceptions, it is assumed that most variation in weight in persons of the same height is a result of fat mass and its distribution. Body mass index (BMI) measured as body weight in kg/height in m^2 is the formula used in most epidemiological studies. BMI allows meaningful comparisons of weight status within and between populations. It also allows for the identification of individuals at risk for adverse outcomes who may warrant intervention. The NIH released classification guidelines for BMI in 1998 (*see* Table 1). However, it is important to recognize that BMI guidelines have not yet been developed for the oldest-old.

Table 1
NIH Guidelines for Classification of Obesity

Weight status	BMI (kg/m^2)
Healthy weight	18.5–24.9
Overweight	25.0–29.9
Obesity class I	30.0–34.9
Obesity class II	35.0–39.9
Obesity class III	≥40.0

4.1.1. WAIST CIRCUMFERENCE AND WAIST-TO-HIP RATIO

Waist circumference and waist-to-hip ratio are also useful in the assessment of obesity because it is an android pattern of abdominal adiposity that is most strongly associated with comorbidities like cardiovascular disease, diabetes, and hypertension *(10)*. With the patient standing, the waist circumference is measured at its narrowest point and the hip circumference at its widest. Increased health risk for comorbid conditions including hypertension, diabetes, and cardiovascular disease has been reported for waist circumference ≥ 35 inches in females and ≥ 40 inches in males *(1)*. An abdominal fat distribution is indicated by a waist-to-hip ratio > 0.80 for females and > 0.95 for males.

5. INTERACTION WITH THE AGING PROCESS

5.1. Mortality

A J-shaped relationship has been detected between BMI and mortality in most observational studies. Individuals with low and high BMIs are at greater risk of mortality *(11)*. A 50–100% increase in risk of death as a result of all causes has been associated with BMI ≥ 30 *(1,11,12)*. Most of the increased mortality was associated with cardiovascular causes. Excess mortality was even detected in those aged 65–74 yr *(13)*. Early studies not adequately controlling for smoking or preexisting illness suggested that weight excess was associated with reduced mortality among the elderly. More rigorous studies have found that excess body weight increases risk of mortality from any cause and that the desirable BMI range for optimal health may be lower than previously thought *(14,15)*. After differences in weight were controlled, loss of body fat has been associated with decreased mortality risk in subjects age 42–58 yr *(16)*. Logically, obesity is a greater relative risk factor for mortality among youth and middle-aged when compared to older adults, likely reflecting a survivorship effect.

5.2. Comorbid Disease

Obesity is associated with increased chronic disease burden, including hypertension, type II diabetes, cardiovascular disease, and osteoarthritis. Increased risk of these comorbidities has been observed with excess body weight and is also associated with moderate weight gain (5 kg or more) in middle age *(13,15,17–20)*.

Hypertension is extremely prevalent in the United States today *(see* Chapter 16). It affects more than 50 million Americans, placing it among the most common chronic diseases in the United States *(21)*. Hypertension is also a known risk factor for premature death from cardiovascular disease, stroke, and renal failure. BMI and weight are the strongest predictors of blood pressure in humans *(22,23)*. This association has been observed in both sexes as well as in all age and ethnic groups *(22,24)*. Weight loss can reduce both blood pressure and the need for medication.

Obesity is also associated with increased risk of type II diabetes *(18,25,26)*. Sixty-seven percent of adults with type II diabetes have a BMI of at least 27 and 46% have a BMI of at least 30. At any given BMI, abdominal adiposity increases the risk for hyperinsulinemia and glucose intolerance *(17,27,28)*. NHANES II data revealed that the relative risk for developing diabetes was 3.8 times greater for obese persons aged 45–75 yr *(29)*. Physical activity and weight loss improve blood glucose control in diabetic patients *(17)* and can even reduce the need for medical management *(27)*. A recent study found that weight loss was associated with a 58% decrease in risk of developing overt diabetes in patients with impaired glucose tolerance *(30)*. Even a weight loss of as little as 5% of body weight has been shown to improve glycemic control *(31)*.

Obese adults are also at a greater risk for the development of cardiovascular disease. An increase in relative risk occurs at levels of being overweight previously considered to be insignificant. Analysis of the Framington cohort suggests that body weight is a significant predictor of coronary heart disease (CHD) independent of other factors *(32)*. In this study, the incidence of CHD increased by a factor of 2.4 in obese women and 2.0 in obese men under age 50 *(32)*. Rimm et al. *(33)* found a 72% increase in risk for fatal or nonfatal CHD in middle-aged men with BMI between 25 and 29 when compared with those having a BMI < 23. Age, sex, ethnicity, body fat distribution, and degree of fitness all affect the relationship between degree of overweight and the development of CHD *(34–36)*. In the Nurse's Cohort Study, women with a BMI between 25 and 28.9 had a twofold increase in risk of CHD, whereas those with BMI > 29 had a 3.6 increase in relative risk in comparison with women with BMI < 21 *(37)*.

Osteoarthritis is the most common type of arthritis, and its prevalence increases with aging. More than 70% of total hip and knee replacements are because of osteoarthritis *(19)*. The risk of developing osteoarthritis is increased by excess body weight resulting from the incremental stress on weight bearing joints *(19,20,38)*. NHANES I (1971–1975) *(19,38)* findings suggested that obese women (BMI 30–35) had a 4 times greater risk of developing osteoarthritis when compared with those having a BMI < 25 in adults ages 35–74 yr. For men in the same BMI range, the increased risk was 4.8. Although being overweight and obesity are risk factors for the development of osteoarthritis, increased body weight is associated with an apparent reduction in risk of developing osteoporosis *(39)*.

5.3. Functional Impairment

In addition to increasing the risk for the development of comorbid medical conditions, elevated BMI is associated with increased prevalence of functional limitation and disability *(40–46)*. In a longitudinal study of 2634 older persons age 65 yr and greater it was observed that women had a higher prevalence of functional decline than men at the upper ranges of BMI categories *(47)*. Both males and females at BMI ≥ 35 were found to be at significantly increased risk of reporting instrumental activities of daily living (IADL) decline or functional decline of any kind. Weight gain of at least 20 lbs over a 4-yr period was associated with increased risk of functional decline *(47)*. Higher BMI may influence the risk for disability by increasing stress on various joints or decreasing the flexibility of movement *(43)*. Associated medical comorbidities like heart disease, diabetes, and pulmonary disorders may also contribute to functional decline.

Sarcopenia is the decline in muscle mass that occurs with aging. Postulated causes of decreased muscle mass in the obese older person include inactivity, immobility, and deconditioning. Sarcopenic obesity may have a profound impact on the functional capacity of older persons. Appreciable muscle mass is required for movement, and limited mobility is the likely outcome of sarcopenia in obese individuals.

Although obesity is associated with functional decline there is the potential that weight loss could diminish these undesirable outcomes. Fine et al. *(48)* conducted a 4-yr follow-up that examined the impact of weight change among women in the Nurses' Health Study. Among a subset of these women who were greater than 65 yr of age they found that a weight loss of 20 lbs or greater was associated with a decline in physical functioning among those older women who had BMI < 25 and with improved physical functioning among those who were obese. Jensen and Friedmann *(47)* found that weight loss of 10 lbs was associated with functional decline among older persons, but the cohort did not include enough obese subjects with weight loss to do a valid subanalysis *(47)*. It is problematic in a cohort study to distinguish volitional weight reduction from that related to underlying disease or inflammatory condition. It is necessary to learn whether older adults should be targeted for moderate weight reduction or weight maintenance.

6. INTERVENTIONS AND TREATMENT

Strong evidence suggests weight loss in obese individuals may reduce risk for diabetes, hypertension, cardiovascular disease, and osteoarthritis. Who should be targeted for counseling or intervention? NIH guidelines suggest that middle aged adults with a BMI of 25–29.9 or greater should be counseled on the principles of weight loss and maintenance *(1)*. It is less clear what should be recommended for the older person. Certainly additional weight gain should be avoided by those who are overweight or obese. It would seem prudent to use an individualized approach and not exclude any patient from weight reduction intervention on basis of age alone.

The goals of weight loss and weight management should include (1) prevention of further weight gain; (2) reduction of body weight; and (3) maintenance of long-term weight loss. Prevention of further weight gain is especially important in older adults who may not be motivated to lose weight and/or those that fall into the BMI range for being overweight. In general, the initial weight loss goal should be losing 10% of current body weight over 6 mo. Once this is achieved, further weight loss attempts can be considered if warranted. The rate of weight loss should ideally be 0.45–0.90 kg/wk. After 6 mo of weight loss therapy, efforts should emphasize weight maintenance. The weight lost will usually be regained unless weight maintenance efforts are rigorously implemented. Reinforcement of diet therapy, physical activity, and behavior modification should be continued indefinitely. It should be emphasized that even modest weight reduction of 5 kg may reduce risk for development of comorbid conditions by 50% or more *(15,18,19,49)*.

6.1. Diet Therapy

In order for weight loss attempts to be successful, an energy deficit must be achieved. A deficit of 500–1000 kcal daily would translate into weight loss of 1–2 lbs weekly. Counseling by a registered dietitian is recommended. Calorie goals of 1200–1800 kcal/d are typical. Total calories consumed should not be less than 800 kcal/d. Very low-calorie diets (less than 800 kcal/d) should be considered only for selected obese middle-aged

Table 2
Low-Calorie Diet Guidelines for Weight Reduction

Nutrient	Recommended intake	
Calories	Approx 1200–1800/d	
Total fat	30% or less of total calories	
Saturated fatty acids	**Step I**	**Step II**
	8–10% of total calories	<7% of total calories
Monounsaturated fatty acids	Up to 15% of total calories	
Polyunsaturated fatty acids	Up to 10% of total calories	
Cholesterol	<300 mg/d	<200 mg/d
Protein	Approx 15% of total calories	
Carbohydrate	55% or more of total calories	
Sodium chloride	No more than 6 g/d	
Calcium	1000–1500 mg/d	
Fiber	20–30 g/d	

persons under close supervision. Experience with these diets among older persons is limited. Depending on the patient's cardiovascular risk status the diet therapy should be consistent with the National Cholesterol Education Program's Step I or Step II diet. Saturated fat intake should be limited to no more than 10% of total calories and no more than 30% of total calories should come from fat (Table 2). Diet therapy should include efforts aimed at ensuring that all of the recommended daily allowances are met and this may require the use of a vitamin supplement. Education should also include emphasis on adequate calcium intake and physical activity. This issue is of great importance in the preservation of bone mass during weight loss especially for middle- and older-aged women who are at risk of losing bone mass because of menopause. Loss of bone mineral has been detected among dieting older persons *(50)*. Adequate intake of calcium-rich foods should be emphasized, and supplementation should be considered in those whose intake is determined to be inadequate. Patients should be educated on food composition, preparation, and portion control and patient food preferences should be considered to improve compliance. Frequent contact with a qualified health care provider during diet therapy helps promote weight loss and maintenance.

Very low-calorie diets (VLCD) (<800 cal/d) are not recommended for general use. The goal of these diets is to severely decrease total energy intake while providing adequate dietary protein to avoid loss of lean body mass. These diets induce ketosis with rapid weight loss. Close monitoring is required as a result of fluid and electrolyte shifts. VLCDs are also associated with increased risk of the development of gallstones. Despite dramatic weight loss, recidivism is common because such diets are not practical for long-term use, and many patients on VLCDs learn little in regard to "real world" lifestyle modifications.

Promises of rapid weight loss are very attractive to consumers, but consumers and health care providers should be aware of the hazards associated with "fad" diets. Such diets often advocate the complete exclusion of certain groups of foods, thus placing consumers at increased risk for the development of nutrient deficiencies. Successful weight loss and maintenance programs should be based on sound scientific rationale, they must be safe and nutritionally adequate, as well as practical and applicable to the patient's social and ethnic background. If these principles do not apply to the prospective weight loss program, it should be avoided.

6.2. Physical Activity

Physical activity is the best predictor of long-term weight loss maintenance *(51,52)*. Additionally, physical activity has benefits with regard to decreased cardiovascular and diabetes risks beyond the benefits associated with weight reduction alone *(30)*. Additional benefits of physical activity include increased energy expenditure, decreased body fat, and maintenance of muscle and bone mass. Physical activity should be initiated slowly and gradually increased in intensity for obese patients. This is especially important in older adults. Physical ability (safety/suitability) can be assessed using a simple questionnaire (e.g., PAR-Q) to assess patient risk factors *(53)* as fear of injury discourages many older persons. Steps should also be taken to increase daily physical activities. These may include such activities as taking the stairs instead of the elevator, walking the dog, or playing with grandchildren. Mall-walking programs are available in many locations. The ultimate goal should be 30 min or more of moderate-intensity physical activity on most (preferably all) days of the week. These activities can be spread throughout the day. Swimming pool arthritis programs are an attractive option for older adults because of reduced burden on painful joints. For the frail older person who is obese, flexibility and resistance exercises can also be helpful to facilitate movement and enhance muscle mass, respectively *(54,55)*. Specific exercises should be closely supervised and prescribed by an exercise physiologist with expertise in this area. The exercises may involve light weights (1–3 lbs) or resistance bands and should be based on the capabilities of the individual.

6.3. Behavior Modification

Behavior modification involves the application of principles of social cognitive theory to modify behaviors that contribute to obesity *(1,56)*. These behavioral changes should be implemented to help achieve weight loss as well as weight maintenance and to facilitate overcoming barriers to both dietary and exercise compliance. Specific strategies may include self-monitoring of dietary intake and physical activity *(57)* as well as stress management. Other behavior modification tools include stimulus control, problem solving, rewards, cognitive restructuring, and social support *(55,58)*. Stimulus control involves identifying cues which seem to encourage undesirable eating behaviors. For example, a major behavioral concern is eating in front of the television, which has been associated with increased BMI *(59)*. Patients may also be encouraged to cognitively restructure unrealistic goals and inaccurate beliefs about weight. Unrealistic weight loss goals are a major contributor to recidivism.

6.4. Pharmacotherapy

Interventions involving diet, physical activity/exercise, and behavior modification are the mainstays of weight reduction therapy. These fundamental interventions should generally be undertaken for a trial period before other therapies are considered. Pharmacotherapy can be an option for patients with BMI ≥ 30 without risk factors and for those with BMI ≥ 27 with risk factors or underlying disease. However, there is only limited published experience with pharmacotherapy among older persons and their application in this population cannot be recommended at this time. Appropriate use of pharmacotherapy requires careful patient selection and close follow up. Patients who are treated with pharmacotherapy should also receive ongoing diet, physical activity/exercise, and behavior modification interventions.

The FDA has approved several medications for weight loss, but only two medications (sibutramine and orlistat) for long-term use greater than 3 mo. For short-term treatment less than 3 mo medications, such as mazindol, diethylpropion, phentermine, benzphetamine, and phendimetrazine may be used.

Two agents, fenfluramine and dexfenfluramine, that act to stimulate serotonin release and block its reuptake were removed from the market in September 1997 because of apparent associations with increased risk for primary pulmonary hypertension (PPH) and for valvular heart disease. Any patients with a history of using these medications should be screened to ensure that a cardiac evaluation was subsequently performed. Recent reports suggest that the risk for progression of valvular disease may be limited *(60)*.

Sibutramine (Meridia) was approved by the FDA in November of 1997 for long-term use (>3 mo) in obesity. Sibutramine inhibits the reuptake of norepinephrine and serotonin. Sibutramine functions as an anorexiant by increasing satiation and decreasing hunger. It moderately enhances weight loss and helps facilitate weight maintenance. Typical side effects may include increased heart rate by 3–6 beats/min and increased blood pressure by 4 mm Hg *(61)*. Sibutramine should not be used in patients with congestive heart failure, arrythmias, uncontrolled hypertension, coronary artery disease, or history of stroke.

Orlistat (Xenical) was approved by the FDA for long-term (>3 mo) in the treatment of obesity in April of 1999. Orlistat is not an appetite suppressant. It acts by inhibiting pancreatic lipase activity and reducing fat absorption. Fat-soluble vitamins should be supplemented in patients taking orlistat. If the patient does not lose 2 kg (4.4 lbs) in the first 4 wk of treatment the likelihood of long-term response is low. Gastrointestinal side effects can include bloating, cramps, and diarrhea.

Various herbal dietary supplements are widely promoted as weight loss aides. These supplements are not regulated by the FDA, therefore their use is not recommended. Certain ephedra alkaloids, including pheylpropanolamine, have been marketed with caffeine for weight loss. These products were banned in 1983 because of increased reports of adverse side effects *(62)*. Other dietary supplements that contain ephedra (ma huang) are widely promoted for weight loss and increased energy. Use of these products has been found to be associated with adverse reactions including cardiovascular symptoms such as hypertension, palpitations, and tachycardia. Central nervous system reactions like strokes and seizures have also been reported. As a result of these complications, the FDA has proposed limits on the dose and duration of use of supplements containing ephedra.

6.5. Weight Loss Surgery

Bariatric surgery is an option for a limited number of carefully selected middle-aged adults with clinically severe obesity. Advanced age (greater than 65 yr) and very serious comorbidities may predispose patients to an increased risk of adverse surgical outcomes. These patients are generally not considered candidates for bariatric surgery, but are evaluated on a case by case basis. In younger patients the goals of bariatric surgery are to increase longevity and improve quality of life. Guidelines for consideration are BMI ≥ 40 or BMI ≥ 35 with comorbid conditions (e.g., hypertension, dyslipidemia, diabetes, sleep apnea, degenerative joint disease) *(1)*. This type of intervention should be reserved only for patients in which multiple treatment efforts have failed and who are suffering from complications associated with severe obesity. Surgery should only be considered in those patients who are highly motivated and have acceptable operative risk. An integrated program to provide counseling on diet therapy, physical activity, and behavior modification with social support must be in place before and after surgery. The primary goal of bariatric surgery is to assist in the management of comorbid conditions associated with obesity. Weight loss associated with bariatric surgery has achieved improvement and even resolution of many comorbid conditions including type II diabetes, hypertension, sleep apnea, and obesity-related cardiomyopathy *(1,63–66)*. Because behavior modification is necessary for long-term success after surgery, patients with significant psychotic disorders, mental retardation, substance abuse, or self-destructive behavior should not be considered. Gastrointestinal surgeries in current use include gastric restriction (e.g., vertical gastric banding) and gastric bypass (e.g., Roux en Y). Gastric bypass can now be performed laparoscopically in some selected cases. Bariatric surgery offers the possibility of achieving and maintaining appreciable weight loss for persons who otherwise have had little success *(67)*. A new procedure called the gastric band is a purely nutrient restrictive procedure that involves placing a tight plastic band around the upper stomach to create a small proximal pouch. There are less operative risks and a shorter recovery period associated with this procedure. Weight loss results are similar to those experienced with vertical gastric banding *(68)*.

7. SUMMARY

Although data is limited, age alone should not preclude treatment for obesity in adult men and women. A clinical decision to forego obesity treatment in older adults should be guided by patient wishes and opportunity for benefit. It remains unclear whether the emphasis for older obese persons should be on weight loss or weight maintenance. It is likely that modest weight reduction can have appreciable health benefits for many middle- and older-aged persons. Steps should be taken to avoid adverse effects on muscle mass and bone density.

Once a moderate weight reduction is achieved, then efforts should focus on weight maintenance. Selected patients that fail conventional medical therapy are candidates for pharmacologic and surgical interventions (Table 3).

8. RECOMMENDATIONS FOR CLINICIANS

1. A complete history and physical and nutritional assessment should be conducted. This assessment should include calculation of BMI (kg/m^2) and waist-to-hip ratio as well as a discussion with the patient regarding these values. Increased health risk is associated with: BMI > 25 kg/m^2, waist circumference greater than 35 inches in females or greater than 40 inches in males, and/or waist-to-hip ratio > 0.80 in females or > 0.95 in males.
2. Additional information collected should include patient's satisfaction with current body weight and BMI, weight history, and previous weight loss attempts.
3. Current lifestyle habits should also be assessed such as current dietary patterns, smoking history, and degree of physical activity.
4. The patient's current state of health should be assessed as should comorbidity risks.
5. The weight loss plan should be individualized according to psychosocial, behavioral, and biological factors. The weight loss goals should be appropriate based on assessment,

Table 3
A Guide to Selecting Treatment

Treatment	BMI category (kg/m²)				
	25–26.9	27–29.9	30–34.9	35–39.9	≥ 40
Diet, physical activity, and behavior therapy	With comorbidities	+	+	+	+
Pharmacotherapy		With comorbidities	+	+	+
Bariatric surgery				With comorbidities	+

⁺Treatment indicated regardless of comorbidities (i.e., hypertension, dyslipidemia, diabetes).

encouraging a weight loss rate of 0.45–0.90 kg/wk with a final program goal of 10% of body weight over 6 mo.

6. The patient should be instructed on a calorie- and fat-restricted diet that includes a variety of foods. Education should also focus on adequate intakes of dietary calcium and fiber. Menus and recipes, restaurant dining, portion control, low-calorie snacking, and food preparation methods should all be discussed. Formal education by and contact with a registered dietitian is recommended.

7. Behavioral therapy should include self-monitoring of nutrient intake and physical activity. Stress management, stimulus control, problem solving, contingency management, and social support should be addressed.

8. Physical activity should be monitored. Reasonable goals are to increase daily activities and to participate in planned physical activity for 30 min daily.

9. Pharmacotherapy may be considered for patients who are compliant with dietary and activity guidelines yet continue to be unsuccessful at achieving weight loss. As a result of the lack of published experience among older persons, pharmacotherapy in this population cannot be recommended at this time.

10. Bariatric surgery for obesity is an option for patients who meet certain risk criteria and have failed multiple weight loss attempts.

11. Once weight loss is achieved weight maintenance efforts should be implemented to avoid weight regain. These efforts should include a healthy, low-calorie diet with physical activity of at least 30 min/d, follow-up encounters with a registered dietitian for accountability and reinforcement, as well as weekly measurement of body weight.

REFERENCES

1. National Institutes of Health. Clinical guidelines on the identification, evaluation, and treatment of overweight and obesity in adults: The Evidence Report. Obes Res 1998;6(suppl 2):51S–209S.

1a. Flegal KM, Carroll MD, Ogden CL, Johnson CL. Prevalence and trends in obesity among U.S. adults, 1999–2000. JAMA 2002;288:1723–1727.

2. Flegal KM, Carroll MD, Kuczmarski RJ, Johnson CL. Overweight and obesity in the United States: Prevalence and trends, 1960–1994. Int J Obes 1998;22:39–47.

3. Jensen G, Kita K, Fish J, Heydt D, Frey C. Nutrition risk screening characteristics of rural older persons: relation to functional limitations and health care charges. Am J Clin Nutr 1997;66:819–828.

4. Valencia ME, Bennett PH, Ravussin E, Esparza J, Fox C, Schulz LO. The Pima Indians in Sonora, Mexico. Nutr Rev 1999;57:S55–S57.

5. Morley J. Anorexia or aging: Physiologic and pathologic. Am J Clin Nutr 1997;66:760–773.
6. McDowell MA, Briefel RR, Alaimo K, Bischof AM, Caughman CR, Carroll MD, et al. Energy and macronutrient intakes of persons age 2 months and over in the United States: Third National Health and Nutrition Examination Survey, phase 1, 1998–1991. Advance Data 1994;255:1–3.
7. Bouchard C, Tremblay A, Despres JP, Nadeau A, Lupien PJ, Theriault G, et al. The response to long-term overfeeding in identical twins. N Engl J Med 1990;322:1477–1482.
8. Farooqi IS, Jebb SA, Langmack G, Lawrence E, Cheetham CH, Prentice AM, et al. Effects of recombinant leptin therapy in a child with congenital leptin deficiency. N Engl J Med 1999;331:879–884.
9. Ludwig DS, Tritos NA, Mastaitis JW, Rohit K, Kokkotou E, Elmquist J, et al. Melanin-concentrating hormone overexpression in transgenic mice leads to obesity and insulin-resistance. J Clin Invest 2001; 107:379–386.
10. Kissebah AH, Krakower GR. Regional adiposity and morbidity. Physiol Rev 1994;74:761–811.
11. Troiano RP, Frongillo EA Jr, Sobal J, Levitsky DA. The relationship between body weight and mortality: A quantitative analysis of combined information from existing studies. Int J Obes Relat Metab Disord 1996;20:63–75.
12. Manson JE, Stampfer MJ, Hennekens CH, Willet WC. Body weight and longevity: A reassessment. JAMA 1987;257:353–358.
13. Stevens J, Cai J, Pamuk ER, Williamson DF, Thun MJ, Wood JL. The effect of age on the association between body mass index and mortality. N Engl J Med 1998;338:1–7.
14. Voorrips LE, Meijers JH, Sol P, Seidell JC, van Staveren WA. History of body weight and physical activity of elderly women differing in current physical activity. Int J Obes Relat Metab Disord 1992; 16:199–205.
15. Huang Z, Willet WC, Manson JE, Rosner B, Stamfer MJ, Speizer FE, Colditz GA. Body change, weight change, and risk for hypertension in women. Ann Intern Med 1998;128:81–88.
16. Allison DB, Zannolli R, Faith MS, Heo M, Pietrobelli A, VanItallie TB, et al. Weight loss increases and fat loss decreases all cause mortality rate: Results from two independent cohort studies. Int J Obes Relat Metab Disord 1999;23:603–611.
17. Pi-Sunyer FX. Weight and non-insulin dependent diabetes mellitus. Am J Clin Nutr 1996;63(suppl): 426S–429S.
18. Colditz GA, Willet WC, Rotnitsky A, Manson JE. Weight gain as a risk factor for clinical diabetes in women. Ann Intern Med 1995;122:481–486.
19. Felson DT. Weight and osteoarthritis. Am J Clin Nutr 1996;63(Suppl):430S–432S.
20. Hochberg MC, Lethbridge-Cejku M, Scott WW, Reichle R, Plato CC, Tobin JD. The association of body weight, body fatness, and body fat distribution with osteoarthritis of the knee: Data from the Baltimore Longitudinal Study of Aging. J Rheumatol 1995;22:488–493.
21. Joint National Committee on Detection, Evaluation, and Treatment of High Blood Pressure. The fifth report of the Joint National Committee on Detection, Evaluation, and Treatment of High Blood Pressure. Arch Intern Med 1993;153:154–183.
22. Stamler R, Stamler J, Riedlinger WF, Algera G, Roberts RH. Weight and blood pressure. JAMA 1978; 240:1607–1610.
23. Dyer AR, Elliot P. The Intersalt Study: relations of body mass index to blood pressure. J Hum Hypertens 1989;3:299–308.
24. Wassertheil-Smoller S, Blaufox D, Oberman AS, Langford HG, Davis BR, Wylie-Rosett J. The trial of antihypertensive interventions and management (TAIM) study. Arch Intern Med 1992;152:131–136.
25. Chan JM, Rimm EB, Colditz GA, Stamfer MJ, Willett WC. Obesity, fat distribution, and weight gain as risk factors for clinical diabetes in men. Diabetes Care 1994;17:961–969.
26. Sowers J. Modest weight gain and the development of diabetes: another perspective. Ann Intern Med 1995;122:548–549.
27. Fitz JD, Sperling EM, Fein HG. A hypocaloric high-protein diet as primary therapy for adults with obesity-related diabetes: Effective long-term use in a community hospital. Diabetes Care 1983;6:328–333.
28. Lean MEJ, Hans TS, Seidell JC. Impairment of health and quality life in people with large waist circumference. Lancet 1998;351:853–856.
29. Van Itallie T. Health implications of overweight and obesity in the United States. Ann Intern Med 1985; 103:983–988.
30. Tuomilheto J, Linstrom J, Eriksson JG, Valle TT, Hamalainen H, Ilanne-prikka P, et al. Prevention of type 2 diabetes mellitus by changes in lifestyle among subjects with impaired glucose tolerance. N Engl J Med 2001;344:1343–1350.

31. Wing RR, Koeske R, Epstein LH, Nowalk MP, Gooding W, Becker D. Long-term effects of modest weight loss in type II diabetic patients. Arch Intern Med 1987;147:1749–1753.
32. Hubert HB, Feinleib M, McNamara P, Castelli WP. Obesity as an independent risk factor for cardiovascular disease: A 26-year follow-up of participants in the Framington Heart Study. Circulation 1983;67: 968–977.
33. Rimm EB, Stamfer MJ, Giovannucci E, et al. Body size and fat distribution as predictors of coronary heart disease among middle-aged and older U.S. men. Am J Epidemiol 1991;141:1117–1127.
34. Eckel RH. Obesity in heart disease. Circulation 1997;96:3248–3250.
35. Lee CD, Blair SN, Jackson AS. Cardiorespiratory fitness, body composition, and all-cause cardiovascular disease mortality in men. Am J Clin Nutr 1999;69:373–380.
36. Kissebah AH, Krakower GR, Sonnenberg GE, Hennes MMI. Clinical manifestations of the metabolic syndrome. In: Handbook of Obesity. Bray GA, Bouchard C, James WPT (eds.), Marcel Dekker, New York, NY, 1998 pp. 601–636.
37. Willett WC, Manson JE, Stamfer MJ, Colditz GA. Weight, weight change and coronary heart disease in women. JAMA 1995;273:461–465.
38. Felson DT. Does excess weight cause osteoarthritis and, if so, why? Ann Rheum Dis 1996;55:668–670.
39. Albala C, Yanez M, Devoto E, Sostin C, Zeballos L, Santos JL. Obesity as a prospective factor for postmenopausal osteoporosis. Int J Obes Relat Metab Disord 1996;20:1027–1032.
40. Hubert HB, Bloch DA, Fries JF. Risk factors for physical disability in an aging cohort: The NHANES I epidemiologic follow-up study. J Rheumatol 1993;20:480–488.
41. Ensrud KE, Nevitt MC, Yunis C, Cauley JA, Seeley DG, Fox KM, Cummings SR. Correlates of impaired function in older women. J Am Geriatr Soc 1994;42:481–489.
42. Galanos AN, Nevitt MC, Yunis C, Pieper CF, Cornoni-Huntley JC, Bales CN, Fillenbaum GG. Nutrition and function: Is there a relationship between body mass index and the functional capabilities of community-dwelling elderly. J Am Geriatr Soc 1994;42:368–373.
43. Launer LJ, Harris T, Rumpel C, Madana J. Body mass index, weight change, and risk of mobility disability in middle-aged and older women. JAMA 1994;271:1093–1098.
44. Coakley EH, Kawachi I, Manson JE, Speizer FE, Willet WC, Colditz GA. Lower levels of physical functioning are associated with higher body weight among middle-aged and older women. Int J Obes 1998;22:958–965.
45. Davis JW, Ross PD, Preston SD, Nevitt MC, Wasnich RD. Strength, physical activity, and body mass index: Relationship to performance based measures and activities of daily living among older Japanese women in Hawaii. J Am Geriatr Soc 1998;46:274–279.
46. Friedmann JM, Elasy T, Jensen GL. The relationship between body mass index and self-reported functional limitation among older adults: a gender difference. J Am Geriatr Soc 2001;49:398–403.
47. Jensen GL, Friedmann JM. Obesity is associated with functional decline among community dwelling rural older persons. J Am Ger Soc 2002;102:918–923.
48. Fine JT, Colditz GA, Coakely EH, Moseley G, Manson JE, Willett WC, Kawachi I. A prospective study of weight change and health-related quality of life in women. JAMA 1999;282:2136–2142.
49. Felson DT, Zhang Y, Anthony JM, Naimark A, Anderson JJ. Weight loss reduces the risk for symptomatic knee osteoarthritis in women. Ann Intern Med 1992;116:535–539.
50. Jensen LB, Kollerup G, Quaade F, Sorensen OH. Bone mineral changes in obese women during a moderate weight loss with and without calcium supplementation. J Bone Miner Res 2001;16:141–147.
51. Pate RR, Pratt M, Blair SN. Physical activity and public health. A recommendation from the Centers for Disease Control and Prevention and the American College of sports Medicine. JAMA 1995;27: 402–407.
52. NIH Consensus Conference. Physical activity and cardiovascular health. JAMA 1996;276:241–246.
53. Thomas S, Reading J, Shepard RJ. Revision of the physical activity readiness questionnaire. Can J Sport Sci 1992;17:338–345.
54. Hurley BF, Roth SM. Strength training in the elderly: Effects on risk factors for age-related disease. Sports Med 2000;30:249–268.
55. Keysor JJ, Jette AM. Have we oversold the benefit of late-life exercise? J Gerontol A Biol Sci Med Sci 2001;56:M412–423.
56. Foreyt JP, Poston WS. What is the role of cognitive-behavior therapy in patient management? Obes Res 1998;(suppl 1):18S–22S.
57. Boutelle KN, Kirschenbaum DS. Further support for consistent self-monitoring as a vital component of successful weight control. Obes Res 1998;6:219–224.

58. Foreyt JP, Poston WS. The role of the behavioral counselor in obesity treatment. J Am Diet Assoc 1998 Oct;98(10 suppl 2):S27–S30.

59. Crespo CJ, Smit E, Troiano RP, Bartlett SJ, Macera CA, Andersen RE. Television watching, energy intake, and obesity in US children: Results from the NHANES III 1988–1994. Arch Pediatr Adolesc Med 2001;155:360–365.

60. Burger AJ, Sherman HB, Charlamb MJ, Kim J, Asinas LA, Flickner SR, Blackburn GL. Low prevalence of valvular heart disease in 226 phentermine-fenfluramine protocol subjects prospectively followed for up to 30 months. J Am Coll Cardiol 1999;34:1153–1158.

61. Bray GA, Ryan DH, Gordon D, Heidingsfelder S, Cerise F, Wilson K. A double-blind randomized placebo-controlled trial of Sibutramine. Obes Res 1996;4:263–270.

62. Haller CA, Benowitz NL. Adverse cardiovascular and central nervous system events associated with dietary supplements containing ephedra. N Engl J Med 2000;343:1833–1838.

63. Pories WJ, Swanson MS, MacDonald KG, Long SB, Morris PG, Brown BM, et al. Who would have thought it? An operation proves to be the most effective treatment for adult-onset diabetes mellitus. Ann Surg 1995;222:339–352.

64. Alpert MA, Singh A, Terry BE, Kelly DL, Villarreal D, Mukerji V. Effect of exercise on left ventricular systolic function and reserve in morbid obesity. Am J Card 1989;63:1478–1482.

65. Foley EF, Benotti PN, Borlase BC. Impact of gastric restrictive surgery on hypertension in the morbidly obese. Am J Surg 1992;186:294–297.

66. Sugarman HJ, Fairman RP, Baron PL, Kwentus JA. Gastric surgery for respiratory insufficiency of obesity. Chest 1986;90:81–86.

67. Maclean LD, Rhode BM, Sampalis J, Forse RA. Results of the surgical treatment of obesity. Am J Surg 1993.165;155–159.

68. Morino M, Toppino M, Garrone C, Morino F. Laparoscopic adjustable silicone gastric banding for the treatment of morbid obesity. Br J Surg 1994;81:1169.

E. Alimentary Tract Disorders

23 Oral Health and Nutrition

Christine Seel Ritchie and Kaumudi Joshipura

1. ORAL HEALTH STATUS IN OLDER ADULTS

Oral health contributes greatly to quality of life in older adults. Oral health can add to or hinder a person's ability to sustain a satisfying diet, participate in interpersonal relationships and maintain a positive self-image. Oral health problems may lead to chronic pain and discomfort and alterations in diet. Deterioration in oral health is not an inevitable consequence of aging but results from the cumulative effects of lifestyle and environmental factors, medication use and disease.

Tooth loss generally results from extractions for periodontal disease or caries. Aging or the cumulative effect of factors over time produces a number of dental changes including wear, attrition, and yellowing of older teeth. The bones of the maxilla and mandible are subject to the same changes seen in other parts of the body, including bone resorption and formation. Jaw or alveolar bone will atrophy with tooth loss, especially when unresolved for long periods, which may make fitting of dentures more difficult. Alveolar bone resorption accelerates with both local disease, such as periodontal disease and systemic conditions like osteoporosis *(1)*. With healthy aging, there is no decrease in salivary production, however, medications and some systemic conditions, such as Sjogren's syndrome (an autoimmune disorder characterized by loss of salivary function) alter saliva production substantially *(2)*. Subtle changes in saliva occur with aging and include alterations in mucin concentration that can lead to decreased lubrication, and changes in the protective ability of salivary secretory IgA antibody *(3)*.

1.1. Common Oral Conditions in Older Adults

1.1.1. DENTAL CARIES, PERIODONTAL DISEASE, AND TOOTH LOSS

Tremendous variation exists in the oral health of older adults. Caries rates, tooth loss and soft tissue lesions vary tremendously by socioeconomic status and region. Although dental caries are generally considered a disease of children and younger adults, recent studies suggest that a significant increase in caries occurs with aging. Decay that is seen with aging may be seen around restorations, at the gingival margin, and at the root following exposure because of gingival recession *(4)*. Nearly one third of people 65 yr or older have untreated dental caries *(5)*.

From: *Handbook of Clinical Nutrition and Aging*
Edited by: C. W. Bales and C. S. Ritchie © Humana Press Inc., Totowa, NJ

Like caries, periodontal diseases are infections caused by bacteria in plaque. Accumulation of plaque and calculus (plaque that calcifies) produces a low-grade inflammatory process of the gingiva or gums. If the inflammatory process is allowed to progress to involve the underlying alveolar (jaw) bone and connective tissue, teeth loosen and eventually extrude resulting from the loss of bony and connective tissues support. Periodontal disease involves the reduction in the connective tissue (known as attachment loss) and alveolar bone supporting the teeth and is common among adults. Because the impact of periodontal disease is cumulative, manifested as loss of attachment and alveolar bone loss, the severity of periodontal disease or prevalence (defined as bone loss or attachment loss greater or equal to a certain threshold) increases with age, however, the incidence of new periodontal disease does not increase with age. Within each ethnic group, the highest proportion of those affected is among those 70 yr and older (6).

Tooth loss commonly occurs because of extractions indicated resulting from severe periodontal disease or dental caries (7). Although the edentulous rate (those who have lost all their natural teeth) increases with aging, wide regional variation exists in the percentages of the population aged 65 and older without teeth. In Hawaii, 13.9% of adults 65 and older are edentulous, whereas in West Virginia, the rate is 47.9% (8). In general, however, older Americans are retaining more of their teeth than ever before, putting them at increased risk for root caries and periodontal disease (9).

1.1.2. SOFT TISSUE LESIONS

Recurrent aphthous ulcers (RAU) is a common mucosal disease. It has been associated with hypersensitivities to specific foods, food dyes, and food preservatives (10). Nutritional deficiencies, especially of iron, folic acid, and various B vitamins, have also been reported to be common in individuals with apthous ulcers, and improvements are noted with suitable dietary supplements (11). Symptomatic treatment includes tetracycline mouth rinse, betamethasone gel, beclomethasone spray, and amlexanox 5% topical paste, all of which significantly reduce ulcer duration and pain (10,12).

Because older adults are often edentulous (without teeth) and wear partial or complete dentures, oral candidiasis is also more common in this population. Candidiasis often causes symptoms of burning and soreness in the mouth, sensitivity to acidic and spicy foods, a foul taste in the mouth, or may be asymptomatic. The most common form of oral candidiasis is denture stomatitis caused by continuous wearing of ill-fitting or inadequately cleaned dental appliances (chronic erythematous candidiasis). Candidal angular cheilosis occurs in folds at the angles of the mouth and is closely related to a denture sore mouth (13). Another common form of Candida infection is pseudomembranous candidiasis (thrush), affecting any of the mucosal surfaces. These infections occur more often among those with protein-calorie malnutrition, resulting from the accompanying alterations in T-cell related immunity that occur with that condition. Candida infections can generally be controlled with antifungal medications used locally or systemically.

The most serious and potentially fatal oral condition among older adults is oral cancer. Each year in the United States, approx 30,200 new cases of oral and pharyngeal cancers are diagnosed and about 7800 people die from these cancers (14). Life expectancy is shortened in oral cancer by an average of 17 yr. The median age at diagnosis is 64, and rates of recurrence rise with age. The overall 5-yr survival rate for people with oral and pharyngeal cancer is 52% and has not changed in the past 25 yr (15).

1.2. Impact of Chronic Disease on Oral Health

Older adults experience a host of chronic diseases, many of which have oral manifestations or adversely affect oral health. In response to chronic diseases, older adults use increasing numbers of medications. Many of these medications have negative consequences on the mouth, most notably in contributing to the development of xerostomia (dry mouth), which may increase risk for dental caries, tooth wear, periodontal disease, pain or inflammation of the tongue, oral injury or infection, and dysfunction of chewing, speech, swallowing, and taste *(16)*.

2. IMPACT OF NUTRITIONAL STATUS ON ORAL HEALTH

2.1. Plaque and Calculus Formation

Bacteria in the mouth, or oral flora, form plaque, a complex community or biofilm that adheres to teeth. These bacteria ferment sugars and carbohydrates and generate acid that can dissolve minerals in tooth enamel and lead to dental caries.

Plaque can be present in subjects who do not consume carbohydrates, but is more prolific and produces more acid in individuals who eat sucrose-rich food. Frequency of carbohydrate consumption, physical characteristics of food (e.g., softness and stickiness), and timing of food intake all contribute to plaque formation *(17,18)*.

Plaque on tooth surfaces mineralizes to form calculus or tartar, which is often covered by unmineralized biofilm. Calculus exacerbates local inflammatory responses and may set up a long-standing gingival infection *(19)*.

2.2. Dental Caries

Although the presence of bacteria is critical to caries initiation, diet plays an important role in caries occurrence and progression. Foods containing fermentable carbohydrates result in acid production by cariogenic plaque bacteria. When plaque pH falls below 5.5 for an appreciable period of time, demineralization is likely to occur, which if left unchecked can advance to form a cavity that can extend through the dentin (the part of the tooth located under the enamel) to the pulp tissue.

Dietary control of dental caries requires modifying the form and quantity of fermentable carbohydrate ingestion (*see* Table 1) and avoidance of foods that are cariogenic. The acidogenic activity of foods determine their cariogenic potential *(20)*. In addition, oral clearance time impacts cariogenicity. The role of frequency of food consumption is not clear. Although the form of sugar may be important, food that may be perceived as "sticky" may not be cariogenic and vice versa *(6)*. The total amount of sugar and fermentable carbohydrates in the diet seems to be the most important consideration, and those with high caries susceptibility should be advised to curtail their intake. Artificial sweeteners, such as aspartame and saccharin and sugar alcohols (e.g., sorbitol) mannitol and xylitol, are noncariogenic in clinical trials *(21)*. Saliva also contains components that can directly attack cariogenic bacteria, and contains calcium and phosphates that help remineralize tooth enamel.

2.3. Periodontal Disease

The role of nutrients in periodontal disease appears related to conditions that lead to increases in dental plaque, impairment of host defenses and weakened integrity of the

Table 1
Dietary Behaviors Affecting Caries Risk

Behaviors promoting caries risk	Behaviors reducing caries risk
• Excessive ingestion of dietary acids such as lemons, oranges, fruit juices, and carbonated beverages (can result in severe dental erosion) • Excessive ingestion of fermentable carbohydrates	• Consumption of green tea • Substitution of sugar with "sugar-free" sweeteners • Ingestion of cheese (reduces oral ph) • Chewing sugar-free gum (increases salivary flow) • Eating carbohydrates with food or water • Good oral hygiene practices

Source: Adapted from Makenin and Philosophy *(22)*.

periodontal tissues. Several surveys suggest that inadequate calcium intake is associated with greater levels of periodontal disease *(23)*. Krall et al. *(24)* showed that calcium supplementation in postmenopausal women with deficient calcium intake protected against tooth loss. Deficiencies of ascorbate and folate have been associated with severity of gingivitis (a precursor of periodontal disease) *(25,26)*, but less closely associated with periodontal disease. Given our current understanding of the role of immune function and inflammatory response in periodontal disease, it is likely that immune-modulating nutrients, such as some antioxidants and omega-three fatty acids, could alter the inflammatory process in periodontal disease.

Recently an interesting association between periodontal disease and obesity has been noted in Saito's study of Japanese adults. Increasing body mass index and waist-hip ratio was associated with increasing risk of periodontitis *(27)*. Given recent evidence regarding adipose tissue as a reservoir for inflammatory cytokines, it is possible that increasing body fat increases the likelihood of an active host inflammatory response in periodontal disease *(28)*.

2.4. Oral Cancer

Oral and pharyngeal cancers (OC) include tumors affecting the oral cavity and pharynx, the majority of which are squamous cell carcinoma. About half a million cases arise annually worldwide *(29)*. The overall 5-yr survival rate is about 52% with early detection the key to improving the survival rate *(14)*. Oral cancer is generally preceded by precancerous lesions, which include oral epithelial dysplasia, erythroplakia, leukoplakia, lichen planus, and submucous fibrosis (rare in Western countries). The major risk factors for OC are tobacco and alcohol use. In Asian countries chewing tobacco, beetle nut and beetle quid are major risk factors. Chewing tobacco use is also increasing in the United States. The relation between nutrition and oral cancer, and the impact of oral cancer on the patient's ability to eat and swallow are discussed below.

2.4.1. FRUITS AND VEGETABLES

A consistent finding across numerous studies is that a diet high in fruits and vegetables is protective against oral precancer *(30,31)* and cancer *(32,33)*. A generous consumption of fruits was associated with a 20–80% reduced risk of OC even when smoking and alcohol intake and other factors including total caloric intake were taken into account *(34–36)*. Vegetables are also protective *(33,37)* although not all studies show a protective effect *(38)*. The inconsistencies may be explained by variation in specific vegetables consumed and there seems a suggestion that raw vegetables may be more protective than cooked. A study evaluating specific fruits and vegetables suggested that green vegetables, salad, and apples were more protective. Tomato shows a strong and consistent protective effect for oral cancer in 12 of 15 studies *(39)*, and in one study on leukoplakia *(30)*. Raw tomatoes were more protective than cooked tomatoes *(39)*. A protective effect was also found for raw vegetables among Japanese adults *(40)*. Glutathione—an antioxidant found in fruits and vegetables was protective only if it was derived from fruit and raw vegetables *(41)*.

2.4.2. ANTIOXIDANTS

Several antioxidants found in vegetables and fruits show a protective effect against oral cancer. Specific antioxidants including vitamin A, vitamin B_{12}, vitamin C, tocopherol (vitamin E), retinoids, carotenoids, lycopene, beta-carotene, folate, glutathione, thiamine, Vitamin B_6, folic acid, niacin, α-tochopherol, and lutein have been shown to be protective against oral cancer *(34,42–47)* and precancer *(30,48–57)* in one more or more studies. Studies that have evaluated subgroups have generally found higher beneficial effects of fruits and vegetables and their constituent micronutrients among smokers and drinkers than among abstainers *(52)*.

Retinoids and beta carotene in controlled therapeutic doses show protective effects, with fewer new primary tumors in persons with previous oral cancers and reversals or reduction in size of premalignant lesions *(53–55)*. High doses of 13-cis-retinoic acid (50–100 mg/m^2 body surface area/d for a year) have been effective in the treatment of oral leukoplakia *(46)*. Sixty-seven percent of patients with this condition showed major decreases in lesion size vs 10% among placebo group and in prevention of second primary tumors *(56)* (2% had secondary tumors after a median follow up of 32 mo vs 12% in placebo group). Trials using beta-carotene supplements (60 mg/d for 6 mo) have shown reduced risk of oral cancers and remission of precancers with an improvement of at least one grade dysplasia in 39% and no change in 61% *(57)*.

2.4.3. OTHER FOOD AND NUTRIENTS

A protective effect of fiber was observed for both oral submucous fibrosis and leukoplakia *(30)* and for oral cancer *(32,47)*. There is a suggestion that meat *(47,58)*, desserts, maize, and saturated fats and/or butter may be risk factors *(58–60)* and that olive oil may be protective *(59)*. Nitrate, nitrite, and nitrate reductase activity in saliva *(61)* and high intake of nitrite containing meats *(32)*, have been linked to increased risk. Iron may be protective against OC *(49)* and leukoplakia *(34)*.

2.5. Nutrient Deficiencies Affecting the Tongue

A number of vitamin deficiencies have oral manifestations, that affect the tongue. Riboflavin deficiency may cause glossitis, swelling and erythema of the oral mucosa. Individuals with niacin deficiency may also present with oral manifestations, including stomatitis and glossitis, with the tongue appearing red, smooth, and raw. Findings with pyridoxine deficiency may be similar to that seen with niacin deificiency. Because these vitamin deficiencies are fairly rare in developed countries, most clinicians may not see patients with a specific vitamin deficiency. Clinicians are more likely to see patients on a "milk toast" diet who have multiple vitamin deficiencies due to poor intake of a number of micronutrients.

In iron-deficiency anemia, the glossitis that occurs has been described as a diffuse or patchy atrophy of the dorsal tongue papillae, in some cases accompanied by pain. Vitamin B_{12} deficiency may be accompanied by oral manifestations including atrophy and erythema of the dorsal tongue and oral mucosa with burning sensations in the affected area. In all of the cases noted previously, treatment is based on identifying and correcting the primary cause that in most cases will alleviate tongue symptoms (62).

3. IMPACT OF ORAL HEALTH ON NUTRITION

3.1. Impact of Altered Dentition on Nutrition

A number of studies have demonstrated an association between tooth loss and dietary intake. Many studies show that edentulous individuals are more likely to eat an unhealthy diet (e.g., ingesting too few nutrient-dense foods and too much calorie-rich, high-fat foods) compared to people with natural teeth. In studies of healthy older adults, edentulous individuals have been noted to consume fewer fruits and vegetables, lower amounts of fiber, and higher amounts of fat (63,64). Joshipura et al. (65) observed that edentulous male health professionals consumed fewer vegetables, less fiber and carotene, more cholesterol, saturated fat and calories than participants with 25 or more teeth after adjusting for age, smoking, exercise, and profession. Edentate individuals are more likely to have lower intakes of micronutrients, such as calcium, iron, pantothenic acid, vitamins C and E than their dentate counterparts (66). In summary, most of the studies relating tooth loss and nutrition suggest that nutrient intake diminishes with fewer teeth. These changes seen in fruit, vegetable, and micronutrient intake with tooth loss may partially explain the recent findings suggesting associations between tooth loss and cardiovascular disease. Thus, patients with tooth loss warrant aggressive counseling regarding methods to maintain dietary quality, such as blending or shredding fresh fruits and vegetables to preserve adequate intake.

Although eating with dentures may be preferable to eating without teeth, most studies suggest that denture use only partly compensates for missing teeth. In Krall et al. (67) study of veterans, individuals with full dentures consumed fewer calories, thiamine, iron, folate, vitamin A and carotene than individuals with other dentitions. Papas et al. (68) evaluated the impact of full dentures and noted both lower intake of protein and 19 other nutrients. In a separate population, Papas et al. (69) reported that subjects who wore dentures consumed more refined carbohydrates, sugar and dietary cholesterol than their dentate counterparts. The above studies suggest that the presence of dentures contributes to poorer intake across multiple nutrients compared to dentate subjects. Poor denture fit may contribute to some of these differences. In a study of denture wearers in Quebec, those that wore dentures providing poor masticatory performance consumed significantly less fruits and vegetables than those with dentures that provided good masticatory performance (70). Likewise in Swedish older adults, poorly fitting upper dentures were associated with decreased intake of vitamin C (71). Among older Australians, women who reported poorly fitting dentures consumed greater amounts of sweets and dessert items (72). Therefore, patients with dentures should be questioned regarding denture fit. If dentures fit poorly, appropriate referrals to dental professionals should be made.

In addition to comparing diets between individuals with natural teeth and individuals with dentures, studies have also examined dietary differences among edentulous subjects with and without dentures. Not surprisingly, edentulous subjects without dentures consumed more mashed food (73) and in a study of Swedish women, edentulous women without dentures consumed more fat (64). Whether the placement of dentures in an edentulous patient makes a substantial difference in the patient's intake remains unclear. Garett et al. (74) conducted a randomized trial of no dentures, fixed partial dentures (FPD) and removable partial dentures (RPD) among the partially edentulous and found no differences in intake between the groups. Sebring et al. (75) studied the affect of conventional maxillary and implant-supported or conventional mandibular dentures on patients who were edentulous with no prostheses. In both groups, calorie intake decreased; percentage of calories from fat also decreased significantly over the subsequent 3 yr. Lindquist (76) evaluated the impact of prosthetic rehabilitation, using optimized complete dentures and then tissue-integrated mandibular fixed prostheses (TIP) on 64 dissatisfied complete denture wearers. There was no change in diet after optimizing complete dentures, but there was a persistent increase in fresh fruit consumption after placement of TIP. Olivier et al. (77) evaluated dietary counseling in addition to prosthetic relining for the edentulous on chewing efficiency, dietary fiber intake from various sources and gastrointestinal esophageal, and colonic symptoms. Chewing ability and fiber intake from fruits and vegetables were significantly improved. However, because all groups received dietary counseling, it was not possible to separate the effect of relining from the counseling. In summary, dietary quality may improve with the placement of dental prostheses, but the changes are not substantial. Dietary counseling at the same time prostheses are fitted may assist patients in behavioral change and optimize the impact of their new chewing capabilities.

The relationship between dental status and weight, weight/height, and body mass index (BMI) varies with the population studied. In Mojon et al. (78) study of nursing home residents, compromised oral functional status was associated with a BMI of less than 21 kg/m^2, after controlling for functional dependence and age. In Hirano et al. (79) study of community-dwelling older adults, the authors reported a similar association between masticatory ability and lower body weight, after controlling for age and sex. However, in Johansson et al. (63) cross-sectional study of healthier older adults, edentulous patients actually had higher BMIs, compared to dentate subjects. In Elwood and Bate's (80) study of older Welsh adults, there was a trend toward higher weight and height/weight among subjects with no teeth or dentures. The differences in findings in these studies may result from the different characteristics of the populations evaluated, with sicker older adults more likely to lose weight in response to altered dentition, and healthier older adults more likely to maintain adequate intake but alter intake to softer foods that are more calorie-dense.

The largest study to date to evaluate blood nutrient status in relation to dental status is the British National Diet and Nutrition Survey (66). In their cross-sectional study of 490 free-living and institutionalized older adults, the authors reported that edentate subjects had significantly lower mean plasma levels of retinol, ascorbate and tocopherol than dentate subjects, after controlling for age, sex, social class, and region of residence.

Among dentate subjects, mean plasma vitamin C levels were positively associated with increased numbers of occlusal pairs of teeth. Another study of adults in Sweden *(63)* reported lower serum high-density lipoprotein (HDL) levels among edentulous individuals compared to those who were dentate.

In summary, individuals with compromised dentition tend to have poorer dietary quality. Clinicians should inquire about dentition status and strategize with patients regarding improving dietary quality in the context of patients' oral health limitations.

3.2. Impact of Oral Cancer on Nutrition

Oral cancer has a major impact on eating and swallowing. The location or progression of the tumor itself and the side effects of treatment hamper feeding and swallowing. Side effects of radiation, primarily a result of damage to the salivary glands and reduction in saliva production, include xerostomia, dental caries, oral mucositis, and bacterial and fungal infections. Side effects of chemotherapy include mucositis, fungal infections, xerostomia, throat and mouth pain, taste changes, food aversions, nausea, and diarrhea. Other complications include aspiration, osteoradionecrosis and trismus (restricted opening of the jaw) *(81)*. Side effects of surgery vary according to location and extent of surgery. The oral phase of swallowing is affected by surgical resection *(82)*. Means to counter common problems faced by OC patients are listed in Table 2. These interventions can improve nutritional intake and overall quality of life.

3.3. Impact of Other Oral Pain on Nutrition

Studies of patients with non-malignancy related chronic oral pain have not focused on nutritional outcomes. The only study of temporomandibular disorder pain dysfunction syndrome (TDPDS) is limited in size and scope with a suggestion that dietary choices are negatively impacted by TDPDS symptoms *(83)*. In a broader study of orofacial discomfort, no relationship was identified between multiple orofacial complaints and dietary intake *(84)*. This relationship warrants more study given the many anecdotal reports associating oral pain with alterations in nutrient intake.

3.4. Impact of Xerostomia on Nutrition

With xerostomia, individuals may have inadequate lubrication and moisture in the mouth to chew food and create an adequate food bolus for swallowing. In addition, xerostomia may contribute to altered taste perception and to food sticking to the tongue or hard palate. Three studies of xerostomia have found that diet/nutrition and the quality of saliva were affected by Sjogren's Syndrome and xerogenic medications. Loesche et al. *(85)* reported that individuals with complaints of xerostomia were more likely to avoid crunchy vegetables (e.g., carrots), dry foods (e.g., bread) and sticky foods (e.g. peanut butter). Rhodus et al. *(86)* studied 28 patients with Sjogren's syndrome and compared them to a group of controls matched on diabetes, depression, cardiovascular disease, arthritis, age, gender and dental health. Caloric and micronutrient intakes were significantly lower among xerostomic patients. Rhodus and Brown *(87)* also evaluated 84 older residents of an extended care facility. Energy, protein, fiber, vitamin A, C, and B_6, thiamine, riboflavin, calcium and iron were significantly lower in the patients with xerostomia than those without. These studies suggest that xerostomia impairs optimal nutrient intake, however, these studies are hampered by

Table 2
Problem of Oral Cancer Patients and Management

Problem	Management
Xerostomia—which could lead to other problems such as caries	Sugar-free mints and gums, artificial saliva, increased intake of water, or induce medically by pilocarpine hydrochloride administration
Increased caries susceptibility	Instruction on oral hygiene and avoidance of food high in sugar, dental referral daily fluoride gel
Trismus makes chewing difficult	Recommend appropriate jaw exercises
Dysphagia	Assess swallowing ability and risk of aspiration, monitor feeding capabilities, modify food consistency as indicated, use alternative route of nutritional support if necessary
Risk of aspiration	Use airway protection techniques and use of feeding devices as indicated
Malnutrition	Obtain a dietary consultation. Consider enteral or parenteral routes for patients who cannot meet their nutritional needs by mouth

Source: Minasian and Dwyer (81).

their small size and cross-sectional design. Rhodus et al. (86) noted that the body mass index for the xerostomic individuals with Sjogren's syndrome was significantly lower than for the control group. In their study of older extended care facility residents, they also noted a significantly lower body mass index among the xerostomic subjects (87). Dormenval et al. (88) evaluated hospitalized older adults and noted that low unstimulated salivary flow rates were associated with low body mass index, triceps skin fold thickness and arm circumference.

4. CONCLUSION

Oral conditions that affect and are affected by nutrition, including dental caries, periodontal disease, xerostomia and oral cancer, are more common in older adults. Dietary behaviors contribute substantially to the development of dental caries throughout life. Avoidance of in-between meal snacks, use of sugar-free candy or gum, and consumption of carbohydrates with meals and water can reduce caries incidence. Nutritional modulation of immune function through the use of antioxidants may reduce progression of periodontal disease, but studies are lacking. Many epidemiologic studies and a few randomized controlled trials have demonstrated the protective effect of fruits and vegetables and antioxidants on oral cancer risk. Studies suggest tooth loss impacts dietary quality and nutrient intake in a manner that may increase risk for several systemic diseases. Further, impaired dentition may contribute to weight change, depending on age and other population characteristics. Attention to dietary quality is particularly important among individuals with chewing disability from tooth loss or edentulousness. Patients with oral cancer experience numerous complications that increase their risk for poor dietary intake. Close attention should be given to prevention of caries in patients with xerostomia, treatment of pain in patients with mucositis, modification of food consistency in patients with dysphagia, and alternative feeding routes if nutritional needs cannot be met orally.

5. RECOMMENDATIONS FOR CLINICIANS

1. Clinicians should advise their dentate patients to restrict between-meal snacks, eat carbohydrates with meals, and limit foods that are cariogenic.
2. Consumption of fruits and vegetables appears to reduce risk for the development of oral cancer.
3. Supplementation with retinoids should be considered for patients at high risk for oral cancer. Beta-carotene has also been demonstrated to reduce oral cancer risk.
4. Vitamin deficiencies of iron, B_{12}, niacin and pyridoxine should be considered in patients with glossitis and poor dietary intake.
5. Patients with poor dentition are at increased risk for poor/inappropriate dietary intake. Clinicians should counsel patients regarding ways to increase intake of nutrient-dense foods and minimize softer calorie-dense, nutrient-poor foods. Pureed or shredded fruits and vegetables may serve as a means of insuring adequate intakes of these food groups. A multivitamin should be considered in this group as well.
6. Patients with oral cancer and radiation-induced xerostomia should be counseled to use sugar-free mints and gums and routinely apply fluoride to teeth to prevent dental caries in.

REFERENCES

1. Bhaskar S. Maxilla and Mandible (Alveolar Process). Orban's Oral Histology and Embryology. Mosby Year Book, St. Louis, MO, 1991, pp. 239–259.
2. Baum B. Age changes in salivary glands and salivary secretions. In: Geriatric Dentistry. Pederson PH, Loe H, eds. Copenhagen, Munksgaard, 1986, pp. 114–122.
3. Navazesh M, Mulligan RA, Kipnis V, et al. Comparison of whole saliva flow rates and mucin concentrations in healthy Caucasian young and aged adults. J Dent Res 1992;71:1275–1278.
4. Beck J, Hunt RJ, Hand JS, Field JM. Prevalence of root and coronal caries in a noninstitutionalized older population. J Am Dent Assoc 1985;111:964–967.
5. Vargas CM, Yellowitz JA. The oral health of older Americans. CDC and Prevention National Center for Health Statistics Aging Trends 2001:1–6.
6. Burt BA. Dentistry, Dental Practice, and the Community. 5th ed. W.B. Saunders Company, Philadelphia, PA, 1999.
7. Phipps KR. Relative contribution of caries and periodnotal disease in adult tooth loss for an HMO dental population. J Public Health Dent 1995;55:250–252.
8. Tomar S. Total tooth loss among persons aged greater than or equal to 65 years—selected states, 1995–1997. MMWR 1997;48:206–210.
9. Douglass CW, Shih A. Denture usage in the United States: A 25 year prediction. J Dent Res 1998;77:209.
10. Ship JA. Recurrent aphthous stomatitis. An update. Oral Surg Oral Med Oral Pathol Oral Radiol Endod 1996;81:141–147.
11. Nolan A, McIntosh WB, Allam BF, Lamey PJ. Recurrent aphthous ulceration: Vitamin B1, B2 and B6 status and response to replacement therapy. J Oral Pathol Med 1991;20:389–391.
12. Khandwala A, Van Inwegen RG, Charney MR, Alfano MC. Five % amlexanox oral paste, a new treatment for recurrent minor aphthous ulcers: II. Pharmacokinetics and demonstration of clinical safety. Oral Surg Oral Med Oral Pathol Oral Radiol Endod 1997;83:231–238.
13. Field EA, Speechley JA, Rugman FR, et al. Oral signs and symptoms in patients with undiagnosed vitamin B12 deficiency. J Oral Pathol Med 1995;24:468–470.
14. Greenlee R, Murray T, Bolden S, Wingo P. Cancer Statistics. CA Cancer J Clin 2000;50:7.

15. Ries LA, Hankey BF, Miller BA, Clegg L, Edwards BK. SEER cancer statistics review, 1973–1996, National Cancer Institute, Bethesda, MD.

16. Atkinson JC. Clinical pathology conference: xerostomia. Gerodontics 1986;2:193–197.

17. Burt BA, Isamil AZ. Diet, nutrition, and food cariogenicity. J Dent Res 1986;65:1475–1484.

18. Gustafsson B, Quensel C-E, e.a. L Swenander Lanke L. The Vipeholm dental caries study. The effect of different levels of carbohydrate intake on caries activity in 436 individuals observed for five years. Acta Odont Scand 1954;11:232–364.

19. Mandel I. Calculus update: prevalence, pathogenecity and prevention. J Am Dent Assoc 1995;126: 573–580.

20. Hefferren JJ, Osborn JC. Foods, consumption factors and dental caries. Gerodontics 1987;3:26–29.

21. Alfin-Slater R, Pi-Sunyer F. Sugar and sugar substitutes. Comparisons and indications. Postgrad Med 1987;82:46–50.

22. Makinen KK, Philosophy L. The role of sucrose and other sugars in the development of dental caries; a review. Int Dent J 1972;22:363–386.

23. Nishida M, Grossi SG, Dunford RG, et al. Calcium and the risk for periodontal disease. J Periodontol 2000;71:1057–1066.

24. Krall E, et al. Postmenopausal estrogen replacement and tooth retention. Am J Med 1997;102:536–542.

25. Leggott P, Robertson PB, Jacob RA, et al. Effects of ascrobic acid depletion and supplementation on perdontal health and subgingival microflora in humans. J Dent Res 1991;70:1531–1536.

26. Pack A. Folate mouthwash: Effects on established gingivitis in periodontal patients. J Clin Periodontol 1984;11:619–628.

27. Saito T, Shimizaki Y, Koga T, et al. Relationship between upper body obesity and periodontitis. J Dent Res 2001;80:1631–1636.

28. Shuldiner A, Yang R, Gong D. Resistin, obesity and insulin resistance—the emerging role of the adipocyte as an endocrine organ. N Engl J Med 2001;345:1345–1346.

29. Sankaranaryanan R, Masuyer E, Swaminathan R, et al. Head and neck cancer: A global perspective on epidemiology and prognosis. Anticancer Res 1998;18:4779–4786.

30. Gupta PC, Herbert JR, Bhonsle RB, et al. Dietary factors in oral leukoplakia and submucous fibrosis in a population-based case control study in Gujarat, India. Oral Dis 1998;4:200–206.

31. Morse DE, Pendrys DG, Katz RV, et al. Food group intake and the risk of oral epithelial dysplasia in a United States population. Cancer Causes Control 2000;11:713–720.

32. Gridley G, McLaughlin JK, Block G, et al. Diet and oral and pharyngeal cancer among blacks. Nutr Cancer 1990;14:219–225.

33. Levi F, Pasche C, La Vecchia, et al. Food groups and risk of oral and pharyngeal cancer. Int J Cancer 1998;77:705–709.

34. Gupta PC, Herbert JR, Bhonsle RB, et al. Influence of dietary factors on oral precancerous lesions in a population-based case-control study in Kerala, India. Cancer 1999;85:1885–1893.

35. Steinmetz KA, Potter JD. Vegetables, fruit, and cancer prevention: A review. J Am Diet Assoc 1996;96:1027–1039.

36. Winn DM. Diet and nutrition in the etiology of oral cancer. Am J Clin Nutr 1995;61:437S–445S.

37. Day GL, Shore RE, Blot WJ, et al. Dietary factors and second primary cancers: A follow-up of oral and pharyngeal cancer patients. Nutr Cancer 1994;21:223–232.

38. McLaughlin JK, Gridley G, Block G, et al. Dietary factors in oral and pharyngeal cancer. J Natl Cancer Inst 1988;80:1237–1243.

39. De Stefani E, Orregia F, Boffetta P, et al. Tomatoes, tomato-rich foods, lycopene and cancer of the upper aerodigestive tract: A case-control in Uruguay. Oral Oncol 2000;36:47–53.

40. Takezaki T, Hirose K, Inoue M, et al. Tobacco, alcohol and dietary factors associated with the risk of oral cancer among Japanese. Jpn J Cancer Res 1996;87:555–562.

41. Flagg EW, Coates RJ, Jones DP, et al. Dietary glutathione intake and the risk of oral and pharyngeal cancer. Am J Epidemiol 1994;139:453–465.

42. Barone J, Taioli E, Herbert JR, Wynder EL. Vitamin supplement use and risk for oral and esophageal cancer. Nutr Cancer 1992;18:31–41.

43. Benner SE, Winn RJ, Lippman SM, et al. Regression of oral leukoplakia with alpha-tocopherol: A community clinical oncology program chemoprevention study. J Natl Cancer Inst 1993;85:44–47.

44. Blot WJ. Nutrition intervention trials in Linxian, China: Supplementation with specific vitamin/mineral combinations, cancer incidence, and disease-specific mortality in the general population. J Natl Cancer Inst 1993;85:1483–1492.

45. Garewal HS. Beta-carotene and vitamin E in oral cancer prevention. J Cell Biochem Suppl 1993: 262–269.
46. Hong WK, Endicott J, Itri LM, et al. 13-cis-retinoic acid in the treatment of oral leukoplakia. N Engl J Med 1986;315:1501–1505.
47. Zheng W, Blot WJ, Diamond EL, et al. Serum micronutrients and the subsequent risk of oral and pharyngeal cancer. Cancer Res 1993;53:795–798.
48. Nagao T, Ikeda N, Warnakulasuriya S, et al. Serum antioxidant micronutrients and the risk of oral leukoplakia among Japanese. Oral Oncol 2000;36:466–470.
49. Negri E, Franceschi S, Bosetti C, et al. Selected micronutrients and oral and pharyngeal cancer. Int J Cancer 2000;86:122–127.
50. Ramaswamy G, Rao VR, Kumaraswamy SV, et al. Serum vitamins' status in oral leucoplakias—a preliminary study. Eur J Cancer B Oral Oncol 1996;32B:120–122.
51. Zain RB, Fukano H, Nagao T, Abang Z, Razak IA, et al. Oral habits, serum micronutrients and oral mucosal lesions among the Indigenous people of Sarawak. Oral Oncol, 1999. 6, Macmillan, India: 185–188.
52. Tavani A, Gallus S, La Vecchia C, et al. Diet and risk of oral and pharyngeal cancer. An Italian case-control study. Eur J Cancer Prev 2001;10:191–195.
53. Khuri FR, Lippman SM, Spitz MR, et al. Molecular epidemiology and retinoid chemoprevention of head and neck cancer. J Natl Cancer Inst 1997;89:199–211.
54. Papadimitrakopoulou VA, Hong WK. Retinoids in head and neck chemoprevention. Proc Soc Exp Biol Med 1997;216:283–290.
55. Zain RB. Cultural and dietary risk factors of oral cancer and precancer—a brief overview. Oral Oncol 2001;37:205–210.
56. Hong WK, Lippman SM, Itri LM, et al. Prevention of second primary tumors with isotretinoin in squamous-cell carcinoma of the head and neck. N Engl J Med 1990;323:795–801.
57. Garewal HS, Katz RV, Meyskens F, et al. Beta-carotene produces sustained remissions in patients with oral leukoplakia: Results of a multicenter prospective trial. Arch Otolaryngol Head Neck Surg 1999; 125:1305–1310.
58. Garrote LF, Herrero R, Reyes RM, et al. Risk factors for cancer of the oral cavity and oro-pharynx in Cuba. Br J Cancer 2001;85:46–54.
59. Franceschi S, Favero A, Conti E, et al. Food groups, oils and butter, and cancer of the oral cavity and pharynx. Br J Cancer 1999;80:614–620.
60. Fioretti F, Bosetti C, Tavani A, et al. Risk factors for oral and pharyngeal cancer in never smokers. Oral Oncol 1999;35:375–378.
61. Badawi AF, Hosny G, el-Hadary M, et al. Salivary nitrate, nitrite and nitrate reductase activity in relation to risk of oral cancer in Egypt. Dis Markers 1998;14:91–97.
62. Herschaft E, Waldron C. Oral and Maxillofacial Pathology. WB Saunders Company, Philadelphia, PA, 1995, pp. 600–604.
63. Johansson I, Tidehag P, Lundberg V, Hallmans G. Dental status, diet and cardiovascular risk factors in middle-aged people in northern Sweden. Community Dent Oral Epidemiol 1994;22:431–436.
64. Norlen P, Steen B, Birkhed D, Bjorn AL. On the relationship bewteen dietary habits, nutrients, and oral health in women at the age of retirement. Acta Odontologica Scand 1993;51:277–284.
65. Joshipura KJ, Willett WC, Douglass CW. The impact of edentulousness on food and nutrient intake. J Am Dent Assoc 1996;127:459–467.
66. Sheiham A, Steele JG, Marcenes W, et al. The relationship among dental status, nutrient intake, and nutritional status in older people. J Dent Res 2001;80:408–413.
67. Krall E, Hayes C, Garcia R. How dentition status and masticatory function affect nutrient intake. J Am Dent Assoc 1998;129:1261–1269.
68. Papas A, Palmer CA, Rounds MC, et al. The effects of denture status on nutrition. Spec Care Dent 1998;18:17–25.
69. Papas A, Joshi A, Giunta, JL, et al. Relationships among education, dentate status, and diet in adults. Spec Care Dent 1998;18:26–32.
70. Laurin D, Brodeur JM, Bourdages J, et al. Fibre intake in elderly individuals with poor masticatory performance. J Can Dent Assoc 1994;60:443–446.
71. Nordstrom G. The impact of socio-medical factors and oral status on dietary intake in the eighth decade of life. Aging (Milano) 1990;2:371–385.
72. Horwath C. Chewing Difficulty and Dietary Intake in the Elderly. J Nutr Elderly 1989;9:17–24.

73. Lamy M, Mojon Ph, Kalykakis G, Legrand R, Butz-Jorgensen E. Oral status and nutrition in the institutionalized elderly. J Dent 1999;24:443–448.
74. Garrett N, Kapur K, Hasse A, Dent R. Veterans Administration Cooperative Dental Implant Study—Comparisons between fixed partial dentures supported by blade-vent implants and removable partial dentures. Part V: Comparisons of pretreatment and posttreatment dietary intakes. J Prosthet Dent 1997; 77:153–160.
75. Sebring N, Guckes A, Li SH, McCarthy G. Nutritional Adequacy of reported intake of edentulous subjects treated with new conventional or implant supported mandibular dentures. J Prosthet Dent 1995; 74:358–363.
76. Lindquist L. Prosthetic Rehabilitation of the Edentulous Mandible. Swed Dent J 1987;48:1–39.
77. Olivier M, Laurin D, Brodeur JM, et al. Prosthetic relining and dietary counselling in elderly women. J Can Dent Assoc 1995;61:882–886.
78. Mojon P, Budtz-Jorgensen E, Rapin C. Relationship between oral health and nutrition in very old people. Age Ageing 1999;28:463–468.
79. Hirano H, Ishiyama N, Watanabe I, Nasu I, et al. Masticatory ability in relation to oral status and general health on aging. J Nutr Health Aging 1999;3:48–52.
80. Elwood P, Bates J. Dentition and nutrition. Dent Pract 1972;22:427–429.
81. Minasian A, Dwyer JT. Nutritional implications of dental and swallowing issues in head and neck cancer. Oncology (Huntingt) 1998;12:1155–1169.
82. Kronenberger MB, Meyers AD. Dysphagia following head and neck cancer surgery. Dysphagia 1994;9:236–244.
83. Irving J, Wood G, Hackett A. Does temporomandibular disorder pain dysfunction syndrome affect dietary intake? Dent update 1999;26:405–407.
84. Yontchev E, Sandstrom B, Carlsson GE. Dietary pattern, energy and nutrient intake in patients with orofacial discomfort complaints. J Oral Rehabil 1989;16:345–351.
85. Loesche W, Abrams J, Terpenning M, Bretz W, Dominguez L, Grossman N, et al. Dental findings in geriatric populations with diverse medical backgrounds. Oral Surg Oral Med Oral Pathol 1995;80: 43–54.
86. Rhodus NL. Qualitative Nutritional Intake Analysis of Older Adults with Sjogren's Syndrome. Gerodontology 1988;7:61–69.
87. Rhodus N, Brown J. The association of xerostomia and inadequate intake in older adults. J Am Diet Assoc 1990;90:1688–1692.
88. Dormenval V, Budtz-Jorgensen E, Mojon P, et al. Nutrition, general health status and oral health status in hospitalised elders. Gerodontology 1995;12:73–80.

Dysphagia Evaluation, Treatment, and Recommendations

Carol Smith Hammond, Candice Hudson Scharver, Lisa W. Markley, Judy Kinnally, Marianne Cable, Linda Evanko, and David Curtis

1. INTRODUCTION TO DYSPHAGIA: IMPACT IN THE ELDERLY

Dysphagia results from bolus flow interruption by an incoordination, obstruction or weakness of the biomechanics of swallowing *(1)*. Impaired swallowing or dysphagia can cause significant morbidity and mortality. Swallowing disorders are especially common in the elderly and can lead to malnutrition, starvation, aspiration pneumonia, and airway obstruction *(2,3)*. There are subtle effects on the anatomy and physiology of the swallowing mechanism that accompany normal aging *(1)*.

Increased life expectancy and incidence of acute and chronic ailments have resulted in a significant number of dysphagic elderly *(4)*. Seventy-five percent of strokes, a condition commonly associated with swallowing problems, occur in people over the age of 65 yr, and the incidence rises with age *(5)*. Stroke often results in dysphagia *(6)*, affecting up to 75% of patients with brainstem level lesions *(7)*. In a study at our facility, over two-thirds of a cohort containing patients referred for dysphagia evaluations were over age 65 yr *(8)*; they came from both acute and long-term care areas of the medical center. Swallowing disorders are reported to affect 10% of acutely hospitalized elderly *(4)* and 30–60% of nursing home patients *(6)*. General population surveys have suggested that up to 10% of individuals older than age 50 yr experience swallowing problems *(9)*.

2. CAUSES OF DYSPHAGIA

Dysphagia may result from neurological disorders, such as stroke and Parkinson's disease, degenerative diseases, like chronic obstructive pulmonary disease (COPD), and cancer (primarily of the head and neck). Swallowing problems can further complicate postsurgical patients' recovery as well *(10)*. We find that some patients are in a state of

From: *Handbook of Clinical Nutrition and Aging*
Edited by: C. W. Bales and C. S. Ritchie © Humana Press Inc., Totowa, NJ

decompensation from various biologically or psychologically based medical conditions and are categorized as moderate to severely dysphagic during the initial phases of medical treatment. Many patients with interdisciplinary team intervention recover swallowing ability as their condition improves.

The medical conditions found to be most often associated with dysphagia are listed in Table 1. The aging patient is at an increased risk for developing dysphagia as a result of age and nutritionally induced physiologic changes, and as a result, nutritional disorders such as malnutrition. Untreated dysphagia may result in protein-energy malnutrition. This nutritional deficit can lead to life-threatening conditions and increased risk of accompanying infections, secondary to immunocompromise *(11)*. Langmore et al. reported predictors of aspiration pneumonia, which is associated with dysphagia and is a major cause of morbidity and mortality among the elderly *(12)*. These are listed in Table 2.

Numerous medications may variably affect swallow function *(13)*. Neuroleptic drugs, for example, can cause "tardive dyskinesia" and sedatives can reduce alertness needed for oral bolus control and result in oropharyngeal dysphagia. Cancer patients undergoing radiotherapy and chemotherapy often develop xerostomia, changes in taste sensation, tongue swelling, mucositis, and necrosis of teeth and gums. Table 3 lists some of the medications and their possible sequelae *(2)*.

3. NORMAL SWALLOW

Swallowing may be defined as bolus flow from the lips to the stomach. Anatomical structures related to swallowing are illustrated in Fig. 1. Swallowing is a complex act that involves the coordinated activity of over 20 muscles innervated by the central and peripheral neural systems of the mouth, pharynx, larynx and esophagus. The swallow has been divided into four phases *(14)*: oral preparatory, oral propulsive, pharyngeal, and esophageal (Fig. 2).

3.1. Oral Preparatory Phase

Food and liquid are prepared during the oral preparatory phase for movement through the digestive system by the muscles of mastication and the teeth. Mastication refers to the grinding of solid food mixed with saliva necessary for bolus formation *(14)*. A bolus is formed in preparation for the swallow stages that follow.

3.2. Oral Propulsive Phase

Once the bolus has been formed, it is ready for transport into the pharynx. The tongue slides the bolus along the hard palate, propelling it under positive pressure into the pharynx *(14)*. Both cortical and brainstem pathways are involved in the coordinated function needed for oral propulsion *(14)*. This phase includes the labial, lingual, and buccal musculature which is innervated by the facial, hypoglossal, and trigeminal cranial nerves, respectively *(10)*.

3.3. Pharyngeal Phase

Upon voluntary propulsion of the bolus into the pharynx, the reflexive pharyngeal swallow is triggered. The pharyngeal phase follows immediately with single bolus swallows. Mastication of solid food requires 5–10 s as the bolus accumulates piecemeal in the valleculae, a space formed by the epiglottis and base of tongue in the oropharynx *(14)*.

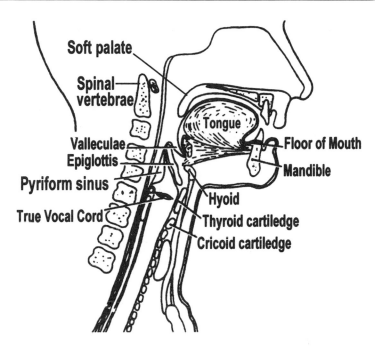

Fig. 1. Anatomical structures related to swallowing.

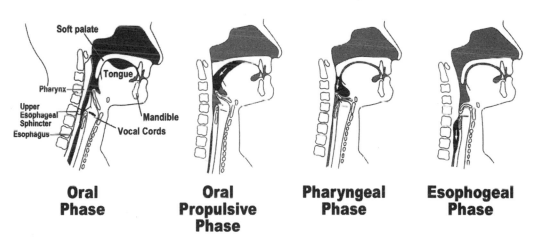

Fig. 2. The swallow has been divided into four phases: oral preparatory, oral propulsive, pharyngeal, and esophageal.

Regardless of the food consistency, the pharyngeal phase involves a rapid sequence of overlapping events. In order to protect the airway, the soft palate elevates and the hyoid bone and larynx move upward and forward. The intrinsic laryngeal musculature constricts to shorten the aryepiglottic folds and close the true and false vocal cords.

Table 1
Dietary Modification Recommendations by Medical Diagnostic Group

Most common diagnostic group	Long-term tube feedings recommended	NPO recommended as all consistencies aspirated	Thickened liquid required (Ensure and thin liquids aspirated). Solid food recommended	Ensure (supplemental, nectar) liquids swallowed without aspiration and solid food recommended
Cerebrovascular accident (CVA) n = 95	12%	9%	23%	4%
Head and neck cancer n = 28	25%	25%	10%	0
Lung disease n = 19	0	19%	10%	3%
Gastrointestinal disorders n = 19	21%	5%	21%	0
s/p coronary artery bypass graft (CABG) n = 5	20%	20%	20%	0
Parkinson's disease n = 7	0	14%	28%	0
Multiple sclerosis n = 6	0	0	50%	0
Cervical spine disease n = 10	11%	11%	11%	0
Dementia n = 5	0	0	20%	0

Source: Smith-Hammond et al. *(50).* NPO, nothing by mouth; s/p status post.
Dietary modification recommendations by medical diagnostic group.
Recommendations for consecutive referrals to the Speech Pathology Service for dysphagia evaluation and treatment are categorized by foods and liquids found to be swallowed without risk of aspiration. All patients were evaluated with the use of radiological or endoscopic procedures. Patients were grouped by primary medical diagnosis as documented in their record.

550

Table 2
Signs and Symptoms of Dysphagia

Clinical signs	Coughing/choking while eating, drinking, or taking meds	Productive cough	Dysphonia or wet, gurgly voice	Food/liquid residue in oral cavity or pharynx	Drooling	Nasal regurgitation	Unintentional weight loss
Clinical and respiratory signs	Aspiration pneumonia	Pneumonia	Shortness of breath paired with fever spike	Not managing oral/pharyngeal secretions	Respiratory rate > 30 breaths per minute prebolus administration	Increased respiratory rate after eating	Recurrent bronchitis
Chest X-ray	Middle and/or lower lobe infiltrate or opacity	Aspiration pneumonia					
Patient report	Food and liquid going down wrong way	Afraid they will choke and stop breathing	Eating smaller meals or change of diet	Multiple swallows to make food go down	Avoids certain foods/hard to chew foods	Tired after the end of a meal; taking more than 45 min	Vomiting after eating
Predictors of aspiration pneumonia	Dependent for feeding	Dependent for oral care	Number of decayed teeth	1 medical medical diagnosis	Smoking	> 3 medications	Tube feeding

Table 3
Medications and Medical Treatments Associated with Dysphagia

Medication or treatment	Affect on swallow function

Sedatives
Neuroleptics
Anticonvulsants
Ethyl alcohol
Barbiturates
Antianxiety
Opiod analgesic
	Reduces alertness needed
	  for control of food
	  and liquids in the pharynx
	Hypofunction
	  of swallowing musculature
	Dystonia

Corticosteriods Lipid-lowering drugs	Myopathy
Anticholinergics Antihypertensives Antihistamines Antipsychotics Narcotics Anticonvulsants Antiparkinsonian agents Antineoplastics Antidepressants Anxiolytics Muscle relaxants Diruetics Decongestants Psychotropic agents	Xerostomia-dry the oral, pharyngeal mucosa
Antibiotics	Inflammation, swelling
Pill irritation	Esophageal inflammation
Chemotherapy Radiotherapy	Change in taste sensation Tongue swelling Mucositis Tooth and gum necrosis Xerostomia
Neuroleptics	Tardive dyskinesia

Mediations and medical treatments associated with dysphagia. Affect of medications and medical treatments on swallow function. *Source*: Buffington et al. *(13)*.

The epiglottis folds over the arytenoid cartilages to protect the airway. The action of the tongue against the contracting pharyngeal musculature drives the bolus inferiorly into the pharynx. Adequate strength of the pharyngeal musculature is necessary for functional constriction of the pharynx behind the tail of the bolus *(15)*. The pharyngeal walls move inward with a progressive wave of contraction from top to bottom providing continuing pressure to move the bolus toward the esophagus. The bolus traverses bilaterally through the pyriform sinuses, spaces formed by the sides of the pharyngeal wall and the larynx pharyngeal recesses. The upper esophageal sphincter relaxes to allow the bolus to pass into the esophagus. An intact neuromuscular system is required for all of the complex movements of the pharyngeal phase to be completed within one to two seconds.

3.4. Esophageal Phase

The upper esophageal sphincter is opened by the combination of cricopharyngeal muscle function along with the cricoid cartilage, forming a rigid ring of muscle and cartilage, that anchors the mechanism during the forward movement of the hyoid bone and larynx (14). The upper esophageal sphincter closes after passage of the food and the pharyngeal structures then return to resting position to prevent regurgitation of swallowed material from reentering the laryngeal area. During the esophageal phase, the bolus is moved by a pressure wave through the esophagus. The lower esophageal sphincter relaxes and allows propulsion of the bolus into the stomach. The lower sphincter closes after the bolus enters the stomach preventing gastroesophageal reflux (14).

4. MEDICAL DIAGNOSES AND DYSPHAGIA PHASE AFFECTS

The following section will present common disorders seen in each phase of the swallow.

4.1. Oral Dysphagia

Disorders affecting the oral preparatory and oral propulsive phases usually result from impaired control of the lingual and/or labial musculature, although dental problems may also be involved. When eating solid food, patients may have difficulty chewing resulting from missing teeth or poor fitting dentures. Weakened or desensitized muscles of mastication can result in "pocketing" of food in the buccal spaces of the oral cavity. Food that remains in the oral cavity for an extended period of time can cause halitosis and present an increased choking risk. Poor lingual strength and coordination may result in poor bolus control. An uncontrolled bolus may fall into an unprotected larynx and can lead to choking and/or passage of material below the vocal folds into the proximal trachea, known as aspiration (16).

Inability to voluntarily initiate a swallow is commonly seen following brain surgery, as well as in advanced stages of dementia, and in chronic stroke patients. Some cognitively impaired patients prepare the bolus, but do not initiate the bolus propulsion phase. The bolus remains sitting in the depression on the ventral surface of the tongue for extended periods of time. Containment of food and liquid in the oral cavity extends feeding time and reduces the amount of food ingested, thus placing patients at risk for malnutrition.

4.2. Pharyngeal Dysphagia

As a result of the complex nature of the pharyngeal phase of swallowing, several factors can negatively impact proper passage of the bolus from the mouth to the esophagus. Weakened constriction of the pharyngeal musculature and decreased base of tongue retraction can result in the retention of bolus material in the pharyngeal musculature after the swallow, placing a patient at risk for subsequent aspiration. If pharyngeal clearance is severely impaired, patients may be unable to ingest sufficient amounts of food and drink.

Inadequate laryngeal elevation, decreased epiglottic retroversion, and incomplete laryngeal closure during the swallow can result in ineffective protection of the airway, and aspiration. Additionally, weakness of the soft palate and pharynx may lead to the nasal regurgitation (nasal reflux) of food causing discomfort and aversion to eating *(17)*. Persons who aspirate are at increased risk for the occurrence of serious respiratory sequelae, including shortness of breath, airway obstruction and aspiration pneumonia *(18–21)*.

Radiation therapy to the head and neck musculature can impair pharyngeal range of motion, resulting decreased movement of the involved structures during the swallow. This fibrosis can place the postradiation patient at risk for aspiration *(10)*.

A pharyngeal diverticulum, or Zenkers, is a pouch formed in a weak area of the pharyngeal wall, which may also impair pharyngeal emptying by diverting the bolus from its normal course *(22,23)*.

4.3. Esophageal Dysphagia

Although the esophagus may be screened during a videofluorographic assessment of oropharyngeal swallowing-function with the help of a radiologist, esophageal dysphagia is usually evaluated by a gastroenterologist. When esophageal dysfunction is suspected, the speech pathologist recommends a gastroenterology referral. Patients with esophageal dysphagia often complain of a globus sensation, reporting that food gets "stuck in their throat," the need for multiple swallows per bolus, coughing on solids and liquids, or vomiting after meals. Esophageal dysphagia generally results from structural abnormalities (e.g., luminal stenosis or deformity), or motor dysfunction (peristaltic or sphincter function abnormalities). Gastroesophageal reflux is a common problem that can result in structural and/or motor dysfunction *(24)*.

5. AGE-RELATED CHANGES IN THE SWALLOW

Changes in the oropharyngeal swallow with normal aging may be negligible, yet if the system is stressed by disease or trauma, dysphagia symptoms may result *(25)*. Increased stiffness and decreased flexibility of the swallowing structures, as well as overall declinations in muscle function reduce maximal strength and pressure within the oral, pharyngeal, and esophageal systems *(1)*. Any disease state in the elderly can place stress on a declining swallowing mechanism and push the system to a pathological state.

5.1. Anatomic and Physiological Changes

Anatomical and physiological changes associated with aging may cause relatively few primary difficulties with swallowing outside of disease context. Ossification of cartilage and the caudal movement of the laryngeal complex in the elderly contribute to anatomical changes that may reduce flexibility during swallowing. Changes in the central nervous system resulting from the aging process may stress the swallowing complex as well. Physiologic changes include increased swallowing transit times, decreased strength of the masticatory, labial and lingual musculature, reduced salivary production, and altered dentition *(1)*.

5.2. Sensory Changes

Sensory changes with age often affect psychosocial issues such as quality of life related to eating (Chapters 8 and 9). Vision may affect the ability to distinguish color and texture of various foods on the plate, thus indirectly affecting appetite. Gustatory changes include decreased taste sensation, which may result in increased use of sugar and salt to enhance flavor. Many elderly wear dentures that cover the hard palate, thereby reducing the number of taste receptors available and reducing the flavor of food. Decline in olfactory function resulting from degeneration of the olfactory nerve and olfactory mucosa is observed in the geriatric population. If the senses of smell and vision are affected, then decreased ability to see and taste food may result in diminished enjoyment and willingness to eat *(1)*.

5.3. Swallow Function Changes in the Elderly

Several reports have indicated a general slowing in the overall transit time for a bolus passing through the oropharynx *(26–29)*. Longer swallow duration before the pharyngeal swallow begins leaves the laryngeal vestibule exposed for longer periods of time, potentially placing elderly adults at greater risk for aspiration *(30)*. Older individuals are able to complete fewer consecutive liquid swallows in 10 s compared to younger individuals, which may be the result of a fatigue factor *(29)*. Decreased pharyngeal and laryngeal sensation may place the elderly at greater risk of aspiration *(31)*. Young (21–32 yr) and old (63–84 yr) healthy individuals were compared using radiological evaluation of swallow and no difference was found between groups for aspiration of material below the level of the vocal folds or penetration of material into the laryngeal area. However, when the swallowing system was stressed, older individuals aspirated and the younger group did not *(26)*.

Anatomic and physiological changes in the hypopharynx and upper esophageal sphincter have been reported with aging. An increased likelihood of esophageal motility problems, achalasia, and presbyesophagus are also associated with age. However, investigators agree that these esophageal problems may reflect the presence of common comorbidities in older individuals, such as neurological disorders and diabetes mellitus *(1)*.

6. EVALUATION OF SWALLOW: INTERDISCIPLINARY COMPONENTS

The evaluation of swallowing function can be optimally performed using an interdisciplinary approach. The first signs and symptoms of a swallowing problem may be identified by the patient, someone in his or her environment, or a medical professional.

Some patients are not consciously aware of their swallowing difficulty. Stroke patients can demonstrate severe dysphagia on objective evaluation of swallow and yet report no swallowing difficulty when questioned *(32)*. Subtle signs and symptoms of dysphagia (Table 2) and the presence of cognitive, speech, language or hearing deficits can make the presence of a swallowing problem difficult to detect. The clinician must often rely on the medical record and history alone in determining the risk factors for dysphagia. In many facilities, the speech pathologist interviews the patients and family regarding swallowing problems during the initial clinical assessment.

6.1. Medical Record Review

A thorough medical record review is conducted to determine if medical history (Table 1) or signs and symptoms (Table 2) indicate increased likelihood of dysphagia. Review of medications should be included in the medical history as some drugs are associated with dysphagia (Table 3).

6.2. Patient Interview

The Dysphagia Disability Index (DDI) *(33)* and the Swallowing Quality of Life Index SWAL QOL *(34)* are two interviewing instruments that probe patients for functional, emotional and physical effects associated with swallowing problems. Patients or their caregivers are interviewed for information about the onset, duration, and severity of the swallowing problem and provide information that is often beneficial in guiding the evaluation process. The reflux symptom index (RSI) is a short nine question rating scale used to indicate patient's subjective symptoms of LPR (larygopharyngeal reflux). For example, the question is asked how the problem has affected a patient in the past month for the "sensation of something sticking in your throat or a lump in your throat." Administration of this index could assist the clinician in differentiating prandial from postprandial swallowing issues based on patient complaints *(34a)*.

6.3. Dietitian Nutritional Assessment

Dietitians often detect dysphagia in patients through observation at mealtime or personal interview during their initial nutritional screening. Suspected dysphagia should be reported to the managing physician, who can then consult the speech pathologist for an evaluation. The dietitian may institute alterations in the diet plan while awaiting further speech pathology evaluation. For patients suspected to be dehydrated, malnourished, or experiencing unintentional weight loss, a full dietary consult with nutritional assessment should be requested.

6.4. Cognitive Evaluation

The cognitive status of a patient should be assessed to determine if the patient can give a reliable medical history, and if he is an appropriate candidate for compensatory techniques during an instrumental swallowing evaluation with possible subsequent dysphagia treatment. The Neurobehavioral Cognitive Status Exam (COGNISTAT) is a screening tool that assesses six domains: level of consciousness, attention, speech and language abilities, memory, calculation, and reasoning *(35)*. The following sections will discuss cognitive domains, which relate to dysphagia evaluation and treatment.

6.4.1. LEVEL OF CONSCIOUSNESS

Patients must be alert, awake, and able to accept food into the mouth. If patients are extremely lethargic or experiencing inconsistent levels of alertness they may exhibit prolonged or inadequate preparation of the bolus, delayed triggering of the pharyngeal swallow, and increased risk of aspiration. Many chronically inattentive, lethargic patients, like many with dementia, are often incapable of oral intake sufficient for nutrition or hydration even if their swallow is functional, resulting from inconsistent levels of alertness, inability to focus on the task, or fatigue. Post-head injury patients or those with severe neurological impairment may exhibit slow oral movements, resulting in a significantly increased length of time to initiation of the swallow and reduced oral intake. Some neurologically impaired patients exhibit abnormal reflexes such as a hyperactive gag, tongue thrusting, or tonic bite. Before proceeding with an objective swallow-evaluation, the patient should be able to remain alert for at least 20–30-min intervals, the time needed to complete an objective swallow evaluation or eat a meal *(10)*.

6.4.2. MEMORY

Memory function must be evaluated to determine if verbal cues, written aids, or supervision are necessary for the patient to follow recommendations given for safe per oral (PO) nutrition. Patients with dementia may need constant supervision during eating to maintain compensatory postures, or would otherwise not be candidates for such techniques.

6.4.3. SPEECH AND LANGUAGE FUNCTION

Functional level of auditory comprehension is evaluated to determine the patient's ability to understand the clinician's interview, directions given during the swallow evaluation process, and treatment recommendations. The ability to speak and express complaints of dysphagia or answer interview questions is also important for evaluation protocols. Recent reports indicate dysarthria (muscle weakness that can affect articulation) and aphasia (language impairment) are correlated with dysphagia following stroke. Expressive and receptive language function should be sampled and the speech pathologist should adapt evaluation and treatment protocols to compensate for speech and language impairment. Additionally, hearing loss is common in the elderly, and if left unaddressed can negatively affect the evaluation and treatment process.

6.4.4. REASONING

Reasoning skills are screened to determine if further psychological evaluation is warranted and should be functional for the patient to make appropriate decisions concerning treatment.

7. SUBJECTIVE OR CLINICAL EVALUATION OF SWALLOWING

The clinical evaluation of swallowing is often initiated at bedside in the acute stage of hospitalization or in the nursing home patient. A cognitive screening is often performed at this time. Spontaneous speech is assessed for the presence of dysphonia (abnormal voice) and dysarthria (abnormal speech articulation), which are signs of dysfunction often associated with oral and pharyngeal dysphagia.

An oral mechanism examination is performed to assess strength, range of motion, and sensation of the oral/facial musculature. The oral cavity and pharynx are inspected for mucosal abnormalities (masses, lesions, and signs of dehydration) and dental integrity. The soft palate is examined for position and symmetry during phonation and at rest. The presence or absence of the gag reflex is determined. Many persons with normal swallowing have an absent gag reflex, and conversely, some patients with dysphagia have a normal gag (36). However, absent gag in addition to a weak voluntary cough, has been correlated with the presence of aspiration in one study of stroke patients (37).

Once the oral motor assessment has been completed, ice chips, water, and other trial boluses are administered to estimate the integrity of the oral and pharyngeal stages of swallowing. Methods used to clinically assess the pharyngeal phase of swallowing include vocal quality assessments following bolus administration, laryngeal palpation to evaluate movement of the larynx during the swallow, and cervical auscultation. Cervical auscultation with a stethoscope is used to detect movement of air and fluid (during the respiration and swallow sequence) through the pharynx and larynx during and after the swallow. For adults with dysphagia, the respiratory pattern is variable and breath sounds are characterized by bubbling, throat clearing or stridor *(38,39)*.

Upon bolus administration, the speech pathologist looks for clinical signs of aspiration. These signs may include decreased oral control of the bolus, coughing, throat clearing, "wet" or dysphonic vocal quality, and may indicate a swallowing problem. After swallowing, the patients should continue to be observed to see if there is a delayed cough or throat clearing response post bolus administration.

Clinicians who work in long-term care settings rely heavily on the clinical dysphagia examination, because instrumental examination procedures, e.g., videofluoroscopy, endoscopy, and manometry are often difficult to obtain. The research literature, however, does not support the confident use of the clinical examination alone as a method of detecting aspiration or planning diet and treatment. Neither individual clinical examination components *(40)* nor clinicians' judgments during the examination *(41,42)* have correlated well with the presence of aspiration on objective evaluation of swallow.

Aspiration normally provokes a strong cough reflex. If sensation is impaired, "silent aspiration" (without reflexive cough or throat clearing) may occur *(43)*, thus limiting what can be detected at bedside. The use of pulse oximetry as a supplement to the clinical evaluation to improve detection of dysphagia has been reported *(44)*. New initiatives that have been proposed to add more objective measures to the clinical evaluation of swallow include measurement of aerodynamic properties of voluntary cough. Clinical report indicates that the rise time of the expulsive phase of the voluntary cough, not reflexive cough, has been correlated with aspiration on radiological evaluation and can be applied clinically *(45)*.

8. OBJECTIVE EVALUATIONS OF SWALLOW

The two methods commonly used by speech pathologists for the instrumental evaluation of oropharyngeal swallowing function are videofluorographic and endoscopic assessment. Research reports indicate they are equally sensitive to aspiration during feeding *(46)*. Both methods have their advantages and disadvantages, however, patient presentation, clinician preference, and availability of equipment are generally the deciding factors in determining which method will be used.

8.1. Radiological Evaluation

The videofluorographic swallow evaluation (VSE) is a technique which offers the advantage of visualization of the oral, pharyngeal and esophageal phases of the swallow *(10)*. In practice, the terms "videofluorographic swallow study," "modified barium swallow," and "pharyngoesophagram," are some examples of terminology used to refer to this exam. The protocol includes transport of the patient to the radiology clinic, or in some cases, the use of a mobile VSE system for nursing home residents. The patient is seated in an upright position, often in a chair designed for this purpose, and given foods and liquids that are mixed with barium sulfate to make them radiopaque. The VSE appears as a moving picture X-ray of the bone, cartilage, and soft-tissue swallowing structures, as the food and liquid mixed with barium passes through all stages of the swallow. The study is recorded for later analysis. In most facilities, a radiologist and speech pathologist jointly conduct this study.

8.2. Fiberoptic Endoscopic Evaluation of Swallow (FEES)

Fiberoptic Endoscopic Evaluation of Swallowing (FEES), is a procedure in which the SLP (or otolaryngologist in some facilities), passes a flexible nasopharyngoscope transnasally to obtain a superior view of the pharynx and larynx *(47)*. Because pharyngeal contraction obstructs the lumen of the scope, motion of the pharynx "during the swallow" is not visualized, as there is a brief period of "white out." However, this procedure can identify laryngeal penetration and aspiration with direct observation of bolus material in the larynx or trachea. Factors that impact aspiration risk such as the ability of the vocal folds to protect the airway, identification of excess pharyngeal secretions, and bolus residue can also be assessed. Esophageal regurgitation into the hypopharynx may be visualized with this method when the inlet to the upper esophageal sphincter is in sight and this is often observed during more lengthy studies.

One advantage of this method is that the patient can be evaluated at bedside on an in-patient ward, in the intensive care unit, in the clinic, or in any skilled nursing facility, therefore eliminating the need for transport to the radiology clinic. Unlike the VSE where the radiation exposure limits the time of the study, the FEES allows the examiner to observe swallowing function for the duration of an entire meal. A patient may then be thoroughly challenged during this time to assess for possible fatigue. Also, this allows time to attempt multiple compensatory techniques when appropriate.

8.3. Additional Diagnostic Studies

Esophagogastroduodenoscopy (EGD), performed by a gastroenterologist, can be used to rule out neoplasia in patients who complain of thoracic dysphagia or odynophagia (pain on swallowing) *(23)*. Esophageal manometry and pH probe studies may be appropriate when a motility disorder or gastroesophageal reflux disease (GERD) is suspected, but they are rarely the first lines of investigation.

9. DYSPHAGIA TREATMENT

The goals of dysphagia therapy focus on reduction of aspiration, improved swallow ability, optimized nutritional status, and quality of life. Dysphagia therapy is individualized based on functional and structural abnormalities and the initial responses to treatment trials are observed at the patient's bedside or during the instrumental swallow study.

Theories of treatment form the basis of compensation for lost function, optimization of residual function, and substitution of intact function *(48)*. Obviously, no "cookbook" methods exist that provide treatment for the wide variety of medical diagnoses that predispose a patient to dysphagia. However, speech pathologists generally make recommendations with ultimate long-term goals in mind, including independent eating unlimited by swallowing function, safe and efficient swallowing of all consistencies, and effective use of compensatory strategies when needed *(49)*.

In many acute care hospitals, long-term care facilities, and outpatient clinics, the following noninvasive treatments and procedures have been emphasized:

1. Dietary consistency modification of liquid viscosities and food textures;
2. Compensatory postures and physiologic exercise programs when appropriate;
3. Patient and family education regarding diet recommendations, aspiration precautions, and reflux precautions;

4. Interdisciplinary dysphagia management;
5. Alternative means of nutrition (e.g., tube feeding).

9.1. Modification of Dietary Consistencies

The results of the instrumental swallowing evaluation make it possible to design an individualized diet for each dysphagic patient. This diet should include foods that can be swallowed with minimal aspiration risk while optimizing PO nutrition *(2)*. During a pilot evaluation of 95 patients at the Durham VAMC, dietary modification therapy was recommended for 54% (28/52) of CVA patients and 37% (16/43) of patients who were dysphagic secondary to any other cause *(50)*.

It has been noted that thick liquids often do not penetrate into the laryngeal vestibule when the laryngeal elevation and closure is incomplete *(51)*. As a result, some dysphagic patients may require diet recommendations that restrict thin liquid, but can include thick liquid for hydration. When such alterations are necessary, it is important that the patient, family, and dietitian are made aware of the liquid viscosity most appropriate for the patient, in an effort to maximize compliance. In contrast to outpatients, hospital inpatients on thickened liquids may have less choice about compliance with thickened liquid diet orders.

The dietitian and physician should closely monitor hydration level as a result of risk for dehydration, particularly when thick liquid has been recommended. Free water intake by dysphagic patients has been controversial. Two groups of stroke patients in a rehabilitation unit who aspirated thin liquids during videofluorographic swallow study were randomized to a study group with thickened liquids and free access to water *(52)*. Only thickened liquids were provided to the control group. No therapy techniques were imposed on either group. Patients with severe cough reflex reaction to aspiration of thin liquids were excluded. Results during the 30-d follow-up period revealed no pneumonia, dehydration, or complication developed by any patient of either group. Patients in the study group all reported satisfaction with access to free water. This recommendation should be made, however, on a patient by patient basis, taking into account each individual's mental status, medical status, and number of risk factors associated with aspiration pneumonia, such as those described by Langmore et al. *(12)*.

Clinicians have been encouraged to rheologically match videofluorographic fluids with mealtime fluids *(10)*. Dantas et al. *(53)*, for example, recommended specification of viscosities in videofluorographic management. Often, test materials that are used during instrumental swallowing evaluations have not been matched to diets available in the institutional kitchen or community environment. Test materials must be carefully and consistently measured, similar to real food viscosities, to increase the likelihood that liquid consumed during the swallow study matches that which the patient receives on the meal tray afterward. The Brookfield viscometer has been utilized to formulate recipes to match the viscosity of the target liquids.

9.1.1. SAMPLE OF CURRENT VIDEOFLUOROGRAPHIC SWALLOWING EVALUATION LIQUID RECIPES

Recipes are included in Table 4.

1. Thin liquid: 90cc (6 oz) water, 2-level tablespoons, E-Z-HD Barium Sulfate for suspension (98% w/w).

Table 4
Evaluation Materials Used in Radiological and Endoscopic Evaluations of Swallow

Type of evaluation material and examples of "real food" liquids which match by viscosity (cP)	Recipes for preparation of radiologic protocol	Recipes for preparation for endoscopic protocol
Thin liquid (3-8 cP): Coffee, soda, milk, juice, punch mixed from flavored powder and water	90 cc (3 oz) water 2 level tB E-Z-HD Barium Sulfate for suspension (98% w/w)	90 cc milk with 5 drops
Ensure liquid (34-50cP): Liquid supplements Nectar thick liquids	90 cc (3 oz) Ensure Plus 2 level tB E-Z-HD Barium Sulfate for suspension (98% w/w)	Ensure liquid with 5 drops food coloring
Thickened liquid (250-300 cP): Milkshake, thick cream soups Honey thick liquids	90 cc premixed thickened Crystal Lite (sugar free) 2 level tB E-Z-HD Barium Sulfate for suspension (93% w/w)	Thickened Crystal Lite and 5 drops food coloring 4 oz applesauce and 5 drops food coloring
Applesauce and pudding	4 oz applesauce and 1 level tB E-Z-HD Barium Sulfate for suspension (98% w/w) 4 oz pudding and 1 level tB E-Z-HD Barium Sulfate for suspension (98% w/w)	4 oz pudding and 5 drops food coloring
Solid food	1/4 Nabisco graham cracker with applesauce or pudding and 1 tB Barium Sulfate mixture	1/4 Nabisco graham cracker and applesauce or pudding and 5 drops food coloring
Bulk thickened liquids Crystal Lite	8 level tBs Thicken-Up 1 level tB Crystal Lite (Kraft) 32 oz water Mix with hand mixer to create a smooth mixture	8 level tBs Thicken-Up 1 level tB Crystal Lite (Kraft) 32 oz water Mix with hand mixer to create a smooth mixture

Recipes developed by the interdisciplinary team for evaluation materials used in radiological and endoscopic evaluations of swallow. Available liquid consistencies served to the patients are listed in each level.

2. Ensure liquid: 90cc (6 oz) Ensure Plus, 2-level tablespoons, E-Z-HD Barium Sulfate for suspension (98% w/w).
3. Thickened liquid: 90cc (6 oz) premixed thickened liquid (honey consistency—*see* bulk recipe), 2-level tablespoons, E-Z-HD Barium Sulfate for suspension (98% w/w).
4. Premixed honey thickened liquid recipe—bulk: 8-level, tablespoons, Thicken-Up; 1-level tablespoon, Crystal Lite (Kraft/sugar-free); 32 oz water. Mix with nonelectric hand mixer or wire whisk to create a smooth mixture.

Viscosity reliability in the evaluation and interdisciplinary treatment of dysphagic patients was the focus for a Geriatric Research, Education, and Clinical Center (GRECC) outreach project funded by the Veterans Administration. Dietitians and speech pathologists from our medical center traveled to selected VA medical centers where speech pathologists were conducting videofluorographic swallow evaluations for viscosity training sessions. Test barium solutions were measured with a Brookfield viscometer and reformulation of recipes for thickened liquids was initiated at the individual centers.

Results indicated that 80% of the sites were using evaluation material consistent with thin liquids only, with no thick liquid represented in their instrumental evaluation protocol. When comparing the liquids available, only one site used any thickened liquid (450 centipoise cP) during the videofluorographic evaluation, although a range of viscosities were served to the patients at mealtime. Based on these findings, it is clear that medical facilities need to develop a barium "testing" recipe consistent with the viscosity of liquids served to patients by their nutrition and food service. These findings provided support for a multidisciplinary program for dysphagia therapy that includes dietary modifications based on radiographic findings as a cornerstone for dysphagia patient management.

9.2. Compensatory Techniques and/or Physiologic Exercise Programs

A speech pathologist's goal when evaluating dysphagia is often recommendation of the least restrictive diet. For appropriate candidates, this may often involve assessing the effectiveness of compensatory postures and maneuvers during instrumental evaluation based on the individual's swallowing deficits. Techniques have been developed to improve opening of the upper esophageal sphincter, increase pharyngeal clearance and minimize aspiration *(54–56)*. Tucking the chin (neck flexion) during the swallow may reduce aspiration in some patients. Turning the head toward the weak side may improve pharyngeal clearance by deflecting the bolus to the strong side in a patient with unilateral pharyngeal weakness *(57)*. Innovative treatment options such as VitalStim™ transcutaneous electrical stimulation *(58)*, surface electromyography biofeedback *(59,60)*, and the Lee Silverman Voice Treatment for idiopathic Parkinson's disease *(61)* have been successfully used with specific populations.

A patient who is a good candidate for use of compensatory techniques should exhibit adequate comprehension and memory, as needed to implement and comply with specific postural maneuvers that may compensate for swallowing dysfunction. An exception can sometimes be made if the patient will have consistent and active supervision by a caregiver for the duration of each meal. The ability to follow commands is necessary for active participation in a swallowing exercise regimen. It is ideal for a patient to be able to implement these exercises several times per day independent of the speech pathologist. However, when memory deficits prevent this, family members (when available) can be educated as to how to lead these "independent" sessions.

9.3. Patient Education/Ethical Dilemmas

Patient and family satisfaction after discharge increases with the amount of time spent with the patient, even if there is no change in test performance *(62)*. Both before and after instrumental swallowing evaluations, patients and caregivers should be educated as to the reason for the assessment, what is involved in the evaluation, and assessment results. On an outpatient basis, they are often shown the videotape of the swallow study and provided with applicable handouts. Compliance with various therapy techniques has been found to be variable despite education, and may be related to patient's perception of the severity of their dysphagia *(63)*.

Speech pathologists and other professionals may become involved in ethical decisions regarding dysphagia management. In this process, patient education regarding the nature of the dysphagia, associated diet recommendations, and risks of noncompliance can be essential. Landes proposes an ethical decision model that may be applied when a patient refuses an alternative source of nutrition and hydration *(64)*. This is based on an unpublished student workbook that is cited in her article *(65)*. The following steps are described:

1. Review the case situation and determine the two courses of action. An example involved a choice between a patient's wishes to remain on an oral diet and recommendations for a nonoral diet as a result of health risks.
2. List the factually based reasons supporting each course of action. Perhaps the patient believes that he would experience a decrease in quality of life on a nonoral diet and the treatment team believes the patient could prolong his life with the nonoral diet.
3. Given the reasons supporting each course of action, identify the ethical principles that support each action.
4. List the factually based reasons for not supporting each course of action. For example, if the patient maintains his oral diet, he risks aspiration and possible pneumonia. If the nonoral diet is implemented, he may experience reduced quality of life, and the literature does not support elimination of pneumonia risk with tube feedings.
5. Given the reasons for not supporting each course of action, identify the ethical principles that would be compromised if each action were taken.
6. Formulate a justification for the superiority of one of the two courses of action by processing all information from the previous five steps. If the patient is competent and has been informed of all the risks of the oral diet, he has the right to make an autonomous decision that may be contrary to the recommendations of the team.

Following proper documentation of the patient's wishes and thorough education as to the possible risks involved with these wishes, the speech pathologist should focus on dysphagia management with the diet posing the least aspiration risk. Court cases have, in general, ruled in favor of honoring patients' rights when patients have completed Advanced Directives or Living Wills.

9.4. Interdisciplinary Intervention

Family and medical caregivers (e.g., physicians, dietitians, rehabilitation personnel and nursing) can play an important role in the identification and management of swallowing problems. The speech pathologist performs the swallow study and often, provides assessment results to the doctor and dietitian. The dietitian, in collaboration with the physician and/or medical team, recommends dietary changes using the diet restrictions indicated on completion of the instrumental swallowing evaluation, with a primary goal of maximizing nutritional intake. The dietitian plays a vital role in observing and monitoring dysphagic patients in both acute and outpatient settings. If a patient aspirates thin liquid, thickened liquids are ordered along with the consistency of solid foods that the patient can best tolerate. If a patient reports difficulty chewing solid food, the dietitian may adjust the diet from regular to soft foods according to patient preference.

The patient is observed at mealtime by the dietitian to determine if food intake is adequate. If adequate intake is in question, or observation is not available for all meals, calorie counts can be ordered and completed by the nursing/dietary staff. The dietitian often prompts the physician to request initial or repeat dysphagia evaluations in the acutely ill, as their medical status changes or improves, or if hydration status is compromised resulting from a need for thickened liquids. Thickeners are provided in patient rooms and on medicine carts to maximize compliance with diet modifications and encourage liquid intake. Once the patient has been discharged from the hospital, the outpatient dietitian can encourage appropriate nutritional follow-up, as they can provide education as needed and monitor changes in weight and laboratory results. Proper nutritional management, especially in the dysphagic elderly, is essential to promote adequate PO intake and prevent additional compromise in swallowing function (11).

The occupational therapist provides adaptive utensils and assists patients with upper extremity difficulties to improve the functional acts of feeding. Position recommendations, especially head flexion during the swallow, may require adaptive cups provided by the occupational therapist. Dental professionals are consulted if chewing problems can be addressed through dental care including denture placement and fit.

Langmore concluded that dependence on feeding and oral care were the best predictors for aspiration pneumonia in the study groups of outpatients, acute (not intensive care) inpatients, and nursing home patients (12). Additionally, the presence of decayed teeth and the need for assistance with brushing teeth was associated with pneumonia, also suggesting the need for intervention by dental professionals when appropriate. Dryness of the mouth, or xerostomia, can result from decreased production of saliva, secondary to medications or radiation treatments. This can further increase swallowing difficulty, promote increased bacterial concentration, and a heightened risk of aspiration pneumonia.

It is important that nurses and aides who feed patients are made aware of the specific recommendations for those with dysphagia. In addition, continued education of nursing staff on aspiration and reflux precautions enables them to consult with speech pathologists when patients show initial signs of dysphagia or exhibit changes that require reevaluation.

Caregivers play an integral part in supervised feeding groups by monitoring several patients at a time who are having difficulty swallowing. These feeding groups are often a collaborative effort involving the speech pathologist, dietitian, and occupational therapist in consultation with the nursing staff that supervises the group and encourages consistent implementation of the recommended dysphagia treatment.

9.5. Alternative Means of Nutrition

When prandial aspiration is a severe risk, more invasive therapies, such as tube feeding, may be necessary for the short or long term. This can be accomplished temporarily via assorted nasogastric tubes, or for extended periods via gastrostomy/PEG or jejunostomy/PEJ tubes (Chapter 26). Patients under an ongoing NPO recommendation would require alternative means of nutrition. Tube feedings are typically the last resort because of the associated risk of complications, such as aspiration of reflux, skin breakdown at the site in insertion, potential for infection, pneumonia, prolonged hospital stay and greater morbidity. The interdisciplinary team will, if appropriate, make treatment recommendations and systematically monitor swallow function with the goal to discharge tube feedings as soon as possible. Alternatively, this team may determine that a feeding tube is not an appropriate choice for an individual, based on the patient's medical condition, cognitive status, overall prognosis, and other complicating factors. Many hospitals have Ethics Committees to provide further consultation.

During a study of 272 Washington state nursing homes using the Minimum Data Set, 5266 residents were identified with chewing and swallowing problems, of which 10.5% also had a feeding tube *(66)*. Those residents who were tube fed were found to have a poorer survival rate after 1 yr than those not tube fed. In another prospective study of 189 VA outpatients, inpatients, and nursing home patients, tube feeding was found to increase risk of aspiration pneumonia *(12)*. Langmore speculated that aggressive oral hygiene and pharyngeal suctioning of excess secretions may help prevent the colonization of oropharyngeal bacteria that can increase risk for pneumonia. Yamaya *(67)* also describes this important consideration, noting increased risk secondary to aspiration of bacteria in oral pharyngeal secretions. Currently, controversy exists regarding the need for an overt, witnessed occurrence of aspiration to precipitate a diagnosis of aspiration pneumonia *(18)*.

In a recent study, 16 nursing home patients with a history of neurogenic dysphagia secondary to single or multiple CVAs, and a 6-mo minimum history of PEG tube placement were enrolled in two dysphagia management groups for a range of 2–16 wk *(68)*. As a result of therapy, all patients received significant PO dietary upgrades, 63% became aspiration free and 37% aspirated only thin liquids. Weight gains were noted in 15 of 16 patients, and the remaining patient was placed on weight reduction for obesity management. Albumin was monitored, with trends increasing toward a normal level. The daily cost of PEG tube feedings, including eight cans of Ultra-cal, a feeding bag, a feeding irrigation tray, and dressing change kits ranged from $27.95 to $41.68. In contrast, daily oral feeding costs were estimated at $5.50 to $7.00. Thus, the annual cost savings for oral feeds compared to tube feeds were computed as 83%. Klor acknowledged cost of speech evaluation and treatment intervention as comprising 21–31% of the nonoral costs *(68)*.

10. RECOMMENDATIONS FOR CLINICIANS

An interdisciplinary team approach to intervention for swallowing disorders is both rewarding to the clinician and advocates optimal patient quality of life. The following recommendations are pertinent to acute and long-term care.

Initial Assessment by the Speech Pathologist:

1. Obtain a thorough case history.
2. Perform a clinical bedside examination of oral motor and swallowing function including bolus administration.
3. Assess adequacy of dentition/oral hygiene.
4. Document respiratory rate/status.
5. Screen cognition; administer Dysphagia Disability Index or Swallowing Quality of Life Index assessments.
6. Perform an objective/instrumental swallow study when appropriate.

Treatment/Intervention Recommendations:

7. The speech pathologist should provide patients with individualized dietary recommendations, viscosity modifications, and compensatory techniques as appropriate.
8. Physician and dietitian should review swallow study results and the dietitian should provide specific dietary instructions. Follow with calorie counts and weight monitoring, as indicated.
9. Initiate or continue aspiration and reflux precautions.
10. Institute and continue vigorous oral hygiene; provide water, ice chips, or pleasurable supplemental boluses such as popsicles or lollipops as appropriate.
11. Educate patients and caregivers regarding evaluation results, treatment goals, and expected outcomes. They should be provided with appropriate handouts, recipes, and resources when necessary.
12. Monitor weight and vital signs dependent on patient medical status.
13. Repeat instrumental swallowing evaluations and outcome measures as needed to assess for changes in swallowing function that may allow for possible dietary upgrades, with an ultimate goal of least restrictive diet recommendations with maximum PO intake.

REFERENCES

1. McCullough GH. Normal swallowing in the geriatric population. SID13 Newsletter on Swallowing and Swallowing Disorders 2001;10:14–18.
2. Palmer JB, DuChane AS. Rehabilitation of swallowing disorders in the elderly. In: Rehabilitation of the Aging and Elderly Patient. Felsenthal G, Garrison SJ, Steinberg FU (eds.), Williams & Wilkins, Baltimore, MD, 1994, pp. 275–287.
3. Siebens H, Trupe E, Siebens A, Cook F, Anshen S, Hanauer R, et al. Correlates and consequences of eating dependency in institutionalized elderly. J Am Genatr Soc 1986;34:192–198.
4. Lugger KE. Dysphagia in the elderly stroke patient. J Neurosci Nurs 1994;26:78–84.
5. Donner, MW, Jones B. Aging and neurological disease. In: Normal and Abnormal Swallowing Imaging in Diagnosis and Therapy. Donner MW, Jones B (eds.), Springer-Verlag, New York, pp. 189–202.
6. Mendez L, Friedman LS, Castell DO. Swallowing disorders in the elderly. Clin Geriatr Med 1991;7: 215–230.
7. Daniels SK, Brailey K, Priestly DH, Harrington LR, Weisberg JA, Foundas AL. Aspiration in patients with acute stroke. Arch Phys Med Rehabil 1998;79:14–19.
8. Readling MJ. Reliability of the Dysphagia Disability Index-revised in determining oropharyngeal and esophageal dysphagia. Thesis submitted to the Faculty of North Carolina Central University, Durham, NC, 2000.
9. Patterson WG. Dysphagia in the elderly. Can Fam Physician 1996;42:925–932.
10. Logemann JA. Evaluation ad treatment of swallowing disorders. College-Hill, San Diego, CA, 1986.
11. Hudson HM, Daubert CR, Mills RH. The interdependency of protein-energy malnutrition, aging, and dysphagia. Dysphagia 2000;15:31–38.
12. Langmore SE, Terpenning MS, Schork A, Chen Y, Murray JT, Lopatin D, Loesche WJ. Predictors of aspiration pneumonia: how important is dysphagia. Dysphagia 13:69–81.
13. Buffington DE, Graham AS, Jackson AJ. Pharmacological considerations. In: Swallowing Intervention in Oncology. Sullivan PS and Guilford AM (eds.), Singular Publishing Group, San Diego, CA, pp. 227–246.
14. Dodds WJ, Stewart ET, Logemann JA. Physiology and radiology of the normal oral and pharyngeal phases of swallowing. A J Roentogenol 1990;154:953–963.
15. Kendall KA, Leonard RJ. Pharyngeal constriction in elderly dysphagic patients compared with young and elderly nondysphagic controls. Dysphagia 2001;16:272–278.
16. Palmer JB, Drennan JC. Evaluation and treatment of swallowing impairments. Am Fam Physician 2000;61:2453–2462.
17. Dodds, WJ, Logemann JA, Stewart ET. Radiologic assessment of abnormal oral and pharyngeal phases of swallowing. AJR Am J Roentgenol 1990;154:965–974.

18. Feinberg MJ, Knebl J, Tully J, Segall L. Aspiration and the elderly. Dysphagia 1990;5:61–71.
19. Kidd D, Lawson, Nesbitt R, MacMagon J. The natural history and clinical consequences of aspiration in acute stroke. QJM 1995;88:409–413.
20. Teasell RW, Mc Rae M, Marchuk Y, Fienston HM. Pneumonia associated with aspiration following stroke. Arch Phys Med Rehabil 1996;77:707–709.
21. Ding R, Logemann JA. Pneumonia in stroke patients: A retrospective study. Dysphagia 2000;15: 51–57.
22. Goyal RK. Disorders of the cricopharyngeus muscle. Otolaryngol Clin North Am 1984;17:115–130.
23. Castell DO. Esophageal disorders in the elderly. Gastroenterol Clin North Am 1990;19:235–254.
24. Ravich WJ. Esophageal dysphagia. In: Dysphagia Diagnosis and Management. Groher M (ed.), Butterworth-Heinemann, Boston, MA, 1992, pp. 85–106.
25. Robbins JA, Levine R, Wood J, Roecker RB, Luschei E. Differentiation of normal and abnormal airway protection during swallowing using the penetration aspiration scale. Dysphagia 1999;14:228–232.
26. Tracy JF, Logemann JA, Kahrilas PJ, Jacob P, Kobara M, Krugler C. Preliminary observations on the effects of age on oropharyngeal deglutition. Dysphagia 1989;4:90–94.
27. Robbins JA, Hamilton JW, Lof GL, Kempster GB. Oropharyngeal swallowing in normal adults of different age groups. Gastroenterology 1992;50A:103:823–829.
28. Shaw DW, Cook IF, Gabb M, Holloway RH, Simula ME, Panagopoulos V, Dent J. Influence of normal aging on oropharyngeal and upper esophageal sphincter function during swallow. Am J Physiol 1995; 268:G389–G396.
29. Sonies BC, Parent LJ, Morrish K, Baum BJ. Durational aspects of the oral-pharyngeal phase of swallow in normal adults. Dysphagia 1988;3:1–10.
30. Barczi SR, Sullivan PA, Robbins JA. How should dysphagia care of older adults differ? Establishing optimal practice records. Semin Speech Lang 2000;21:347–361.
31. Aviv JE. Effects of aging on sensitivity of the pharyngeal and supraglottic areas. Am J Med 1997; 103:745–765.
32. Horner J, Massey EW. Silent aspiration following stroke. Neurology 1988;38:317–319.
33. Jacobson B, Silbergleit A, Sumlin T, Johnson A. Dysphagia Disability Index-Revised (DDD). September 2000; unpublished outcome measure. Henry Ford Hospital, Detroit, MI.
34. McHorney CA, Robbins J, Lomax, Rosenbek JC, Chignell K, Kramer AE, Bricker, DE. The SWAL-QOL and SWAL-CARE outcomes tool for oropharyngeal dysphagia in adults: III. documentation of reliability and validity. Dysphagia 2002;17:97–114.
34a. Belafsky PC, Postma GN, Koufman JA. Validity and reliability of the reflux symptom index (RSI). J Voice 2002;16:274–277.
35. Kiernan RJ, Mueller J, Langston JW, Van Dyke C. The neurobehavioral cognitive status examination: A brief but differentiated approach to cognitive assessment. Amer Coll Physic 1987;107:481–485.
36. Leder SB. Gag reflex and dysphagia. Head Neck 1996;18:138–141.
37. Horner J, Massey EW, Riske JE, Lathrop DL, Chase KN. Aspiration following stroke. Clinical correlates and outcomes. Neurology 1988;38:1359–1362.
38. Selley WG, Flack FC, Brooks WA. Respiratory patterns associated with swallowing, part 2. Neurologically impaired dysphagic patients. Age Ageing 1989:18;173–176.
39. Vice FL, Heinz JM, Giuriati G, Hood M, Bosma JF. Cervical auscultation of suckle feeding in newborn infants. Dev Med Child Neurol 1990:32;760–768
40. Linden, P, Siebens A. Dysphagia: Predicting laryngeal penetration. Arch Phys Med Rehabil 1983; 64:281–284.
41. Sortin R, Somers S, Austin W, Bester S. The influence of vdieofluoroscopy on the management of the dysphagic patient. Dysphagia 1988 2:127–135.
42. Splanigard M, Hutchins B, Sulton L, Chaudhuri G: Aspiration in rehabilitation patients: videofluoroscopy vs bedside clinical assessment. Arch Phys Med Rehabil 69:637–640.
43. Horner J, Massey WE. Silent aspiration following stroke Neurology 1988;38:317–319.
44. Smith HA, Lee SH, O'Neill PA, Connolly MJ. The combination of bedside swallowing assessment and oxygen saturation monitoring of swallowing in acute stroke: a safe and humane screening tool. Age Ageing 2000;29:495–499.
45. Smith Hammond C, Davenport PW, Hutchison AA, Otto RA. Motor innervation of the cricopharyngeus muscle by the recurrent laryngeal nerve. J Appl Physiol 1997;83:89–94.
46. Kidder TM, Langmore SE, Martin BJ. Indications and techniques of endoscopy in evaluation of cervical dysphagia: comparison with radiographic techniques. Dysphagia 1994;9:256–261.

47. Langmore SE, Schatz K, Olsen N. Fiberoptic endoscopic evaluation of swallow safety: A new procedure. Dysphagia 1988;2:216–219.
48. Logemann JA. Ninth Annual Dysphagia Research Society Meeting, Efficacy and Outcomes of Dysphagia Management: Where are we? October 26–28, 2000.
49. American Speech-Language-Hearing Association National Outcomes Measurement System (NOMS) Training Manual 1998.
50. Smith-Hammond CA, Scharver CH, Galanos AN, Evanko L, Heard MA, Daubert C, et al. Real Food Viscosity Recommendations by Medical Diagnostic Grouping Based on Radiologic and Endoscopic Evaluations, poster presentation American Speech-Language Hearing Association, San Antonio, TX, 1998.
51. Pouderoux P, Kahrilas PJ. Deglutitive tongue force modulation by volition, volume, and viscosity. Gastroenterology 1995;108:1418–1426.
52. Garon BR, Engle M, Ormiston CJ. A randomized control study to determine the effects of unlimited oral intake of water in patients with identified aspiration. Neuro Rehab 1997;11:139–148.
53. Dantas RO, Dodds WJ, Massey BT, Kern MK. The effect of high- vs low-density barium preparations on the quantitative features of swallowing. Am J Roentgenol 1989;153:1191–1195.
54. Shaker R, Kern M, Bardan E, Taylor, A, Stewart ET, Hoffmann RG, et al. Augmentation of deglutitive upper esophageal sphincter opening in the elderly by exercise. AJP 1997;272:G1518–G1522.
55. Fujiu M, Logemann J. Effect of a tongue-holding maneuver on posterior pharyngeal wall movement during deglutition. Am J Speech Lang Pathol 1996;5:23–30.
56. Kahrilas PJ, Logemann JA, Krugler C, Flanagan E. Volitional augmentation of upper esophageal sphincter opening during swallowing Am J Physiol 1991;62.
57. Rasley A, Logemann JA, Kahrilas PJ, Rademaker AW, Pauloski BR, Dodds WJ. Prevention of barium aspiration during videofluoroscopic swallow studies: Value of change in posture. AJR 1993;160:1005–1009.
58. Freed ML. Electrical stimulation for swallowing disorders caused by stroke. Respir Care 2001;46:446–474.
59. Huckabee ML, Cannito MP. Outcomes of swallowing rehabilitation in chronic brainstem dysphagia: A retrospective evaluation. Dysphagia 1999;14:93–109.
60. Ding R, et al. Surface electromyographic and electroglottographic studies in normal subjects under two swallow conditions: Normal and during the mendelsohn maneuver. Dysphagia 2002;17:1–12.
61. Sharkawi AE, Ramig L, Loemann JA, Pauloski BR, Rademaker AW, Smith CH, et al. Swallowing and voice effects of Lee Silverman Voice Treatment (LSVT): A pilot study. J Neurol Neurosurg Psychiatr 2002;72:31–36.
62. McAdams S. Presentation. Functional Assessment and Goal Setting in Neurogenic Disorders. Raleigh, NC, March 16, 2002.
63. Lieter AE, Windsor J. Compliance of geriatric dysphagic patients with safe-swallowing instructions. J Med Speech-Language Pathol 1996;4:289–300.
64. Landes TL. Ethical issues involved in patients' rights to refuse artificially administered nutrition and hydration and implications for the speech-language pathologist. Amer J Speech-Language Pathol 1999;8:109–117.
65. Rubin SE, Wilson CA, Fischer J, Vaughn B. Ethical practices in rehabilitation: A series of instructional models for rehabilitation education programs. Unpublished student workbook, Southern Illinois University-Carbondale, 1992.
66. Mitchell SL. Does artificial enteral nutrition prolong the survival of institutionalized elders with chewing and swallowing problems? J Gerontol Series A, Biol Sci Med Sci 1998;53:207–213.
67. Yamaya M, Yanai M, Ohrui T, Arai H, Sasaki H. Interventions to prevent pneumonia among older adults. J Amer Geriatr Soc 2001;49:85–90.
68. Klor BM, Milanti FJ. Rehabilitation of neurogenic dysphagia with percutaneous endoscopic gastrostomy. Dysphagia 1999;14:162–164.

25 Gastrointestinal Senescence and Digestive Diseases of the Elderly

Gerald W. Dryden and Stephen A. McClave

1. INTRODUCTION

In the absence of disease, the function of the gastrointestinal system is altered very little during aging. Few processes may be designated as inevitable, predictable, biological changes associated with normal aging independent of specific disease states *(1)*. A reserve capacity exists for the gastrointestinal system minimizing the effect of most of the changes that occur with aging. A growing body of literature involving human studies has helped define the effect of age on gastrointestinal function, and has disproved myths and misconceptions when changes seen in animal models were extrapolated to the human condition. With the exception of reduced absorption of certain vitamins (A, D, K, and B_6) and minerals (calcium and zinc), the aging process alone should not result in malnutrition, deterioration of nutritional status, or clinical symptomology resulting from dysfunction of the gastrointestinal system. However, a number of disease processes have an increased incidence with aging. Although these disease processes have nutritional implications for the geriatric population, they do not always require specific changes in nutritional therapy.

This chapter reviews many of the normal changes in the gastrointestinal system that occur with aging, and describes the common disorders of the digestive system which occur more frequently in the elderly population. Focus will be placed on nutritional implications of these processes, and on recommendations for the optimal nutritional interventions to assist in the management of these difficult problems.

2. ESOPHAGUS

2.1. Physiology

Presbyesophagus describes a multitude of motility defects purportedly associated with the aging esophagus. These defects included decreased contractile amplitude, polyphasic multi-peaked (nonpropulsive) waves, incomplete relaxation of the lower and upper esophageal sphincters, and esophageal dilation *(2)*. Extensive studies have shown that these changes do not occur in the asymptomatic, healthy geriatric population. When present,

From: *Handbook of Clinical Nutrition and Aging*
Edited by: C. W. Bales and C. S. Ritchie © Humana Press Inc., Totowa, NJ

these manometric abnormalities are usually the result of specific pathologic processes such as diabetes, neurologic disease, or side effects from medications *(2)*.

True defects in motility occurring as an effect of normal aging turn out to be relatively mild or minor in magnitude. Upper esophageal sphincter (UES) pressure is slightly decreased and there is a delayed relaxation of the UES in response to swallowing. The sensory threshold for initiation of swallowing may increase, and synchronous nonperistaltic contractions increase slightly in frequency. Although the contraction amplitude does not change, the frequency that a swallow successfully induces an esophageal contraction decreases. The number of myenteric neurons in the esophageal wall decreases by 20–60% *(1)*, but these changes do not correlate with the development of symptoms. Whereas esophageal sensitivity decreases with age, there is no change in acid secretion or the duration and frequency of acid reflux episodes *(1,2)*. Lower esophageal sphincter pressure remains unchanged, as does gastric emptying.

2.2. Disease Processes

Dysphagia (difficulty swallowing), found frequently in the geriatric population, occurs in over 10% of the population >50 yr of age *(2)*. Symptoms of dysphagia encompass two categories of disease processes. Oropharyngeal transfer dysphagia relates to abnormalities of transfer of the food bolus from the oropharynx to the body of the esophagus, and is more often associated with cognitive/perceptive changes and neurologic deficits *(2)* (Chapter 24). The term *esophageal dysphagia* describes symptoms caused by abnormalities in the body of the esophagus impairing movement of the food bolus to the stomach. The causes of esophageal dysphagia can be divided into structural abnormalities, such as peptic strictures or obstructive luminal malignancies (esophageal carcinoma), and motility disorders, such as achalasia. Elderly patients are more likely to develop motility disorders than structural abnormalities *(2)*. Although none of the changes in motility ascribed to aging alone account for primary disorders of motility, aging is associated with an increased incidence of several disease processes which may contribute to abnormal motility (e.g., diabetes, Parkinson's Disease, scleroderma, and neuropathies) *(2)*. Patients afflicted with these diseases also have an increased risk for drug-induced esophageal dysfunction. A small percentage of elderly patients develop unexplained aperistalsis, others develop primary motility disorders such as achalasia or diffuse esophageal spasm.

Gastroesophageal reflux disease (GERD) occurs commonly throughout adult life, but becomes even more prevalent with aging *(2)*. Although the reasons for a 20% prevalence of GERD in the elderly population are not clear, concomitant disease processes and medications affecting lower esophageal sphincter pressure, esophageal motility abnormalities, delays in gastric emptying, and decreases in salivary flow contribute *(2)*. Symptoms of GERD in the geriatric population may be underreported (resulting from decreased sensitivity of the esophagus), atypical (regurgitation, vomiting, and chest pain may occur more commonly than classic heartburn), and may be confused with symptoms of coexistent disorders, such as chronic obstructive pulmonary disease (COPD) and coronary heart disease. Increasing problems with GERD in the elderly population may contribute to exacerbation of concomitant disease process such as asthma, chronic bronchitis, COPD, or angina associated with coronary heart disease *(2)*. The prevalence of Barrett's esophagus, a complication of chronic GERD in which the esophagus becomes lined with columnar intestinal metaplasia, increases with age and actually plateaus in the 7th decade *(2)*.

Barrett's esophagus is the key risk factor for development of adenocarcinoma of the esophagus. The recent trend for increased incidence of adenocarcinoma of the GE junction seen over the past decade may in part be related to the increased incidence of Barrett's with the aging population. With the expected expansion of the geriatric population as the "baby boomer" generation ages, further increases in the prevalence of adenocarcinoma of the esophagus in the elderly may be seen in the future (2).

2.3. Nutritional Implications/Therapy

The development of dysphagia contributes to increased morbidity and mortality in the elderly population (2). Importantly, the development of dysphagia should not be attributed to normal aging; instead, symptoms of dysphagia should prompt the initiation of a full workup and management effort. Dysphagia diets, in which mechanically soft food replaces solid food (e.g., meat, raw apples, and fresh bread which are prone to impaction), may be helpful in a patient with mechanical stricture before the patient can undergo complete dilation therapy. Dysphagia diets are more likely to benefit patients with malignant strictures or difficult benign strictures requiring frequent dilation, and should not be expected to benefit the management of patients with disorders of esophageal motility. Ultimately, patients with esophageal carcinoma are often unfit for surgical resection; instead, they may be treated by endoscopic therapy such as photodynamic therapy, endoscopic mucosal resection, or palliative stents (2). Elderly patients with primary disorders of motility, such as achalasia, are more likely to respond to pneumatic dilation than to medical therapy (2). Surprisingly, elderly patients respond better to injection of botulinum toxin into the lower esophageal sphincter in achalasia than younger adults.

In elderly patients with GERD, higher levels of acid suppression may be needed to relieve symptoms and heal esophagitis (2). With active inflammation in the esophagus, strategies to reduce the symptoms of chest pain and heartburn include avoidance of acidic or irritating food substances (e.g., orange juice, tomato juice, or apple juice) or corrosive medications, such as doxycycline, potassium chloride or nonsteroidal antiinflammatory drugs. Likewise, reduction of GERD symptoms may be accomplished by avoiding agents that decrease the lower esophageal sphincter pressure (e.g., high fat, alcohol, chocolate, nicotine, and peppermint). Weight loss may also reduce symptoms of GERD.

3. STOMACH

3.1. Physiology

No significant change in basal or stimulated gastric acid output from the stomach occurs with normal aging (3). A mild decrease in basal and stimulated pepsin activity occurs, as a result of a decrease in either chief cell mass or function (1). Therefore, no significant increase in the aggressive factors of acid or pepsin occurs to contribute to the development of peptic ulcer disease in the elderly population. However, mucosal defense alterations occurring with normal aging may increase the risk of mucosal injury to elderly patients. Both the content and synthesis of prostaglandins in the gastric mucosa decrease with age, possibly accounting for some of the risk (1). Aging associated reductions in gastric mucosal blood flow and bicarbonate production may also contribute to the development of peptic ulcer disease. Sodium ion and nonparietal cell fluid secretion also diminish with aging. Alterations seen in animal models (such as decreased gastric mucous content and reduced regenerative capacity of the gastric mucosa) have not been confirmed in humans to date *(4)*. Gastric motility changes found in normal aging are limited to a slowing of vagally-mediated liquid emptying by the fundus, while antral emptying of solid foods is preserved *(5)*. As a result of the abnormalities in liquid emptying, mixed meal emptying may be slightly delayed. Decreased nitric oxide production in the fundus may account for the decreased fundic adaptive relaxation that leads to earlier satiation in the elderly *(6)*.

3.2. Disease Processes

Chronic gastritis resulting in reduced acid secretion occurs commonly in the geriatric population, with an overall prevalence of 11–50% *(5)*. Patients should be evaluated to determine which of two separate disease processes may be involved in generating the chronic gastritis. Type A gastritis occurs less commonly (<5% of persons over the age of 60), involves the body and fundus of the stomach, and is associated with pernicious anemia *(5)*. This process is actually an autosomal-dominant inherited disease and involves antiparietal cell, anti-intrinsic factor, and antithyroid antibodies. Type A gastritis is less likely to generate symptoms and is associated with more profound loss of acid secretion, including achlorhydria, than type B gastritis. Type B gastritis is associated with *Helicobacter pylori* infection and occurs much more commonly in the geriatric population. The prevalence of *H. pylori* is age-related, and increases from a 24% prevalence in the 6th decade, to a 37% prevalence in the 8th decade of life *(5)*. Type B gastritis is more likely to generate symptoms of dyspepsia or abdominal pain, and tends to affect the antrum and body of the stomach with a mild superficial, but chronic, inflammatory process *(5)*.

Susceptibility to peptic ulcer disease increases with age *(7)*. The reasons for the increased susceptibility of the geriatric population may be related to a combination of factors, including decreased mucosal defense (occurring naturally with aging), increased prevalence of *H. pylori*, and increased use of nonsteroidal anti-inflammatory drugs (NSAIDs) *(8)*. The incidence, prevalence, rate of hospitalization, and mortality from peptic ulcer disease all increase in persons older than 65 yr of age *(7)*. In fact, 85–90% of the mortality seen in peptic ulcer disease occurs in patients > 65 yr of age *(7)*.

Clinically significant delayed gastric emptying should not occur as a result of the aging process alone. However, problems may be precipitated by development of concomitant disorders, such as diabetes, or by the increased use of drugs (e.g., anticholinergic agents or tricyclic antidepressants), which can lead to delayed gastric emptying *(1)*. The combination of delayed gastric emptying and age related satiety changes (geriatric patients develop a greater degree of satiation after meals) may be the contributory factors behind the physiologic anorexia of aging *(6)*.

3.3. Nutritional Implications/Therapy

Type A atrophic gastritis, ensuing from an autoimmune process where antibodies develop to the parietal cell and intrinsic factor, results in pernicious anemia and clinically significant malabsorption of vitamin B_{12}. The lack of intrinsic factor production is complicated by the development of achlorhydria, as the presence of acid is necessary to absorb protein-bound vitamin B_{12}. Achlorhydria leads to a diminished capacity for food-bound B_{12} absorption in type A atrophic gastritis (7). In type B antral gastritis, associated with *H. pylori*, levels of intrinsic factor production are rarely low enough to cause B_{12} deficiency (5).

Achlorhydria, or severe hypochlorhydria, contributes to significant problems in the absorption of certain vitamins and minerals. Bacterial overgrowth, which commonly develops in the face of decreased gastric output, interferes with absorption of vitamin B_{12}. The bacteria in the small bowel can actually take up or bind vitamin B_{12}. Achlorhydria slows the gastric emptying of solids and may actually accelerate liquid emptying (5). Achlorhydria may interfere with the pH-dependent uptake mechanism of certain minerals, particularly ferric iron and calcium (5). Achlorhydria similarly decreases absorption of folic acid. However, an interesting paradox in vitamin B_{12} and folate levels occurs in the setting of severely reduced gastric acid output and bacterial overgrowth. The bacteria in the small bowel can actually digest vitamin B_{12}, resulting in decreased vitamin B_{12} levels. In contrast, serum folate levels may rise as a result of active bacterial synthesis of folic acid within the lumen of the gut (5). Folate and vitamin B_{12} are required to convert homocystine to methionine. Therefore, deficiencies of either or both of these vitamins can contribute to increased homocystine levels, which by itself is a risk factor for accelerated atherosclerosis in the geriatric population (9). Large doses of oral vitamin B_{12} supplementation (100–1000 µg/d) may be effective in lowering the elevated methylmalonic acid levels seen in patients with hyperhomocysteinemia (10).

For patients with type B antral gastritis combined with hypochlorhydria, supplements of unbound, free oral B_{12} may be adequate to prevent deficiencies. For patients with type A atrophic gastritis with achlorhydria, parenteral injections or pharmacologic doses of B_{12} may be required (5). In some situations, oral supplementation with high doses of vitamin B_{12} may overwhelm the lack of intrinsic factor, helping to maintain adequate serum levels.

Patients with peptic ulcer disease rarely require a change in diet. The bland diet previously recommended in the pre-*H. pylori* era, in which patients avoided spicy or highly seasoned foods, is not needed to control symptoms or promote healing, and should be relegated to the past. Only in the situation of a food intolerance, wherein a patient experiences episodes of dyspepsia with repeated challenges, should a specific food be eliminated from the diet.

In patients with upper gastrointestinal bleeding from peptic ulcer disease, resumption of oral intake depends on the findings on endoscopy. Patients found to have a clean ulcer base may resume feeding immediately following endoscopy. Patients found to have a visible vessel in the ulcer bed requiring endoscopic therapy (where some risk of rebleeding is still present), should be started back on clear liquids at 24 h, followed by resumption of full diet at 48 h.

4. SMALL BOWEL

4.1. Physiology

Overall structure of the small bowel does not change with aging. Although some studies in humans report shortening of the villi in the elderly, consensus seems to indicate that upper small bowel mucosal histology does not change (7). Lactase activity frequently decreases with age, but sucrase and maltase activity remain unchanged. Sodium and glucose cotransport activity decrease with age *(5)*. Although small bowel transit appears intact, blood flow may be reduced *(1)*. Small bowel permeability does not change with age. Although the ability of B lymphocytes and plasma cells to produce immunoglobulins may decrease with aging, the overall number of plasma cells increases, such that secretory immunoglobulin levels (especially IgA and IgG) actually increase with age *(11)*. Intestinal absorption of drugs changes very little with aging *(7)*. The rise in cholecystokinin (CCK) levels resulting from infusion of fat into the duodenum increases with age. Elevated CCK levels may contribute to early satiety and decreased gastric emptying *(1)*.

In general, carbohydrate metabolism remains intact with increasing age *(5)*, although there is some evidence of a slight, but insignificant, decrease in absorptive capacity for carbohydrates in the geriatric population *(7)*. Although upper extremes of age do not alter D-xylose test results, hydrogen breath test results following ingestion of >200 g of carbohydrate are more likely to be abnormal in the geriatric population than in younger adults. This difference may be attributed to either slightly decreased absorption or bacterial overgrowth *(7)*. No significant defects occur in protein metabolism, although small increases in nitrogen spillage into the stool may be noted with excessive protein loading in the elderly *(5)*. Likewise, fat metabolism is well maintained in the elderly population at levels of normal fat ingestion (<100 g/d). High-fat ingestion (>115 g/d) in the elderly may result in slight decreases in fat absorption, as well as decreased fat resynthesis within the intestinal mucosa *(1)*.

Alterations in the absorption of some vitamins and minerals occur as a natural consequence of aging. Absorption and metabolism of fat-soluble vitamins tend to be affected more by aging than that of water-soluble vitamins. Clearance of vitamin A from the circulation decreases in the elderly, and can contribute to the unexpectedly high levels of vitamin A sometimes found in the serum of elderly patients. In contrast, vitamin D levels may be reduced in elderly patients, resulting from reduced dietary intake and reduced renal and skin synthesis of vitamin D. Compounded by reduced intestinal absorption related to a decrease in intestinal vitamin D receptors, all these factors can contribute to clinically significant vitamin D deficiency. The synthesis of vitamin K by intestinal bacteria from fermented foods (menaquinones) remains intact *(5)*, while a slight decrease in the ingestion of vitamin K derived from green leafy vegetables (phylloquinones) may be seen. Of the water-soluble vitamins, only the absorption of vitamin B_6 in the proximal small bowel has been shown to be decreased by advancing age. Even with supplementation, deficiencies can occur in up to 40% of the elderly population *(5)*. Of trace minerals, only the absorption of calcium is reduced with aging in both sexes. This deficiency can be compounded by lactase deficiency, often leading to reduced ingestion of dairy products and lower intake of dietary calcium.

4.2. Disease Processes

The development of bacterial overgrowth occurs with increased frequency in the geriatric population. Normal intestinal motility, gastric acid production, undisrupted intestinal anatomy, and secretory immunoglobulins usually act together to prevent bacterial overgrowth *(5)*. Achlorhydria/hypochlorhydria from chronic gastritis, motility abnormalities precipitated by the onset of diabetes or scleroderma, or disruption of intestinal continuity by intestinal surgery place geriatric patients at increased risk for bacterial overgrowth. The typical bacteria colonizing the small bowel include coliforms and anaerobes that contribute to nutritional abnormalities by actively binding or metabolizing vitamins, or by deconjugating bile salts, leading to steatorrhea and fat malabsorption. Symptoms of bacterial overgrowth in the geriatric patient can be nondescript or atypical, ranging from abdominal bloating to diarrhea, weight loss, steatorrhea, or clinical malnutrition (5).

Decreased lactase activity seen with aging, places geriatric patients at increased risk for lactose intolerance (5). Although virtually all infants can digest lactose, the majority of adults in most ethnic groups cannot. Although over 75% of adults worldwide show evidence of lactase deficiency, approx 25% of adults in the United States cannot digest lactose (5). As with bacterial overgrowth, the symptoms of lactose intolerance may be nonspecific, including abdominal bloating, gas, and diarrhea.

Inflammatory bowel diseases (IBD) have been shown to have a bimodal peak of incidence. This means that in addition to a high incidence of new cases in the second decade of life, a second rise in new diagnoses of these diseases occurs during the sixth decade. In general, geriatric patients with Crohn's disease are more likely to develop nutritional sequelae, such as protein–calorie malnutrition, than patients with ulcerative colitis. Severity of the disease processes varies. Risk factors leading to impaired nutritional status include the extent of bowel affected, the length of bowel resected during surgical procedures, and the type of medical therapy required to achieve remission.

4.3. Nutritional Implications/Therapy

Overall, no specific alterations to the standard Recommended Daily Allowance (RDA) for fat, carbohydrate, and protein intake exist for the normal geriatric population. Given the few abnormalities in the absorption and metabolism of these macronutrients, certain recommendations can be made (5) (see Table 1). Fat should comprise <30% of total calories. Intake of monounsaturated fats should comprise 10–15% of calories, and the intake of saturated and polyunsaturated fat should comprise <10% each of the total caloric intake. In geriatric populations, protein intake <1.0 g/kg/d may be insufficient to achieve nitrogen balance in the absence of a high caloric intake (>40 kcal/kg/d) (5). Ingestion of carbohydrates should comprise 55–60% of total calories, and elderly patients should be encouraged to increase the ratio of complex carbohydrates to simple sugars.

The elderly patient avoiding dairy products because of symptoms of lactose intolerance may be at increased risk for development of osteopenia. Use of lactobacillus or acidophilus, taken in conjunction with dairy products, may allow elderly patients to continue to satisfy their dietary needs of calcium and vitamin D. Most studies have shown low-lactose or lactose-free milk to be better tolerated than lactose-containing milk, but the controversial results of the most recent, well-controlled studies revealed no difference in the tolerance of these products (12).

In the specific case of bacterial overgrowth, bacterial deconjugation of bile salts results in passive absorption of free bile acids, leading to impaired micelle formation, and ultimately fat malabsorption. In this scenario, nutrients at greatest risk of malabsorption include the fat-soluble vitamins A, D, E and K. Adequate levels of vitamin A may be better achieved by increasing the intake of carotene-containing fruits and vegetables, as opposed to the intake of preformed supplemental vitamin A. Requirements for supplemental vitamin D may be higher in a home-bound or institution-bound geriatric patient than in a younger adult (who would tend to have greater sun exposure).

Table 1
Nutrients Altered by Aging Alone

Nutrient	Alteration
Vitamin A	↑
Vitamin D	↓
Vitamin B_6	↓
Calcium	↓

The reduction of vitamin B_6 absorption, which occurs naturally with advancing age, increases the risk of developing elevated levels of homocysteine. Vitamin B_6 is required for enzymatic conversion of homocysteine to cystathionine *(5)*. Vitamin B_6 supplementation may be beneficial in maintaining normal levels of homocysteine *(10)*.

5. COLON

5.1. Physiology

As with most other aspects of the gastrointestinal system, colonic function remains intact with advancing age *(12)*. Despite an aging-related decrease in neuronal density in the colon, no change in transit time occurs *(1)*. Following a meal, segmental contractions and mass movements increase similarly in the elderly compared to younger controls, but these actions are less likely to be associated with propulsive activity in the sedentary geriatric adult *(12)*. An increase in collagen deposition is associated with aging, resulting in an age-related decrease in wall elasticity of the rectum and descending colon *(11)*. Ironically, the strength of the bowel wall decreases with age *(7)*. Although patients maintain their subjective sensation of rectal volume, manometry studies demonstrate a decrease in resting pressure of the anal sphincters. Additionally, the rectal volume at which external sphincter tonic activity is lost decreases with advanced age *(13)*. Elderly women may experience additional pudendal nerve damage due to perineal descent *(13)*. Overall, effective colonic motility remains intact in the geriatric patient, as long as they remain physically active.

5.2. Disease Processes

While constipation is four to eight times more common in the elderly adult than in younger controls *(7)*, it is not more common in healthy, ambulatory elderly citizens *(13)*. The reduced wall elasticity, impaired subjective sensation of rectal volume, and the diminished efficacy of colonic propulsion seen in sedentary elderly individuals all contribute to the development of constipation. Specific causes of constipation are numerous and include functional etiologies (e.g., depression, confusion, immobility), drugs (iron, opiates, calcium antagonists, antidepressants, and diuretics), endocrine causes (hypothyroidism, hypercalcemia), dietary factors (low fiber, poor fluid intake), and mechanical reasons (diverticulosis, ischemia, cancer, and inflammatory bowel disease) *(13)* (*see* Table 2).

The presence of diverticulosis increases linearly with advancing age, occurring in part as a result of a progressive decrease in mechanical integrity of the gut, decreased resistance to pressure (because of increased collagen deposition), and reduced wall elasticity *(3,11)*.

Table 2
Conditions of Aging Associated with Constipation

Poor social function
    Depression
    Confusion
    Immobility
Medications

    Opiates
    Iron supplements
    Calcium channel blockers
    Antidepressants
    Diuretics
Endocrine abnormalities

    Hypothyroidism
    Hypercalcemia
Dietary factors

    Low levels of fiber intake
    Poor fluid intake
Mechanical factors

    Colonic ischemia
    Colon cancer
    Inflammatory bowel disease

Angiodysplastic lesions, which are small vascular lesions of the gastrointestinal mucosa, occur more commonly with aging. Their overall incidence in the geriatric population ranges from 0.2% to 6.2%, with most patients showing a peak incidence in the 7th to 8th decade *(14)*. Angiodysplasias are thought to result from degenerative changes over time, with repeated partial intermittent obstruction of submucosal veins as they pierce the muscularis of the bowel wall. Precapillary sphincter tone is lost, creating arterio-venous malformations *(14)*. Angiodysplasias tend to be more frequent on the right side of the colon where the wall pressures are higher *(14)*. Approximately 50–100% of angiodysplasias are found in the cecum and ascending colon, whereas 21–46% are found in the descending and sigmoid colon *(14)*. Fortunately, massive lower GI bleeding from angiodysplasias is fairly rare in the geriatric population (occurring in <15% of cases) *(14)*. Iron deficiency anemia may result from slow blood loss by the angiodysplasias over time, affecting approx 10–15% of the geriatric population *(14)*. Although little data exists on changes in stool evacuation associated with increasing age, fecal incontinence is not thought to comprise a part of the natural aging process *(1)*. Fecal incontinence may be a pathologic process resulting from anal sphincter dysfunction, impaired rectal sensation from neurologic disease, and/or reduced rectal distensibility *(1)*.

Colonic neoplasia increases with advancing age *(3)*. This age-dependent increase in colonic carcinoma may be the result of altered metabolism of carcinogens, cumulative exposure to carcinogens over time, and/or altered cell proliferation in response to exposure to environmental factors *(3)*.

5.3. Nutrition Implications/Therapy

Important management strategies in the elderly patient with constipation include increasing water intake to 6–8 glasses/d and increasing overall fiber content of the diet. Insoluble fiber (e.g., wheat bran) is more effective than soluble fiber because it tends to trap water, increase fecal bulk, decrease transit time, and is easily fermented by colonic bacteria *(13)*. Osmotic laxatives like sorbitol and lactulose are recommended over stimulant laxatives, such as senna, phenolphthalein, and Dulcolax. Long-term complications (e.g., enteric neuropathy) may be associated with use of the latter agents.

Recent studies utilizing dietary fiber supplementation to reduce risk of subsequent colonic neoplasia failed to demonstrate a benefit over control subjects, as did studies examining the effect of dietary supplementation with vitamins C, E, beta carotene and calcium *(15–19)*. Fiber supplementation failed to impact the recurrence rate of colorectal adenomas in colonoscopic surveillance programs *(15,16)*. Although these studies have been criticized for the short term of followup and the failure to factor in life-long patterns of fiber ingestion, firm recommendations for high-fiber diets to specifically prevent colorectal carcinoma cannot be made at this time.

6. LIVER

6.1. Physiology

In general, measures of liver biochemistry do not change with aging. Blood tests for bilirubin, AST, ALT, and alkaline phosphatase should remain unchanged throughout the aging process *(20)*. However, studies have documented decreases in liver size, splanchnic blood flow, and liver perfusion associated with aging, as well as a reduction in dynamic liver function (documented by specific tests, such as galactose elimination and caffeine clearance) *(1)*. Studies have also shown age-related decreases in regenerative capacity and liver cell proliferation in response to injury *(20)*. Protein synthesis (especially albumin) remains preserved, and gall bladder contractions are not affected by age *(1)*.

6.2. Disease Processes

Overall, no specific age-related diseases of the liver have been documented *(20)*. However, the prevalence of clinically apparent viral hepatitis C may be increasing in the geriatric population over the next few decades. The current prevalence of anti-HCV antibodies is higher in the elderly than in younger adults *(20)*. In general, the disease course from hepatitis C may be more benign in the elderly population. Concomitant ethanol abuse worsens mortality and speeds the progression to cirrhosis. The increasing incidence of viral hepatitis C in the geriatric population may lead to a significant increase in hepatocellular carcinoma over the next 10–20 yr. These changes may soon give the false impression that hepatocellular carcinoma is associated with aging as well *(20)*.

While autoimmune hepatitis is usually a disease of young persons, 20% of patients with this disease present after the age of 65 yr *(20)*. Primary biliary cirrhosis (PBC) may be slightly more prevalent in the elderly population, with the mean age of onset at 60 yr of age *(20)*. Alcoholic liver disease may occur more frequently in the elderly population, resulting from an age-related decline in the rapid metabolism of ethanol. In the United States, the peak age of presentation in some studies has been as late as the 7th decade *(20)*. Unfortunately, increasing age is associated with increased severity of symptoms and increased mortality from alcoholic liver disease.

6.3. Nutritional Implications/Therapy

The deleterious nutritional implications from liver disease usually do not manifest until the patient progresses to cirrhosis. At that time, reduced protein synthesis, hypoalbuminanemia, cachexia, and loss of muscle mass (often despite increasing actual body weight from fluid retention, edema, and ascites) may complicate the progression to cirrhosis. In respect to nutritional recommendations, patients should be placed on a high-calorie, high-protein diet (as much as is tolerated). Efforts should be made to discourage limitations in protein intake, even in the face of encephalopathy. Encephalopathy may be treated aggressively with lactulose and neomycin. Even in end-stage liver disease it is rarely necessary to restrict protein intake. Proteins from vegetable source (peanuts, beans, lentils) are less likely to cause encephalopathy than proteins from animal sources. Patients should be placed on a low sodium diet. Restriction of free-water intake is required only in end-stage liver disease, when hyponatremia is accompanied by edema and ascites. Patients with advanced liver disease should be monitored for fasting hypoglycemia, and may require more frequent meals to reduce symptomatology from the low serum glucose levels. Eliminating further ethanol intake is of paramount importance for patients with alcoholic liver disease. Abstinence is particularly important for patients with chronic hepatitis C infection.

7. PANCREAS

7.1. Physiology

Overall, although a number of changes within the pancreas have been documented to occur with advancing age, no disease process per se may be directly attributed to aging. The weight or mass of the pancreas gland decreases with age, by as much as 33% (5). Histologically, studies have shown that ductular epithelial dysplasia and patchy lobular fibrosis may occur as a consequence of aging (1). The pancreatic duct may become dilated up to 10 mm, and there may be associated ductular ectasia. Ductular changes rarely progress to fibrosis and atrophy (5). Parenchymal changes within the gland may lead to lipoatrophy, lipofuscin deposition, and further fibrosis (5). Exocrine secretion of enzymes and pancreatic juices remains intact with advancing age. Therefore, fat maldigestion should not be expected under normal circumstances. Only with repeated stimulation can elderly patients be shown to have a slight decrease in pancreatic enzyme output when compared to younger adults (5). With regard to endocrine function of the pancreas, hyperinsulinemia may occur after meals in the elderly, resulting from increased proinsulin levels and decreased insulin clearance (1).

7.2. Disease Processes

Theoretically, decreased insulin sensitivity and mild pancreatic beta-cell dysfunction may predispose the elderly adult to glucose intolerance in comparison to younger controls (1).

8. CONCLUSIONS

Overall, few dietary alterations are required for the management of the healthy elderly adult. Although there are changes in the gastrointestinal system that occur with aging, the changes are relatively minor, clinically inconsequential, and rarely generate symptoma-

Table 3
Gastrointestinal Changes of Senescence by Segment

Segment of GI tract	Age-related alterations in the GI tract	Diseases with nutritional consequences
Esophagus	Minor alterations in UES	Dysphagia GERD
Stomach	↓ Pepsin activity ↓ Prostaglandin synthesis ↓ Mucosal blood flow ↓ Gastric fluid secretion	Gastritis type A Gastritis type B Delayed gastric emptying Achlorhydria
Small intestine	↓ Lactase activity ↓ Intestinal blood flow ↓ Sodium/glucose co-transport	Bacterial overgrowth Lactose intolerance Inflammatory bowel disease

Colon	↓ In neuronal density
	↓ Wall elasticity
	    from collagen deposition
	↓ Resting pressure
	    of internal anal sphincter
		Constipation
		Diverticulosis
		Angiodysplasia

Liver	↓ Liver size and blood flow
	↓ Dynamic liver function
		Hepatic encephalopathy
		    cirrhosis (hepatitis C,
		    ethanol, primary biliary
		    cirrhhosis)

Pancreas	↓ Pancreatic mass Ductular changes/fibrosis	Pancreatic cancer Chronic pancreatitis Diabetes

tology. In fact, the development of clinical signs or symptoms should not be attributed to normal aging; more likely, they reflect the onset of a new disease and warrant a full diagnostic evaluation. Most alterations in nutritional status that occur in the geriatric adult generally reflect the consequence of a specific disease process (see Table 3). Knowledge of those disease processes for which the elderly are at risk leads to successful evaluation and management of the disease and its corresponding nutritional derangements.

9. RECOMMENDATIONS FOR CLINICIANS

1. Dysphagia in an older adult warrants a full evaluation to detect possible anatomic or motility disorders; dysphagia diets are more beneficial for patients with structural disorders than for those with motility disorders.
2. Reduction of GERD symptoms may be accomplished by avoiding agents that decrease the lower esophageal sphincter pressure (e.g., high-fat foods, alcohol, chocolate, nicotine, and peppermint), avoidance of acidic or irritating food substances such as orange juice, tomato juice, or apple juice, and weight loss if indicated.

3. For patients with type B antral gastritis with hypochlohydria and vitamin B_{12} deficiency, supplements of unbound, free oral vitamin B_{12} may be adequate to prevent deficiencies.
4. Patients with peptic ulcer disease rarely require changes in their diet.
5. Reductions in intestinal absorption of vitamin B_6 and vitamin D may warrant their oral supplementation.
6. Older patients with constipation should increase water intake to 6–8 glasses/d, along with increasing the overall fiber content of the diet. Insoluble fiber (e.g., wheat bran) is particularly useful.
7. Patients with liver disease should be placed on a high-calorie, high-protein diet (as much as is tolerated, even in the setting of encephalopathy).

REFERENCES

1. Dharmarajan TS, Pitchumoni CS, Kokkat AJ. The aging gut. Pract Gastroent 2001;25:13–28.
2. Tack J, Vantrappen G. The aging oesophageus. Gut 1997;41:422–424.
3. Majumdar APN, Jaszewski R, Dubick MA. Effect of Aging on the Gastrointestinal Tract and the Pancreas. Proc Soc Exp Biol Med 1997;215:134–144.
4. Lee, M, Feldman M. The aging stomach: Implications for NSAID gastropathy. Gut 1997;41:425–426.
5. Saltzman JR, Russell RM. Nutritional, physiologic, and pathophysiologic considerations of the gastrointestinal tract. The aging gut. Gastroenterol Clin 1998;27:309–324.
6. Morley JE. Anorexia of aging: Physiologic and pathologic. Amer J Clin Nutr 1997;66:760–763.
7. Holt PR. Editorial: Are gastrointestinal disorders in the elderly important? J Clin Gastroenterol 1993; 16:186–188.
8. Cullen D, Hawkey GM, Greenwood DC, Humphreys H, Shepherd V, Logan RFA, Hawkey CJ. Peptic ulcer bleeding in the elderly: Relative roles of Helicobacter pylori and non-steroidal anti-inflammatory drugs. Gut 1997;41:459–462.
9. Jacobsen DW. Homocysteine and vitamins in cardiovascular disease. Clin Chem 1998,44:1833 1843.
10. Stabler SP, Lindenbaum J, Allen RH. Vitamin B-12 deficiency in the elderly: Current dilemmas. Amer J Clin Nutr 1997;66:741–749.
11. Hosoda S, Bamba T, Nakago S, Fujiyma Y, Senda S, Hinata M. Age-related changes in the gastrointestinal tract. Nutr Rev 1992;50:374–377.
12. Vesa TH, Marteau P, Korpela R. Lactose intolerance. J Amer Coll Nutr 2000;19:165S–175S.
13. Baslon R, Gibson PR. Lower gastrointestinal tract. Med J Aust 1995;162:155–157.
14. Sharma R, Gorbien MJ. Angiodysplasia and lower gastrointestinal tract bleeding in elderly patients. Arch Intern Med 1995;155:807–812.
15. Alberts DS, Martinez ME, Roe DJ, et al. Lack of effect of a high-fiber cereal supplement on the recurrence of colorectal adenomas. N Engl J Med 2000;342:1156–1162.
16. Schatzkin A, Lanza E, Corle D, et al. Lack of effect of a low-fat, high-fiber diet on the recurrence of colorectal adenomas. N Engl J Med 2000;342:1149–1155.
17. MacLennan R, Macrae F, Bain C, et al. Randomized trial of intake of fat, fiber, and beta carotene to prevent colorectal adenomas. J Natl Cancer Inst 1995;87:1760–1766.
18. Hofstad B, Almendingen K, Vatn M, et al. Growth and recurrence of colorectal polyps: A double-blind 3-year intervention with calcium and antioxidants. Digestion 1998;59:148–156.
19. Bonithon-Kopp C, Kronborg O, Giacosa A, et al. Calcium and fibre supplementation in prevention of colorectal adenoma recurrence: A randomized trial. Lancet 2000;356:1300–1306
20 James OFW. Parenchymal liver disease in the elderly. Gut 1997;41:430–432.

26

Provision for Enteral and Parenteral Support

Mark H. DeLegge and David A. Sabol

1. INTRODUCTION

The Centers for Disease Control and Prevention (CDC) estimate that 20% of Americans will be 65 yr or older by the year 2050. Currently, those aged 85 yr or older are among the fastest growing segments of the population. The aging process affects multiple organ functions. With aging, changes in body composition, most notably a decrease in skeletal muscle mass and an increase in total body fat with greater visceral fat stores, are noted *(1)*. These are just a few changes in physiology, metabolism, and function of the aged that result in altered nutritional requirements.

Nutrition is viewed as a cornerstone of therapy in the treatment of various disease states such as hypertension, diabetes, coronary artery disease, and obesity. Nutrition is also tied to our social events and celebrations symbolizing health, vitality, and happiness *(2)*. Risks of malnutrition include fatigue, weakness, and impaired immune function *(1)*. Thus, the road to recovery from simple diseases, such as an upper respiratory infection, incorporates the provision of adequate nutrition as no disease process improves significantly with starvation. The challenge in overcoming various disease states in the elderly is, therefore, a combination of age-related changes resulting in altered nutritional requirements and the provision of providing nutrition in those who cannot or will not eat. In addition, there are a number of ethical issues concerning aggressive nutritional intervention, especially for a terminal disease process *(2)*.

2. ENTERAL NUTRITION

2.1. Introduction to Percutaneous Endoscopic Gastrostomy

The field of enteral nutrition has expanded dramatically over the past 15–20 yr *(3)*. However, the benefit of enteral feeding in the terminally ill has not been well established. As a society, we associate eating with health and life. Many families are unwilling to withhold feedings, even faced with the imminent death of a loved one *(2)*.

Enteral access must be obtained for tube feedings to begin (Table 1). Temporary access may include a nasogastric tube or naso-small bowel feeding tube. These tubes are easily

From: *Handbook of Clinical Nutrition and Aging*
Edited by: C. W. Bales and C. S. Ritchie © Humana Press Inc., Totowa, NJ

Table 1
Routes of Enteral Access

1. Nasogastric tube (NGT)
2. Naso-small bowel feeding tube
3. Percutaneous endoscopic gastrostomy (PEG) tube
4. Percutaneous endoscopic jejunostomy (PEJ) tube
5. Percutaneous endoscopic gastrostomy/jejunostomy (PEG/J) tube
6. Surgical gastrostomy tube
7. Surgical jejunostomy tube

placed at the bedside and can also be easily removed. Unfortunately, these tubes often fail secondary to clogging or inadvertent dislodgment and do not provide a secure access route for the provision of calories, medications, or fluids (4). More permanent access can be obtained either endoscopically or surgically via either a gastrostomy or jejunostomy. Percutaneous endoscopic gastrostomy (PEG) has developed into a very common procedure to obtain gastric access; accounting for approx 100,000 procedures/yr in the United States (2,5).

The development of the PEG procedure and standardized PEG kits was an important technological advance in the enteral access field. The ethics of PEG placement and feeding in patients with a perceived poor quality of life, however, continues to pose a difficult question. Decisions regarding enteral nutrition should not be relegated to the specialist providing enteral access. Rather, decisions regarding enteral nutrition should be made after extensive discussions between the primary clinician and the patient or proxy. These discussions should address treatment goals and the benefits and risks of the procedure given the patients' underlying condition.

2.2. Indications for PEG Placement

2.2.1. CANCER

Weight loss has been associated with poor performance status in cancer patients (1). One area of oncology in which PEG tubes are proven is in patients with head and neck cancer. Head and neck cancers are commonly diagnosed in advanced stages. Aggressive chemotherapy and radiotherapy can lead to dysphagia, odynophagia, dehydration, and malnutrition that may interrupt treatment and lead to more frequent hospitalizations (7). The benefit of PEG tubes in this setting was illustrated in a retrospective study that included 88 patients of whom 32 (40%) received a prophylactic gastrostomy tube prior to radiotherapy and chemotherapy. Patients who received a PEG had an average of 3.1 kg of weight loss when compared to 7 kg of weight loss for patients without a PEG. In addition, the PEG group required significantly fewer hospitalizations for dehydration and malnutrition and had no interruption in treatment compared to interruptions in 18% of patients in the non-PEG group (8). The PEG tube, especially in these instances, also serves as a medication and hydration delivery port.

2.2.2. CNS DISORDERS

Available data support the use of PEG tubes in patients with central nervous system (CNS) disorders that are associated with dysphagia (9). Studies in patients with dysphagic strokes have demonstrated improved nutrition and rehabilitative gains following

PEG placement *(2,10)*. In one study, the most common CNS indication was hemispheric stroke. This study subsequently showed that the majority of patients (85%) were discharged to a nursing home. The authors reported a 1-, 18-, and 48-mo survival of 78%, 35%, and 27%, respectively *(2)*. PEG tubes also can provide reliable long-term enteral access for patients with traumatic brain injury and in patients with neurodegenerative diseases such as amyotrophic lateral sclerosis *(9,11–13)*. The rehabilitation potential improves and possibly accelerates the recovery of swallowing without aspiration in appropriate patients. This, in turn, can improve a clinical response to other medical therapies by a convenient and relatively low-cost means of providing nutrition *(9)*.

2.2.3. DEMENTIA

Dementia is a common disorder of the elderly that may frequently lead to anorexia, dysphagia, and weight loss *(2)*. As a result, it is a frequent diagnosis indicated for referring patients for PEG. It has been estimated that 36,000 elderly patients with dementia receive a PEG each year *(14)*. However, the role of PEG tubes in patients with dementia is controversial. Patients who require a PEG tube because of dementia are usually severely impaired and frequently near death. The benefit of providing artificial nutrition in such patients is unclear *(15)*. No large randomized trials have demonstrated a survival difference between patients with dementia with or without a PEG. Such a study, however, is likely not feasible as a result of its ethical considerations. Retrospective studies attempting to answer this question are limited because variations in the severity of illness in patients may have influenced the decision to place a PEG. One study in nursing home patients with dementia suggested a reduction in long-term mortality amongst those who received PEG *(16)*. However, Finucane et al. reviewed the evidence from a 33-yr Medline search and concluded that the widespread practice of tube feeding for severely demented patients should be discouraged on clinical grounds *(17)*.

2.3. Complications of PEG Placement

The complication rate of PEG varies based on the criteria and cohorts used and ranges from 3% to 14% overall, with a mortality rate approaching 1% *(18–21)*. A multitude of complications have been described using this technique and include both problems that arise during PEG placement as well as those occurring postprocedure (Table 2) *(19,22)*. Most delayed complications result from an individual patient's comorbidities, such as poor wound healing, aspiration, or coagulopathy *(22,23)*. The most commonly reported complication is peristomal wound infection *(19,21)*. Other minor complications include peristomal leakage, pneumoperitoneum, tube extrusion/migration, cutaneous or gastric ulceration, fever, transient ileus, and volvulus *(21,22,24–26)*. Major complications are rare and include gastric or colonic perforation, gastrocolic or colocutaneous fistula, hematoma, peritonitis, and necrotizing fasciitis *(21–24)*. Aspiration and bleeding are not infrequent and may be minor or life-threatening *(21,22,24)*.

To limit the risk of tube feed aspiration with gastric feeding, caregivers must raise the head of the patient's bed 30–45 degrees during and one hour after feeding. One may also use an intermittent or a continuous feeding regimen rather than the rapid bolus method. This will eliminate the delivery of a large volume of feeding over a short period of time. In all cases, gastric residuals should be checked regularly and signs of feeding intolerance should be monitored. Gastric residuals greater than 200 mL are worrisome. Small bowel feedings may be used to prevent tube feed aspiration although this data is controversial.

Table 2
Complications of PEG Placement

1. Peristomal wound infection
2. Peristomal leakage
3. Pneumoperitoneum
4. Tube extrusion/migration
5. Cutaneous/gastric ulceration
6. Fever
7. Transient ileus
8. Volvulus
9. Gastric/colonic perforation
10. Gastrocolic/colocutaneous fistula
11. Hematoma
12. Peritonitis
13. Necrotizing fasciitis
14. Aspiration
15. Bleeding

To limit the risk of aspiration with small bowel feeding, the feeding port of the nasoenteric tube, PEJ, or PEG/J should be close to or beyond the ligament of Treitz. Radiographs may be needed to confirm tube position as severe vomiting or coughing may displace them *(3)*.

Diarrhea is a common, though poorly defined, complication resulting from many etiologies during tube feeding. Etiologies may include antibiotics or sorbitol-containing products, formula osmolality, rate of infusion, bacterial overgrowth, hypoalbuminemia, bacterial contamination of the enteral fluid, and disease-associated physiological disturbances. In instances where an infectious source is contemplated, the presence of fecal leukocytes will be helpful. Obtaining such tests as a Clostridium difficile toxin, enteric stool pathogens, stool osmolality, and various breath tests should all be ordered in the proper clinical context. An abdominal radiograph and a digital rectal exam will help to rule out a stool obstruction with leakage of liquid stool. Though universal recommendations are not available for preventing or eliminating this complication, it is possible to pay careful attention to fluid and electrolyte management in order to minimize any metabolic complications *(3)*.

2.4. Outcomes and Quality of Life Following PEG Placement

PEG tube feedings can be accomplished safely in severely and chronically ill older adults *(27)*. Long-term care facilities (LTCF) account for a large percentage of patients requiring care after receiving a PEG in the hospital setting. In LTCFs, PEG tubes are often preferred as the enteral access device because of their reliability when compared to nasogastric tubes. The decision to place a PEG in patients in LTCFs relies, oftentimes, with the opinions of patients' families and health care workers. A prospective series of 70 patients in a LTCF with a PEG suggested a trend toward weight stabilization and an increase in serum albumin *(4)*.

Several studies have attempted to describe survival following PEG in patients with a multitude of disease processes. Survival defined at one month is a common endpoint in PEG studies. Few studies have described survival with longer follow-up. The largest of these studies focused on 80,000 Medicare patients who underwent PEG placement or surgical gastrostomy. Seventy-five percent of these patients were older than 75 yr of age. Common indications for enteral access were neoplasms, cerebrovascular disorders, and aspiration pneumonia. Overall in-hospital mortality was 15%. Mortality at 1 and 3 yr was 63% and 81%, respectively. Late mortality and healing of pressure ulcers, an indication of nutritional status, improved in those who received a PEG (3,28,29).

The previous studies indicate that the overall 30-d survival is 70% to 80% following PEG placement. Short-term mortality is often related to the underlying comorbidities rather than from the placement of the PEG tube. The severe disability and comorbidities in the patients who receive PEG tubes are often reflected in the high long-term mortality following PEG placement (3).

Few well-designed studies have evaluated quality-of-life following PEG placement. One study noted a positive effect on quality of life by 55% of patients and 80% of their caregivers (30). Another evaluated quality of life in 100 consecutive nursing home patients (median age was 76) who received a PEG. By a validated quality-of-life scale, 35% improved, 37% showed no change, and 28% worsened after PEG placement (31).

As a general rule, the effectiveness of PEG tubes should only be determined from studies that properly measure realistic and achievable outcomes. Whether PEG tubes improve quality of life has not been established. These issues are difficult to measure or assess in patients who are often demented or neurologically impaired. However, patients in long term care facilities who develop swallowing disorders may benefit from PEG placement and the subsequent benefits of nutrition therapy as with regards to mortality (28). Family and patient input is paramount to establishing reasonable goals.

The decision to place a PEG in the LTCF often relies on the opinion of health care workers and patients families regarding the appropriateness of PEG insertion. The opinion of the family appears to be weighted heavily in this decision (31–33). This was illustrated by 180 physicians who were interviewed regarding their decision to start tube feedings in a hypothetical patient population. Ninety percent of the physicians felt that initiating tube feedings was the correct decision if family members were in agreement with this decision. However, only 50% of the same physicians believed that initiating tube feedings was the right decision if the family members or the patient were not in favor of tube feedings. Physicians concerned with the legal aspects of nutrition were more inclined to believe that tube feedings should be initiated. However, those physicians more concerned with health care costs were more likely not to initiate tube feedings (32). Therefore, it is reasonable to assume that realistic expectations of what PEG tubes can accomplish should be a factor in the decision-making process of placing PEG tubes in nursing home patients (34).

3. PARENTERAL NUTRITION

3.1. Introduction to Total Parenteral Nutrition

A subset of patients cannot tolerate oral or enteral feeding and thus may require more calories than can be provided by these means resulting from severe metabolic stress or gastrointestinal dysfunction or obstruction. The development of total parenteral nutrition (TPN) and its clinical application in the early 1970s was a milestone of modern medicine. Previously, patients with congenital intestinal anomalies, short bowel syndrome, or complications from abdominal surgery would often die of starvation. However, its effect on

Table 3
Reasons and Examples for Initiating TPN

1. Bowel obstruction when surgery is delayed	Obstructing tumor
2. High-output enterocutaneous fistula	Crohn's disease
3. Prolonged postoperative ileus	Cholecystectomy
4. Severe mucositis	Chemotherapy
5. Severe burns or trauma	3rd degree burns
6. Critical illness	Necrotizing pancreatitis
7. Intestinal failure	
8. Motility disorder	Scleroderma

morbidity and mortality in conditions, such as cancer therapy and critical illness, for which TPN is most commonly used, is much less certain (35).

3.2. Indications

The most common reasons for starting TPN in hospitalized patients include: bowel obstruction when surgery is delayed; high-output enterocutaneous fistula; prolonged postoperative ileus; severe mucositis; severe burns or trauma; critical illness, and; intestinal failure (see Table 3) (35,36).

Patients with extensive intestinal resections usually require early TPN support until bowel adaptation occurs. In all patients, attempts should be made to stop TPN by adjusting the diet and using an oral rehydration solution and antimotility agents. Outpatients who may require parenteral nutrition include those with severe pancreatitis, those who do not tolerate jejunal feeding, those with an intestinal obstruction from cancer or stricture, those with a high intestinal bypass fistula or high-volume diarrhea, or those with severe abdominal pain worsened with eating. Patients who are critically ill with comorbid diseases such as renal failure, brittle diabetes, and heart failure usually are not candidates for long-term parenteral nutrition because of a high incidence of related complications (35).

Consideration of when to begin TPN should take into account the number of days fasting, the nutritional state, and the catabolic disease. Subjective global assessment taking into account weight change, oral intake, strength, metabolic demand, gastrointestinal symptoms, and physical findings is as reliable and reproducible as any nutritional assessment (35).

Once TPN is started, patients must be monitored for tolerance, nutritional adequacy, and complications. A management team consisting of a dedicated physician, nurse, nutritionist, and pharmacist is cost-effective for patients receiving parenteral nutrition and has been shown to be associated with reduced complications (35,37). This approach optimizes setting calorie and protein goals based on the Harris-Benedict equation or indirect calorimetry and the patient's urine urea nitrogen (UUN) in order to maintain a positive nitrogen balance. The catheter site should be inspected daily for signs of inflammation. Blood glucose and electrolytes should be checked daily until stable. Maintaining glucose levels less than 200 mg/mL is optimal. Liver function tests and triglyceride levels should be drawn monthly. Serum albumin is a poor marker of nutrition in sick patients resulting from its decrease in metabolically stressed patients caused by capillary leak. Therefore, a low albumin is a better marker for poor outcome than nutritional state in the setting of stress (35).

The choice of the location and device for delivering TPN should be based on the patient's medical condition and activity requirements. The subclavian vein is often chosen for long-term access because of its reduced incidence of complications. Multilumen catheters allow for the infusion of a number of fluids and medications at the same time as well as for blood to be drawn from patients with poor peripheral venous access. In general, the risk of central venous catheter infection increases in direct proportion to the number of lumens. Tunnelled, silastic catheters, such as the Hickman and Broviac catheters, are also commonly used for long-term vascular access. With these catheters, fibrotic tissue adherence is induced by a Dacron cuff. This cuff is important for preventing bacterial migration along the catheter tract. A final common central venous access device is the peripherally inserted central catheter (PICC). A PICC line is inserted into a peripheral vein with the tip of the catheter directed into the superior vena cava. These catheters are available as single or double lumen *(38)*. They can help avoid the complications related to central venous access such as pneumothorax.

3.3. Complications

The effects of total parenteral nutrition on the gastrointestinal tract include decreases in brush-border hydrolase and nutrient-transporter activity, an increase in mucosal permeability, and a slight decrease in microvillus height. The splanchnic response to endotoxin appears to be exaggerated in normal subjects fed parenterally, suggesting that TPN may amplify the metabolic derangements that develop during sepsis. The incidence of pneumonia and sepsis is increased in patients receiving parenteral nutrition as compared to enteral nutrition. Catheter-related complications include pneumothorax, artery or nerve injury, hemothorax, air emboli, infection, and venous thrombosis. Dedicating a catheter solely to the administration of TPN decreases the incidence of infection. Line infection is mostly the result of *Staphylococcus aureus*, *Staphylococcus epidermidis*, and *Candida* species. Patients who require short-term nutritional support may benefit from peripheral parenteral nutrition (PPN). This therapy is limited by the concentration of dextrose provided to the patient with the overall solution containing a dextrose concentration of less than 10%. Phlebitis occurs more commonly with peripheral parenteral nutrition (PPN) but also can happen with centrally placed lines if the catheter is misplaced or migrates into a smaller vein. This is a result of damage in peripheral veins by hypertonic solutions because of their low blood flow. Therefore, most of the calories provided as PPN must be from fat in order to minimize the potential for venous inflammation *(35,38)*.

Parenteral feeding can lead to hyperglycemia, hypophosphatemia, hypokalemia, hypomagnesemia, hyponatremia, and fluid overload. Blood glucose is difficult to control in those with severe pancreatitis and stressed diabetics. Blood glucose should be maintained at 200 mg/dL or less. Hyponatremia is usually the result of inappropriate antidiuretic hormone secretion. Urine tests for sodium and osmolality aids in the diagnosis. In this instance, the urine sodium is <10 and the urine osmolality is inappropriately increased. Treatment involves either increasing the sodium in the formula or restricting free water *(35,38)*.

Refeeding syndrome is a complication of rapid overfeeding in the severely malnourished that is potentially lethal. In this situation, glucose stimulates an accelerated uptake of phosphate, potassium, magnesium, and water into cells which results in possible arrhythmias, muscle weakness, and myocardial swelling resulting in cardiorespiratory failure. Initially, 20 kcal/kg or less of actual body weight should be given daily in order to avoid this complication. Moreover, corresponding electrolytes should be added to the formula and be monitored daily. Once the serum electrolytes stabilize, calories may then be slowly increased (35,38). It is thought that refeeding syndrome occurs more frequently in the elderly population.

Hepatic abnormalities are common and most likely secondary to infection, medication, and shock. Patients started on parenteral nutrition may have transient elevations of the transaminases and alkaline phosphatase. In adults, the absence of enteric stimulation of bile flow and gallbladder contractility because of a lack of oral intake may be a primary factor for the development of gallstones, biliary sludge, and cholestasis. Cholestasis is an etiology that is poorly understood, yet rare in adults (35,38,39). Bacterial translocation resulting from gut mucosal hypoplasia and impaired mucosal immunity may provide an additional mechanism where loss of oral intake induces hepatic injury (39). Many times it is necessary to decrease the carbohydrate component as hepatic steatosis, a complication of long-term parenteral nutrition, is believed to be related to insulin responses to carbohydrate infusions.

3.4. Outcomes of Total Parenteral Nutrition

The elderly generally tolerate parenteral nutrition well. They do not appear to be at greater risk for complications than younger adults; yet, they are just as susceptible to the same complications (40). It is not, therefore, appropriate to exclude the elderly as potential candidates for parenteral nutrition on the sole basis of age (1).

Parenteral nutrition has been proven to be helpful in patients with intestinal failure and high-output enterocutaneous fistulas (1,35). Home parenteral nutrition may improve the quality of life in patients with carcinomatosis and chronic partial bowel obstruction. Quality of life issues have not been studied in hospitalized patients. However, its overall benefit, is uncertain and may cause harm in patients with AIDS, critical illnesses, bone marrow transplant, cancer therapy, wasting illnesses, and those who are perioperative (see Table 4). The cost effectiveness of parenteral nutrition has been difficult to measure because it is unclear to what extent malnutrition contributes to a poor outcome (35).

A recent study from Italy showed that enteral feeding following major abdominal surgery failed to demonstrate a reduction in postoperative complications and mortality when compared to parenteral nutrition (41). Blondin et al. looked retrospectively at hemodialysis patients with malnutrition who received parenteral nutrition. They concluded that there were significant decreases in the number of hospitalizations and days in the hospital among TPN recipients (42). Parenteral nutrition also proved efficacious in those who received it for 7–10 d prior to an operation, in those needing nutritional support to promote wound healing and to enhance muscle strength, and in those severely ill surgical patients who receive glutamine-supplemented TPN (43).

However, Powell-Tuck et al. showed that glutamine supplementation of parenteral feeds is not always beneficial. A consensus was made stating that it may have advantages in surgical patients and in those with a hematological malignancy (44). It has also been shown that the probability of survival in intestinal failure in those with short bowel syndrome after 2 yr of TPN is 94% (45). Finally, Kalfarentzos et al. concluded that early enteral nutrition should be used instead of parenteral nutrition in patients with severe pancreatitis (46,47).

There is a paucity of information regarding the use of parenteral nutrition in the elderly. However, outcome data suggests that we should be using the same criteria as we

Table 4
Parenteral Nutrition

Helpful	May not be helpful
1. Bowel obstruction	1. AIDS
2. High-output enterocutaneous fistula	2. Bone marrow transplant
3. Prolonged postoperative ileus	3. Cancer therapy
4. Severe mucositis	4. Wasting illnesses
5. Intestinal failure	5. Perioperative period
6. Critical illness	6. Critical illness
7. Motility disorder	

currently do for our younger patients including short-bowel syndrome, small bowel obstruction, gastrointestinal motility disorders, gastrointestinal fistulas, and pancreatitis.

4. ENTERAL VS PARENTERAL NUTRITION

Enteral feeding, as opposed to parenteral nutrition, improves epithelial structure and function, enhances mucosal immunity, and provides rapid advancement of feeds. A combined approach is necessary when the total energy needs of a patient are not met by enteral nutrition alone (36). Intragastric feeds are generally preferable from a more physiologic nature, but feeds administered beyond the ligament of Treitz should be used in patients at risk for aspiration (3,47).

Instances when the gastrointestinal tract is not accessible or functional, as in patients with obstruction, necrotizing or inflammatory enterocolitis, or short gut syndrome, necessitate the use of parenteral nutrition. However, it has been shown that the use of preoperative TPN should be limited to those who are severely malnourished unless there are other indications (3,36). In these patients, the parenteral nutrition should be continued for 7–10 d after surgery. Associated complications of parenteral nutrition are related not only to the solution, but also to the central venous access device. Bauer et al. have also shown that TPN has no clinically relevant outcome in ICU patients during the early phase of nutritional support despite correcting nutritional parameters, such as retinol-binding protein and prealbumin, more rapidly than enteral nutrition (49).

5. CONCLUSIONS

Considering the available data and our clinical experience, we believe that enteral nutrition in the elderly should be used whenever possible as it is proven to be more cost-effective and likely safer. Nutrition support teams are a valuable adjunct that may significantly improve care and decrease related complications.

In most elderly patients, nutritional support should be started after 7–14 d without nutrient intake (1). However, patients with preexisting malnutrition should be started on nutritional support earlier. Mechanical bowel obstruction is the only absolute contraindication to enteral feeding. Nasogastric or nasoenteric tubes are preferred over gastrostomy or jejunostomy tubes for periods of <30 d as they are minimally invasive. Various methods of nasogastric tube placement, endoscopically or fluoroscopically, should be reserved for those in whom bedside techniques have been unsuccessful (3).

Tubes placed beyond the third portion of the duodenum, especially past the ligament of Treitz, may have a decreased risk of aspiration. The risk for aspiration can be limited for gastric feeding by raising the head of the bed 30–45 degrees during and 1 h after feeding, by using continuous feeding regimens, by checking gastric residuals regularly, and by considering jejunal access in patients with a history of related aspiration pneumonia or gastroesophageal reflux and in those with gastric motility dysfunction from head trauma injuries. Prokinetic drugs given before placement of smaller nasoenteric tubes beyond the pylorus may be beneficial. For small bowel feeding, episodes of severe vomiting or coughing may displace some nonsurgical tubes. Also, the feeding port of the nasoenteric tube or PEJ should be as close to the ligament of Treitz as possible or beyond (3).

Intermittent gravity feeding is sufficient for most patients with nasogastric or gastrostomy tubes. For jejunal and gastrostomy feedings, pump-controlled infusions given continuously to decrease gastroesophageal reflux are recommended. Standard isotonic, polymeric tube feeding formula is appropriate, including jejunal feeding, for most situations. Currently, specialty feeding formulations have a limited clinical role. However, the use of elemental formulations should be reserved for patients with severe dysfunction of small-bowel absorption (3).

Although metabolic abnormalities may be more common with parenteral nutrition as compared to enteral nutrition, careful management of fluid and electrolytes can minimize metabolic complications from common conditions such as diarrhea. In fact, fiber probably has little role in controlling tube feeding-related diarrhea (3).

Parenteral nutrition should be reserved for those patients with a dysfunctional gastrointestinal tract where it is impossible to feed enterally. The same inclusion criteria for receiving parenteral nutrition applies to older patients and younger patients. Close monitoring is required for this interventional nutrition therapy. The determination of reasonable goals for nutrition, the avoidance of personal bias of physicians regarding its use, and sensitivity to families' needs and desires will ensure appropriate delivery of nutrition (2).

Nutritional support is widely used for several reasons. There is an association between malnutrition, common in hospitalized patient, and increased morbidity and mortality. Intuitively, well-nourished patients will respond most favorably to treatment. Nutritional support can be administered safely to most patients, and clinical trials indicate that it is beneficial in selected patients. The plethora of relatively small, retrospective, uncontrolled trials focusing on various patient populations have limited the development of evidence-based guidelines. Guidelines need to incorporate reasonable goals and objectives. Weight gain, survival, or improvement in functional status may be unrealistic goals in the elderly. Maintaining or improving a patient's health-related quality of life, reducing a patient's pain and suffering, and providing an access for hydration or medication delivery may be obtainable, reasonable goals, even in the short term, in patients with ultimately terminal diseases (2,35,48). Family goals are very important in order to reach realistic decisions regarding nutrition interventions and support.

6. RECOMMENDATIONS FOR CLINICIANS

1. Enteral nutrition should be the nutritional support modality of choice if a patient is unable to maintain adequate nutrition orally.

2. Enteral and parenteral nutrition should only be initiated after discussion with the patient and/or their proxy about treatment goals and potential benefits or complications of these forms of nutritional support.

3. In well-nourished patients, nutritional support should be started after 7–10 d without nutrient intake.

4. In malnourished patients, nutritional support should be initiated immediately.

5. Contraindications to enteral feeding include mechanical bowel obstruction, ileus, hypotension, or conditions predisposing to hemodynamic instability

6. Older adults should be screened for malnutrition, especially prior to elective surgery. Individuals with malnutrition or at a high risk for malnutrition should be referred to a multidisciplinary team for further evaluation and intervention.

7. Given the relative decrease in proportion of lean body mass in older adults, careful attention should be paid to maintaining nitrogen balance and minimizing muscle breakdown. Appropriate body mass measurements should be followed.

8. Preoperative nutrition supplementation should occur in malnourished cancer patients scheduled for surgery.

9. Enteral feeding is preferred to parenteral nutrition because of the maintenance of epithelial structure, epithelial function, mucosal immunity, and overall cost.

REFERENCES

1. Jensen GL, McGee M, Binkley J. Nutrition in the elderly. Gastroenterol Clin North Amer 2001;30: 313–334.
2. DeLegge MH. PEG placement: Justifying the intervention. UpToDate 2001;9(1).
3. Kirby DF, DeLegge MH, Fleming CR. American Gastroenterological Association technical review on tube feeding for enteral nutrition. Gastroenterology 1995;108:1282–1301.
4. Park RHR, Allison MC, Lang J, Spence E, Morris AJ, Danesh BJZ, et al. Randomised comparison of percutaneous endoscopic gastrostomy and nasogastric tube feeding in patients with persisting neurological dysphagia. BMJ 1992;304:1406–1409.
5. Steigman G, Goff J, VanWay C, et al. Operative versus endoscopic gastrostomy: Preliminary results of a prospective, randomized trial. Am J Surg 1988;155:88–91.
6. Angelini F. Technology, development, stewardship, and ethical considerations. Ann NY Acad Sci 1988; 534:858–862.
7. Pajak TF, Laramore GE, Marcial VA, et al. Elapsed treatment days— a critical item for radiotherapy quality control review in head and neck trials. RTOG report. Int J Radiat Oncol Biol Phys 1991;20: 13–20.
8. Lee JH, Machtay M, Unger LD, Weinstein GS, Weber RS, Chalian AA, et al. Prophylactic gastrostomy tubes in patients undergoing intensive irradiation for cancer of the head and neck. Arch Otolaryngol Head Neck Surg 1998;124:871–875.
9. Harbrecht BG, Moraca RJ, Saul M, Courcoulas AP. Percutaneous endoscopic gastrostomy reduces total hospital costs in head-injured patients. Am J Surg 1998;176:311–314.
10. James A, Kapur K, Hawthorne AB. Long-term outcome of percutaneous endoscopic gastrostomy feeding in patients with dysphagic stroke. Age Ageing 1998;27:671–676.
11. D'Amelio LF, Hammond JS, Spain DA, et al. Tracheostomy and percutaneous endoscopic gastrostomy in the management of head-injured patient. Ann Surg 1994;60:180–185.
12. Chio A, Finocchiaro E, Meineri P, Bottacchi E, Schiffer D, et al. Safety and factors related to survival after percutaneous endoscopic gastrostomy in ALS. Neurology 1999;53:1123–1125.
13. Kasarskis EJ, Scarlata D, Hill R, Fuller C, Stambler N, Cedarbaum JM, et al. A retrospective study of percutaneous endoscopic gastrostomy in ALS patients during the BDNF and CNTF trials. J Neurol Sci 1999;169:118–125.
14. Gillick MR. Rethinking the role of tube feeding in patients with advanced dementia. New Engl J Med 2000;342:206–210.

15. Sanders DS, Carter MJ, D'Silva J, James G, Bolton RP, Bardhan KD. Survival analysis in percutaneous endoscopic gastrostomy feeding: A worse outcome in patients with dementia. Am J Gastroenterol 2000; 95:1472–1475.

16. Mitchell SL, Kiely DK, Lipsitz LA. The risk factors and impact on survival of feeding tube placement in nursing home residents with severe cognitive impairment. Arch Intern Med 1997;157:327–332.

17. Finucane TE, Christmas C, Travis K. Tube feeding in patients with advanced dementia. JAMA 1999;282:1365–1370.

18. Levine GM, Deren JJ, Steiger E, Zinno R. Role of oral intake and maintenance of gut mass and disaccharide activity. Gastroenterology 1974;647:975.

19. Steiner M, Bourges HR, Freedman LS, Gray SJ. Effect of starvation on tissue composition of the small intestine in the rat. Am J Physiol 1968;215:75.

20. Haskel Y, Xu D, Lu Q, Deitch EA. The modulatory role of gut hormones in elemental diet and intravenous total parenteral nutrition-induced bacterial translocation in rats. J Parenter Enteral Nutr 1994;18: 159–166.

21. Moore EE, Jones TN. Benefits of immediate jejunostomy feeding after major abdominal trauma: A prospective, randomized study. J Trauma 1986;26:874.

22. Alverdy J, Chi HS, Sheldon GF. The effect of parenteral nutrition on gastrointestinal immunity: The importance of enteral stimulation. Ann Surg 1985;202:681.

23. Adams S, Dellinger EP, Wertz MF, et al. Enteral versus parenteral nutritional support following laparotomy for trauma: A randomized prospective trial. J Trauma 1986;26:883.

24. Deitch EA, Ma WJ, Ma L, et al. Protein malnutrition predisposes to inflammatory-induced gut-origin septic states. Ann Surg 1990;211:560.

25. Moore FA, Moore EE, Jones TN, et al. TEN versus TPN following major abdominal trauma: Reduced septic morbidity. J Trauma 1989;29:916.

26. Kudsk KA, Croce MA, Fabian TC, et al. Enteral versus parenteral feeding: Effects on septic morbidity after blunt and penetrating abdominal trauma. Ann Surg 1992;215:503.

27. Callahan CM, Haag KM, Weinberger M, Tierney WM, Buchanan NN, Stump TE. Outcomes of percutaneous endoscopic gastrostomy among older adults in a community setting. J Am Geriatr Soc 2000; 48:1048–1054.

28. Rudberg MA, Egleston BL, Grant MD, Brody JA. Effectiveness of feeding tubes in nursing home residents with swallowing disorders. J Parenter Enteral Nutr 2000;24:97–102.

29. Grant MD, Rudberg MA, Brody JA. Gastrostomy placement and mortality among hospitalized medicare beneficiaries. JAMA 1998;279:1973–1976.

30. Bannerman E, Pendlebury J, Phillips F, Ghosh S. A cross-sectional and longitudinal study of health-related quality of life after percutaneous gastrostomy. Eur J Gastroenterol Hepatol 2000;12:1101–1109.

31. Weaver JP, Odell P, Nelson C. Evaluation of the benefits of gastric tube feeding in an elderly population. Arch Fam Med 1993;2:953–956.

32. Von Preyss-Friedman SM, Uhlmann RF, Cain KC. Physicians' attitudes toward tube feeding chronically ill nursing home patients. J Gen Int Med 1992;7:46–51.

33. Van Rosendaal GMA, Verhoef MJ, Kinsella TD. How are decisions made about the use of percutaneous endoscopic gastrostomy for long-term nutritional support? Am J Gastroenterol 1999;94:3225–3228.

34. Kaw M, Sekas G. Long-term follow-up of consequences of percutaneous endoscopic gastrostomy (PEG) tubes in nursing home patients. Dig Diseases Sci 1994;39:738–743.

35. Semrad CE. Parenteral nutrition. Clin Persp Gastroenterol 2000;3:307–314.

36. Collier S, Duggan C. Overview of parenteral and enteral nutrition. UpToDate 2001;9(1).

37. Ochoa JB, Magnuson B, Swintowsky M, Loan T, Boulanger B, McClain C, et al. Long-term reduction in the cost of nutritional intervention achieved by a nutrition support service. Nutr Clin Prac 2000;15: 174–180.

38. DeLegge MH. Home parenteral nutrition: A physician's perspective. Infusion 1998;4:31–36.

39. Quigley EMM, Marsh MN, Shaffer JL, Markin RS. Hepatobiliary complications of total parenteral nutrition. Gastroenterology 1993;104:286–301.

40. DeLegge MH, Ireton-Jones CI. Outcomes of parenteral nutrition use in the elderly as compared to a younger population. Submitted to Nutrition Week; San Diego, CA, 2002.

41. Pacelli F, Bossola M, Papa V, Malerba M, Modesti C, Sgadari A, et al. Enteral vs parenteral nutrition after major abdominal surgery. Arch Surg 2001;136:933–936.

42. Blondin J, Ryan C. Nutritional status: A continuous quality improvement approach. Am J Kidney Dis 1999;33:198–202.

43. Wilmore DW. Postoperative protein sparing. World J Surg 1999;23:545–552.
44. Powell-Tuck J, Jamieson CP, Bettany GEA, Obeid O, Fawcett HV, Archer C, Murphy DL. A double blind, randomized, controlled trial of glutamine supplementation in parenteral nutrition. Gut 1999;45:82–88.
45. Messing B, Crenn P, Beau P, Boutron-Ruault MC, Rambaud JC, Matuchansky C. Long-term survival and parenteral nutrition dependence in adult patients with the short bowel syndrome. Gastroenterology 1999;117:1043–1050.
46. Kalfarentzos F, Kehagias J, Mead N, Kokkinis K, Gogos CA. Enteral nutrition is superior to parenteral nutrition in severe acute pancreatitis: results of a randomized prospective trial. Br J Surg 1997;84:1665–1669
47. The veterans affairs total parenteral nutrition cooperative study group. Perioperative total parenteral nutrition in surgical patients. New Engl J Med 1991;325:525–532.
48. Souba WW. Nutritional support. New Engl J Med 1997;336:41–48.
49. Bauer P, Charpentier C, Bouchet C, Nace L, Raffy F, Gaconnet N. Parenteral with enteral nutrition in the critically ill. Intensive Care Med 2000;26:838–840.

F. Renal Disorders

27 Nutrition in Chronic Renal Disease and Renal Failure

Giuliano Brunori

1. INTRODUCTION

In the next several decades, older adults will represent the fastest growing cohort; in fact, by 2041, 60% of the total population will be older than 60 yr, and one-third older than 70 yr in the United States. Women will be predominant in this population, particularly in the oldest age group. Poverty, loneliness, and isolation will be the major problems this older population will continue to face *(1,2)*.

2. IMPACT OF AGING ON PHYSIOLOGY AND RENAL FUNCTION: INTERACTION WITH NUTRITION

Growing older is not a disease process, but is associated with many physiological modifications. The most important changes affect homeostasis. The reduction in homeostasis or reserve capacity represents the loss of the body's capacity to handle nutrient loads, toxins, insults, and stressors (e.g., injury or infection) *(3)*. For instance, glomerular filtration rate and hepatic blood flow decrease with age; however, function, is not reduced unless intercurrent stress ensues.

Chronic diseases (e.g., cardiovascular disease, renal disease, and diabetes) and disabilities are often more present in older adults, being commonly associated with renal insufficiency. Patients with advanced renal disease tend to be older. In fact, in the United States, approx 50% of patients initiating maintenance dialysis are over the age of 65 yr *(4)*.

Older patients suffering from renal disease or affected by end-stage renal disease (ESRD) and treated by dialysis, either hemo- or peritoneal dialysis, are at risk of developing malnutrition. Several cross-sectional studies, primarily performed in patients on dialysis treatment, have reported that these patients frequently present with protein-calorie malnutrition (PCM); the incidence varies between 8% to 40% *(5,6)*. PCM has been reported to be more common in elderly patients than in young patients. In a study published by Cianciaruso and Brunori *(6)*, the incidence of malnutrition evaluated on the basis of Subjective Global Nutritional Assessment (SGA) was higher in men and woman undergoing peritoneal dialysis (PD) when compared to patients on hemodialysis (MHD).

From: *Handbook of Clinical Nutrition and Aging*
Edited by: C. W. Bales and C. S. Ritchie © Humana Press Inc., Totowa, NJ

PCM occurred in 42.3% of PD patients when compared to 30.8% of MHD patients. The SGA data referred to three different age ranges (18–40 yr, 41–64 yr, and 65 yr or older) and indicated a greater prevalence of malnutrition in both men and woman undergoing PD in comparison with MHD for patients who were 18–40 or 41–64 yr of age. For the 65 yr and older group, the SGA was not different between hemo- and peritoneal dialysis in either men or women: the incidence of PCM was 48% in PD patients and 51% in MHD patients.

In older adults with advanced chronic renal failure *not* receiving dialysis treatment, few data are available on the incidence of malnutrition. Some authors *(7–9)* have observed that patients with advanced renal failure can maintain a neutral or positive nitrogen balance during the period of a recommended low-protein diet. In the Modification of Diet in Renal Disease (MDRD) study, baseline evaluation of these predialysis patients revealed an average glomerular filtration rate (GFR) of 39.8 mL/min/1.73 m^2. Among these patients, 11%–16% had a dietary protein intake of <0.75 g/kg/d and 10% had a body weight <90% of standard. Nutritional parameters worsened as GFR decreased *(10)*. Although these observations were not stratified for patient age, it is reasonable to suggest that the prevalence of malnutrition is higher in elderly patients on dialysis treatment, but these data need to be confirmed by more extensive studies. In a recent paper, Garg et al. evaluated 1113 older patients with chronic renal insufficiency (evaluated as a GFR < 60 mL/min). Malnutrition was present in 4% of patients with moderate chronic renal failure (CRF) (GFR between 30 to 60 mL/min) and in 14.6% of patients with more pronounced CRF (GFR < 30 mL/min) *(11)*.

Malnutrition has important adverse effects on morbidity and mortality in ESRD patients *(12)*. Despite wide variability in mortality rates of ESRD patients in different countries, 24% in the United States *(13)*, 11% in Europe *(14)*, and < 10% in Japan *(15)*, malnutrition remains a common risk factor for mortality in each of these populations.

The following sections will discuss nutrition assessment in chronic renal disease, protein and energy requirements, and how to treat or prevent PCM in this group of patients.

3. NUTRITION ASSESSMENT IN PATIENTS WITH CHRONIC RENAL DISEASE

In recent years, many efforts have been made to identify reliable methods for assessing nutritional status of ESRD patients, to correlate dialysis dose with nutrition and to define the factors that might accelerate or exacerbate malnutrition in uremia.

Nutrition assessment is multifaceted and, for older patients, requires the involvement of many members of a geriatric team (e.g., dietitian, speech and language therapist, physician, and so on). Repeated assessments are needed to permit the monitoring of therapeutic interventions. Once patients at risk of malnutrition have been identified, appropriate nutritional interventions can be defined to treat the causes of PCM. Early and repeated nutritional screening to identify patients at risk or those with early malnutrition with appropriate interventions to correct nutritional deficits should be an integral clinical goal in older patients with chronic renal disease.

3.1. Definition of Nutritional Status in Patients with Chronic Renal Disease

The clinical history serves as the foundation for nutritional assessment. In particular, problems relating to eating difficulties, weight loss, bowel habits, presence of other

or drug–nutrient interactions, and coexisting diseases (e.g., diabetes, chronic heart failure, hypertension) will affect various biochemical indices.

Serum albumin is only minimally altered by aging; the range of values broadens, but the distribution remains normal. Many publications on MHD or PD patients showed a strong correlation between patients' morbidity and mortality and serum albumin concentrations (12,21,22). The lower the concentration, the higher the risk. Similarly, serum prealbumin strongly correlates with nutritional status and dialysis outcomes (23). These biochemical parameters represent suitable tools for the follow-up of the nutritional status of ESRD patients. Having a short half-life (2–3 d) and a small body pool (0.01 g/kg body weight), serum prealbumin, in particular, is a more sensitive indicator than albumin of visceral protein status and responds more rapidly to changes in nutrition.

Recently, in a French survey of 7000 ESRD patients, 20% were reported having a serum albumin lower than 35 g/L, and 36% having a serum prealbumin <300 mg/L, despite a mean value for solute removal (Kt/V), indicating an adequate dose of dialysis. Moreover, the mean normalized protein nitrogen appearance was higher than 1 g/kg/d in 65% of the patients (24).

However, it must be recognized that low-serum concentrations of albumin may be the result of nonnutritional factors, as certain enteropathies, nephrotic syndrome, liver disease, heart failure, and (in PD patients) high peritoneal losses, particularly during episodes of peritonitis. Serum concentrations of acute-phase reactant proteins, such as C-reactive protein (CRP), have been shown to be very high in some ESRD patients and to correlate inversely with serum albumin. In the presence of an inflammatory state, synthesis of albumin is reduced, whereas that of the acute-phase reactant protein is increased (25).

Many factors can induce an inflammatory state, including the quality of dialysis water, dialysis fluid back filtration, and infections of graft or fistula. In these conditions, the inflammatory process leads to an increase in IL-6 production and the liver, in response to this situation, increases the synthesis of CRP and decreases that of albumin. It must be pointed out that the correlation between acute-phase reactants and nutritional parameters is low with r values ranging from 0.2 to 0.5, and in most patients on dialysis, CRP levels are low (25,26).

Although serum albumin often serves as an indicator of concurrent illness or inflammation, in the renal literature, serum albumin concentration has remained as a useful indicator of protein-energy malnutrition. The large body of literature, in individuals with or without chronic renal failure, relating albumin to nutritional status and the powerful association between low concentration of albumin and morbidity or mortality risk in elderly patients with CRF or on renal replacement therapy strongly support this assertion (27).

Serum cholesterol is a valid and clinically useful marker of protein-energy nutritional status in patients on dialysis. Predialysis serum cholesterol is generally reported to exhibit a high degree of collinearity with other nutritional markers such as albumin, prealbumin, and creatinine, as well as age. The relationship between serum cholesterol and mortality has been described as either "U-shaped" or "J-shaped", with mortality increasing as the serum cholesterol concentrations rise above the 200–300 mg/dL range or fall below approx 200 mg/dL (28). A low-serum cholesterol concentration may represent a reduced protein intake, or the presence of comorbid conditions, including inflammation. Elderly patients with low, low-normal (<150–180 mg/dL), or declining serum cholesterol levels should be investigated for possible nutritional deficits.

Twenty-four hour urinary excretion of creatinine is often used to assess lean body mass. As a result of the loss of lean body mass associated with normal aging, creatinine excretion decreases. However, in elderly patients with CRF, urinary creatinine excretion is not a reliable measure for assessing lean body mass because of reduced renal excretion. In patients on dialysis, the serum creatinine levels before dialysis reflect the sum of dietary protein (foods rich in creatine and creatinine, e.g., skeletal muscle) and endogenous (skeletal muscle) creatinine production minus the urinary excretion, dialyitic removal and endogenous degradation. Patients with low predialysis serum creatinine (approx 10 mg/dL) should be evaluated for PEM and wasting of skeletal muscle. A low serum creatinine concentration, in particular in the absence of substantial endogenous urinary creatinine clearance, suggests low dietary protein intake and/or reduced skeletal muscle mass and is associated with increased mortality rates *(29)*.

In clinically stable dialysis patients, the rate of urea nitrogen appearance (UNA) in the dialysate and urine is assumed to closely reflect dietary protein intake and is called the protein equivalent of nitrogen appearance (PNA). PNA normalized to desirable body weight correlates with other measures of nutritional status *(30)*. The National Kidney Foundation Disease Outcomes Quality Initiative Nutrition Work Group recommends use of the normalized PNA for monitoring protein status in stable dialysis patients *(27)*.

3.5. Tests of Body Composition

Some instrumental tests using direct and indirect methods, have been proposed for assessing body composition and body protein status.

The first methods measure a specific chemical or anatomic constituent of body composition. They are accurate, but frequently invasive, expensive, and difficult to justify and apply in all patients and are primarily investigational. The most popular tests are neutron activity, computed tomography, magnetic resonance imaging, dual-energy X-ray absorptiometry, and total-body water. A detailed description of these methods has been made elsewhere *(31)*.

The indirect methods include measures of body weight and volume, and bioelectric impedance (BIA). These methods are based on assumptions regarding the density of body tissue and the concentration of water and electrolyte in fat-free mass (FFM). The errors inherent in these methods are greater than those of direct methods and are affected by the problems of sample specificity.

BIA can estimate FFM. It is easy to perform even in out-patient departments and does not require much patient collaboration, and the data are reproducible *(32)*. The most important limitation results from significant intermachine differences among manufactures, the inappropriate placement and different types of electrodes, contact between body parts, and the assumption of a constant electrolyte concentration in tissue among individuals.

The whole-body dual-energy X-ray absorptiometry (DEXA) is a reliable, noninvasive method to assess the three main components of body composition: fat mass, fat-free mass, and bone mineral mass and density. The accuracy of DEXA is less influenced by the variation of hydration that commonly occurs in ESRD patients. Studies of DEXA in CRF, MHD or PD patients reported a higher precision and accuracy of DEXA as compared with anthropometry, total-body potassium counting, creatinine index, and BIA *(33)*. The main limitations to DEXA are the cost of the instrument, the need of dedicated space to house a DEXA unit, and the cost of any single test. Furthermore, DEXA does not distinguish well between intracellular and extracellular water compartments.

A variety of methods are available for the assessment of nutrition status of patients with CRF or ESRD on dialysis. Some are easy to perform; others are more sophisticated, precise, and expensive. The selection of methods depends on what we want to know about our patients and why. We have a wide number of methods, and we describe the "state of the art" about assessing nutritional status. But, we need the development of methods that are concurrently accurate, inexpensive, and noninvasive. Once these methods have been established, reliable and representative reference data for epidemiologic and clinical studies can be developed.

4. NUTRITIONAL STATUS OF OLDER PATIENTS WITH CRF WITH AND WITHOUT DIALYSIS

Longitudinal and cross-sectional data indicate that patients with CRF, either on conservative treatment or in dialysis, have low energy intake and are underweight *(34,35)*. Garg and colleagues reported the result of the National Health And Nutrition Examination Survey (NHANES) III, a cross sectional survey conducted from 1988 to 1994. Demographic information was collected for all persons 60 yr of age or older, invited to participate ($N = 8357$), and of these, 79% were interviewed ($N = 5724$), and 63% had a measurement of serum creatinine ($N = 5248$) *(11)*. The patients were stratified into three groups of GFR, by serum creatinine (GFR < 30, 30–60 and > 60 mL/min/1.73 m^2). A GFR lower than 30 mL/min/1.73 m^2 was present in 2.3% of men and 2.6% of women; these participants demonstrated low energy and protein intake and higher serum markers of inflammation. Dietary and nutritional factors were estimated from 24-h dietary recall, biochemistry measurements, anthropometry and bioelectrical impedance.

Participants were defined "malnourished" if they demonstrated at least three of the following five criteria:

Parameter	
Serum albumin	≤ 37 g/L
Weight (kg)	≤ 63.9 (male)
	≤ 51.8 (female)
Serum cholesterol	< 4.1 mmol/L
Energy intake	< 15 kcal/kg/d
Protein intake	< 0.5 g/kg/d

Among the patients defined as malnourished by the criteria used to assess malnutrition, 88% showed a protein intake <0.5 g/kg/d, 86.6% an energy intake <15 kcal/kg/d, and 77.7% a serum albumin <37 g/L.

In multivariate analysis, a GFR < 30 mL/min/1.73 m^2 was independently associated with malnutrition (odds ratio 3.6 [2.0–6.6]) after adjustment for relevant demographic, social, and medical conditions. Ikizler and colleagues evaluated the relationship between the progression of renal failure and spontaneous dietary protein intake (DPI) and other indices of malnutrition *(36)*. In this study, the authors showed that the mean protein intake (± standard deviation [SD]) was 1.01±0.21 g/kg/d for patients with a

GFR >50 mL/min and decreased to 0.85±0.23 g/kg/d for patients with a GFR between 25 to 50 mL/min. The DPI further decreased to a level of 0.70±0.17 g/kg/d for patients with a GFR between 10 and 25 mL/min and was only 0.54±0.16 g/kg/d for patients with a GFR lower than 10 mL/min. A similar trend was reflected in measures of serum cholesterol, transferrin, and total creatinine excretion. The authors concluded that the progression of renal failure is associated with a spontaneous decrease in DPI, especially at GFRs below 25 mL/min, and that most nutritional indices in CRF patients worsen as GFR and DPI decrease. As a consequence, dietary protein restriction should be used cautiously when GFR falls below 25 mL/min. Also, because of the large effect of malnutrition on subsequent survival, the initiation of dialysis therapy should be considered if the patient's DPI is <0.7 g/kg/d in spite of adequate nutritional counselling.

Lorenzo and colleagues performed a study for evaluating the incidence of hypoparathyroidism in elderly patients on hemodialysis *(37)*. The authors attempted to analyze whether the spontaneous decrease in protein intake in elderly, as suggested by Movilli et al. *(38)* and by Cancarini et al. *(39)*, favors a better control of serum phosphorus and parathyroid hormone levels. The results showed that elderly patients had the lowest energy and protein intake. Patients in the age group of 60–69, had a DPI of 0.88±0.29 g/kg/d and a dietary energy intake (DEI) of 21.8±5.9 kcal/kg/d. The oldest group (70–80 yr of age) showed a DPI of 0.84±0.36 and a DEI of 22.8±7.4 kcal/kg/d. This study clearly showed that in elderly hemodialysis patients, the dietary intake (both protein and energy intake) is dramatically decreased far below the recommended daily intake.

As low body weights, (adjusted for age, gender, height) are associated with increased morbidity and mortality in patients on dialysis, it seems important to aggressively attempt to maintain adequate energy intakes in the elderly.

5. FACTORS CAUSING MALNUTRITION IN ELDERLY PATIENTS WITH CRF OR ON DIALYSIS

There are many factors that induce calorie-protein malnutrition in elderly patients with CRF or on dialysis. Table 2 lists the most relevant.

Many patients starting dialysis, present with malnutrition. In some patients this can be the result of reduced dietary intake, as a result of the use of low-protein diet without adequate diet counseling, or to the referral of patients never seen by a nephrologist or dietitian at the time of starting dialysis. Those patients with malnutrition starting dialysis therapy are more likely to remain malnourished and have courses complicated by higher rates of hospitalizations and infections than those patients starting dialysis well nourished.

In patients on dialysis, there are many causes for PCM (Table 2). We must keep in mind that these patients may be exposed to the risk of inadequate diet counselling or self-induced dietary restrictions. Self-induced dietary restrictions may be a consequence of a lack of information after the shift from a conservative dietary therapy to dialysis. Moreover, frequent hospitalizations can induce disturbances in dietary habits and reduce nutrient intake. This is more dangerous when hospitalization is from an acute catabolic illness.

Anorexia plays a mayor role in inducing PCM in ESRD patients. It can be induced by many factors, including uremic toxins, GI disorders, esophagitis, peptic ulcers, gastritis, delayed gastric empyting, unpalatable drugs, and psychosocial disorders (e.g., loneliness and poverty commonly observed in elderly patients). Recent studies report that PCM

Table 2
Factors Causing Malnutrition in Elderly Patients with CRF or on Dialysis

1. Previous malnutrition from inadequate low-protein diet

2. *Dialysis-related factors*
   Inadequate Kt/V
   Intradialytic losses of amino acids and protein
   Glucose absorption (in PD patients)
   Chronic inflammation
   Bioincompatible membranes
   Blood losses
   Endotoxin back-filtration

3. *Metabolic and endocrine disorders*
   Acidosis
   Hyperparathyroidism
   Anemia
   Insulin, growth hormone, and IGF-1 resistance

4. *Gastrointestinal diseases*
   Anorexia
   Gastroparesis (diabetic patients)
   Taste disturbances
   Digestive side effects of drugs

5. *Miscellaneous*
   Depression
   Low socioeconomic status/poverty
   Loneliness
   Edentulous
   Frequent hospitalization
   Inadequate diet counseling
   Loss of mobility, independence
   Alcohol abuse
   Mental impairment, confusion

CRF, chronic renal failure; Kt/V, solute removal, PD, peritoneal dialysis; IGF-1, insulin-like growth factor-1.

begins when the GFR is closer to 30 mL/min/1.73 m^2, and continues to fall with decreasing GFR *(36)*. As reported by Walser et al. *(40)* and by our group *(41)*, patients following low- or very low-protein diets do not present with PCM if they are regularly followed by a nephrologist and dietitian, receive adequate caloric intake, and start dialysis with very low-residual renal function. Correct dietary counseling can dramatically reduce the risk of malnutrition.

Recently, Lim and Kopple *(42)* reported that a daily protein intake of 0.9 g/kg/d for patients on chronic hemodialysis and 1.0 g/kg/d for peritoneal dialysis patients can be enough to maintain neutral or slightly positive nitrogen balance. This value is lower than that suggested previously; in fact, a more generous protein intake is recommended, at least 1.2 g/kg/d for patients on hemodialysis and 1.3–1.4 g/kg/d for patients in PD. A more important question raised by the authors concerns the recommended intake of calories. The recommended dietary energy allowance for person older than 51 yr is 30 kcal/kg/d.

All dietary surveys in the ESRD patients showed that energy intake is lower, ranging from 23 to 29 kcal/kg/d *(43)*. A sufficient energy intake is needed to spare the protein necessary to maintain a neutral or slightly positive nitrogen balance, because less dietary protein will be needed for energy and thus degradated by oxidation. Moreover, a higher daily carbohydrate intake will induce an increase in secretion of insulin, one of the most anabolic hormones. Only when patients are eating a diet sufficient in calories can the daily protein intake be fixed at the value recently suggested by Lim and Kopple *(42)*.

The progressive decrease in dietary intake of protein and calories has been related to the effects of taste disturbances, delayed gastric emptying, poorly palatable diet resulting from salt and electrolyte restriction, postdialysis malaise, and finally, to uremic toxins that could affect appetite directly. Anderstam and colleagues infused uremic ultrafiltrate into the peritoneal cavity of rats, and in a second group of rats infused saline or plasma ultrafiltrate of normal subjects. The rats infused with uremic ultrafiltrate reduced their daily spontaneous food intake *(44)*. The molecular weight of the substances that might induce anorexia was reported to be between 1000 and 5000 D.

Leptin, with a molecular weight of 15 kD, has been indicated as an anorexiant compound in renal patients. It regulates body composition by lowering food intake and increasing metabolic rate. Several sudies in ESRD patients have reported an increase in the absolute plasma leptin level or the ratio of plasma leptin to some measure of body fat *(45)*. Anorexia and weight loss are frequently observed in malnourished uremic patients and the effects of leptin coincide with relevant findings in this group of patients. In patients on renal replacement therapy losing lean body mass we demonstrated elevated serum levels of leptin compared to patients who increased LBM (Brunori G, unpublished data, year). This polypeptidic hormone is synthesized by adipocytes and has been shown to reduce appetite in rats and to induce weight loss when, in obese subjects, it is used as a recombinant product *(46)*.

The dose of dialysis may affect daily nutrient intake through its impact on removal of uremic toxins. Some authors reported an increase in appetite after increasing Kt/V *(47–49)*. Lindsay *(50)* showed a direct relation between Kt/V and protein nitrogen appearance (PNA) in a prospective randomized study in which in a group of patients Kt/V was increased from 0.9 to 1.3 for 3 mo. In this group, PNA rose from 0.81 g/kg/d to 1.02, whereas PNA did not change in the second group in which Kt/V was maintained low.

Many patients with an adequate dialysis dose, i.e., ≥1.3 in HD and ≥2.0 in PD, have a very poor PNA and, hence, a low daily nutrient intake. This is not surprising because many patients present comorbid conditions that may lead to a reduced nutrient intake independent of their uremic status.

Metabolic acidemia, a common complication of chronic renal failure, can also promote protein catabolism *(51–55)*. The acidemia induces an increased proteolysis in skeletal muscle, by the enhanced activity of the ATP dependent ubiquitin pathway *(52)*. Based on evidence supporting this increased proteolysis, we recommend patients with metabolic acidosis the use of oral sodium bicarbonate supplements, usually approx 2–4 g/d (25–50 mEq/d) in order to maintain serum bicarbonate at or above 22 mmol/L. However, the effects of acidemia may depend on its severity.

Chauveau et al. studied 7132 French subjects on dialysis and reported that better nutritional parameters were observed in patients who had mild metabolic acidosis than in those who had predialysis bicarbonate concentration within the normal range *(56)*. Patients were adequately dialyzed, with Kt/V > 1.3. The authors hypothesized that, within certain limits, the magnitude of metabolic acidosis was linked to patients' protein intake, with sulfur-containing amino acids being the main cause of acid production and accumulation of hydrogen ions in the intradialytic period. The improved nutritional status observed in mild metabolic acidosis patients suggests that the higher protein intake could overcome the usual catabolic effects of acidosis.

Other factors affecting nutritional status are protein losses during dialysis and protein breakdown induced by dialysis *(57,58)*. For example, in patients treated with bio-incompatible membranes, the resulting release of cytokines, such as interleukin-1, may cause enhanced protein catabolism. During dialysis using a low flux cuprophane membrane, 4–9 g of free amino acids are lost per day. With high-flux dialyzers (in fasting patients) the loss of free amino acids is about 8 g. In PD patients the daily loss of protein is also about 8 g, but it can reach a level of 20–25 g/d during episodes of peritonitis. Reuse of dialyzers, as routinely performed in the United States *(59)*, has been reported to be a cause of increased loss of proteins when polysulfone membranes were reprocessed many times with bleach of formaldehyde *(60)*. Finally, deficiency of water-soluble vitamins in MHD patients, resulting from low nutrient intake and losses during dialysis, can induce PCM.

6. MANAGEMENT OR FLUID AND ELECTROLYTE DISTURBANCES IN OLDER ADULTS WITH RENAL DISEASE

In aged persons, fluid and electrolyte balance becomes an important factor in homeostasis and deserves serious consideration as part of nutritional monitoring. Usual requirements of fluid are estimated at 1 mL/kcal ingested or 30 mL/kg of body weight. In elderly individuals, inadequate fluid intake to compensate for normal observable output (sweat, feces, urine) and insensible losses (lung, skin) may lead to problems associated with dehydration.

6.1. Renal Handling of Sodium and Fluids

Profound changes take place with age in the structure and function of the kidneys *(61)*. Some of these are of great clinical importance and others are of physiological interest. Furthermore, handling of drugs by the aged individual and by the aging kidney changes over time.

In general, the aged kidney is quite capable of maintaining normal plasma electrolyte concentrations *(62)* and pH under usual circumstances. The functional deficits appearing with age usually relate to a reduction in the capacity of the kidney to change in response to extreme stresses. This may be the result of blunted maximal tubular secretory and resorptive capability. It can be explained by the progressive loss of functioning nephrons alone (more pronounced in patients with glomerular nephropathy), a decrease in the number of energy-producing mitochondria, lower concentrations of adenosine triphosphatase activity or other enzyme levels, or decreased tubular cell transport capacity (as observed in kidneys of old animals) *(63)*.

Hypernatremia and hyponatremia are probably the most common disturbances in older adults. It is well known that there is a reduced capacity to conserve sodium with increasing age, consistent with clinical observations that high sodium excretion and depletion rates are frequently found in patients on geriatric wards *(64–66)*.

The capacity of the aging kidney to adapt to a low-salt intake is also clearly blunted. In a study published by Macias-Nunez *(65)*, young people achieved sodium balance in 5 d, whereas the elderly were unable to reach sodium balance in 10 d. It has become fairly routine medical practice to restrict dietary sodium for patients who have hypertension, congestive heart failure, chronic renal disease or cirrhosis. However, many of the conditions for which dietary sodium is restricted can be treated with drugs that reduce the need for more than mild sodium intake reduction.

In spite of the lower sodium tubular load, 24-h urinary sodium output and fractional excretion of sodium are significantly greater in the elderly. This suggests that the renal tubule of the elderly subjects is unable to retain sodium adequately, either in absolute terms or when corrected for glomerular filtration.

The renal management of sodium by the aging kidney can be influenced, apart from the tubular incompetence, by several pathological factors, such as obstructive uropathy, urinary infections, surreptitious diuretics intake, and pyelonephritis. Furthermore, significant reductions in plasma and urinary aldosterone concentrations (67), lower renin concentrations (68), the exaggerated response to atriopeptin characterized by a greater increase in natriuresis, calciuresis, diuresis, and changes in urinary and plasma cGMP concentrations can be responsible for the inability of elderly people to maintain plasma sodium under normal concentrations.

Hypernatremia (plasma sodium >150 mmol/L) occurs in 1% of hospital admissions of patients aged over 60 yr. In these patients, mortality is 40% (69). From a practical point of view, there are four clinical situations leading to hypernatremia: water deficiency, water deficiency in excess to salt deficiency, salt excess, and redistribution (normal water, normal salt).

Water deficiency can occur through inadequate access to water (confusion, dementia, cerebro-vascular accident, immobility, dysphagia), and the frequent fluid loss that occurs in the course of infectious disease with fever. The increase of 1°C of body temperature requires 1 L of water to maintain a stable fluid volume. In this situation, sick older adults have an increased need for fluids, but may not receive adequate replacement fluids. Furthermore, elderly people lose their sense of thirst and may become confused and disoriented when ill, which may contribute to anorexia or decreased dietary intake of fluids (70).

Water deficiency in excess of salt deficiency is seen in situations of urinary loss, such as osmotic diuresis caused by hyperglycaemia, i.v., or nasogastric feeding, radiological contrast media, and loop diuretics. Other causes are gastrointestinal losses owing to diarrhea, laxative abuse and vomiting, skin losses through sweating in hot climates, and burns or exfoliative dermatitis.

Hypernatremia mediated by salt excess is produced by administration of excess hypertonic saline or sodium bicarbonate, or by dialysis error (high Na content in the bath solution). The most common causes of hypernatremia in the elderly are water deficiency (insufficient intake) and excessive gastrointestinal and urinary loss of fluids. To prevent this clinical situation, it is necessary to ensure that elderly patients consume ≥2 L of fluid/d. In patients with chronic renal failure, water deficiency followed by hypotension can significantly reduce the residual renal function and, in some cases, can be the reason to start chronic dialysis treatment. In patients with CRF, careful surveillance of fluid balance is mandatory.

The incidence of hyponatremia (plasma sodium < 130 mmol/L) is another common problem in elderly patients and generally is associated with poor prognosis. The incidence of hyponatremia ranges between 7% to 11% of hospital admissions; severe hyponatremia occurs in 1–4% of hospitalizations (71). Nearly half of the cases result from the use of diuretics. Common causes of hyponatremia in patients admitted to geriatric wards are; 47% water overload, 27% salt and water depletion, 22% salt and water overload, and 6% mixed aetiology (71).

Hyponatremic states may be produced in cases either of acute water overload, such as volume replacement with solutions lacking electrolytes, particularly postoperatively, or chronic overload as in cases of hypothyroidism and ADH inappropriate secretion syndrome. Other causes are nephrotic syndrome, liver cirrhosis, and congestive heart failure.

6.2. Renal Handling of Potassium

Potassium requirements in elderly persons do not seem to be mediated by age per se, but rather, are more related to changes resulting from diseases and their treatments. In normal subjects, the kidney continues to maintain external potassium balance and normal serum potassium concentration until very late in the course of chronic renal disease by increasing the rate of kaliuresis per nephron. Severe hyperkalemia is uncommon in patients with chronic renal failure unless they are taking an angiotensin-converting enzyme inhibitor or an angiotensin receptor antagonist.

Hypokalemia may occur in elderly people receiving diuretic therapy and is compounded by an inadequate intake of dietary potassium. Although this is the most common cause of hypokalemia in elderly people, vomiting, diarrhea, excessive use of purgatives, renal tubular acidosis, and other causes may also contribute to an abnormal decrease in serum potassium levels.

The most important consequences of hypokalemia are electrocardiographic abnormalities and arrhythmia, depression, anorexia, fatigue, disorientation, confusion, abdominal distension, paralytic ileus, and glucose intolerance. Many of these conditions are present in patients with chronic renal failure resulting from other causes; thus hypokalemia may exacerbate these pathological conditions.

Hyperkalemia in elderly people, as previously reported, is related to impaired renal failure and may result in severe cardiac arrhythmia, leading to sudden death. This electrolyte disturbance is frequent when elderly patients are treated either alone or in combination with angiotensin-converting enzyme inhibitors, potassium-sparing diuretics (diabetics), nonsteroidal anti-inflammatory drugs, or when metabolic acidosis is not corrected by sodium bicarbonate supplements.

7. ENERGY AND PROTEIN REQUIREMENTS IN OLDER ADULTS WITH RENAL DISEASE

7.1. Chronic Renal Failure Without Dialysis

It is critical that patients on low-protein diets receive adequate caloric intake in order to minimize muscle wasting. In 2000, the National Kidney Foundation published the "Kidney Disease Outcomes Quality Initiative Practice Guidelines" for nutrition in chronic renal failure (72). In these guidelines, it has been suggested that in elderly patients (>60 yr), either on low-protein diet or in dialysis, a dietary energy intake of 30–35 kcal/kg/d should be prescribed.

The recommended dietary protein intake for patients with CRF (GFR lower than 25 mL/min) who are not undergoing maintenance hemodialysis, should be 0.6 g protein/kg/d. For individuals who do not accept such a diet or who are unable to maintain adequate dietary energy intake, a higher daily intake (up to 0.75 g protein/kg/d) may be prescribed. In some highly compliant patients, some reports suggest that a very low protein diet (0.3 g protein/kg/d) supplemented with a mixture of amino acids and keto acids may be prescribed *(40,41,73)*. In these patients a close follow-up is necessary in order to monitor any risk of malnutrition and to detect the point at which dialysis can not be longer postponed.

7.2. Chronic Renal Failure on Dialysis

The energy expenditure in patients with CRF is similar to that of healthy subjects when measured at rest, while sitting quietly, and during prescribed exercise *(74)*. Available data indicates that a diet providing approx 30–35 kcal/kg/d in patients 60 yr of age or older, who tend to be less physically active, is sufficient to maintain neutral nitrogen balance, to promote higher serum albumin concentration and more normal anthropometric parameters, and to reduce urea nitrogen appearance (i.e., to improve protein utilization) *(75)*.

Although in elderly patients with CRF energy requirements have not been well studied, the suggested value is based, in part, on the recommended dietary allowances of older normal adults (RDA) *(76)*. The DEI, for patients 60 yr of age or older, on maintenance dialysis or on peritoneal dialysis is similar to the intake suggested for nondialyzed patients. For patients on renal replacement therapy, the recommended protein intake is 1–1.2 g/kg/d for patients on hemodialysis and 1.2–1.4 g/kg/d for patients on peritoneal dialysis.

8. MANAGEMENT OF PCM

When elderly patients with CRF or ESRD not yet on dialysis, display signs or symptoms related to PCM, or are at risk for developing malnutrition, the proposed steps in Table 3 for managing PCM should be followed.

There are many reasons why some older people are unable to meet their physiological needs for nutrients *(77)*. These are, in particular:

- Assistance with feeding, ranging from 2% (age class 65–84) to 7% (>85 yr-old)
- Food preparation, ranging from 3.5% (age class 65–84) to 26% (>85 yr-old)
- Difficulty shopping, ranging from 2% (age class 65–84) to 37% (>85 yr-old)
- Not shopping, ranging from 2% (age class 65–74) to 30% (>75 yr-old)
- Not cooking, ranging from 6% (age class 65–74) to 12% (>75 yr-old)
- Financal limitations

Before starting any nutrition support therapy, these reasons should be eliminated and treated when possible. Otherwise, it is likely that more sophisticated medical and pharmacologic approaches will simply be wasting time and money.

Other important pratical questions include the following: Is the patient able to chew? Has the patients impaired swallowing? In fact, eating can be impaired by local oral pathology, such as pain from gingivitis, fractured and decayed teeth, loss of dentition, impaired salivation, or candidiasis. An Italian study has characterized the way in which food intake differs between elderly subjects with adequate natural dentition or inadequate natural dentition, with or without dentures. Dietary intake was determined by the number of functional units (i.e., opposable teeth) not the number of teeth, and dentures were a fully effective replacement for natural teeth *(78)*.

The normal swallow that occurs in almost all young individuals is a symmetric and synchronized act which may be present in only 16% of those older than 70 yr, who

Table 3
Management of PCM

Medical history and social history. Physical examination. Pay attention to dialysis adequacy, acidemia.

Identify the main causes of the declining nutritional status, in particular the presence of catabolic illnesses.

Assess nutritional requirements (vitamins, steroid therapy, liver failure).

Teach patients, families or significant others concerning appropriate nutritional intake.

If, despite all these maneuvers, the nutrient intake remains inadequate, further nutritional treatment may include:

Oral nutritional supplement

Tube feeding

Intradialytic parenteral nutrition

Hormone therapy: rhGH, IGF-1, rhEPO

Megesterol acetate (appetite stimulant)

---

rhGH, recombinant human growth factor; IGF-1, insulin-like growth factor-1; rhEPO, recombinant human erythropoietin.

otherwise have no evidence of dysphagia (79). In advancing age, nerve conduction velocity slows, tongue muscle strength reduces, the pharyngo-esophagael segment of the pharynx presents a reduced compliance, resulting in variability in the swallowing process. Oropharyngeal dysphagia may often be mild and its detection requires good observation of the way patients eat. Oral incontinence (dribbling, spillage of food from the mouth) is embarrassing and may lead older people to decide not to eat in social occasion, where food is available, because of anxiety.

After a clear evaluation of these situations, in patients at risk or presenting with malnutrition a nutrition support can be started. Many elderly patients can be managed using nutritional support methods that include oral supplementation, enteral feeding, or parenteral nutrition.

While it may be reasonable, humane, ethical, moral and legal to attempt to correct malnutrition in elderly, evidence is increasing that nutritional supplementation improves nutritional indices, but may not affect outcome. The variety of the problems that impair eating in elderly patients are the main causes for these disappointing results.

When the cause of undernutrition have been identified, it is essential to coordinate and integrate the patient's medical treatment with his/her nutritional needs and other goals of care. It is important to pay attention to the presentation of food, particularly if it is thickened or pureed. Thickened drinks do not taste pleasant, and pureed food is often presented as an amorphous mass. Altering the presentation of pureed food as real food can often recreate interest.

Many therapeutic diets for common comorbid conditions (e.g., low-salt, low-fat, low-carbohydrate diets) significantly reduce the palatability of meals. The problems they address may be managed with alternate therapies permitting the use of normal diets (and not a specific diet for uremic patient), and thus improving nutrition intake. General strategies include frequent small meals (for those who are easily fatigued), favorite foods, and oral nutritional supplements.

In patients with CRF, a spontaneous reduction in dietary intake is frequently observed with the progression of renal failure. The progressive decline in nutritional intake is the cause of the appearance of malnutrition in these patients. Because the presence of malnutrition at the initiation of renal replacement therapy is predictive of future mortality, interventions that maintain or improve nutritional status during progressive renal failure are mandatory. A regular monitoring (1–3-mo interval) of the patients' nutritional status should be a routine component of the care for the patient with CRF.

A low daily nutrient intake can be improved by the use of oral supplements. There are different supplements available at present. It must be kept in mind that, after a first period of patient compliance with this therapy, patients, may spontaneously reduce their intakes as a result of the low palatability of the products. Based on the authors' experience, the highest compliance is observed when the oral supplements are used as partial source of daily protein and calorie intake, and not as total daily nutritional intake.

Tube feeding may be an effective method for nourishing patients with PCM. This method has been show to be effective in the treatment of the pediatric dialysis population (80). One survey, performed in our hospital, demonstrated that at least 50% of hospitalized patients aged ≥60 yr required enteral or tube feeding (unpublished data). Only a few studies have been conducted on elderly patients with CRF or ESRD receiving tube nutrition. The data obtained in pediatric patients suggests the use of tube feeding may be applied in malnourished elderly patients. Elderly patients require careful monitoring to assure adequate intake and to avoid any complications associated with tube feeding. The most commonly encountered complication in elderly patients is fluid and electrolyte imbalance. Fluid shifts may occur rapidly in these patients, potentially resulting in peripheral edema or, at the most severe, cardiac failure.

If tube feeding is not tolerated by patients, parenteral nutrition (PN), either intradialytic parenteral nutrition or total parenteral nutrition, should be proposed in response to failure of increasing oral nutrient intake. However, there are no convincing data, (from well-designed randomized studies) supporting the use of PN. Furthermore, this method can present side effects, including nausea, malaise, liver failure and sepsis. In one published study on the use of PN in malnourished patients, the worst outcomes were reported in patients with a serum albumin greater than 35 g/dL (81).

The addition of amino acids to solutions for hemo- (82) or peritoneal dialysis (83) has been reported to be effective in increasing amino acid uptake, and therefore, protein synthesis. Further studies, on larger groups for patients, are necessary to demonstrate whether this treatment will improve the nutritional and clinical status of malnourished patients.

Finally, a number of studies have evaluated the potential benefits of hormone therapy. Recombinant human growth hormone (rhGH) or recombinant human insuline-like growth factor-1 (IGF-1) has been tested in experimental trials. Recombinant human growth hormone may promote protein synthesis, decrease protein degradation, and improve nitrogen balance during acute and chronic administration in uremic patients (84–86). IGF-1 is the active compound of rhGH and in ESRD patients were found to produce anabolic effects (87). Presently, long-term studies are not available, in particular in elderly patients, and data are needed to validate this therapy. Anemia is related with fatigue, low physical activity and, as a consequence, low-nutrient intake. CRF or ESRD elderly anemic patients treated with rherythropoietin show an improvement of daily

Table 4
Protocol for Nutritional Monitoring of Elderly Patients with Chronic Renal Failure

Monthly

Anthropometry
1. Subject nutritional global assessment
2. Predialysis weight (in MHD patients)
3. Intradialytic weight gain
4. Previous month weight (in CRF patients and in PD patients)

Serum chemistries
1. Serum urea
2. Urinary urea (in patients on dialysis with residual renal function and in patients with CRF)
3. Creatinine
4. Urinary creatinine (in patients on dialysis with residual renal function and in patients with CRF)
5. Calcium
6. Phosphorus
7. Potassium
8. Venous bicarbonate
9. Albumin
10. Cholesterol
11. Hemoglobin

Serum chemistries, every 3 mo
1. Prealbumin
2. Transferrin
3. Iron
4. CRP
5. Kt/V
6. Weekly creatinine clearance (in PD patients)
7. Urea reduction ratio
8 Urea nitrogen appearance

Every 6 mo
1. Dietary history
2. Anthropometry
3. DEXA
4. BIA (?)

activity and of well being. In addition, patients displayed an improvement of nutritional status. The maintenance of hemoglobin levels in the suggested range (9.5–12 g/dL) is another step in the prevention of malnutrition.

Because malnutrition can be insidious, the nutritional status of elderly patients should be frequently monitored. It should be assessed during the low-protein diet period in patients with CRF and at the start of dialysis treatment, at regular intervals of 1–6-mo (Table 4). Once the patient has been evaluated and any degree of malnutrition has been identified, a specific and correct nutritional therapy should be started. A reduction in morbidity and mortality of the group of elderly patients with CRF should be observed. Elderly individuals, being more different from each other than any other group of people, present constant challenges for their caregivers. Because the elderly are the most rapidly growing segment of the Western countries, even among patients starting dialysis therapy and are the users of the greatest portion of the health care resources, it is imperative that information regarding aging and nutrition in patients with chronic renal failure be gathered through scientific endeavor and be disseminated to all health care practitioners.

9. RECOMMENDATIONS FOR CLINICIANS

1. Regular nutrition monitoring and counseling is critical in chronic renal failure patients to prevent the development of malnutrition.
2. Common etiologies of malnutrition related to CRF that should be evaluated include a poor understanding of dietary recommendations, inadequate dialysis dose, bio-incompatible membranes, acidosis, uremia-associated anorexia, delayed gastric emptying and early satiety in the case of peritoneal dialysis.
3. Severe restriction of sodium or water should be avoided unless absolutely necessary. Most older patients should consume ≥ 2 L of fluid/d.
4. In patients with CRF not on dialysis, daily energy intake should be 30–35 kcal/kg/d and daily protein intake should be 0.6 g/kg/d. For individuals who do not accept such a diet or who are unable to maintain adequate dietary energy intake, a higher daily intake of protein should be prescribed.
5. In patients with CRF on dialysis, daily energy intake should be 30–35 kcal/kg/d and daily protein intake should be 1.0–1.2 g/kg/d for patients on hemodialysis and 1.2–1.4 g/kg/d for patients on peritoneal dialysis.

REFERENCES

1. Grundy E. Ageing, ill health and disability. In: Increasing Longevity. Tallis RC (ed.), Royal College of Physicians, London, 1998.
2. Warnes MA. Population ageing over the next decades. In: Increasing Longevity. Tallis RC (ed.) Royal College of Physicians, London, 1998.
3. Horan MA. Advances in understanding the concept of biological ageing. In: Increasing Longevity. Tallis RC (ed.) Royal College of Physicians, London, 1998.
4. US Ren Data Syst. USRDS 2000 Annual Data Report. US Dep Public Health Hum. Serv., Public Health Serv., Natl. Inst. Health, Bethesda, MD, 2000.
5. Young GA, Kopple JD, Lindholm B, et al. Nutritional assessment of continuous ambulatory peritoneal dialysis patients: an international study. Am J Kidney Dis 1991;17:462–471.
6. Cianciaruso B, Brunori G, Kopple JD, et al. Cross-sectional comparison of malnutrition in continuous ambulatory peritoneal dialysis and hemodialysis patients. Am J Kidney Dis 1995; 26:475–486.
7. Kopple JD. Treatment with low protein and amino acid diets in chronic renal failure. In: Proceedings of the VII International Congress of Nephrology. Montreal. Karger S (ed.), Basel, 1978, pp. 497–507.
8. Kopple JD, Swendseid ME. Nitrogen balance and plasma amino acid levels in uremic patients fed an essential amino acid diet. Am J Clin Nutr 1974;27:806–812.
9. Bergstrom J, Furst P, Noree LO. Treatment of chronic uremic patients with protein poor diet and oral supply of essential amino acids. I. Nitrogen balance studies. Clin Nephrol 1975;3:187–194.
10. Modify Diet Renal Disease Study Group. Relationship between nutritional status and the glomerular filtration rate: results from the MDRD study. Kidney Int 2000;57:1688–1703
11. Garg AX, Blake PG, Clark WF, et al. Association between renal insufficiency and malnutrition in older adults: Results from the NHANES III. Kidney Int 2001;60:1867–1874.
12. Lowrie EG, Lew LN. Death risk in hemodialysis patients: the predictive value of commonly measured variables and an evaluation of death rate differences between facilities. Am J Kidney Dis 1990;15: 458–482.
13. Held PJ, Brunner FB, Okada M, et al. Five-year survival for end stage renal disease patients in the United States, Europe and Japan. 1982 to 1987. Am J Kidney Dis 1990;15:451–457.

14. Valderrabano F, Berthoux F, Jones E, Mehls O. Report on management of renal failure in Europe, XXV, 1994: End stage renal disease and dialysis report. Nephrol Dial Transplant 1996;11(suppl 1):S2–S21.

15. Shinzato T, Nakai S, Akiba T, et al. Survival in long term hemodialysis patients: Results of the annual survey of the Japanese society for dialysis therapy. Nephrol Dial Transplant 1997;12:884–888.

16. Guarneri G, Toigo G, Situlin R, et al. Nutritional status in patients on long term low protein diet or with nephrotic syndrome. Kidney Int 1989;36(suppl 27):S195–S200.

17. Maroni BJ, Steinman TI, Mitch WE. A method for estimating nitrogen intake of patients with chronic renal failure. Kidney Int 1985;27:58–65.

18. Nelson EE, Hong CD, Pesce AL, et al. Anthropometric norms for the dialysis population. Am J Kidney Dis 1990;16:32–37.

19. Detsky AS, McLaughlin JR, Baker JP, et al. What is the subjective global assessment of nutritional status? JPEN 1987;11:8–13.

20. Enia G, Sicuso C, Alati G, Zoccali C. Subjective global assessment of nutrition in dialysis patients. Nephrol Dial Transplant 1993;8:1094–1098.

21. Maiorca R, Brunori G, Zubani R, et al. Predictive value of dialysis adequacy and nutritional indices for mortality and morbidity in CAPD and HD patients. Nephrol Dial Transplant 1995;10:2295–2305.

22. Churchill DN, Taylor DW, Cook RJ, et al. Canadian hemodialysis morbidity study. Am J Kidney Dis 1992;23:214–234.

23. Sreedhara R, Avram MM, Blanco M, et al. Prealbumin is the best nutritional predictor of survival in hemodialysis and peritoneal dialysis. Am J Kidney Dis 1996;28:937–924.

24. Aparicio M, Cano N, Chauveau P, et al. Nutritional status of hemodialysis patients: A French national cooperative study. Nephrol Dial Transplant 1999;14:1679–1686.

25. Kaysen GA, Rathore V, Shearer GC, Depner TA. Mechanism of hypoalbuminemia in hemodialysis patients. Kidney Int 1995;48:510–516.

26. Owen WF, Lowrie EG. C-reactive protein as an outcome predictor for maintenance hemodialysis patients. Kidney Int 1998;54:627–636.

27. National Kidney Foundation. Kidney Disease Outcomes Quality Initiative Update, 2000.

28. Lowrie EG, Huang WH, Lew NL. Death risk predictors among peritoneal dialysis and hemodialysis patients: A preliminary comparison. Am J Kidney Dis 1995;26:220–228.

29. Avram MM, Mittman N, Bonomini L, et al. Markers for survival in dialysis: A seven-year prospective study. Am J Kidney Dis 1995;2:209–219.

30. Kloppenburg WE, Stegman CA, deJong PE, Huisman RM. Relating protein intake to nutritional status in hemodialysis patients: How to normalize the protein equivalent of total nitrogen appearance. Nephrol Dial Transplant 1999;14:2165–2172.

31. Brunori G. Comparison of nutritional status in PD and HD patients. Nieren und Hochdruckkrankheiten 1994;23(suppl 2):S121–S125.

32. Chumela WG, Guo S. Bioelectrical impedance: Present status and future directions. Nutr Rev 1994;52:123–131.

33. Woodrow G, Oldroyd B, Smith MA, Turney JH. Measurements of body composition in chronic renal failure: Comparison of skinfold anthropometry and bioelectrical impedance with dual energy X-ray absorptiometry. Eur J Clin Nutr 1996;50:295–301.

34. Dwyer JT, Cunniff PJ, Maroni BJ, et al. The hemodialysis pilot study: Nutrition program and participant characteristic at baseline. The HEMO study group. J Ren Nutr 1998;8:11–20.

35. Thunberg BJ, Swamy AP, Cestero RV. Cross-sectional and longitudinal measurements in maintenance hemodialysis patients. Am J Clin Nutr 1981;34:2005–2012.

36. Ikizler TA, Greene JH, Wingard RL, Parker Ra, Hakim RM. Spontaneous dietary intake during progression of chronic renal failure. J Am Soc Nephrol 1995;6:1386–1391.

37. Lorenzo V, Martin M, Rufino M, et al. Protein intake, control of serum phosphorus, and relatively low levels of parathyroid hormone in elderly hemodialysis patients. Am J Kidney Dis 2001;37:1260–1266.

38. Movilli E, Filippini M, Brunori G, et al. Influence of protein catabolic rate on nutritional status, morbidity and mortality in elderly ureaemic patients on chronic hemodialysis: a prospective 3-year follow-up study. Nephrol Dial Transplant 1993;8:735–739.

39. Cancarini G, Costantino E, Brunori G, et al. Nutritional status in long-term CAPD patients. In: Advances in Peritoneal Dialysis, vol. 8. Peritoneal Dialysis Bulletin, Inc., Toronto, Canada, 1992, pp. 84–87.

40. Walser M. Does prolonged protein restriction preceding dialysis lead to protein malnutrition at the onset of dialysis? Kidney Int 1993;44:1139–1144.

41. Brunori G, Viola BF, Zubani R, et al. Can a very low protein diet (VLPD) postpone the start of dialysis in elderly uremic patients? Abstracts book 10th Int Congress on Nutrition and Metabolism in renal disease, Lyon, 2000, 36.
42. Lim VS, Kopple JD. Protein metabolism in patients with chronic renal failure: Role of uremia and dialysis. Kidney Int 2000;58:1–10.
43. Kopple JD. Dietary protein and energy requirements in ESRD patients. Am J Kidney Dis 1996;32 (suppl 4):S97–S104.
44. Anderstam B, Mamoun AH, Sodersten P, Bergstrom J. Middle-sized molecule fractions isolated from uremic ultrafiltrate and normal urine inhibit ingestive behavior in the rat. J Am Soc Nephrol 1996;7: 2453–2460.
45. Clark WR, Gao D. Low molecular weight proteins in end stage renal disease: Potential toxicity and dialytic removal mechanism. J Am soc Nephrol 2002;13:S41–S47.
46. Heymsfield SB, Greenberg AS, Fujioca K, et al. Recombinant leptin for weight loss in obese and lean adult. A randomised, controlled, dose-escalation trial. JAMA 1999;282:1568–1575.
47. Lindsay R, Spanner E. A hypothesis: The protein catabolic rate is dependent upon the type and amount of treatment in dialyzed uremic patients. Am J Kidney Dis 1989;8:382–389.
48. Hakim RM, Breyer T, Ismail N, Schlman G. Effects of dose of dialysis on morbidity and mortality. Am J Kidney Dis 1994;23:661–669.
49. Yang CS, Chen SW, Chiang CH, et al. Effect of increasing dialysis dose on serum albumin and mortality in hemodialysis patients. Am J Kidney Dis 1996;27:380–386.
50. Lindsay RM, Spanner E, Heidenhiem AP et al. Which comes first, Kt/V or PCR—chicken or egg? Kidney Int 1992;42(suppl 38):S32–S36.
51. Papadoyannakis NJ, Stefanides CJ, McGeown M. The effect of the correction of metabolic acidosis on nitrogen and protein balance of patients with chronic renal failure. Am J Clin Nutr 1984;40:623–627.
52. Mitch WE, Medina R, Greiber S, et al. Metabolic acidosis stimulates muscle protein degradation by activating the ATP-dependent pathway involving ubiquitin and proteosomes. J Clin Invest 1994;93: 2127–2133.
53. Ballmer PE, McNurlan MA, Hulter HN, et al. Chronic metabolic acidosis decreases albumin synthesis and induces negative nitrogen balance in humans. J Clin Invest 1995;95:39–45.
54. Movilli E, Zani R, Carli O, et al. Correction of metabolic acidosis increases serum albumin concentrations and decreases kinetically evaluated protein intake in hemodialysis patients: a prospective study. Nephrol Dial Transplant 1998;3:1719–1722.
55. Garibotto G, Russo R, Sofia A, et al. Skeletal muscle protein synthesis and degradation in patients with chronic uremia: the influence of metabolic acidosis. Kidney Int 1994;45:1432–1439.
56. Chaveau P, Foque D, Combe C, et al. Acidosis and nutritional status in hemodialyzed patients. Semin Dial 2000;13:241–246.
57. Borah M, Schoenfeld PY, Gotch FA, et al. Nitrogen balance in intermittent hemodialysis therapy. Kidney Int 1978;14:497–500.
58. Gutierrez A, Alvestrand A, Wahren J, Bergstrom J. Effect of in vivo contact between blood and dialysis membranes on protein catabolism in humans. Kidney Int 1990;38:487–494.
59. Levin NW. Dialyzer reuse: A currently acceptable practice. Semin Dial 1996;6:89–90.
60. Kaplan AA, Halley SE, Lapkin RA, Graeber CW. Dialysate protein losses with bleach processed polysulphone dialyzer. Kidney Int 1995;47:573–578.
61. Macais-Nunez JF, Cameron JS. Renal function and disease in the elderly. Butterworths, London, 1987.
62. Refoyo A, Macias-Nunez JF. The maintenance of plasma sodium in the healthy aged. Geriatr Nephrol Urol 1991;1:65–68.
63. Barrows DH Jr, Falzone JH Jr, Shock NW. Age differences in the succinoxidase activity in homogenates and mitochrondia from livers and kidneys of rats. J Gerontol 1960;15:130–133.
64. Epstein M, Hollenberg NH. Age as a determinant of renal sodium conservation in normal man. J Lab Clin Med 1976;87:411–417.
65. Macias-Nunez JF. Renal handling of sodium in old people: A functional study. Age Ageing 1978;7:178–181.
66. Macias-Nunez JF, Garcia-Iglesias C, Tabernero-Romo JM, et al. Renal management of sodium under indomethacin and aldosterone in the elderly. Age Ageing 1980;9:165–172.
67. Crane M, Harris JJ. Effect of ageing on renin activity and aldosteron excretion. J Lab Clin Med 1976;87:947–959.
68. Wiedmann P. Interrelations between age and plasma rennin, aldosterone and cortisol, urinary cathecolamines, and the sodium/volume state in normal man. Klin Wochenschr 1977;55:723–733.

69. Solomon LR, Lye M. Hypernatremia in the elderly patient. Gerontology 1990;36:171–179.
70. Rowe JW. Health and disease in old age. In: Aging. Rowe JW, Besdine RW (eds.), Boston, Little, Brown and Co, 1982.
71. Solomon LR, Sangster G, Lye M. Hypernatremia in the elderly patient. Geriatr Nephrol Urol 1992;2:63–74.
72. K/DOQI Clinical practice guidelines for nutrition in chronic renal failure. Am J Kidney Dis 2000; 35(suppl 2):S1–S140.
73. Aparicio M, Chauveau P, De Pregigout V, et al. Nutrition and outcome on renal replacement therapy of patients with chronic renal failure treated by a supplemented very low protein diet. J Am Soc Nephrol 2000;11:708–716.
74. Monteon FJ, Laidlow SA, Shaib JK, Kopple JD. Energy expenditure in patients with chronic renal failure. Kidney Int 1986;30:741–747.
75. Kopple JD, Monteon FJ, Shaib JK. Effect of energy intake on nitrogen metabolism in nondialyzed patientswith chronic renal failure. Kidney Int 1986;229:734–742.
76. Food and Nutrition Board NRCN: Recommended Daily Allowances (ed 10). National Academy, Washington, DC, 1989.
77. Smithard DG, Blandford G, Grimble GK. Nutrition support in the elderly. In: Artificial nutrition support in clinical practice, 2nd ed. Payne-James J, Grimble G, Silk D (eds), Greenwich Medical Media Ltd., London, 2001, pp. 681–700.
78. Apollonio I, Carabelelse C, Frattola A, Trabucchi M. Influence of dental status on dietary intake and survival in community-dwelling elderly subjects. Age Ageing 1997;26:445–456.
79. Ekberg O, Fienberg MJ. Altered swallowing function in elderly patients without disphagia: Radiologic findings in 56 cases. Br J Radiol 1982;55:253–257.
80. Coleman JE, Norman LJ, Watson AR. Provision of dietetic care in children on chronic peritoneal dialysis. J Renal Nutr 1999;9:145–148.
81. Chertow GM, Ling J, Lew NL, et al. The association of intradialytic parenteral nutrition administration with survival in hemodialysis patients. Am J Kidney Dis 1994;24:912–920.
82. Chazot C, Shahmir E, Matias B, Kopple JD. Provision of amino acids by dialysis during maintenance haemodialysis (MHD). (Abstract). J Am Soc Nephrol 1995;6:574.
83. Kopple JD, Bernard D, Messana J et al. Treatment of malnourished CAPD patients with an amino acids based dialysate. Kidney Int 1997;52:1663–1670.
84. Ikizler TA, Wingard RL, Flakoll PJ, et al. Effects of recombinant human growth hormone on plasma and dialysate amino acid profiles in CAPD patients. Kidney Int 1996;50:229–234.
85. Iglesias P, Diez JJ, Fernandez Reyes MJ, et al. Recombinant human growth hormone therapy in malnourished dialysis patients: A randomized controlled study. Am J Kidney Dis 1998;32:454–463.
86. Johannson G, Bengtoss BA, Ahlmen J. Double-blind, placebo-controlled study of growth hormone treatment in elderly patients undergoing chronic hemodialysis: Anabolic effect and functional improvement. Am J Kidney Dis 1999;33:709–717.
87. Foque D, Peng SC, Shahmir E, Kopple JD. Recombinant human IGF-1 induces an anabolic response in malnourished CAPD patients. Kidney Int 2000;57:646–654.

G. MUSCULOSKELETAL DISORDERS

28 Osteoarthritis

Timothy E. McAlindon

1. INTRODUCTION

Osteoarthritis (OA) is the most common form of joint disease and a major cause of disability in the elderly. The disorder is strongly associated with increasing age and has been estimated to affect between two and ten percent of all adults (1,2). It is responsible for some 68 million work loss days/year and for more than 5% of the annual retirement rate (3). Furthermore, osteoarthritis is the most frequent reason for joint replacement at a cost to the community of billions of dollars per year (4).

OA is characterized pathologically by focal damage to articular cartilage (5). This may range in severity from minor surface roughening to complete cartilage erosion. The process is generally noninflammatory and is often described as being "degenerative" or resulting from "wear and tear." The cartilage damage is usually accompanied by some form of "reaction" in the surrounding bone. Osteophytes are an early bony response to cartilage damage. These consist of outgrowths of bone from the peripheral margin of the joint. They may confer some protection to an osteoarthritic joint by reducing instability (6). The trabeculae in the bone adjacent to an area of osteoarthritic cartilage become thickened, and are susceptible to microscopic fracturing. This gives rise to the appearance of "subchondral sclerosis" on a radiograph. In severe disease, particularly where full thickness cartilage has occurred, circumscribed areas of bony necrosis may develop in the subchondral bone. These may be filled with marrow fat, or with synovial fluid which has tracked from the joint space through the cartilage defect into the subchondral bone. They give rise to the radiographic appearance of "cysts." Ultimately the subchondral bone itself may be eroded, or may collapse. In some cases, a low-level synovitis develops resulting from the presence of crystal or other cartilaginous "detritus," which may contribute to damage in the joint.

Biochemically, cartilage consists of a network of collagen fibrils (predominantly type II) which constrain an interlocking mesh of proteoglycans that resist compressive forces through their affinity for water. The tissue is relatively avascular and acellular. Turnover in healthy cartilage is slow and represents a balance between collagen and proteoglycan synthesis and degradation by enzymes such as metalloproteinases. In early osteoarthritis, the chondrocytes (cartilage cells) proliferate and become metabolically active. These hypertrophic chondrocytes produce cytokines (e.g., IL-1, TNF-α), degradative enzymes

From: *Handbook of Clinical Nutrition and Aging*
Edited by: C. W. Bales and C. S. Ritchie © Humana Press Inc., Totowa, NJ

Table 1
Established Risk Factors Associated with Osteoarthritis

Constitutional factors
    Increased age
    Female gender
    Obesity
Mechanical factors
    Heavy/repetitive occupations
    Heavy physical activity
    Major joint injury
Endocrine factors
    Hemachromatosis
Genetic factors
    Mutations in the type II collagen gene

(e.g., metalloproteinases) and other growth factors. Proteoglycan production is increased in early OA, but falls sharply at a later stage when the chondrocyte "fails."

1.1. Risk Factors for Osteoarthritis

The striking relationship of OA with increasing age and with heavy physical work has led to its characterization as a "degenerative" disorder (1). In fact, this paradigm is inaccurate because a variety of mechanical, metabolic, and genetic disorders may lead to osteoarthritis (7). A more contemporary view is that OA results from dynamic interaction between destructive and reparative processes within a joint. Established risk factors for OA are listed in Table 1.

1.2. Osteoarthritis and Diet

There is enormous public interest in the relationship between diet and arthritis, but there has been relatively little focus in traditional scientific studies on the relationship between nutritional factors (other than obesity) and OA. This is surprising given the large numbers of studies of osteoporosis, another widespread age-related skeletal disorder, which have shown widely accepted associations with dietary factors. A more important reason to study the relationship between dietary factors and OA, however, is that there are many mechanisms by which certain micronutrients can be hypothesized to influence osteoarthritis processes. Furthermore, there have been several recent studies that have shown apparent effects of various micronutrients on the natural history of this disorder.

2. MECHANISMS THROUGH WHICH MICRONUTRIENTS CAN BE HYPOTHESIZED TO INFLUENCE OSTEOARTHRITIS PROCESSES

2.1. Antioxidant Effects

There is considerable evidence that continuous exposure to oxidants contributes to the development or exacerbation of many of the common human diseases associated with aging (8). Such oxidative damage accumulates with age and has been implicated in the pathophysiology of cataract (9), coronary artery disease (10) and certain forms of cancer

(11). As the prototypical age-related "degenerative" disease, OA may also be a product of oxidative damage to articular tissues.

Reactive oxygen species are chemicals with unpaired electrons. These are formed continuously in tissues by endogenous and some exogenous mechanisms *(8)*. For example, it has been estimated that 1–2% of all electrons which travel down the mitochondrial respiratory chain leak, forming a superoxide anion ($O_2^{•-}$) *(12)*. Other endogenous sources include release by phagocytes during the oxidative burst, generation by mixed function oxidase enzymes, and in hypoxia-reperfusion events *(13)*. Reactive oxygen species are capable of causing damage to many macromolecules including cell membranes, lipoproteins, proteins and DNA *(14)*. Because these reactive oxygen species are identical to those generated by irradiation of H_2O, "living" has been likened to being continuously irradiated *(8)*.

Furthermore, there is evidence that cells within joints produce reactive oxygen species, and that oxidative damage is physiologically important *(15)*. In laboratory studies, animal and human chondrocytes have been found to be potent sources of reactive oxygen species *(15,16)*. Hydrogen peroxide production has been demonstrated in aged human chondrocytes after exposure to the proinflammatory cytokines, interleukin-1 and tumor necrosis factor-α, and has been observed in live cartilage tissue *(17)*. Superoxide anions have been shown to adversely affect collagen structure and integrity in vitro, and appear to be responsible, in vivo, for depolymerization of synovial fluid hyaluronate *(16–19)*.

In fact, the human body has extensive and multilayered antioxidant defense systems *(8)*. Intracellular defense is provided primarily by antioxidant enzymes including superoxide dismutase, catalase and peroxidases. In addition to these enzymes, there are a number of small molecule antioxidants which play an important role, particularly in the extracellular space, where antioxidant enzymes are sparse *(20)*. These include the micronutrients alpha-tocopherol (vitamin E), beta-carotene (vitamin A precursor), other carotenoids, and ascorbate (vitamin C). The concentrations of these antioxidants in the blood are primarily determined by dietary intake. The concept that micronutrient antioxidants might provide further defense against tissue injury when intracellular enzymes are overwhelmed, has led to the hypothesis that high dietary intake of these micronutrients might protect against age-related disorders. Because higher intake of dietary antioxidants appears beneficial in respect to outcomes such as cataract extraction and coronary artery disease *(9–11,21)* it is also plausible that they may confer similar benefits for OA.

2.2. Effects on Collagen Metabolism

In addition to being an antioxidant, vitamin C plays several functions in the biosynthesis of cartilage molecules. First, through the vitamin C-dependent enzyme lysylhydroxylase, vitamin C is required for the posttranslational hydroxylation of specific prolyl and lysyl residues in procollagen, a modification essential for stabilization of the mature collagen fibril *(9–11,21–23)*. Vitamin C also appears to stimulate collagen biosynthesis by pathways independent of hydroxylation, perhaps through lipid peroxidation *(24)*. In addition, by acting as a carrier of sulfate groups, vitamin C participates in glycosaminoglycan synthesis *(25)*. Thus, relative deficiency of vitamin C may impair not only the production of cartilage, but also its biomechanical quality.

The results of in vitro and in vivo studies are concordant with this possibility. Studies of adult bovine chondrocytes have shown that addition of ascorbate acid to the tissue culture results in decreased levels of degradative enzymes, and increased synthesis of type II collagen and proteoglycans *(25,26)*. Peterkovsky et al. observed decreased synthesis of cartilage collagen and proteoglycan molecules in guinea pigs deprived of vitamin C. They also reported high levels of IGF-1-binding proteins, which normally inhibit the anabolic effects of IGF-1, a potent growth factor *(27)*. This suggests that vitamin C may also influence growth factors through pathways which remain to be elucidated.

2.3. Effects on Chondrocyte Metabolism

Vitamin D might have direct effects on chondrocytes in osteoarthritic cartilage. During bone growth, vitamin D regulates the transition from growth plate cartilage to bone. Normally, chondrocytes in developing bone lose their vitamin D receptors with the attainment of skeletal maturity. It has recently become apparent, however, that the hypertrophic chondrocytes in osteoarthritic cartilage can redevelop vitamin D receptors *(28)*. These chondrocytes are metabolically active and appear to play an important role in the pathophysiology of osteoarthritis *(29)*. Although this evidence is indirect, it raises the possibility that vitamin D may influence the pathologic processes in osteoarthritis through effects on these cells.

2.4. Effects on Bone

Reactive changes in the bone underlying, and adjacent to, damaged cartilage are an integral part of the osteoarthritic process *(30–36)*. Sclerosis of the underlying bone, trabecular micro-fracturing, attrition and cyst formation are all likely to accelerate the degenerative process as a result of adverse biomechanical changes *(37,38)*. Other phenomena, such as osteophytes (bony spurs) may be attempts to repair or stabilize the process *(6,39)*. It has also been suggested that bone mineral density may influence the skeletal expression of the disease with a more erosive form occurring in individuals with "softer" bone *(40)*. Although some cross-sectional studies have suggested a modest inverse relationship between OA and osteoporosis, recent prospective studies have suggested that individuals with lower bone mineral density are at increased risk for OA incidence and progression *(41)*. The idea that the nature of bony response in OA may determine outcome has been further advanced by the recent demonstration that patients with bone scan abnormalities adjacent to an osteoarthritic knee have a higher rate of progression than those without such changes *(42)*.

Normal bone metabolism is contingent on the presence of vitamin D, a compound that is largely derived from the diet or from cutaneous exposure to ultraviolet light. Suboptimal vitamin D levels may have adverse effects on calcium metabolism, osteoblast activity, matrix ossification and bone density *(43,44)*. Low-tissue levels of vitamin D may, therefore, impair the ability of bone to respond optimally to pathophysiological processes in osteoarthritis, and predispose to disease progression.

2.5. Anti-Inflammatory Properties

Vitamin E has diverse influences on the metabolism of arachadonic acid, an antiinflammatory fatty acid found in all cell membranes. Vitamin E blocks formation of arachidonic acid from phospholipids and inhibits lipoxygenase activity, although it has little effect on cyclooxygenase *(45)*. It is, therefore, possible that vitamin E reduces the modest synovial inflammation that may accompany osteoarthritis.

3. STUDIES OF THE EFFECTS OF NUTRIENTS IN OSTEOARTHRITIS

3.1. Obesity and Osteoarthritis

Overweight people are at considerably increased risk for the development of OA in their knees, and may also be more susceptible to both hip and hand joint involvement *(46)*. Furthermore, weight loss appears to both reduce the risk for development of knee OA and improve symptoms in those with prevalent disease *(46)*. Because overweight individuals do not necessarily have increased load across their hand joints, investigators have wondered whether systemic factors, such as dietary factors or other metabolic consequences of obesity, may mediate some of this association. Indeed, early laboratory studies using strains of mice and rats appeared to suggest an interaction between body weight, genetic factors and diet, although attempts to demonstrate a direct effect of dietary fat intake proved inconclusive *(47,48)*.

3.2. The Case for Vitamin C and Other Antioxidant Micronutrients

3.2.1. ANIMAL STUDIES

OA can be induced in animals by various surgical procedures. Schwartz and Leveille treated guinea pigs prior to such surgery with either a high (150 mg/d) or low (2.4 mg/d) dose of vitamin C *(49)*. Guinea pigs treated with the higher dose of vitamin C (corresponding to vitamin C in humans of at least 500 mg/d) showed, "consistently less severe joint damage than animals on the low level of the vitamin." Features of OA were significantly less frequent in the animals treated with the high dose of vitamin C. Similar findings were reported by Meacock et al. in another surgically-induced guinea pig model of OA. In this study, they supplemented the feeds of half of the animals with vitamin C after the surgical procedure *(50)*. They reported, "Extra ascorbic acid appeared to have some protective effect ($p = 0.008$) on the development of spontaneous [osteoarthritis] lesions…"

3.2.2. EPIDEMIOLOGIC STUDIES

We investigated the association of self-reported dietary intake of antioxidant micronutrients among participants followed longitudinally in the Framingham Knee OA Cohort Study *(51)*, a population-based group derived from the Framingham Heart Study Cohort. Participants had knee X-rays taken at a baseline examination performed during 1983–1985, and had follow-up X-rays approx 8 yr later, during 1992–1993. Knee OA was classified using the Kellgren and Lawrence grading system *(52)*. Knees without osteoarthritis at baseline (Kellgren and Lawrence grade ≤1) were classified as incident osteoarthritis if they had developed grade 2 or greater by follow-up. Knees with osteoarthritis at baseline were classified as progressive osteoarthritis if their score increased by 1 or more.

Nutrient intake, including supplement use, was calculated from dietary habits reported at the midpoint of the study using a food frequency questionnaire. In our analyses, we ranked micronutrient intake into sex-specific tertiles and looked specifically to see if higher intakes of vitamin C, vitamin E and beta-carotene, compared with a panel of nonantioxidant "control" micronutrients, were associated with reduced incidence and reduced progression of knee OA. The lowest tertile for each dietary exposure was used as the reference category. Odds ratios (OR) were adjusted for age, sex, BMI, weight change, knee injury, physical activity, energy intake, and health status.

Six-hundred forty participants (mean age 70.3 yr) had complete assessments. Incident and progressive knee osteoarthritis occurred in 81 and 68 knees, respectively. We found no significant association of incident radiographic knee OA with any micronutrient (e.g., adjusted OR for highest vs lowest tertile of vitamin C intake = 1.1, 95% CI 0.6–2.2). On the other hand, for progression of radiographic knee OA, we found a threefold reduction in risk for those in the middle and highest tertiles of vitamin C intake (adjusted OR for highest vs lowest tertile = 0.3; 95% CI 0.1–0.6). It is notable that those in the highest tertile for vitamin C intake also had reduced risk of developing knee pain during the course of the study (OR = 0.3; 95% CI 0.1–0.8). Reduction in risk of progression was also seen for β-carotene (OR = 0.4; 95% CI 0.2–0.9) and vitamin E but was less consistent, as the beta-carotene association diminished substantially after adjustment for vitamin C, and the vitamin E effect was seen only in men (OR = 0.07; 95% CI 0.01–0.6). No significant associations were observed for any of the micronutrients among the nonantioxidant "panel."

Thus, this study does not support the hypothesis that diets high in antioxidant micronutrients reduce the risk of incident knee OA. On the other hand, the data suggest that some of these micronutrients, vitamin C in particular, may reduce the risk of osteoarthritis progression among those who already have some radiographic changes.

If antioxidants are, indeed, protective for individuals with osteoarthritis, we are left with questions about why the effect appears to be confined to those with existing radiographic changes. One possible explanation relates to differences in the intra-articular environment between healthy and osteoarthritis knees. For example, several pathologic mechanisms, including raised intra-articular pressure (14), low grade inflammation (53) and increased metabolic activity (13) increase the opportunity for oxidative damage in an osteoarthritic knee. Therefore, antioxidants could have a greater role in preventing progression rather than incidence, which can result from a variety of nonmetabolic insults such as knee injury (54).

Another important observation in this study was that the effect of vitamin C was stronger and more consistent than those for β-carotene and vitamin E. Vitamin C is a water-soluble compound with a broad spectrum of antioxidant activity resulting from its ability to react with numerous aqueous-free radicals and reactive oxygen species (8). The extracellular nature of reactive oxygen species-mediated damage in joints, and the aqueous intra-articular environment, may favor a role for a water-soluble agent such as vitamin C, rather than fat-soluble molecules like β-carotene or vitamin E. In addition, it has been suggested that vitamin C may "regenerate" vitamin E at the water–lipid interface by reducing α-tocopherol radical back to α-tocopherol. Whether this occurs in vivo, however, appears controversial. An alternative explanation is that the protective effects of vitamin C relate to its biochemical participation in the biosynthesis of cartilage collagen fibrils and proteoglycan molecules, rather than its antioxidant properties.

3.2.3. Clinical Trials

Benefit from vitamin E therapy has been suggested by several small studies of human osteoarthritis (55–58), of which the most rigorous was a company-sponsored 6-wk double-blind placebo-controlled trial of 400 mg α-tocophorol (vitamin E) in 56 OA patients in Germany (59). Vitamin E treated patients experienced greater improvement in every efficacy measure including pain at rest (69% better in vitamin E vs 34% in placebo, $p < 0.05$), pain on movement (62% better on vitamin E vs 27% on placebo,

$p < 0.01$) and use of analgesics (52% less on vitamin E ; 24% less on placebo, $p < 0.01$). The rapid response in symptoms observed in this study precludes a structural effect in this disorder, and suggests the beneficial effect might be result from some metabolic action such as inhibition of arachidonic acid metabolism.

Selenium has also been tested in a clinical trial as a therapy for osteoarthritis symptoms *(60)*. Hill and Bird conducted a 6-mo double-blind placebo controlled study of Selenium-ACE, a proprietary nutritional supplement in the UK, among thirty patients with unspecified osteoarthritis. The "active" treatment contained on average 144 µg of selenium, and contained unspecified quantities of vitamins A, C and E. In fact, the "placebo" also contained 2.9 µg of selenium. Pain and stiffness scores remained similar for the two groups at all timepoints. The authors concluded that their data did not support efficacy for selenium-ACE in relieving osteoarthritis symptoms.

3.3. Vitamin D

In a separate investigation we tested the association of vitamin D status on the incidence and progression of knee OA among the cohort of participants in the Framingham OA Cohort Study described above *(61)*. The methodology for this investigation was essentially identical except that the analysis was confined to the subset of individuals who both participated in the dietary assessment and provided serum for assay of 25-hydroxy vitamin D ($N = 556$). Dietary intake of vitamin D and serum 25-hydroxy vitamin D levels were modestly correlated in this sample ($r = 0.24$), and, as in the previous study, were unrelated to OA incidence. Risk of progression, however, increased threefold for participants in the middle and lower tertiles of both vitamin D intake (OR for lowest vs highest tertile = 4.0, 95% CI 1.4–11.6) and serum level (OR = 2.9, 95% CI 1.0–8.2). Low-serum vitamin D level also predicted cartilage loss, assessed by loss of joint space (OR = 2.3, 95% CI 0.9–5.5) and osteophyte growth (OR = 3.1, 95% CI 1.3–7.5). We concluded that low serum level, and low intake, of vitamin D were each associated with a highly significant increase in the risk of knee OA progression.

Lane et al. subsequently examined the relationship of serum 25- and 1,25-hydroxy vitamin D with the development of radiographic hip OA among Caucasian women over 65 yr of age who were participating in the Study of Osteoporotic Fractures *(62)*. They measured serum vitamin D levels in 237 subjects randomly selected from 6051 women who had pelvic radiographs taken at both the baseline examination and after 8-yr follow-up.

Radiographs in this study were graded using a validated scoring system for hip OA based on individual radiographic features (osteophytes and joint space narrowing). The investigators analyzed the association of vitamin D levels (ranked in tertiles) with the occurrence of joint space narrowing and with the development of osteophytosis, and with changes in the mean joint space width and individual radiographic feature scores (treated as continuous variables) during the study period. Multivariate analyses were adjusted for age, clinic, weight at age 50, and health status. They found a significantly increased risk for development of joint space narrowing among those in the lowest tertile for 25-hydroxy vitamin D (OR = 2.5, 95% CI 1.1–5.3) as well as associations with continuous measures of progression ($\beta = -0.1$, 95% CI -0.2 to -0.02). An increased risk for development of joint space narrowing among those in the middle tertile for 25-hydroxy vitamin D was also apparent, but did not reach statistical significance.

Therefore, there are two independent epidemiologic studies demonstrating an inverse association of vitamin D status with risk for OA. Both of these studies used a prospective design and included relatively robust measures of vitamin D status. The findings of Lane et al. are of considerable importance because of their remarkable similarity to those found for knee OA in the Framingham Study, and because they additionally suggest that vitamin D may be protective in respect of OA incidence, at least at the hip. Taken together, these studies provide the most compelling evidence for the role of any nutritional factor in the development of OA. One important implication of these findings is that individuals with the lowest risk were in the highest tertile for 25-hydroxy vitamin D, corresponding to levels of over 30 ng/mL.

3.4. Folic Acid and Cobalamin

Flynn et al. performed a 2-mo double-blind randomized three-arm crossover clinical trial of 6400 µg folate vs 6400 µg folate with 20 µg cyanocobalamin vs a placebo among 30 individuals with symptomatic hand osteoarthritis (63). Participants were assessed for tender joints, grip strength, symptoms and analgesic use. In their analyses, the authors stratified the participants according to their baseline grip strength. Ultimately some benefits were found among some strata for certain measures of grip strength and tender joints favoring the folate/cyanocobalamin arm. Few differences, however, were noted in pain scores, global assessments or analgesic use suggesting that this intervention had limited, if any, efficacy.

Dietary intake of folate was also tested as a nonantioxidant control micronutrient in the Framingham Osteoarthritis study described previously. In this observational study, we found no convincing effect of this micronutrient on knee OA incidence or progression.

3.5. Selenium and Iodine: Studies of Kashin-Beck Disease

Kashin-Beck disease is an osteoarthropathy of children and adolescents, which occurs in geographic areas of China in which deficiencies of both selenium and iodine are endemic. Strong epidemiologic evidence exists supporting the environmental nature of this disease (64). Although the clinical and radiologic characteristics of Kashin-Beck disease differ from OA, its existence raises the possibility that environmental factors also play a role in the occurrence of this disorder.

Selenium deficiency together with pro-oxidative products of organic matter in drinking water (mainly fulvic acid) and contamination of grain by fungi have been proposed as environmental causes for Kashin-Beck disease. The efficacy of selenium supplementation in preventing the disorder, however, is controversial. Because selenium is an integral component of iodothyronine deiodinase as well as glutathione peroxidase, Moreno-Reyes et al. studied iodine and selenium metabolism in 11 villages in Tibet in which Kashin-Beck disease was endemic and 1 village in which it was not (65). They found iodine deficiency to be the main determinant of Kashin-Beck disease in these villages, although it should be noted that selenium levels were very low in all the subgroups examined. In an accompanying editorial, Utiger inferred that Kashin-Beck disease probably results from a combination of deficiencies of both of these elements, and speculated that growth plate cartilage is both dependent on locally produced triiodothyronine and sensitive to oxidative damage.

It should be noted that there is little evidence, if any, to suggest that Kashin-Beck disease has any similarities with OA. Further, the single published clinical trial of supplemental selenium (Selenium-ACE) in the treatment of symptoms associated with OA demonstrated no efficacy from this product *(60)*. Thus, there is currently no evidence that selenium offers any benefit to individuals with OA.

4. STUDIES OF OTHER NUTRIENTS IN OA

4.1. Glucosamine and Chondroitin Sulfate

The idea that glucosamine and chondroitin might have therapeutic effects in treating osteoarthritis by providing substrate for reparative processes in cartilage has been around since at least the 1960s. In fact, glucosamine has been used for decades in veterinary medicine for the symptomatic relief of arthritis. Two enticing properties of these "nutraceuticals" are their excellent safety profile and the assertion that they may reduce progression of cartilage damage *(66)*.

4.1.1. LABORATORY STUDIES

Laboratory studies have suggested that both glucosamine and chondroitin can be absorbed through the gastrointestinal tract *(67)*. Radioisotope studies of glucosamine show rapid distribution throughout the body with selective uptake by articular cartilage *(68,69)*. In vitro studies have indicated that glucosamine can stimulate synthesis of cartilage molecules *(70–72)*. The biologic fate of orally administered chondroitin sulfate is less clear, but some evidence exists to suggest that the compound may be absorbed, possibly as a result of pinocytosis *(73)*. Chondroitin sulfate is able to cause an increase in RNA synthesis by chondrocytes *(74)*, which appears to correlate with an increase in the production of proteoglycans and collagens *(75–78)*. Such effects may partly result from competitive inhibition of degradative enzymes *(79)*. In addition, there is evidence that chondroitin sulfate partially inhibits leukocyte elastase *(80)*. Although these data are encouraging, it is clear that these compounds have not been subjected to the systematic level of research and development enjoyed by pharmaceutical products, and that many important questions remain unaddressed. It is uncertain whether these compounds are absorbed intact, whether they are metabolized to any degree, and what role they actually play in vivo. Currently, there remains no theoretical or empirical evidence to support the original supposition that these compounds provide substrate for articular cartilage repair.

4.1.2. CLINICAL STUDIES

4.1.2.1. Placebo-Controlled Trials. In contrast, the clinical efficacy of both glucosamine and chondroitin has been tested in numerous clinical trials. We recently performed a meta-analysis and quality evaluation of trials of glucosamine and chondroitin products for symptoms from knee and/or hip OA *(81)*. We searched for published or unpublished double-blind randomized placebo-controlled trials, of 4 or more weeks duration that reported extractable data on the effect of treatment on symptoms. We found six eligible glucosamine and nine chondroitin trials. Quality scores ranged from 12.3 –55.4% of maximum possible with mean 35.5%. Only two studies described adequate allocation concealment, whereas three reported an intent-to-treat analysis. All were supported to some extent by a manufacturer. Statistical evaluation suggested publication bias resulting from underrepresentation of small null, or negative trials ($p < 0.02$). We calculated an effect size for each trial from the difference in mean outcome value between the treatment and placebo arms, divided by the standard deviation of the outcome value in the placebo group. A scale for effect sizes has been suggested, with 0.8 reflecting a large effect, 0.5 a moderate effect, and 0.2 a small effect. The aggregated effect sizes were moderate for glucosamine and large for chondroitin, but were diminished when only high-quality trials or large trials were considered. We concluded that trials of these preparations for OA symptoms demonstrate moderate to large effects, but that quality issues, and likely publication bias, suggest that these effects may be exaggerated.

A number of further trials have emerged since the publication of the meta-analysis, some of which have had less compelling results. Houpt et al. conducted a 2-mo double-blind randomized placebo-controlled trial (RCT) of glucosamine hydrochloride among 118 participants with knee OA and found trends in favor of active treatment, but did meet the primary endpoint (statistically significant change in the WOMAC pain scale) *(82)*. A 6-mo placebo-controlled RCT of glucosamine among 80 participants with knee OA in the United Kingdom found no difference at all between the groups *(83)*. Rindone et al. also concluded from their 2-mo RCT among 98 VA patients with knee that glucosamine was no better than placebo in reducing knee pain *(84)*. In contrast, a 2-mo RCT of a glucosamine/chondroitin combination among a group of 34 military recruits with knee or spinal OA found significantly greater improvements in selected outcome measures *(85)*. Most recently, Reginster et al. published the results of a 3-yr industry-sponsored placebo-controlled clinical trial of glucosamine, whose primary focus was the influence of treatment on radiographic progression of knee OA. This trial of 200 participants used the WOMAC questionnaire to assess the effect of glucosamine on pain and function. Although the magnitude of effect on symptoms was modest, it is notable that this benefit was present even after 3 yr of treatment *(66)*.

4.1.2.2. Comparator Trials: Glucosamine. Glucosamine has been compared to an NSAID in the treatment of OA in a number of trials *(86–88)*. Muller-Fassbender et al. enrolled 199 hospitalized patients with knee OA into a 4-wk randomized trial of glucosamine sulfate 500 mg 3 times/d, vs ibuprofen 400 mg 3 times/d *(87)*. Participants receiving ibuprofen responded more quickly to treatment but, by the 4-wk time-point, both groups had experienced an identical reduction in their baseline Lequesne Index score. Most notable is the difference in adverse experience rates between the two groups. Thirty five participants in the ibuprofen group reported adverse effects (with seven dropouts) when compared with only six in the glucosamine group (1 dropout). Most of these were gastro-intestinal in nature. The authors concluded that glucosamine and ibuprofen have comparable short-term efficacy, albeit with a slower onset for glucosamine. No power calculations were performed to determine the magnitude of difference that this size of study might be able to detect, nor is information presented about how the 4-wk study duration was determined.

Qiu et al. compared glucosamine with ibuprofen in a 4-wk double-blind RCT of 178 patients with knee OA *(88)*. Both groups responded equally to the treatments, with an approx 50% reduction in scores. Adverse event and dropout rates were strikingly greater ($p = 0.002$) in the ibuprofen arm. Lopes-Vaz compared the efficacy of oral glucosamine 1.5 g/d with ibuprofen 1.2 g/d in an 8-wk double-blind RCT among 38 patients with knee OA *(86)*. Both groups improved, but the scores intersected at the 4-wk time-point, improvement was significantly greater in the glucosamine arm by the end of the trial ($p < 0.05$). There were no power calculations presented in the report. Based on number projections in other NSAID trials *(89)*, it is surprising that any difference was found in this small clinical trial.

4.1.2.3. Comparator Trials: Chondroitin. Morreale et al. performed a 6-mo RCT comparing chondroitin sulfate with diclofenac (a nonsteroidal anti-inflammatory drug) in 146 patients with knee OA *(90)*. The design was rather complex in that participants assigned to the chondroitin took this for 3 mo, whereas those assigned to the NSAID group received diclofenac for 1 mo only. All participants took placebo during months 3–6. A double-dummy approach was used to preserve blinding with all participants observed for the full 6-mo period. Participants were allowed acetaminophen for breakthrough pain. During the first month, both groups showed a fall in the Lequesne Index score, but this was significantly greater in the diclofenac group. The Lequesne Index scores then rebounded following cessation of diclofenac in the NSAID group, but continued to decline in those receiving chondroitin demonstrating significant differences at days 60 and 90 favoring chondroitin. This benefit appeared to persist for 2–3 mo after the chondroitin had been stopped. There were three adverse events in each group thought possibly related to treatment, all of mild or moderate severity. These results contribute to the description of chondroitin as a "symptomatic slow acting drug" for treating OA.

4.1.3. Human Disease-Modification Studies

4.1.3.1. Glucosamine. The most enticing aspect of these compounds is the claim that they may have disease-modifying properties in OA. Reginster et al. recently published the results of the first human RCT designed to investigate this possibility *(66)*. They enrolled 200 knee OA patients into a 3-yr placebo-controlled trial whose primary outcome measure was radiographic joint space width (JSW) in the medial compartment of the knee, a proxy measurement for cartilage thickness. At the end of the trial they found that those who had receiving placebo sustained a mean decrease in JSW of 0.31 (95% confidence limits 0.48–0.13), when compared to only 0.06 (0.22–0.09) among the treated group ($p = 0.04$, for difference). Although these results are intriguing, there are some puzzling aspects to this study. Clinical studies have consistently shown poor correlation between JSW at the knee and the clinical impact of the disease in terms of pain and disability. Another difficulty is that adequacy of radiographic positioning could be influenced by knee symptoms resulting in an underestimation of JSW in those with more severe pain. There is also considerable variability around each of the mean JSW estimates which will reduce expected statistical power in future trials hoping to replicate their findings.

4.1.3.2. Chondroitin. Uebelhart et al. performed a 1-yr RCT trial of chondroitin sulfate (800 mg/d) among 42 participants with knee OA *(91)*. Computer-generated joint space measurements were used to evaluate radiographic progression. They found progression of joint space loss among the placebo group, but no change in those taking chondroitin sulfate. This study has been criticized for short duration of follow-up. Verbruggen et al. evaluated progression of radiographic hand OA during a 3-yr period among 34 patients taking chondroitin sulfate 400 mg 3 times/d when compared to 85 patients taking placebo *(92)*. They found reduced development of erosive OA in the treated group. Limitations of this study include small numbers of participants, unbalanced treatment assignment and questions about the methodology used to obtain radiographs.

4.1.4. Safety Issues

The more rigorous controlled clinical trials of oral glucosamine and chondroitin preparations published as manuscripts in peer-reviewed journals include 600 participants taking oral glucosamine or chondroitin sulfate *(81)*, for up to 3 yr duration *(66)*. These have shown minor or moderate adverse rates similar to those taking placebo. Reported adverse events have generally been gastrointestinal in nature. Comparator studies suggest that glucosamine is substantially safer than NSAIDs, particularly in respect of GI toxicity. Perhaps more problematic is the suggestion that glucosamine may interfere with glucose tolerance. This observation is based on studies administering intravenous glucosamine to laboratory animals *(93)*. Exacerbation, or development, of diabetes has not been reported in clinical trials of oral glucosamine. In particular, no evidence was found of any influence of glucosamine on fasting blood glucose levels in the recent 3-yr trial *(66)*. Thus, it remains doubtful that the laboratory findings are relevant to oral therapy in humans. Further research is needed into the influence of long-term oral glucosamine ingestion on glucose tolerance.

4.2. Other Nutritional Products

A large number of nutritional products are touted for their purported benefits in arthritis and it is encouraging that some of these are now being scientifically evaluated. Blotman et al. recently tested the efficacy and safety of avocado/soybean unsaponifiables (ASU) among 164 individuals with symptomatic osteoarthritis of the knee or hip *(94)*. ASU is thought to have anti-inflammatory and antioxidant effects that might benefit OA. The primary outcome measure in this three-month randomized controlled trial was requirement for analgesics. The treated arm fared modestly better with reduced analgesic requirement (43% vs 67%) and slightly greater improvement on a composite measure of pain and function.

An ayurdevic remedy, prepared from certain herbs and roots, has also been tested in an industry-sponsored placebo-controlled clinical trial, presented recently as abstract *(95)*. The mechanism of action of this patented formulation is unclear, but might involve anti-inflammatory effects. The 32-wk study of 90 participants appeared to show a greater rate of improvement in many of the outcomes tested, including a validated OA assessment instrument.

5. RECOMMENDATIONS FOR CLINICIANS

1. Achieve or maintain ideal body weight. Even modest weight loss in overweight individuals with knee OA may reduce the risk of incident or progressive disease.
2. Optimize vitamin D status. For individuals not at risk of vitamin D deficiency, supplements of 400–800 IU/d are recommended. In the event that either deficiency or toxicity is suspected, measurement of serum 25-hydroxyvitamin D is appropriate—healthy persons have levels of 25–40 ng/mL.
3. Encourage a generous intake of fruits and vegetables, especially those rich in vitamin C.
4. Clinical trials of glucosamine and chondroitin products suggest efficacy in treating OA symptoms, although these effects may be exaggerated. Definitive results are anticipated from a large National Institute of Health (NIH)-funded study which is in progress.

REFERENCES

1. Lawrence JS, Bremner JM, Bier F. Osteo-arthrosis. Prevalence in the population and relationship between symptoms and x-ray changes. Ann Rheum Dis 1966;25:1–24.
2. Cooper C. Osteoarthritis: epidemiology. In: Rheumatology. Klippel JH, Dieppe PA (eds.), Mosby, London, UK, 1994, pp. 7.3.1–7.3.5.
3. Mankin HJ. Clinical features of osteoarthritis. In: Textbook of Rheumatology, 4th ed. Kelly WN, Harris EDJ, Ruddy S, Sledge CB (eds.), W.B. Saunders Co., Philadelphia, PA, 1993, pp. 1374–1384.
4. The Incidence and Prevalence Database for Procedures. Timely Data Resources, Sunnyvale, CA, 1995.
5. Hough AJ. Pathology of osteoarthritis. In: Arthritis and Allied Conditions, 13 ed. Koopman WJ (ed.), Williams & Wilkins, Baltimore, MD, 1997, pp. 1945–1968.
6. Pottenger LA, Philips FM, Draganich LF. The effect of marginal osteophytes on reduction of varus-valgus instability in osteoarthritis knees. Arthritis Rheum 1990;33:853–858.
7. Creamer P, Hochberg MC. Osteoarthritis [see comments]. Lancet 1997;350:503–508.
8. Frei B. Reactive oxygen species and antioxidant vitamins: mechanisms of action. Am J Med 1994; 97(suppl 3A):5S–13S.
9. Jacques PF, Chylack LT, Taylor A. Relationships between natural antioxidants and cataract formation. In: Natural Antioxidants in Human Health and Disease. Frei B (ed.), Academic, San Diego, CA, 1994, pp. 515–533.
10. Gaziano JM. Antioxidant vitamins and coronary artery disease risk. Am J Med 1994;97(suppl 3A):18S–21S.
11. Hennekens CH. Antioxidant vitamins and cancer. Am J Med 1994;97(suppl 3A):2S–4S.
12. Boveris A, Oshino N, Chance B. The cellular production of hydrogen peroxide. Biochem J 1972;128: 617–630.
13. Blake DR, Unsworth J, Outhwaite JM, et al. Hypoxic-reperfusion injury in the inflamed human. Lancet 1989;11:290–293.
14. Ames BN, Shigenaga MK, Hagen TM. Oxidants, antioxidants and the degenerative diseases of aging. Proc Natl Acad Sci USA 199390:7915–7922.
15. Henrotin Y, Deby-Dupont G, Deby C, Franchimont P, Emerit I. Active oxygen species, articular inflammation, and cartilage damage. Exs 1992;62:308–322.
16. Henrotin Y, Deby-Dupont G, Deby C, Debruin M, Lamy M, Franchimont P. Production of active oxygen species by isolated human chondrocytes. Brit J Rheumatol 1993;32:562–567.
17. Rathakrishnan C, Tiku K, Raghavan A, Tiku ML. Release of oxygen radicals by articular chondrocytes: A study of luminol-dependent chemoluminescence and hydrogen peroxide secretion. J Bone Miner Res 1992;7:1139–1148.
18. Greenwald RA, Moy WW. Inhibition of collagen gelation by action of the superoxide radical. Arthritis Rheum 1979;22:251–259.
19. McCord JM. Free radicals and inflammation: protection of synovial fluid by superoxide dismutase. Science 1974;185:529–530.
20. Briviba K, Seis H. Non-enzymatic antioxidant defense systems. In: Natural antioxidants in human health and disease. Frei B (ed.), Academic, San Diego, CA, 1994, pp. 107–128.
21. Hankinson SE, Stampfer MJ, Seddon JM, et al. Nutrient intake and cataract extraction in women: A prospective study. Bmj 1992;305:335–339.
22. Peterkofsky B. Ascorbate requirement for hydroxylation and secretion of procollagen: Relationship to inhibition of collagen synthesis in scurvy. Am J Clin Nutr 1991;54:1135S–1140S.
23. Spanheimer RG, Bird TA, Peterkofsky B. Regulation of collagen synthesis and mRNA levels in articular cartilage of scorbutic guinea pigs. Arch Biochem Biophys 1986;246:33–41.
24. Houglum KP, Brenner DA, Chijkier M. Ascorbic acid stimulation of collagen biosynthesis independent of hydroxylation. Am J Clin Nutr 1991;54:1141S–1143S.
25. Schwartz ER, Adamy L. Effect of ascorbic acid on arylsulfatase activities and sulfated proteoglycan metabolism in chondrocyte cultures. J Clin Invest 1977;60:96–106.
26. Sandell LJ, Daniel LC. Effects of ascorbic acid on collagen mRNA levels in short-term chondrocyte cultures. Connect Tiss Res 1988;17:11–22.
27. Peterkofsky B, Palka J, Wilson S, Takeda K, Shah V. Elevated activity of low molecular weight insulin-like growth factor binding proteins in sera of vitamin C deficient and fasted guinea pigs. Endocrinology 1991;128:1769–1779.
28. Bhalla AK, Wojno WC, Goldring MB. Human articular chondrocytes aquire AU -,25(OH)2 vitamin D-3 receptors. Biochim Biophys Acta 1987;931:26–32.

29. Poole RA. Imbalances of anabolism and catabolism of cartilage matrix components in osteoarthritis. In: Osteoarthritis Disorders. Kuettner K, Goldberg VM (eds.), Amer Acad Orthop Surgeons, Rosemont, IL, 1995, pp. 247–260.

30. Radin EL, Paul IL, Tolkoff MJ. Subchondral changes in patients with early degenerative joint disease. Arth Rheum 1970;13:400–405.

31. Layton MV, Golstein SA, Goulet RW, Feldkamp LA, Kubinski DJ, Bole GG. Examination of subchondral bone architecture in experimental osteoarthritis by microscopic computed axial tomography. Arthritis Rheum 1988;31:1400–1405.

32. Milgram JW. Morphological alterations of the subchondral bone in advanced degenerative arthritis. Clin Orthop Rel Res 1983;173:293–312.

33. Kellgren JH, Lawrence JS. The Epidemiology of Chronic Rheumatism: Atlas of Standard Radiographs. Blackwell Scientific, Oxford, UK, 1962.

34. Anonymous. Cartilage and bone in osteoarthrosis. Brit Med J 1997;62:4–5.

35. Dequecker J, Mokassa L, Aerssens J. Bone density and osteoarthritis. J Rheumatol 1995;22(suppl 43): 98–100.

36. Dedrick DK, Goldstein SA, Brandt KD, O'Connor BL, Goulet RW, Albrecht M. A longitudinal study of subchondral plate and trabecular bone in cruciate-deficient dogs with osteoarthritis followed up for 54 months. Arthritis Rheum 1993;36:1460–1467.

37. Ledingham J, Dawson S, Preston B, Milligan G, Doherty M. Radiographic progression of hospital-referred osteoarthritis of the hip. Ann Rheum Dis 1993;52:263–267.

38. Radin EL, Rose RM. Role of subchondral bone in the initiation and progression of cartilage damage. Clin Orthop Rel Res 1986;213:34–40.

39. Perry GH, Smith MJG, Whiteside CG. Spontaneous recovery of the joint space in degenerative hip disease. Ann Rheum Dis 1972;31:440–448.

40. Smythe SA. Osteoarthritis, insulin and bone density. J Rheumatol 1987;14(suppl):91–93.

41. Zhang Y, Hannan M, Chaisson C, McAlindon T, Evans S, Felson D. Low bone mineral density (BMD) increases the risk of progressive knee osteoarthritis (OA) in women. Arthritis Rheum 1997;40:1798.

42. Dieppe P, Cushnaghan J, Young P, Kirwan J. Prediction of the progression of joint space narrowing in osteoarthritis of the knee by bone scintigraphy. Ann Rheum Dis 1993;52:557–563.

43. Kiel DP. Vitamin D, calcium and bone: Descriptive epidemiology. In: Nutritional assessment of elderly populations: Measurement and function. Rosenberg IH (ed.), Raven, New York, 1995, pp. 277–290.

44. Parfitt AM, Gallagher JC, Heaney RP, Neer R, Whedon GD. Vitamin D and bone health in the elderly. Am J Clin Nutr 1982;36:1014–1031.

45. Pangamala RV, Cornwell DG. The effects of vitamin E on arachidonic acid metabolism. Ann NY Acad Sci 1982;393:376–391.

46. Felson DT. Weight and osteoarthritis. J Rheumatol 1995;22(suppl 43):7–9.

47. Sokoloff L, Mickelsen O. Dietary fat supplements, body weight and osteoarthritis in DBA/2JN mice. J Nutr 1965;85:117–121.

48. Sokoloff L, Mickelsen O, Silverstein E, Jay GE, Jr., Yamamoto RS. Experimental obesity and osteoarthritis. Am J Physiol 1960;198:765–770.

49. Schwartz ER, Leveille C, Oh WH. Experimentally induced osteoarthritis in guinea pigs: Effect of surgical procedure and dietary intake of vitamin C. Lab Animal Sci 1981;31:683–687.

50. Meacock SCR, Bodmer JL, Billingham MEJ. Experimental OA in guinea pigs. J Exp Path 1990;71: 279–293.

51. McAlindon TE, Jacques P, Zhang Y, Hannan MT, Aliabadi P, Weissman B, et al. Do antioxidant micronutrients protect against the development and progression of knee osteoarthritis? Arthritis Rheum 1996;39:648–656.

52. Kellgren J, Lawrence JS. The epidemiology of chronic rheumatism: atlas of standard radiographs. vol 2. Blackwell Scientific, Oxford, 1963.

53. Schumacher HR, Jr. Synovial inflammation, crystals and osteoarthritis. J Rheumatol 1995;22(suppl 43): 101–103.

54. McAlindon TE, Hannan MT, Naimark A, Weissman B, Felson DT. Comparison of risk factors for tibiofemoral and patellofemoral osteoarthritis. Arthritis Rheum 1994;37(suppl):1254.

55. Hirohata K, Yao S, Imura S, Harada H. Treatment of osteoarthritis of the knee joint at the state of hydroarthrosis. Kobe Med Sci 1965;11(suppl):65–66.

56. Doumerg C. Etude clinique experimentale de l'alpha-tocopheryle-quinone en rheumatologie et en reeducation. Therapeutique 1969;45:676–678.

57. Machetey I, Quaknine L. Tocopherol in osteoarthritis: a controlled pilot study. J Am Ger Soc 1978; 26:328–330.

58. Scherak O, Kolarz G, Schodl C, Blankenhorn G. Hochdosierte vitamin-E-therapie bei patienten mit aktivierter arthrose. Z Rheumatol 1990;49:369–373.

59. Blankenhorn G. Clinical efficacy of spondyvit (vitamin E) in activated arthroses. A multicenter, placebo-controlled, double-blind study. Z Orthop 1986;124:340–343.

60. Hill J, Bird HA. Failure of selenium-ace to improve osteoarthritis. Br J Rheumatol 1990;29:211–213.

61. McAlindon TE, Felson DT, Zhang Y, et al. Relation of dietary intake and serum levels of vitamin D to progression of osteoarthritis of the knee among participants in the Framingham Study. Ann Intern Med 1996;125:353–359.

62. Lane NE, Gore LR, Cummings SR, et al. Serum vitamin D levels and incident changes of radiographic hip osteoarthritis: A longitudinal study. Study of Osteoporotic Fractures Research Group. Arthritis Rheum 1999;42:854–860.

63. Flynn MA, Irvin W, Krause G. The effect of folate and cobalamin on osteoarthritic hands. J Am Coll Nutr 1994;13:351–356.

64. Utiger RD. Kashin-Beck disease—expanding the spectrum of iodine-deficiency disorders [editorial; comment]. N Engl J Med 1998;339:1156–1158.

65. Moreno-Reyes R, Suetens C, Mathieu F, et al. Kashin-Beck osteoarthropathy in rural Tibet in relation to selenium and iodine status [see comments]. N Engl J Med 1998;339:1112–1120.

66. Reginster JY, Deroisy R, Rovati LC, et al. Long-term effects of glucosamine sulphate on osteoarthritis progression: A randomised, placebo-controlled clinical trial. Lancet 2001;357:251–256.

67. Tesoriere G, Dones F, Magistro D, Castagnetta L. Intestinal absorption of glucosamine and N-acetylglucosamine, Experientia 1972;28:770–771.

68. Setnikar I, Giachetti C, Zanolo G. Absorption, distribution and excretion of radio-activity after a single I.V. or oral administration of [14C]glucosamine to the rat. Pharmatherapeutica 1984;3:358.

69. Setnikar I, Giachetti C, Zanolo G. Distribution of glucosamine in animal tissues. Arzneimittel forschung/Drug Research 1986;36:729.

70. Vidal Y, Plana RR, Bizzarri D, Rovati AL. Articular cartilage pharmacology: In vitro studies on glucosamine and NSAIDs. Pharmacol Res Commun 1978;10:557.

71. Vidal y Plana RR, Karzel K. Glucosamine: its importance for the metabolism of articular cartilage. 2. Studies on articular cartilage. Fortschr Med 1980;98:801–806.

72. Karzal K, Domenjoz R. Effects of hexosamine derivatives on glycosaminoglycan metabolism of fibroblast cultures. Pharmacology 1971;5:337.

73. Theodore G. Untrsuchung von 35 arhrosefallen, behandelt mit chondroitin schwefelsaure. Schweiz Rundschaue Med Praxis 1977;66.

74. Vach J, Pesakova V, Krajickova J, Adam M. Efect of glycosaminoglycan polysulfate on the metabolism of cartilage RNA. Arzneim Forsch/Drur Res 1984;34:607–609.

75. Ali SY. The degradation of cartilage matrix by an intracellular protease. Biochem J 1964;93:611.

76. Baici A, Salgam P, Fehr K, Boni A. Inhibition of human elastase from polymorphonuclear leucocytes by a GAG-polysulfate. Biochem Pharm 1979;29:1723–1727.

77. Hamerman D, Smith C, Keiser HD, Craig R. Glycosaminoglycans produced by human synovial cell cultures collagen. Rel Res 1982;2:313.

78. Knanfelt A. Synthesis of articular cartilage proteoglycans by isolated bovine chondrocytes. Agents Actions 1984;14:58–62.

79. Bartolucci C, Cellai L, Corradini C, Corradini D, Lamba D, Velona I. Chondroprotective action of chondroitin sulfate. Competitive action of chondroitin sulfate on the digestion of hyaluronan by bovine testicular hyaluronidase. Int J Tissue React 1991;13:311–317.

80. Bartolucci C, Cellai L, Iannelli MA, et al. Inhibition of human leukocyte elastase by chemically and naturally oversulfated galactosaminoglycans. Carbohydr Res 1995;276:401–408.

81. McAlindon TE, LaValley MP, Gulin JP, Felson DT. Glucosamine and chondroitin for treatment of osteoarthritis: a systematic quality assessment and meta-analysis. JAMA 2000;283:1469–1475.

82. Houpt JB, McMillan R, Paget-Dellio D, Russell A, Gahunia HK. Effect of glucosamine hydrochloride (GHcl) in the treatment of pain of osteoarthritis of the knee. J Rheumatol 1998;25(suppl 52):8.

83. Hughes RA, Carr AJ. A randomized double-blind placebo-controlled trial of glucosamine to control pain in osteoarthritis of the knee. Arthritis Rheum 2000;43(9 suppl):S384.

84. Rindone JP, Hiller D, Collacott E, Nordhaugen N, Arriola G. Randomized, controlled trial of glucosamine for treating osteoarthritis of the knee. West J Med 2000;172:91–94.

85. Leffler CT, Philippi AF, Leffler SG, Mosure JC, Kim PD. Glucosamine, chondroitin, and manganese ascorbate for degenerative joint disease of the knee or low back: A randomized, double-blind, placebo-controlled pilot study. Mil Med 1999;164:85–91.

86. Lopes Vaz A. Double-blind clinical evaluation of the relative efficacy of ibuprofen and glucosamine sulphate in the management of osteoarthrosis of the knee in out-patients. Curr Med Res Opin 1982;8: 145–149.

87. Muller-Fassbender H, Bach GL, Haase W, Rovato LC, Setnikar I. Glucosamine sulfate compared to ibuprofen in osteoarthritis of the knee. Osteoarthritis Cartilage 1994;2:61–69.

88. Qiu GX, Gao SN, Giacovelli G, Rovati L, Setnikar I. Efficacy and safety of glucosamine sulfate versus ibuprofen in patients with knee osteoarthritis. Arzneimittelforschung 1998;48:469–474.

89. Bellamy N, Buchanan WW, Chalmers A, et al. A multicenter study of tenoxicam and diclofenac in patients with osteoarthritis of the knee. J Rheumatol 1993;20:999–1004.

90. Morreale P, Manopulo R, Galati M, Boccanera L, Saponati G, Bocchi L. Comparison of the antiinflammatory efficacy of chondroitin sulfate and diclofenac sodium in patients with knee osteoarthritis. J Rheumatol 1996;23:1385–1391.

91. Uebelhart D, Thonar EJ, Delmas PD, Chantraine A, Vignon E. Effects of oral chondroitin sulfate on the progression of knee osteoarthritis: A pilot study. Osteoarthritis Cartilage 1998;(6 suppl A):39–46.

92. Verbruggen G, Goemaere S, Veys EM. Chondroitin sulfate: S/DMOAD (structure/disease modifying anti- osteoarthritis drug) in the treatment of finger joint OA. Osteoarthritis Cartilage 1998;(6 suppl A): 37–38.

93. Giaccari A, Morviducci L, Zorretta D, et al. In vivo effects of glucosamine on insulin secretion and insulin sensitivity in the rat: possible relevance to the maladaptive responses to chronic hyperglycaemia. Diabetologia 1995;38:518–524.

94. Blotman F, Maheu E, Wulwik A, Caspard H, Lopez A. Efficacy and safety of avocado/soybean unsaponifiables in the treatment of symptomatic osteoarthritis of the knee and hip. A prospective, multicenter, three-month, randomized, double-blind, placebo-controlled trial. Rev Rhum Engl Ed 1997; 64:825–834.

95. Chopra A, Lavin P, Chitre D, Patwardhan B, Polisson R. A clinical study of an ayrudevic medicine (Asian medicine) in OA knees. Arthritis Rheum 1998;41:S992.

29 Nutritional and Pharmacological Aspects of Osteoporosis

John J. B. Anderson and David A. Ontjes

1. INTRODUCTION

Osteoporosis is a disease characterized by low bone mass and an increased risk of fracture. It is typically a chronic multifactorial disease occurring in late adulthood, following menopause in women and a decade or so later in men. Osteoporosis may appear in younger individuals who may be at high risk because of hypogonadism, malabsorptive gastrointestinal disorders, and exposure to excessive glucocorticoids or other drugs capable of causing a negative calcium balance.

Both hereditary and environmental factors contribute to the multifactorial nature of this disease. Individual differences in constitutional factors as well as lifestyle/environmental determinants influence bone density. In terms of lifestyle, both regular physical activities and a healthy diet remain two of the more important contributors to bone health and the maintenance of its functions into late life. The major function ambulation needs to be preserved as long as possible through exercise and diet. When calcium intake is not adequate, the adaptive role of the calcium regulatory system operates in an attempt to preserve skeletal structure for its functional uses. If the adaptation is not sufficient, loss of both bone mass and density, will lead to fragility fractures. This review focuses on dietary risk factors for osteoporosis and it also considers both nutritional and drug therapies.

2. BONE STRUCTURE

Each individual bone contains two types of bone tissue: Trabecular (cancellous) and cortical (compact). Trabecular tissue is the more metabolically active because it has about 8–10 times more total surface area than a similar mass of cortical tissue. These surfaces are all largely covered by bone cells, including osteoblasts that are responsible for new bone formation and osteoclasts that are involved in resorption of existing bone. In a typical bone, such as a vertebra, trabecular bone is located within the interior, adjacent to the marrow cavity, whereas cortical bone is located more peripherally just beneath the periosteal surface. Each specific bone contains both types of bone tissue, but in different

From: *Handbook of Clinical Nutrition and Aging*
Edited by: C. W. Bales and C. S. Ritchie © Humana Press Inc., Totowa, NJ

proportions. For example, long bones, such as the femur, contain much more trabecular tissue at either end near the hip joint or knee joint and a much greater proportion of cortical bone in the shaft that connects the two ends. This distinction is important because most fractures occur where more metabolically active trabecular bone tissue predominates.

3. BONE GAIN AND BONE LOSS THROUGH THE LIFE CYCLE

In early life, during the growth periods of the skeleton, bone acquisition through new bone formation dominates. This phase represents the making of the skeletal model, i.e., modeling, and it typically ends by 16–18 yr in females and 18–22 yr in males. Modeling is characterized by greater formation than resorption and results in a net gain of bone mass or bone mineral content (BMC) by the end of the growth phase. Modeling is completed at the end of linear growth. In remodeling of the skeleton, resorption of bone equals formation. In this phase, the net amount of bone mass remains fairly constant, though some modest gain may still occur until the mid-20s or beyond. At the end of the modeling phase, fusion of the epiphyses of the long bones causes cessation of growth in length. By age 30 most individuals have achieved a maximum bone mass that will serve as a "healthy norm" for the rest of life. Beyond age 30, a very slow loss of bone mass typically occurs with normal aging. In the definitions of osteopenia and osteoporosis, the mean bone density measurements of a population of 20–29 yr-old males or females are taken as the standards of comparison for determining whether osteoporosis is present later in life.

In late life (i.e., after the menopause in women and a decade or so later in men) imbalances in the remodeling of the skeleton result in more rapid bone losses, so that reductions in both bone mineral content (BMC) and bone mineral density (BMD) occur. The loss of estrogens after menopause and probably the later decline of androgens in men contribute to the increase in resorption, the reduction of formation, or both. The increase in resorption is triggered by increased activity of osteoclasts, and the decline in formation is directly related to decreased activity of osteoblasts. An increase in bone turnover, i.e., increased rates of resorption and formation with resorption dominating formation, greatly accelerates the rate of bone loss. Most individuals are slow or moderate losers of bone, although only a small fraction are "fast losers." Bone turnover is assessed by measurement of chemical markers of degraded matrix proteins, such as collagen, resulting from bone resorption and of hormones, especially parathyroid hormone, involved in calcium homeostasis.

The changes in the skeleton over the life cycle reflect early-life gains and late-life losses. When the losses become sufficient to deteriorate the skeleton to the state of osteoporosis, an individual becomes at risk for fragility fractures of bones such as the lumbar vertebrae and proximal femur (hip). The hip fractures are the most severe and debilitating, and many individuals never recover.

4. MEASUREMENT OF BMC AND BMD

BMC and BMD are measured today using a technique called dual energy X-radiographic analysis (DXA). Osteopenia, or too little bone, is followed by osteoporosis, or even greater bone loss, which places an individual at great risk of a fracture. Quantitative definitions of osteopenia and osteoporosis have been established by the World Health Organization as follows: Osteopenia is between –1 and 2.5 standard deviations (SDs) below the 20–29 yr-old mean values for women or men; and osteoporosis is greater than –2.5 SDs below the 20–29 yr-old means. (These values of individuals at any adult age when compared to means of healthy young adults are known as T-scores.) According to this definition, a postmenopausal 60-yr-old woman with a BMD 3.0 SDs below the mean at different skeletal measurement sites may not have any clinically diagnosed fractures, but she is likely to have fractures over the next few years without any drug (or drug and diet) therapy.

In addition to the DXA determination of bone status, biochemical markers, such as collagen N-telopeptides and bone-specific alkaline phosphatase, may also be used to assess the severity of bone turnover and the potential risk of fracture. Therefore, both clinical observations, e.g., loss of height and pain in the lower back, and biochemical marker data may increase the diagnostic significance of DXA measurements that classify an individual in the osteoporotic range or > 2.5 SDs below the healthy means.

5. ETIOLOGIES AND TYPES OF OSTEOPOROSIS

No single cause predisposes an individual to osteoporosis, but rather a variety of inherited and acquired factors. Some of the most common clinical risk factors are summarized below. Osteoporosis results when too much bone resorption occurs, too little formation exists, or a combination of both coexists. The most common cause of increased bone resorption (often termed "type 1" osteoporosis) results from estrogen deficiency associated with menopause in normal women. Accelerated bone loss continues for about 10 yr after menopause, then the rate of decline subsides to near the rate that exists for normal aging. Estrogen replacement in the postmenopausal period reduces the rate of resorption and stabilizes bone mass. Men with hypogonadism have accelerated bone loss similar to that of postmenopausal women. Other conditions that cause increased bone resorption include hyperparathyroidism and hyperthyroidism.

Age-related bone loss (also known as "type 2" osteoporosis) is characterized by low rates of bone formation. This type of osteoporosis affects both men and women. Although the causation of age-related bone loss is poorly understood, it may be related to decreased intestinal absorption of calcium. Other factors besides advanced age that may cause impaired bone formation include exposure to certain drugs, such as glucocorticoids, and immobilization or lack of mechanical stress on bone itself.

Genetic factors undoubtedly play a major role in determining both the peak bone mass of young adults, and the rate of bone loss in older individuals. In population-based studies, natural variations (polymorphisms) in genes for the vitamin D receptor, the estrogen receptor, and for type 1 collagen matrix protein all appear to affect bone mass.

6. NONDIETARY RISK FACTORS IMPLICATED IN ETIOLOGY OF OSTEOPOROSIS

Several nondietary risk factors—all potentially adverse or harmful—promote the loss of bone and the onset of fractures. Seven of these environmental/lifestyle factors are listed in Table 1.

Each of these factors has a risk associated with it, but when two or three exist together at the same time, the risk of an osteoporotic fracture may increase exponentially rather than additively. For example, the small-framed older postmenopausal woman who

Table 1
Risk Factors: Nondietary

Body thinness with lean body mass (LBM)
Cigarette smoking
Excessive alcohol consumption
Insufficient physical activity
Drugs—over-the-counter and prescription
Decline of sensory perceptions
Falls

Table 2
Risk Factors: Dietary

Low-calcium intake
High-phosphorus intake
Inadequate vitamin D status
High-animal protein and acid load
High-sodium snacks
Vegetarian diet
Poor diet in general

smokes a pack of cigarettes/d, drinks 2–3 servings of alcohol/d, and who has little physical activity in her daily life will typically be at great risk of an early hip fracture (i.e., by age 70 yr or younger). When the old-old (i.e., >80) suffer declines of acuity of their senses, such as vision and equilibrium, or take medications that result in the same effects, they are much more likely to fall and break their hip.

The most important of these adverse factors, in general, may be the decline in regular physical activity that results in the loss of lean body mass (LBM), characterized by declines in muscle strength and tone, because bone loss follows closely the loss of LBM.

7. DIETARY RISK FACTORS IMPLICATED IN ETIOLOGY OF OSTEOPOROSIS

In addition to adverse environmental/lifestyle factors, numerous dietary factors may also have adverse effects on skeletal tissue. These deleterious factors are thought to operate throughout the life cycle, not just during late life. The major variables are given in Table 2, but this list is not exhaustive.

7.1. Calcium and Phosphorus

The most common dietary problem associated with the development of osteoporosis has been an inadequate consumption of calcium at least among Caucasians in Western nations, including pediatric populations (1). Low-calcium intakes in these nations are typically accompanied by high-phosphate consumption because of both the ingestion of naturally occurring phosphorus in foods, especially animal proteins, and also of phosphorus from food fortification. Phosphorus fortification is fairly common in western nations because of the widespread use of processed foods—foods modified with the many applications that utilize phosphate salts of one type or another. Cola-type soft-drink beverages also fit in this category, although technically they are not foods. The net result of consuming phosphate-rich foods may be a low-calcium (Ca) relative to a high-phosphate (P) intake; this effect is worsened when individuals consume little milk or cheese in their usual diets.

If the Ca:P ratio declines to approx 1–4, the serum parathyroid hormone (PTH) concentration becomes elevated (but remains within the normal range). A constantly elevated PTH leads to bone loss and a gradual decline in BMD that eventually becomes osteoporosis *(2)*. How many years bone takes to get into the osteoporotic range, according to WHO definitions, is not clear, but a long-term dietary pattern of low calcium–high phosphate may even contribute to low bone mass in females before they reach 20 yr of age, if fractures among girls and pubertal females are a valid index of low bone mass *(3,4)*.

7.2. Vitamin D

Coupled with limited skin exposure to vitamin D-promoting sunlight, a low intake of vitamin D from foods, especially fortified dairy products in the United States and various deep-sea fish species in much of the world, is now considered a risk factor for low bone mass. The mechanism for this condition is not entirely clear, but a low circulating concentration of 25-hydroxyvitamin D is linked with both a decline in intestinal calcium absorption and an increase in bone turnover with a resultant loss of bone.

7.3. Protein and Acid Load

An usual high-animal protein intake has been reported by some investigators to contribute to bone loss and an increase in risk for osteoporosis. The mechanism is considered to reside in the increased production of acids (i.e., phosphoric and sulfuric) from the degradation of phosphorus- and sulfur-containing amino acids that are considerably greater in animal than plant proteins, such as those derived from soy. The net effect is an increased loss of calcium ions in urine. This loss has been shown acutely and in short-term experiments, but it has not been established in long-term studies.

7.4. Sodium

High-sodium snack foods have become very popular in Western nations and they contribute additional sodium to an already high intake derived from so many foods processed with sodium or salt. Renal losses of calcium increase on high-sodium intakes because the kidneys favor sodium reabsorption at the expense of calcium ions. The net loss of calcium comes from bone, and therefore a loss of bone mass may be associated with excessive consumption of sodium-rich snack foods.

7.5. Other Dietary Factors

Vegetarian diets may also compromise bone health through a number of possible mechanisms *(5)*, but the low calcium and vitamin D intakes from a vegan dietary pattern may be largely responsible for lower bone mass among vegetarians.

Finally, a poor diet, especially one based on a limited intake of fruits and vegetables, may be deficient in other bone-essential nutrients, such as magnesium, vitamin K, zinc, antioxidant nutrients, and probably a dozen others. Any one or a combination of these deficits may inhibit efficient bone formation. Adverse effects include loss of protection against oxidants, and poor regulation of acid–base balance, thus impacting bone as a

Table 3
Recommended Daily Intakes of Selected Nutrient Variables for the Elderly *

| | 51–70 yr | | >70 yr | |
	Male	Female	Male	Female
Energy (kcal)	2300	1900	2300	1900
Protein (g)	63	50	63	50
Calcium (mg)	1200	1200	1200	1200
Phosphorus (mg)	700	700	700	700
Vitamin D (μg)	10	10	15	15
Vitamin D (IU)	400	400	600	600

*Source: Institute of Medicine, Dietary Reference Intakes, National Academy Press, 1997 (1).

major buffering store. Whatever the mechanisms may be, bone health requires a wide variety of nutrients that are best supplied by a varied diet consisting of the recommended numbers of servings of foods each day (6).

Recommended intakes for energy and several nutrients impacting on bone health are listed for the elderly in Table 3.

8. ADAPTATION TO LOW-CALCIUM INTAKES

Several adaptations to dietary intake occur after each meal in healthy individuals; a number of these adaptations directly affect calcium homeostasis by impacting on serum PTH and 1,25-dihydroxyvitamin D concentrations. For example, low calcium intake, especially when coupled with a high phosphate consumption pattern, stimulates PTH secretion via a calcium-sensor on the membranes of parathyroid gland cells. A chronic elevated PTH, in turn, stimulates the removal of calcium from bone and the loss of bone mass and density.

In addition, low-calcium stimulates the vitamin D regulatory mechanism by increasing the renal production of the hormonal form of vitamin D, i.e., 1,25-dihydroxyvitamin D, which leads to an increase in intestinal calcium absorption and bone utilization of calcium. The potential problem in older women, and perhaps men, is that the intestinal adaptation declines, and less calcium can be absorbed with the hormonal stimulus.

Finally, excessive, continuous PTH secretion that may develop late in life with a low Ca/high P ratio diet and low circulating 25-hydroxyvitamin D concentration contributes to bone loss almost across the 24 h/d. It is now recognized that persistent and continuous treatment with PTH causes significant bone loss, whereas a discontinuous treatment with PTH (i.e., once daily or once weekly) increases bone mass and density by stimulating osteoblasts to make new bone tissue. So, any type of low calcium intake that generates a continuous secretion and elevation of PTH in blood will have serious negative consequences on the maintenance of bone mass.

9. DIETARY PREVENTION AND TREATMENT—FOODS AND SUPPLEMENTS

The general principles of both primary and secondary prevention of osteoporosis are similar: (1) increase calcium intake through foods and supplements to 1000 or more mg/d in order to suppress PTH secretion (*see* Section 10.1.1.) *(2)*. Individuals need to obtain sufficient amounts of vitamin D through both foods and supplements to maintain optimal calcium absorption: 800 IUs or more are recommended. Sunshine exposure is also encouraged, depending on geographic latitude and time of the year *(3)*. A healthy overall diet containing virtually all nutrients from foods makes sense from a nutritional perspective. For the elderly, a daily supplement that contains a wide range of nutrients at recommended intake levels is both safe and inexpensive. The current Dietary Reference Intakes (DRIs) should be used to guide consumers in maintaining appropriate amounts of nutrients each day *(1)*.

10. DRUGS AND OTHER AGENTS USED IN THE PREVENTION AND TREATMENT OF OSTEOPOROSIS

The objectives of therapy in osteoporosis include prevention of further excessive bone loss, promotion of bone formation, prevention of fractures, reduction or elimination of pain, and restoration of physical function. Over the last two decades, a number of antiosteoporotic drugs have been developed. The mechanisms of action of these agents vary, as shown in Fig. 1. In simple terms, the agents may be characterized as acting to increase the availability of calcium from the gastrointestinal tract, to decrease the rate of resorption of existing bone, or to increase the rate of formation of new bone. Most of the drugs mentioned below have been shown to improve bone density, and several have also been shown to reduce the incidence of fractures in placebo-controlled clinical trials. Some agents, including calcium, vitamin D supplements, and estrogens, are widely recommended for the prevention of osteoporosis. Estrogens are commonly used to relieve menopausal symptoms in women, whether osteoporosis is present or not. Drugs approved by the Food and Drug Administration for the treatment of osteoporosis in the United States are generally indicated for use in patients having either documented osteoporotic fractures or bone densities at least two SDs below the normal young adult levels *(2)*. At the beginning of therapy it is important to obtain quantitative measurements of bone density at one or more sites of interest (e.g., the lumbar spine and proximal femur). Such measurements can serve as a baseline for evaluating the effects of therapy after 1 or 2 yr. Biochemical markers of bone turnover, particularly breakdown products of bone collagen, may also be used to monitor a therapeutic effect.

10.1. Antiresorptive Agents

Most of the drugs in current use are considered to be antiresorptive agents, acting to reduce rates of bone resorption, rather than to stimulate bone formation. When bone resorption is inhibited and bone formation continues, a modest gain in bone mass, typically 2–5%, can occur. The overall gain tends to be limited because bone formation is eventually down-regulated to match the lowered rate of resorption. Antiresorptive drugs are generally more effective in increasing the mass of trabecular bone than cortical bone because of the higher rate of resorption existing in trabecular bone.

10.1.1. CALCIUM AND VITAMIN D

Patients with severe vitamin D deficiency are unable to mineralize bone matrix normally, and develop osteomalacia. Most individuals with moderately limited vitamin D stores do not have osteomalacia, but they do have mild secondary hyperprathyroidism and a higher bone turnover. Supplementation with calcium and vitamin D serves to

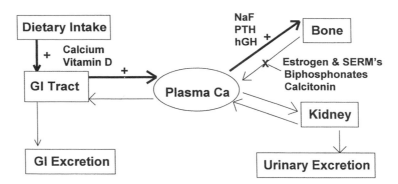

Fig. 1. Effects of therapeutic agents on calcium balance. Increases in dietary calcium and vitamin D result in increased gastrointestinal (GI) absorption . Anabolic agents increase bone formation (heavy arrow from plasma calcium [Ca] to bone). Estrogen and other molecules inhibit bone resorption. Abbreviations: NaF, sodium fluoride; PTH, parathyroid hormone; hGH, human growth hormone; SERMs, selective estrogen receptor modulators.

increase the quantity of calcium absorbed by the gastrointestinal tract, raise serum levels of ionized calcium, and reduce the secretion of parathyroid hormone *(7)*. Rates of bone resorption are thus decreased. In some clinical trials, administration of calcium and vitamin D supplements to older populations in whom prevailing vitamin D stores and calcium intake are low has produced improvements in bone density *(8,9)* and decreased fracture rates *(8,10)*. Other observational studies of large populations have failed to show a relationship between dietary calcium intake, calcium supplements and fracture rates *(11,12)*. The outcomes of these studies may reflect varying intakes of calcium and vitamin D in the study populations prior to entry. In spite of the uncertainty about the efficacy of calcium and vitamin D alone for treatment of osteoporosis, it is widely held that a sufficient intake of both is required as part of any antiosteoporotic regimen.

The requirement for dietary calcium is not precisely defined, but will depend on the age and health status of the individual. The Institute of Medicine of the National Academy of Sciences has recommended an elemental calcium intake of at least 1000 mg/d for adults between 19 and 50 yr of age and 1200 for adults over 50 *(1)*. An intake of 1500 mg/d has been recommended in the past (but not currently) for postmenopausal women not taking estrogen replacement. To reach these levels, calcium supplements will be required in most individuals. Calcium carbonate is widely used and is the least expensive supplement. It is poorly absorbed in individuals with achlorhydria, because it is soluble only in an acidic medium. Calcium citrate is soluble at any pH, and may be better absorbed in achlorhydric individuals *(13)*.

The desirable dietary intake of vitamin D required for bone health is also poorly defined. Results vary depending on the population studied and the degree of sun exposure. The Institute of Medicine has recommended intakes of 5 µg/d (200 IU/d) for adults aged 31–50, 10 µg/d (400 IU/d) for adults aged 51–70, and 15 µg/d (600 IU/d) for those 71 and older *(1)*. The adequacy of dietary supply of vitamin D is reflected in serum levels of 25-hydroxyvitamin D [25(OH)D]. At 25(OH)D serum levels below 80–90 nmol/L, serum levels of parathyroid hormone and rates of bone resorption begin to rise. Thus, a state of vitamin D sufficiency may be defined as having serum levels of 25(OH)D above this threshold. A study of older adults in Boston showed that <50% reached the desired threshold with an average dietary intake of 5 μg (200 IU)/d. When supplemented with vitamin D to an intake of 20 μg (800 IU)/d, 90% reached the targeted 25(OH)D threshold of 80 nmol/L *(14)*. In summary, a vitamin D supplement of approx 20 μg (800 IU)/d is desirable in older adults with limited sun exposure.

10.1.2. ACTIVE METABOLITES OF VITAMIN D

Vitamin D is converted in the body to two active metabolites, 25-hydroxyvitamin D and 1,25-dihydroxyvitamin D (calcitriol). Calcitriol, the most active metabolite, has been evaluated for treatment of osteoporosis because of its potent effects in improving gastrointestinal calcium absorption. The results of several clinical trials have been inconclusive. In one of the largest trials, 622 women with one or more vertebral compression fractures were randomized to receive either a calcium supplement or calcitriol (0.25 μg 2 times/d). The number of new vertebral fractures was significantly reduced in the subjects receiving calcitriol during the second and third years of treatment *(15)*. In other smaller trials, calcitriol failed to reduce the incidence of fractures *(16)*. Hypercalcemia and hypercalciuria are recognized complications of higher doses of calcitriol, particularly when combined with calcium supplements *(17)*. Because of the lack of conclusive evidence of benefit and the potential risk, calcitriol is not considered to be a first line therapy in the treatment of osteoporosis.

10.1.3. ESTROGENS

Estrogen replacement in postmenopausal women prevents excessive bone loss due to estrogen deficiency. Estrogens should be given together with a progestin in women who have an intact uterus to avoid the increased risk of endometrial cancer due to estrogens alone. A large number of clinical studies have shown that both orally and transdermally administered estrogens increase spine BMD in postmenopausal women *(18)*. The evidence for a reduction in fracture risk had not been clearly established in large, prospective randomized clinical trials *(19,20)* until 2002 *(21)*. Estrogens convey both benefits and risks apart from their skeletal effects. The Women's Health Initiative has recently reported results of a trial of conjugated equine estrogens plus medroxyprogesterone vs placebo in 16,608 women, ages 50–79 *(21)*. The relative risk of hip fracture in the estrogen-treated group over 5 yr was reduced to 0.66 (confidence interval 0.45–0.98). This amounted to five fewer hip fractures per 10,000 person years of estrogen therapy. The risk of breast cancer, stroke, and venous thromboembolism was increased with estrogen/progestin replacement, whereas the risk of colorectal cancer was decreased. The study was terminated because the overall health risks of long-term estrogen/progestin replacement appeared to exceed the health benefits.

10.1.4. SELECTIVE ESTROGEN RECEPTOR MODULATORS (SERMs)

These synthetic analogs have the ability to act on the estrogen receptor to produce a variable spectrum of estrogen effects. SERMs are capable of replicating biological effects of natural estrogen in some target tissues, but may act as estrogen antagonists in other tissues. The basis for the observed effects may depend in part on the existence of two types of estrogen receptors existing in different tissues. In bone tissue ERβ is the more abundant whereas in reproductive tissues ERα predominates. Drugs in this class include tamoxifen, a drug used to treat breast cancer, and raloxifene, a drug approved for the treatment of osteoporosis. Raloxifene acts as an estrogen agonist with respect to bone and lipoprotein metabolism. It increases bone density and lowers serum cholesterol when given to postmenopausal women. Raloxifene does not stimulate the endometrium, and like tamoxifen, it acts as an estrogen antagonist in breast tissue. Thus, raloxifene is a good choice as an anti-osteoporosis drug in women at high risk for breast cancer. A large clinical trial has demonstrated that raloxifene therapy reduces vertebral fracture risk in postmenopausal women with osteoporosis (22).

10.1.5. ISOFLAVONES

These naturally occurring phytoestrogens are derived from plant materials and include include genistein and daidzein. Isoflavones appear to act like SERMs or weak estrogen agonists in bone. Phytoestrogens in soy beans may help prevent loss of vertebral BMD in adult life and, hence, may delay the occurrence of osteoporosis (23). Only a few clinical trials in peri- and postmenopausal women have been conducted. Two different groups of investigators used doses of approx 90 mg/d of isoflavones to obtain small increases in vertebral density after 6 mo of treatment (24,25). These studies were not designed to determine whether isoflavones could reduce fracture risk. A recent study of ipriflavone, an artificial derivative of a natural compound found in soy protein, failed to demonstrate improvement in bone density or in biochemical markers of bone metabolism in 474 postmenopausal women. In additional to having no measureable effect on bone mass, approx 13% of women receiving the experimental compound showed a significant decrease in white blood cells (26). Further research will be needed to demonstrate which isoflavones may have beneficial effects on bone and whether fracture incidence is decreased.

10.1.6. BISPHOSPHONATES

These useful drugs are analogs of pyrophosphate, a substance that occurs naturally in bone. Nitrogen-containing bisphosphonates are taken up by osteoclasts resulting in reduced osteoclast activity and survival. They are among the most potent antiresorptive drugs known. Clinical trials of several bisphosphonates, including etidronate, alendronate, and risedronate indicate that bone density is increased in postmenopausal women after two or more years of treatment. Further trials with alendronate (27) and risedronate (28) provide strong evidence that these drugs can reduce fracture risk by 40% to 60% at various skeletal sites, including the spine and hip. These drugs are effective in men with osteoporosis as well as women, making them useful for the treatment of almost all patients with osteoporosis. Alendronate and risedronate are the only bisphosphonates currently approved in the United States for treatment of osteoporosis, but other drugs of this class are likely to be approved in the near future.

10.1.7. CALCITONIN

This natural peptide hormone is produced in small quantities by the parafollicular cells of the normal thyroid gland. Synthetic peptides having the amino acid sequence of either human or salmon calcitonin have been approved for the treatment of osteoporosis. This hormone binds directly to cell surface receptors on osteoclasts, leading to reversible inhibition. The administration of synthetic human or salmon calcitonin in patients with osteoporosis causes a reduction in bone resorption and a modest increase in bone density. Clinical trials have found that intranasal calcitonin therapy reduces the occurrence of vertebral fractures in postmenopausal women (29). Large doses of calcitonin may have an analgesic effect through an independent action on the central nervous system.

10.1.8. Osteoprotegerin

This natural cytokine, osteoprotegerin, also known as OPG, is a recently discovered member of the tumor necrosis factor (TNF) family. It is secreted by several types of cells, including osteoblasts. OPG acts by binding and inactivating an osteoclast-activating factor known as RANK ligand, thus inhibiting osteoclast activation and bone resorption. OPG is detectable in the serum of adult humans and may have an important regulatory role in bone metabolism. When given as a single injection to postmenopausal women, OPG causes long-lasting inhibition of bone resorption, indicating that it is a potentially useful agent for the treatment of osteoporosis *(30)*. Clinical trials examining the effects of OPG on bone mass and fracture risk have not yet been reported.

10.2. Anabolic Agents

All of the currently approved therapies for osteoporosis inhibit bone resorption. However, a great interest has arisen in experimental therapies that promise to stimulate bone formation.

10.2.1. Sodium Fluoride

Fluoride has long been known to be a potent stimulator of bone formation. When taken in higher doses of 50–100 mg/d it causes marked increases in BMD, especially in cancellous bone. Clinical trials with sodium fluoride, however, have produced conflicting results. Earlier studies indicated that although bone density was increased, bone strength was not. Treated patients showed no decrease in vertebral fractures, and an increase in nonvertebral fractures, suggesting that the quality of fluoride-containing bone might be impaired *(31)*. Another group, giving a slow release formulation at a dose of 50 mg/d together with calcium citrate did find that this agent reduced new but not recurrent vertebral fractures *(32)*. Fluoride is not currently approved for use as an antiosteoporosis drug because of continuing concerns about its effectiveness and safety.

10.2.2. Parathyroid Hormone (PTH)

This natural peptide hormone is a primary regulator of calcium homeostasis and bone metabolism in humans and other mammals. Its effects are complex, because it can activate both bone formation and bone resorption, depending on the conditions. Its primary target is the osteoblast, where it can induce proliferation and maturation, thus increasing bone collagen synthesis. These anabolic effects predominate when PTH is present intermittently and in low concentrations. At higher, more sustained concentrations the predominant effect of PTH favors increased osteoclast activity and bone resorption. Osteoclast activation by PTH is probably mediated by cytokines, such as IL-6 and RANK ligand. These cytokines are produced by osteoblasts under the influence of PTH and promote the recruitment and activation of osteoclasts. When recombinant human PTH is given as a daily subcutaneous dose of 50–100 μg/d blood levels are only intermittently elevated. Recent clinical trials have shown that intermittent PTH administration can cause a marked 10–15% increase in spine BMD over a period of 24 mo, with smaller increases in the femoral neck. In the largest PTH trial to dates treatment reduced the risk of both vertebral and nonvertebral fractures in postmenopausal women with osteoporosis *(33)*. The drug is effective in men as well as women *(34)*. Preliminary studies indicate that PTH can be successfully combined with antiresorptive drugs, including estrogens, bisphosphonates, and calcitonin to achieve marked increases in BMD *(35)*.

10.2.3. GROWTH HORMONE AND INSULIN-LIKE GROWTH FACTOR-1 (IGF-1)

These natural peptides play a critical role in determining bone growth and the achievement of optimal bone mass. Growth hormone acts on target tissues to stimulate the formation and release of IGF-1. After the liver, bone is the second richest source of IGF-1 in the body. IGF-1 acts locally in bone to promote chondrocyte and osteoblast differentiation and growth. IGF-1 also circulates in the blood, where its concentration reflects the rate of secretion of growth hormone. Two recent studies have suggested that lower serum levels of IGF-1 are associated with a higher risk of hip and spine fractures *(36,37)*. There have been several small clinical trials determining the effects growth hormone or IGF-1 on bone metabolism and bone density, but none have been designed to examine fracture rates. In one trial involving men over age 65, treatment with recombinant human growth hormone (rhGH) caused a 1.6% increase in lumbar BMD after 6 mo, but the changes were not sustained after 1 yr *(38)*. A more recent study in frail elderly men and women reported a dose-dependent decrease in bone mass after 1 yr of treatment with rhGH despite increases in serum IGF-1 and osteocalcin *(39)*. Both growth hormone and IGF-1 activate the entire bone remodeling system, causing increased bone resorption as well as bone formation. Thus far, the net anabolic effects of these agents on bone have been modest. Their use in elderly individuals is also limited by side effects, including weight gain, edema, carpal tunnel syndrome and glucose intolerance.

11. SUMMARY

Both the incidence and prevalence of osteoporosis are increasing as populations are aging, and greater expenditures for the care of fracture patients are certain to occur. Many hip fracture victims will not survive the first postfracture year. Preventive strategies, either primary or secondary, that are cheap and effective must be identified and implemented. Diet and drug therapy represent the two major approaches, but exercise programs should not be overlooked. Improving the diet with respect to calcium and vitamin D intake may be one of the most easily modifiable approaches for the prevention of osteoporosis. Walking and maintaining activities of daily living by the elderly are also critical for the prevention of osteoporosis. Any type of minimal exercise program should also yield some benefit to the retention of musculoskeletal function.

When osteoporotic fractures occur, or when bone density declines into the osteoporotic range, drug therapy is usually indicated. With the emergence of new pharmacologic agents many choices are now available. Even more choices will be available in the future. Table 4 summarizes the efficacy of the agents currently available, as demonstrated in published clinical trials. Choice of an appropriate agent should depend not only on demonstrated efficacy in reducing fracture risk, but also on patient risk factors and individual side effects. A combination of good nutrition, including sufficient calcium and appropriate exercise will continue to be important, even as antiosteoporotic drugs become more widely used.

12. IMPLICATIONS AND CONCLUSIONS

When ambulation becomes compromised or BMD T-scores of individuals fall within the osteoporotic range, drug therapy, either as prevention or treatment, should be initiated. The choice of drug or drugs for the prevention or treatment of osteoporosis will

Table 4
Efficacy of Antiosteoporotic Therapies in Randomized Clinical Trials

	Increased BMD	Spine fractures	Nonspine fractures	Hip fractures
Calcium and vitamin D preparations				
Calcium monotherapy	+/–	NA	NA	NA
Vitamin D monotherapy	+/–	NA	NA	NA
Calcium + vitamin D	+	NA	+/–	+/–
Calcitriol	+/–	+/–	+/–	NA
Estrogens and SERMs				
Estrogen replacement	+	NS	+/–	NS
Raloxifene	+	+	NS	NS
Bisphosphonates				
Alendronate	+	+	+	+
Risedronate	+	+	+	+
Calcitonin				
Intranasal calcitonin	+	+	NS	NS
Anabolic agents				
Human PTH	+	+	+	NA
Human growth hormone	+/–	NA	NA	NA

NA, data not available; NS, no significant difference in published clinical trials; +, significant difference in one or more clinical trials; +/–, inconsistent results in more than one study.

depend not only on individual risk factors, but also on physician experience. With the emergence of new pharmacologic agents, many choices are now available, including the bone-promoting activity of intermittent PTH. A combination of good nutrition, including sufficient calcium, plus drugs and other modalities should become more commonplace in the armamentarium against osteoporosis.

13. RECOMMENDATIONS FOR CLINICIANS

1. Dual-energy X-radiographic analysis (DXA) is used to measure bone mineral density (BMD). Clinical observations, such as loss of height or back pain, and biochemical measurements (e.g., collagen *N*-telopeptides) used to indicate severity of bone turnover may corroborate the diagnosis of osteoporosis by DXA.
2. Primary and secondary prevention of osteoporosis emphasize (1) increased calcium intake to 1200 mg/d for those over age 50 and (2) intake of sufficient vitamin D to assure optimal calcium absorption (800 IU if sun exposure is limited). The intakes of adequate calcium and vitamin D are requisite parts of any antiosteoporotic regime.
3. Drug therapy is usually indicated when fractures occur or when BMD declines into the osteoporotic range. Most available drugs are antiresorptive, but proformation agents may soon be available.
4. Estrogen replacement therapy helps prevent excessive bone loss resulting from the decline of estrogen production following the menopause and has been linked to reduced relative risk of fracture. However, newly reported concerns about long-term estrogen use indicate that the health risks of this treatment may overshadow its skeletal benefits.

5. Other drug therapies currently approved which reduce bone resorption include bisphosphonates (alendronate, risedronate) and calcitonin (intranasal).

6. Parathyroid hormone given intermittently and at low doses is the only anabolic agent currently recommended for use in patients with osteoporosis.

7. Maintaining physical activity is also a key component of any regimen aimed at preventing osteoporosis or treating osteoporotic patients.

8. Good nutrition from foods, including recommended amounts of calcium and vitamin D, should accompany the use of drugs or other therapeutic modalities. If sufficient calcium or vitamin D cannot be obtained from foods, supplements will be necessary.

REFERENCES

1. Institute of Medicine (IOM), Food and Nutrition Board, National Academy of Sciences. Dietary Reference Intakes for Calcium, Phosphorus, Magnesium, Vitamin D, and Fluoride. National Academy Press, Washington, DC, 1997.
2. Anderson JJB, Sell ML, Garner SC, Calvo MS. Phosphorus. In: Present Knowledge in Nutrition, 8th ed. Russell R, Bowman B (eds.), ILSI Press, Washington, DC, 2003, in press.
3. Goulding A, Cannan R, Williams SM, et al. Bone mineral density in girls with forearm fractures. J Bone Miner Res 1998;13:143–1148.
4. Wyshak G. Teenaged girls, carbonated beverage consumption, and bone fractures. Arch Pediatr Adolesc Med 2000;154:610–613.
5. Anderson JJB. Plant-based diets and bone health: Nutritional implications. Am J Clin Nutr 1999;70: 539s–542s.
6. New SA, Robins SP, Campbell MK, et al. Dietary influences on bone mass and bone metabolism: Further evidence of a positive link between fruit and vegetable consumption and bone health? Am J Clin Nutr 2000;71:142–151.
7. Riggs BL, O'Fallon WM, Muhs J, et al. Long-term effects of calcium supplementation on serum parathyroid hormone level, bone turnover and bone loss in elderly women. J Bone Miner Res 1998;13:168.
8. Chapuy MC, Arlot ME, Duboeuf F, et al. Vitamin D_3 and calcium to prevent hip fractures in elderly women. N Engl J Med 1992;327:1637.
9. Dawson-Hughes B, Harris SS, Krall EA, Dallal GE. Effect of calcium and vitamin D supplementation on bone density in men and women 65 years of age or older. N Engl J Med 1997;337:670.
10. Recker RR, Hinders SK, Davies M, et al. Correcting calcium nutritional deficiency prevents spine fractures in elderly women. J Bone Miner Res 1996;11:1961.
11. Cumming RG, Cummings SR, Nevitt MC, et al. Calcium intake and fracture risk: Results from the study of osteoporotic fractures. Am J Epidemiol 1997;145:926.
12. Owusu W, Willett WC, Feskanich D, et al. Calcium intake and the incidence of forearm and hip fractures among men. J Nutr 1997;127:1782.
13. Recker RR. Calcium absorption and achlorhydria. N Engl J Med 1985;313:70.
14. Dawson-Hughes B, Harris SS. Definition of the optimal 25(OH)-D status for bone. In: Vitamin D Endocrine System. Norman AW, Bouillon R, Thomasset M (eds.), University of California Riverside, Berkeley, 2000, pp. 909–914.
15. Tilyard MW, Spears GF, Thomson J, Dovey S. Treatment of postmenopausal osteoporosis with calcitriol or calcium. N Engl J Med 1992;326:357.
16. Ott SM, Chesnut CH III. Calcitriol treatment is not effective in postmenopausal osteoporosis. Ann Intern Med 1989;110:267.
17. Aloia JF, Vaswani A, Yeh JK, et al. Calcitriol in the treatment of postmenopausal osteoporosis. Am J Med 1988:84:401.
18. Bush TL, Wells HB, James MK, et al. Effects of hormone therapy on bone mineral density: results from the Postmenopausal Estrogen/Progestin (PEPI) Trial. JAMA 1996;276:1389.
19. Rodan GA, Martin TJ. Therapeutic approaches to bone disease. Science 2000;289:1508.
20. Hochberg M. Preventing fractures in postmenopausal women with osteoporosis: A review of recent controlled trials of anti-resorptive agents. Drugs Aging 2000;17:317.
21. Writing Group. Risks and benefits of estrogen plus progestin in healthy postmenopausal women: principal results from the Women's Health Initiative randomized controlled trial. JAMA 2002;288:321.

22. Ettinger B, Black DM, Mitlak BH, et al. Reduction of vertebral fracture risk in postmenopausal women with osteoporosis treated with raloxifene. JAMA 1999;282:1344.

23. Anderson JJB, Garner SC. Phytoestrogens and bone. In: Balleire's Clinical Endocrinology and Metabolism. Adlercreutz HL (ed.), Balliere Tyndall, London, 1998:1–16.

24. Potter SM, et al. Soy protein and isoflavones: Their effects on blood lipids and bone density in postmenopausal women. Am J Clin Nutr 1998;68(suppl):1375S.

25. Alekel DL, et al. Isoflavone-rich soy protein isolate attenuates bone loss in the lumbar spine of perimenopausal women. Am J Clin Nutr 2000;72:844.

26. Alexandersen P, et al. Ipriflavone in the treatment of postmenopausal osteoporosis: A randomized controlled trial. JAMA 2001;285:1482.

27. Black DM, Thompson DE, Bauer DC, et al. Fracture risk reduction with alendronate in women with osteoporosis: The Fracture Intervention Trial. J Clin Endocrinol Metab 2000;85:4118.

28. Harris ST, Watts NB, Genant HB, et al. Effects of risedronate treatment on vertebral and non-vertebral fractures in women with postmenopausal osteoporosis. JAMA 1999;282:1344.

29. Chesnut CH, Silverman S, Andriano K, et al. A randomized trial of nasal spray salmon calcitonin in postmenopausal women with established osteoporosis: The Prevent Recurrence of Osteoporosis Fractures Study. Am J Med 2000;109:267.

30. Bekker PJ, Holloway D, Nakanishi A, et al. The effect of a single dose of osteoprotegerin in postmenopausal women. J Bone Miner Res 2001;16:348.

31. Riggs BL, Hodgson SF, O'Fallon MW, et al. Effect of fluoride treatment on the fracture rate in postmenopausal women with osteoporosis. N Engl J Med 1990;322:802.

32. Pak CYC, Sakhaee K, Adams-Huet B, et al. Treatment of postmenopausal osteoporosis with slow-release sodium fluoride: Final report of a randomized controlled trial. Ann Intern Med 1995;123:401.

33. Neer RM, et al. Effect of parathyroid hormone (1–34) on fractures and bone mineral density in postmenopausal women with osteoporosis. N Engl J Med 2001;344:1434–1441.

34. Kurland ES, Cosman F, McMahon DJ, et al. Therapy of idiopathic osteoporosis in men with parathyroid hormone: Effects on bone mineral density and bone markers. J Clin Endocrinol Metab 2000;85:3069.

35. Rosen CJ, Bilezekian JP. Anabolic therapy for osteoporosis. J Clin Endocrinol Metab 2001;86:957.

36. Sugimoto T, Nishiyama K, Kuribayshi F, Chihara K. Serum levels of IGF-1, IGFBP-2, and IGFBP-3 is osteoporotic patients with and without spine fractures. J Bone Miner Res 1997;12:1272.

37. Bauer DC, Rosen C, Cauley J, Cummings SR. Low serum IGF-1 but not IGFBP-3 predicts hip and spine fracture: The Study of Osteoporotic Fractures. J Bone Miner Res 1998;23:S561.

38. Rudman DV, Feller AG, Nagrog HS, et al. Effect of human growth hormone in men over age 60. N Engl J Med 1990;323:52

39. Rosen CJ, Friez J, MacLean D, et al. The RIGHT study: A randomized placebo controlled trial of recombinant human growth hormone in frail elderly: dose response effects on bone mass and bone turnover. J Bone Miner Res 1999;14:S208.

H. Infectious Diseases and Immunity

30 Aging and Immunity

Shirish Barve, Christine Seel Ritchie, and Craig J. McClain

1. INTRODUCTION

Several clinical and experimental studies have examined age-related changes in immune responses and have associated aging with a decline in immune responses (immunosenescence) *(1–3)*. The most important aspect of age associated immune dysfunction may involve the progressive decline in T lymphocyte functions and cell-mediated immunity. The impairment of T-cell function primarily involves diminished T-cell proliferative responses and IL-2 synthesis and changes in T-cell subsets, namely decreases in naive T cells *(4–6)*. This age-associated decline in immunocompetence is likely a major contributing factor for the increased infection and cancer rates observed in the elderly. These changes in the T-cell functioning may reflect cumulative effects of antigenic exposure, which occurs throughout life. In addition to antigenic exposure, nutritional changes (over- and underfeeding) occur throughout life and can affect organ functions. Several studies have established that nutritional status plays a significant role in immune response and decreases in nutritional status have been associated with impaired immune responses *(7)*. Considerable evidence links immune dysfunction with undernutrition, ranging from such global nutritional problems as protein–energy malnutrition *(8–10)* to specific micronutrient deficiencies, including those of trace elements (e.g., zinc and selenium) and vitamins (e.g., pyridoxine) *(9–12)*. Even "healthy elderly" may be deficient in certain micronutrients, and hence nutritional status may have an important bearing on the age-associated effects on immune responsiveness *(13–15)*.

This review initially describes age-associated declines in immunity, including potential mechanisms, focusing on T-cell subset distribution and functioning. Next we evaluate the influence of nutritional factors, showing the consequences of both global (protein–energy malnutrition) and relatively selective (decreased micronutrient) nutritional deficits. Finally, we focus on supplementation studies that demonstrate the immunopotentiating effects of different nutrients and their potential application in improving the immune status in the elderly.

From: *Handbook of Clinical Nutrition and Aging*
Edited by: C. W. Bales and C. S. Ritchie © Humana Press Inc., Totowa, NJ

2. AGING AND IMMUNITY

2.1. T-Cell Function and Aging: Overview

In the peripheral lymphoid tissue of the aged, the total number of T cells as well as the ratio of CD4 to CD8 T cells remains relatively unchanged. However, there is a gradual change characterized by a decline in naive CD45 RA+, CD44[hi] cells, and an increase in memory cells represented by the CD45 RO+, CD62L (L-selectin) cells *(16–18)*. The age-related change to a higher proportions of cells with a memory phenotype affects both the CD4 and CD8 populations. The factors that contribute to this gradual transition from a predominantly naive cell to a predominantly memory cell population include the reduction in the supply of newly emerging naive cells from the thymus (resulting from age-related thymic involution) and continual antigen-driven conversion of naive to memory cells *(19,20)*. The quantitative changes in the naive and memory cells are also accompanied by qualitative functional changes in these cell compartments.

2.2. Thymus

A major change occurring with age is the shrinkage of the thymic tissue mass or thymus involution. Age-dependent involution of the thymus has been recognized to contribute to the loss of T-cell differentiation and T-cell immunity. However, this assumption may not be universally applicable to all individuals under all circumstances. As indicated in the studies on centenarians, it appears that the thymus continues to generate T cells through old age *(21)*. Evaluation of thymic output using a newly established assay that measures episomal circular DNA generated during excisional rearrangements of the T-cell receptor (TCR) genes (TRECs), has shown the presence of high levels of TRECs in the thymocytes of elderly individuals, showing that old thymi can still generate functional T-cells with actively rearranged TCR genes *(22,23)*. Although high levels of TRECs are observed in the elderly and correlate with the anatomical measurements of lymphoid mass, it is also possible that the large number of TRECs may arise by extrathymic differentiation *(24)*. In fact, altered thymic function in aging may be compensated by alternative sites and pathways of T-cell development. For example, T-cell differentiation has been observed in vitro in the absence of thymic stromal tissue *(25)*. Normal T-cell development has also been demonstrated in the bone-marrow environment *(26)*, and bone-marrow stromal cells have been shown to have the capacity to support T-cell differentiation in vitro *(27)*. The ability of aging human thymic emigrants to respond to costimulatory signals and of adult thymic stroma to support thymocyte viability in organ culture *(28)* suggests that the thymus is able to execute normal T lymphopoiesis during advanced age. The interaction between T cells and the thymus may be important for the maintenance of thymic integrity in aging *(29)*. This possibility is supported by studies on CD4 T cells, which appear to be the most effective at maintaining thymic function *(29,30)*.

2.3. T Lymphocyte Activation

There is a distinct decline in T-cell responses of the aged accompanied by major changes in T-cell function. These changes include both decreased proliferation and secretion of IL-2 upon stimulation of the TCR *(31–34)*. The decline in T-cell responsiveness associated with aging has been attributed to the marked diminution in the early events in T-cell activation. This is reflected by the fact that the necessary early influx of calcium is reduced, and the earliest cell surface alterations associated with activation (e.g., CD69 and CD71) are reduced, leading to a marked reduction of activation-induced IL-2 *(35,36)*. In T cells, compromised function can occur as a result of aberrations in signal transduction through some or all of the TCR components or costimulatory receptors or growth factor receptors. There is evidence for age-dependant impairments at all three levels.

Contact of a quiescent T cell with an antigen-presenting cell (APC) initiates several extra-cellular membrane events, leading to full activation and the induction of the TCR signaling machinery. The first stage is adhesion, facilitated by integrins and adhesion molecules, which provide the essential framework needed for the initial APC T-cell contact. The subsequent stage is the aggregation of the signaling complex that allows the TCR to initiate signal transduction. Induction of T-cell activation in the T-cell–APC conjugates is effected by glycolipid-enriched microdomains in the cell membrane that facilitate the organization of several interactive molecules *(37,38)*. Age-associated defects in cell–cell binding leading to altered activation capacity of the integrin, leuko-cyte-function-antigen-1 (LFA-1), have been observed *(39)*. Only protein kinase C (PKC) ζ, not any other PKC isoforms, selectively localizes to the interfacial membranes of T cells that have formed conjugates with APC, leading to T-cell activation. T-cell–APC conjugates that do not lead to T-cell activation also fail to relocalize PKCζ. Recent studies have shown that although there is no change with age in the proportion of CD4 or CD8 cells that could form conjugates with APC, there is an age-related significant decline in the proportion of conjugates that show relocalization of PKCζ *(4)*.

2.4. Costimulation: CD28 Signaling Enhancing

Upon activation, TCR signaling causes the initial activation of Fyn and Lck and phosphorylation of immunoreceptor tyrosine-based activation motifs (ITAM) on CD3-zeta *(40–42)*. These events lead to the recruitment and activation of the ZAP-70 component, which specifically binds to the phosphorylated ITAMs *(43–45)*. The ZAP-70 protein is further phosphorylated on tyrosine, and the accumulation of phosphotyrosine on proteins of the TCR complex sets the stage for all subsequent signaling interactions. Several studies, both in mouse and man, have examined these events in relation to T-cell activation. Although data on the effect of age on these signaling events have been variable, considerable evidence suggests that they are altered in old cells *(46,47)*. Human studies have shown that Fyn (p59 fyn) enzymatic activity, but not the Lck (p56 lck) activity, is reduced in a large proportion of T cells from the older population in comparison to the young *(46)*. In a different study, reduction in both the amount and degree of phosphory-lation of p56 lck was observed in T cells from the elderly *(48)*. In another study, age-related diminution of p56 lck as well as ZAP-70 activity, but not the levels of either protein, were observed in CD3-stimulated T cells from the elderly *(49)*. The reasons for these discrepancies are not clear, but could possibly arise as a result of variations in the age-dependent T-cell subset distribution.

The consequence of these alterations is a reduction in Zap-70 and subsequently CD3-zeta activation. The amount of Zap-70 or CD3-zeta are not diminished, nor is the association between the two altered, but their degree of phosphorylation after T-cell activation declines with age *(47,50,51)*. Although variable alterations in the early TCR signaling in old T cells have been observed, a decrease in calcium influx has consistently been noted as one of the earliest observed changes.

2.5. Aging, T-Cell Activation, and Clonal Expansion: Proliferative Senescence and Susceptibility to Activation-Induced Cell Death

After the T cells have received appropriate stimulatory/costimulatory signals during antigen presentation, mounting an effective T cell response requires clonal expansion followed by contraction when antigen is no longer present, and reexpansion on repeat contact with antigen. Hence, deficits in the proliferative capacity of the T-cell clones can have a negative impact on the overall immune response. The phenomenon of replicative senescence first described by Hayflick (52) is the loss of the ability to undergo cell division after a finite number of cell doublings. The proposed molecular mechanism involved in this phenomenon is loss of telomeric DNA and gradual shortening of telomeres with each cell division to the point that chromosomal replication cannot occur, thus rendering cells incapable of replicating again (53). Additionally, the loss of other cellular processes such as DNA repair, which decreases with age, may also contribute to telomere shortening (54). The role for telomere loss has been observed in immuno-senescence because lymphocytes reach critical telomere length and undergo replicative senescence (55,56). Support for the role of telomere shortening in aging and T-cell senescence comes from the data on memory T cells, which were observed to have shorter telomeres than naive T cells (57), and lymphocytes from older individuals, which were found to have shorter telomeres than young individuals (58).

T cell proliferation, clonal expansion and survival may also be influenced by the susceptibility of the lymphocytes to activation-induced cell death (AICD). During their progress through many cycles of divisions, memory CD4+ T cells (critical for responses to recall antigens) shift from CD45RBhi+ to CD45RBlo+ phenotype. This shift is accompanied by a gradual loss of Bcl-2 (which is antiapoptotic) and acquisition of Fas (which is apoptotic) expression, as well as gradual loss of the ability to secrete enough IL-2 to maintain autocrine proliferation (59). Examination of CD45RB in vivo in elderly subjects demonstrated and confirmed that CD4+ T cells from old donors have significantly decreased CD45RB expression.

2.6. Aging and Humoral Immunity

Although impairment in the qualitative and quantitative T-cell responses is a major component of immune dysfunction observed in the elderly, aging also has significant negative impact on humoral immunity. One of the initial studies that documented the changes in age-related humoral immunity observed that the quantity of serum antibodies specific for foreign antigens declined with age (60). Experimental and clinical studies show that the effects of aging on humoral immunity are largely the result of changes in the B lymphocyte repertoire (61). Alterations in the B-cell repertoire during aging include a shift from the antibody response to foreign T-dependent antigens produced by B-2 lymphocytes to autologous T-independent antigens stimulated by B-1 lymphocytes (61). Hence, the observed alteration in the B-cell repertoire, not a decrease in humoral immune responsiveness, contributes to the decrease in antibody response to foreign antigens. Studies evaluating the autoantibody response associated with aging have shown that autoantibodies are detected at increased concentrations in the serum of the elderly and consist mainly of auto-anti-idiotype antibodies *(62,63)*. The important clinical consequence of these autoantibodies is that they inhibit the secretion of antibodies to foreign antigens. Aging also affects the diversity of the antibody response, as seen by the preferential loss of IgG antigen-specific antibodies *(64)*. This age-associated loss of IgG correlates with a defect in isotype switching, likely caused by impaired T-cell function that is needed for the generation of germinal centers and isotype switching *(65)*. Overall, the alterations in the humoral immunity during aging play a causal role in the increased susceptibility and sensitivity to infection and the decreased efficacy of vaccines and subsequent diminished protection from infections.

3. NUTRITIONAL MODULATION OF IMMUNE FUNCTION

A major goal in aging is to maintain functionality and to age "successfully." Many strategies have been evaluated concerning maintaining/enhancing immune function in the elderly, and nutritional intervention appears to be the most likely immediate therapeutic target. As reviewed earlier in this book, the elderly are at risk for malnutrition because of multiple physiological, social, psychological, and economic factors (*see* Chapters 1–3, 5, and 11) *(66–68)*. The elderly have a higher incidence of chronic diseases and associated intake of medications, which may affect nutrient utilization. For example, diuretic use can cause increased urinary loss of trace metals (e.g., zinc). Social and economic conditions can adversely affect dietary choices and eating patterns. Some physiological functions naturally decline with age, and this may influence absorption and metabolism. Loneliness and reluctance to eat may complicate an already marginal situation. Nutritional deficiencies can cause immune dysfunction, and nutritional supplementation can improve immune function in some settings in the elderly. We review the effects of specific vitamin or mineral deficiencies and global effects of protein calorie malnutrition on immune function as they relate to the elderly, as well as the potential role of nutritional supplements in improving immune function.

3.1. Selected Individual Minerals/Vitamins and Immune Function

3.1.1. ZINC

Zinc plays a vital role in normal immune function. Initial in vitro studies show zinc to be a potent T-lymphocyte mitogen for both man and animals over a narrow range of concentrations *(69)*. Zinc deficiency in animals causes thymic and lymph node atrophy and impaired cell-mediated cutaneous hypersensitivity *(70)*. Lymphocytes isolated from zinc deficient animals show impaired response to phytohemagglutinin and depression of T-cell-dependent antibody production *(70–72)*. The effect of zinc deficiency on immune function in humans was studied initially in children with acrodermatitis enteropathica, a congenital disorder characterized by both impaired zinc absorption and immunodeficiency. Leukocyte function and cell-mediated immunity are impaired in these children and reversed with zinc supplementation *(73)*. Golden et al. described thymic atrophy in children with protein energy malnutrition and zinc deficiency *(74,75)*; this thymic atrophy was reversed with zinc supplementation. Several groups then documented immune dysfunction in small groups of patients with various disease processes (e.g., short-bowel syndrome, renal failure, sickle cell anemia) associated with zinc deficiency, in which immune function improved with zinc supplementation *(76–78)*. Importantly, zinc supplementation was also shown to decrease the incidence of infection and hospitalization in zinc deficient patients with sickle cell disease *(79)*. Prasad et al. also recently reported decreased duration of cold symptoms in patients of varying ages who were treated with zinc acetate lozenges, but the role of zinc in reducing cold symptoms remains controversial *(80)*.

Recent studies explored mechanisms of zinc deficiency-induced immune dysfunction. Critical research from Fraker et al. documented the association between glucocorticoid activity, lymphocyte apoptosis, and zinc deficiency *(77)*. She has postulated that large amounts of zinc are required to produce billions of lymphocytes daily. Many of these lymphocytes die without being gainfully used in an immune response, and are nutritionally expensive. Thus, from an adaptive stress response, it may make sense to have increased glucocorticoid-mediated lymphocyte apoptosis during zinc deficiency.

With aging, there is a distinct decline in T-cell responses accompanied by major changes in T-cell function including decreased proliferation and secretion of IL-2 on stimulation of the TCR (mimicking changes in zinc deficiency). This knowledge stimulated a number of studies evaluating zinc supplementation on immune function/infections in the elderly *(81)*. Initial studies, such as those by Duchateau, showed beneficial effects when zinc sulfate (220 mg bid × 1 mo) was administered to 15 subjects over the age of 70 *(82)*. Prasad et al. *(83)* demonstrated a high frequency of mild zinc deficiency in ambulatory elderly as assessed by blood cell zinc concentrations. Zinc supplementation in a selected zinc-deficient population improved serum thymulin levels, cutaneous/skin testing, taste acuity, monocyte interleukin-1 (IL-1) production, and lymphocyte ecto 5'-nucleotidase activity. Girodon et al. evaluated trace element and vitamin supplementation on infectious complications over a 2-yr period *(84)*. Patients receiving trace metals (zinc 20 mg/d + selenium 100 μg/d) or trace metals + antioxidants had fewer infections. A study by this group in a large population of institutionalized elderly found that trace metal supplementation significantly improved antibody response to influenza vaccine, and a decrease in respiratory infections approached statistical significance ($p = 0.06$) *(85)*. If zinc supplementation is undertaken, very high doses of zinc should be avoided as they may actually cause immunosuppression *(86)*. High-dose oral zinc therapy can also induce copper deficiency with subsequent anemia and neutropenia *(87)*. Thus, if zinc is to be administered, it should be done in "low levels" (<40–50 mg/d of elemental zinc).

3.1.2. Selenium

Low serum selenium concentrations are well documented in elders and in disease processes, such as type II diabetes (the incidence of which increases with aging) *(88,89)*. Selenium is incorporated as selenocysteine at the active sites of multiple selenoproteins *(90,91)*. The best recognized of these are the glutathione peroxidase enzymes, which play a critical role in antioxidant defense systems.

Micronutrient deficiencies are normally thought to cause increased susceptibility to infection as a result of impairment in host defense systems as described with zinc deficiency. Selenium deficiency appears to act in a highly novel fashion in relation to viral infections. Beck et al. initially showed that selenium-deficient mice develop an inflammatory cardiomyopathy when infected with normally avirulent or benign strains of Coxsackie virus *(92,93)*. Control mice fed a selenium-sufficient diet do not develop cardiac pathology when infected with this same virus. Of great importance, these investigators demonstrated that this new viral virulence was the result of mutations in the viral genome itself. Thus, the avirulent virus mutated to a virulent strain. These virulent strains continue to cause pathology even when administered to mice fed a normal diet. Similar findings were then reported in vitamin E deficient animals, and this change in virulence was clearly linked to oxidative stress. This same group has made similar observations with the influenza virus (94). These observations have great implications for how host nutritional status may influence mutational changes in a viral genome. This may have important implications for the elderly, particularly the institutionalized elderly where viral infections may be easily transmitted from one subject to another. At this point, however, these studies have only been performed in experimental animals and not in humans.

There is also a great interest in the potential role of selenium in carcinogenesis (95,96). For many types of cancer, there is an inverse relation between cancer incidence and the selenium content of the soil. Selenium is being used as a therapeutic agent in certain types of cancer, with the best publicized being prostate cancer (95). There are epidemiologic data suggesting that men with high selenium and vitamin E intakes have a lower risk for prostate cancer. A large randomized trial (SELECT study) is currently enrolling over 30,000 men in a prostate cancer prevention trial, with two of the arms being selenium alone or selenium with vitamin E. Impaired immune surveillance is one possible mechanism for the increase in certain cancers with selenium deficiency.

3.1.3. Vitamin E

In the early 1980s, studies were initiated to investigate the effect of single vitamins on immune function. Chavance et al. (97) performed one of the first retrospective epidemiological studies examining the association of vitamin E levels with immune function in the elderly. This study showed a significant association between higher plasma vitamin E levels and a lower incidence of infections in healthy adults over the age of 60. Evaluation of short-term vitamin E supplementation by Meydani et al., in two placebo-controlled double-blind studies established that vitamin E supplementation alone can significantly enhance DTH responses, antibody titers to certain vaccines and proliferative responses, and IL-2 activities in the elderly (98,99). In the study where the elderly subjects were administered a daily diet containing approximately the recommended daily allowances (RDA) of all nutrients, vitamin E supplementation (800 mg D,L-α-tocopheryl acetate for 30 d), caused an increase in the levels of vitamin E in the lymphocytes by more than threefold and correlated with the enhanced immune responses (98). Additionally, vitamin E supplementation showed no adverse health effects and decreased production of immunosuppressive prostaglandin E2, and decreased levels of serum lipid peroxides (100). Importantly, these studies, where the diets and the environments of the placebo and vitamin E groups were carefully monitored in a metabolic research unit, showed that a single-nutrient supplement has the potential to enhance immune responsiveness in healthy elderly subjects consuming the recommended amounts of all other nutrients.

Meydani et al. (100) further extended their previous findings by examining the effects of supplementation with 60, 200, or 800 IU/d of vitamin E for 6 mo in a placebo-controlled, double-blind study in healthy free-living elderly. In addition to DTH responses, in vitro proliferation and ex vivo antibody titers to clinically relevant vaccines were also determined. Significant enhancement in the DTH responses above placebo levels was observed in all three supplemented groups with the greatest response observed in the 200-IU group. In comparison, in vitro proliferative responses were the highest in the

800-IU group. Examination of the responsiveness to clinically relevant vaccines showed that antibody titers to tetanus were unaffected by vitamin E supplementation, but titers to hepatitis B vaccine were enhanced with the maximum response in the 200-IU group. Similar studies were performed by Pallast et al. *(101)* who investigated the effects of vitamin E supplementation at 50 and 100 mg doses daily for 6 mo in healthy older men (aged 65–80 yr). In this study the dose-related impact of vitamin E on DTH responses was observed mostly in those subjects with initially low responses, indicating that mostly healthy elderly having low-vitamin E status might derive the benefit from vitamin E supplementation.

3.1.4. Vitamin C

An important aspect of the antioxidant role of vitamin C, is that it functions to regenerate the antioxidant form of vitamin E *(102)*. However, in comparison to the extensive studies on the effects of vitamin E on T-cell function and immunity, there is a paucity of studies evaluating the effects of vitamin C in the elderly. One placebo-controlled study *(103)* tested the effect of vitamin C supplementation (500 mg/d im for 1 mo) in the elderly. Enhancement in the T lymphocyte proliferative responses and the tuberculin skin hypersensitivity in comparison to the placebo control was observed. In another study of oral vitamin C supplementation (2 g/d) in an elderly population, enhanced in vitro lymphoproliferative responses were observed, but the vitamin C did not alter the DTH responses *(104)*.

3.2. Effect of Multivitamins in the Elderly

The effects on the immune system of a one-a-day type multivitamin/mineral supplement for 12 mo in healthy elderly were compared with placebo group *(105)*. Significant enhancement of delayed hypersensitivity skin testing >60%) was noted in the supplemented group as compared with the placebo group (<10% increase). Because multivitamins included β-carotene (approx 1 mg), vitamin E (30 IU), vitamin C (60 mg) and other vitamins as well as several minerals, the study did not allow the determination of the contribution made by antioxidants or other components in the multivitamin supplement. However, the significant changes in the serum micronutrient contents were observed only for vitamins E, C, B6, β-carotene, and folic acid.

In similar placebo-controlled intervention trials employing a multivitamin/mineral supplement for 1 yr in healthy elderly, it was observed that micronutrient supplementation can play an important role in the maintenance of normal T-cell function and natural killer (NK) cells and decrease the risk of infection *(106,107)*.

3.3. Undernourishment and Immune Responses in the Elderly

Undernutrition, even mild and short-term, may influence the immune system, and the elderly may react differently than younger individuals. For example, neutrophil chemotaxis decreases modestly with starvation in younger individuals, but then rebounds with refeeding. However, in the elderly, chemotaxis continues to decrease even after initial refeeding *(108)*.

Decreased nutritional status (as established by levels of serum albumin that are decreased, but within the normal range [35–40 g/L]) has important consequences for different T-cell subsets and T-cell functions. Assessment of serum albumin levels in healthy elderly showed that lower levels of albumin correlated with lower levels of CD3+ mature T cells, lower levels of CD8+, higher levels of CD2+CD4-CD8-double negatives and of CD2+CD3-immature T lymphocytes, higher levels of CD57+ NK cells, and decreased CD45RO memory but increased CD45RA naive T lymphocytes *(12,109)*. In addition to these T cell subsets, all elderly subjects expressing low levels of albumin had diminished levels of CD4+ T cells. T-cell functions, as measured by proliferative responses and mitogen (phytohemagglutinin)-induced IL-2 production, were also found to be decreased in healthy elderly as compared to elders with higher serum albumin levels (>40g/L). Hence, the available data suggest that relatively small changes in the protein nutritional status as reflected by lowered albumin levels in elderly subjects can lead to alterations in T lymphocyte subsets accompanied by a general decrease in immune functions.

Protein–energy malnutrition (PEM) has been demonstrated to have a significant influence on the immune responses in the aged individuals. Virtually all aspects of the cell mediated immunity are decreased in the elderly population with PEM as compared with their healthy or even apparently healthy counterparts. Importantly, a very high correlation with the intensity of the nutritional deficit and decrease in immune functions has been reported with profound immunodeficiency displayed by elderly subjects with severe PEM. In addition to lymphopenia and lowered CD4+ T cell counts, PEM is also associated with significantly lowered vaccine antibody responses in the elderly population. The relevance of PEM and its influence on the immune responses is further underscored by many studies in critically ill patients of all ages who showed improvement in immune function with either enteral or parenteral nutritional supplementation *(8,12)*. Similarly, there are limited studies indicating that the decreases in immune responses in the undernourished elderly subjects can also be improved by refeeding therapy *(108)*.

4. CONCLUSIONS

The elderly have well documented changes in immune function, with the dominant alterations relating to thymic atrophy and T-cell dysfunction. There is a diminished number of T-cells, thus limiting the response to new foreign antigens. Humoral immunity may also be altered, with diminished effectiveness against new foreign antigens, but exaggerated response to autologous antigens (with auto anti-idiotipic antibody production). Therefore, the elderly are less able to mount an effective immune response to vaccination or bacterial/viral pathogens. The elderly are also susceptible to malnutrition (both global and isolated nutrient deficiencies). Nutritional deficiencies may impact immune function adversely; thus, nutritional supplementation represents one potential target for immune enhancement. Examples of beneficial effects of vitamins (e.g., vitamin E) and minerals (e.g., zinc supplementation) on immune function are well documented. Moreover, correction of global protein malnutrition with enteral supplements may also improve immune function in the elderly. Lastly, limited studies suggest that vitamin mineral supplements may decrease infections/morbidity in the elderly.

5. RECOMMENDATIONS FOR CLINICIANS

1. Zinc deficiency is common among older adults. Supplementation may reduce infectious complications and improve antibody response to influenza vaccine. If zinc supplementation is elected, a maximum of 40–50 mg/d of elemental zinc should be given in order to avoid the possibility of immunosuppression or copper deficiency seen with high dose zinc supplementation (220 mg zinc sulfate = 50 mg elemental zinc).

2. Inadequate data exists to recommend selenium supplementation.
3. Vitamin E supplementation (with doses ranging between 60–800 IU/d enhances DTH responses and antibody titers to some vaccines (including Hepatitis B).
4. Multivitamins can enhance T cell function and decrease risk of infection and may be advisable whenever dietary intakes are marginal. The multivitamin should meet RDI requirements and include zinc but not iron.
5. Cell mediated immunity decreases with protein energy malnutrition and may be improved with improvement in nutritional status achieved through aggressive feeding.

REFERENCES

1. Makinodan T, Kay MM. Age influence on the immune system. Adv Immunol 1980;29:287–330.
2. Miller RA. Aging and immune function. Int Rev Cytol 1991;124:187–215.
3. Miller RA. The aging immune system: Primer and prospectus. Science 1996;273:70–74.
4. Miller RA. Effect of aging on T lymphocyte activation. Vaccine 2000;18:1654–1660.
5. Pawelec G, Hirokawa K, Fulop T. Altered T cell signalling in ageing. Mech Ageing Dev 2001;122: 1613–1637.
6. Pawelec G, Effros RB, Caruso C, Remarque E, Barnett Y, Solana R. T cells and aging. Front Biosci 1999; 4:D216–D269.
7. Castle SC. Clinical relevance of age-related immune dysfunction. Clin Infect Dis 2000;31:578–585.
8. Chandra RK, Kumari S. Effects of nutrition on the immune system. Nutrition 1994;10:207–210.
9. Lesourd BM. Nutrition and immunity in the elderly: Modification of immune responses with nutritional treatments. Am J Clin Nutr 1997;66:478S–484S.
10. Chandra RK. Grace A. Goldsmith Award lecture. Trace element regulation of immunity and infection. J Am Coll Nutr 1985;4:5–16.
11. Chandra RK, McBean LD. Zinc and immunity. Nutrition 1994;10:79–80.
12. Lesourd B, Mazari L. Nutrition and immunity in the elderly. Proc Nutr Soc 1999;58:685–695.
13. Bailey AL, Maisey S, Southon S, Wright AJ, Finglas PM, Fulcher RA. Relationships between micronutrient intake and biochemical indicators of nutrient adequacy in a "free-living" elderly UK population. Br J Nutr 1997;77:225–242.
14. Haller J. The vitamin status and its adequacy in the elderly: An international overview. Int J Vitam Nutr Res 1999;69:160–168.
15. Ames BN. Micronutrient deficiencies. A major cause of DNA damage. Ann NY Acad Sci 1999;889: 87–106.
16. Linton P, Thoman ML. T cell senescence. Front Biosci 2001;6:D248–D261.
17. Globerson A. T lymphocytes and aging. Int Arch Allergy Immunol 1995;107:491–497.
18. Utsuyama M, Hirokawa K, Kurashima C, Fukayama M, Inamatsu T, Suzuki K, et al. Differential age-change in the numbers of CD4+CD45RA+ and CD4+CD29+ T cell subsets in human peripheral blood. Mech Ageing Dev 1992;63:57–68.
19. Hirokawa K, Makinodan T. Thymic involution: Effect on T cell differentiation. J Immunol 1975;114:1659–1664.
20. Scollay RG, Butcher EC, Weissman IL. Thymus cell migration. Quantitative aspects of cellular traffic from the thymus to the periphery in mice. Eur J Immunol 1980;10:210–218.
21. Franceschi C, Bonafe M, Valensin S. Human immunosenescence: The prevailing of innate immunity, the failing of clonotypic immunity, and the filling of immunological space. Vaccine 2000;18:1717–1720.
22. Livak F, Schatz DG. T-cell receptor alpha locus V(D)J recombination by-products are abundant in thymocytes and mature T cells. Mol Cell Biol 1996;16:609–618.
23. Douek DC, McFarland RD, Keiser PH, Gage EA, Massey JM, Haynes BF, et al. Changes in thymic function with age and during the treatment of HIV infection. Nature 1998;396:690–695.
24. Rodewald HR. The thymus in the age of retirement. Nature 1998;396:630–631.
25. Barda-Saad M, Rozenszajn LA, Globerson A, Zhang AS, Zipori D. Selective adhesion of immature thymocytes to bone marrow stromal cells: relevance to T cell lymphopoiesis. Exp Hematol 1996;24: 386–391.
26. Garcia-Ojeda ME, Dejbakhsh-Jones S, Weissman IL, Strober S. An alternate pathway for T cell development supported by the bone marrow microenvironment: recapitulation of thymic maturation. J Exp Med 1998;187:1813–1823.

27. Pawelec G, Muller R, Rehbein A, Hahnel K, Ziegler BL. Extrathymic T cell differentiation in vitro from human CD34+ stem cells. J Leukoc Biol 1998;64:733–739.

28. Jamieson BD, Douek DC, Killian S, Hultin LE, Scripture-Adams DD, Giorgi JV, et al. Generation of functional thymocytes in the human adult. Immunity 1999;10:569–575.

29. Pawelec G and Solana R. Immunosenescence. Immunol Today 1997;18:514–516.

30. Mehr R, Perelson AS, Fridkishareli M, Globerson A. Feedback regulation of T cell development: Manifestations in aging. Mech Ageing Dev 1996;91:195–210.

31. Gillis S, Kozak R, Durante M, Weksler ME. Immunological studies of aging. Decreased production of and response to T cell growth factor by lymphocytes from aged humans. J Clin Invest 1981;67:937–942.

32. Murasko DM, Goonewardene IM. T-cell function in aging: mechanisms of decline. Annu Rev Gerontol Geriatr 1990;10:71–96.

33. Nagel JE, Chopra RK, Chrest FJ, McCoy MT, Schneider EL, Holbrook NJ, Adler WH. Decreased proliferation, interleukin 2 synthesis, and interleukin 2 receptor expression are accompanied by decreased mRNA expression in phytohemagglutinin-stimulated cells from elderly donors. J Clin Invest 1988;81:1096–1102.

34. Whisler RL, Beiqing L, Chen M. Age-related decreases in IL-2 production by human T cells are associated with impaired activation of nuclear transcriptional factors AP-1 and NF-AT. Cell Immunol 1996;169:185–195.

35. Gupta S. Membrane signal transduction in T cells in aging humans. Ann NY Acad Sci 1989;568:277–282.

36. Whisler RL, Newhouse YG, Donnerberg RL, Tobin CM. Characterization of intracellular ionized calcium responsiveness and inisitol phosphate production among resting and stimulated peripheral blood T cells from elderly humans. Aging: Immunology and Infectious Disease 1991;3:27–36.

37. Xavier R, Brennan T, Li Q, McCormack C, Seed B. Membrane compartmentation is required for efficient T cell activation. Immunity 1998;8:723–732.

38. Montixi C, Langlet C, Bernard AM, Thimonier J, Dubois C, Wurbel MA, et al. Engagement of T cell receptor triggers its recruitment to low-density detergent-insoluble membrane domains. EMBO J 1998;17:5334–5348.

39. Jackola DR, Hallgren HM. Diminished cell-cell binding by lymphocytes from healthy, elderly humans: evidence for altered activation of LFA-1 function with age. J Gerontol A Biol Sci Med Sci 1995;50:B368–B377.

40. van Oers NS, Killeen N, Weiss A. Lck regulates the tyrosine phosphorylation of the T cell receptor subunits and ZAP-70 in murine thymocytes. J Exp Med 1996;183:1053–1062.

41. Watts JD, Affolter M, Krebs DL, Wange RL, Samelson LE, Aebersold R. Identification by electrospray ionization mass spectrometry of the sites of tyrosine phosphorylation induced in activated Jurkat T cells on the protein tyrosine kinase ZAP-70. J Biol Chem 1994;269:29,520–29,529.

42. Gauen LK, Zhu Y, Letourneur F, Hu Q, Bolen JB, Matis LA, Klausner RD, Shaw AS. Interactions of p59fyn and ZAP-70 with T-cell receptor activation motifs: Defining the nature of a signalling motif. Mol Cell Biol 1994;14:3729–3741.

43. van Oers NS, Killeen N, Weiss A. ZAP-70 is constitutively associated with tyrosine-phosphorylated TCR zeta in murine thymocytes and lymph node T cells. Immunity 1994;1:675–685.

44. Wange RL, Malek SN, Desiderio S, Samelson LE. Tandem SH2 domains of ZAP-70 bind to T cell antigen receptor zeta and CD3 epsilon from activated Jurkat T cells. J Biol Chem 1993;268:19,797–19,801.

45. Iwashima M, Irving BA, van Oers NS, Chan AC, Weiss A. Sequential interactions of the TCR with two distinct cytoplasmic tyrosine kinases. Science 1994;263:1136–1139.

46. Whisler RL, Bagenstose SE, Newhouse YG, Carle KW. Expression and catalytic activities of protein tyrosine kinases (PTKs) Fyn and Lck in peripheral blood T cells from elderly humans stimulated through the T cell receptor (TCR)/CD3 complex. Mech Ageing Dev 1997;98:57–73.

47. Utsuyama M, Wakikawa A, Tamura T, Nariuchi H, Hirokawa K. Impairment of signal transduction in T cells from old mice. Mech Ageing Dev 1997;93:131–144.

48. Guidi L, Antico L, Bartoloni C, Costanzo M, Errani A, Tricerri A, et al. Changes in the amount and level of phosphorylation of p56(lck) in PBL from aging humans. Mech Ageing Dev 1998;102:177–186.

49. Fulop T Jr, Gagne D, Goulet AC, Desgeorges S, Lacombe G, Arcand M, Dupuis G. Age-related impairment of p56lck and ZAP-70 activities in human T lymphocytes activated through the TcR/CD3 complex. Exp Gerontol 1999;34:197–216.

50. Whisler RL, Karanfilov CI, Newhouse YG, Fox CC, Lakshmanan RR, Liu B. Phosphorylation and coupling of zeta-chains to activated T-cell receptor (TCR)/CD3 complexes from peripheral blood T-cells of elderly humans. Mech Ageing Dev 1998;105:115–135.

51. Whisler RL, Chen M, Liu B, Newhouse YG. Age-related impairments in TCR/CD3 activation of ZAP-70 are associated with reduced tyrosine phosphorylations of zeta-chains and p59fyn/p56lck in human T cells. Mech Ageing Dev 1999;111:49–66.

52. Hayflick L. Intracellular determinants of cell aging. Mech Ageing Dev 1984;28:177–185.

53. Harley CB, Futcher AB, Greider CW. Telomeres shorten during ageing of human fibroblasts. Nature 1990;345:458–460.

54. Kruk PA, Rampino NJ, Bohr VA. DNA damage and repair in telomeres: Relation to aging. Proc Natl Acad Sci USA 1995;92:258–262.

55. Effros RB, Walford RL. The effect of age on the antigen presenting mechanism in limiting dilution precursor cell frequency analysis. Cell Immunol 1984;88:531–539.

56. Conconi M, Friguet B. Proteasome inactivation upon aging and on oxidation-effect of HSP 90. Mol Biol Rep 1997;24:45–50.

57. Anselmi B, Conconi M, Veyrat-Durebex C, Biville F, Alliot J, Friguet B. Dietary self-selection can compensate an age-related decrease of rat liver 20 S proteosome activity observed with standard diet. J Gerontol Ser A Biol Sci Med 1998;53:B173–B179.

58. McLachlan JA, Serkin CD, Morreyclark KM, Bakouche O. Immunological functions of aged human monocytes. Pathobiology 1995;63:148–159.

59. Salmon M, Pilling D, Borthwick NJ, Viner N, Janossy G, Bacon PA, Akbar AN. The progressive differentiation of primed T cells is associated with an increasing susceptibility to apoptosis. Eur J Immunol 1994;24:892–899.

60. Thomsen O, Kettel K. Die starke der menschlichen Issoagglutninne und entsperchenden Blut-korperperchenrezeptoren im vershiedenenen Lebensaltern. Z. Immunitatsforsch 1929;63:67–93.

61. Weksler ME. Changes in the B-cell repertoire with age. Vaccine 2000;18:1624–1628.

62. Hallgren HM, Buckley CE 3rd, Gilbertsen VA, Yunis EJ. Lymphocyte phytohemagglutinin responsiveness, immunoglobulins and autoantibodies in aging humans. J Immunol 1973;111:1101–1107.

63. Lacroix-Desmazes S, Mouthon L, Kaveri SV, Kazatchkine MD, Weksler ME. Stability of natural self-reactive antibody repertoires during aging. J Clin Immunol 1999;19:26–34.

64. Goidl EA, Innes JB, Weksler ME. Immunological studies of aging. II. Loss of IgG and high avidity plaque-forming cells and increased suppressor cell activity in aging mice. J Exp Med 1976;144:1037–1048.

65. Weksler ME, Russo C, Siskind GW. Peripheral T cells select the B-cell repertoire in old mice. Immunol Rev 1989;110:173–185.

66. Boosalis M, Stuart M, McClain CJ. Zinc in the elderly. In: Morley Geriatric Nutrition, 2nd Ed. Morley JE, Glick Z, Rubenstein LZ, (eds.), Raven, New York, 1995, pp. 115–121.

67. Morley JE. Protein-energy malnutrition in older subjects. Proc Nutr Soc 1998; 57:587–592.

68. Thomas DR, Ashmen W, Morley JE, Evans WJ. Nutritional management in long-term care: development of a clinical guideline. Council for Nutritional Strategies in Long-Term Care. J Gerontol A Biol Sci Med Sci 2000;55:M725–M734.

69. Williams RO, Loer LA. Zinc requirement for DNA replication in stimulated human lymphocytes. J Cell Biol 1973;58:594–601.

70. Brummerstedt E, Flagstad T, Basse A, Andresen E. The effect of zinc on calves with hereditary thymus hypoplasia (lethal trait a 46). Acta Path Microbiol Scand 1971;79:686–687.

71. Gross RL, Osdin N, Fono L, Newberne PM. Depressed immunological function in zinc-deprived rats as measured by misogen response of spleen, thymus, and peripheral blood. Am J Clin Nutr 1979;32:1260–1266.

72. Luecke RW, Simonel CE, Fraker PJ. The effect of restricted dietary intake on the antibody mediated response of the zinc deficient a/j mouse. J Nutr 1978;108:881–887.

73. Oleske JM, Westphal ML, Shore S, Gorden D, Bogden JD, Nahmias A. Zinc therapy of depressed cellular immunity in acrodermatitis enteropathica: its correction. Am J Dis Child 1979;133:915–918.

74. Golden MHN, Golden BE, Harland PSEG, Jackson AA. Zinc and immunocompetence in protein-energy malnutrition. Lancet 1978;2:1226–1227.

75. Golden MHN, Jackson AA, Golden BE. Effect of zinc on thymus of recently malnourished children. Lancet 1977;2:1057–1059.

76. Allen JI, Kay NE, McClain CJ. Severe zinc deficiency in humans: Association with a reversible T-lymphocyte dysfunction. Ann Intern Med 1981;95:154–157.

77. Fraker PJ, King LE, Laskko T, Vollmer TL. The dynamic link between the integrity of the immune system and zinc status. J Nutr 2000;130:1399S–1406S.

78. McClain CJ, Kasarskis EJ, Allen JJ. Functional consequences of zinc deficiency. Prog Food Nutr Sci 1985;9:185–226.

79. Prasad AS, Beck FW, Kaplan J, Chandrasekar PH, Ortega J, Fitzgerald JT, Swerdlow P. Effect of zinc supplementation on incidence of infections and hospital admissions in sickle cell disease (SCD). Am J Hematol 1999;61:194–202.

80. Prasad AS, Beck FW, Grabowski SM, Kaplan J, Mathog RH. Zinc deficiency: Changes in cytokine production and T-cell subpopulations in patients with head and neck cancer and in noncancer subjects. Proc Assoc Am Physicians 1997;109:68–77.

81. High KP: Nutritional strategies to boost immunity and prevent infection in elderly individuals. Clinical Infectious Diseases 2001;33:1892–1900.

82. Duchateau J, Delepesse G, Vrijens R, Collet H. Beneficial effects of oral zinc supplementation on the immune response of old people. Am J Med 1981;70:1001–1004.

83. Prasad AS, Fitzgerald JT, Hess JW, Kaplan J, Pelen F, Dardenne M. Zinc deficiency in elderly patients. Nutrition 1993;9:218–224.

84. Girodon F, Lombard M, Galan P. Brunet-Lecomte P, Monget AL, Arnaud J, et al. Effect of micronutrient supplementation on infection in institutionalized elderly subjects: A controlled trial. Ann Nutr Metab 1997;1:98–107.

85. Girodon F, Galan P, Monget AL, Boutron-Ruault MC, Brunet-Ruault MC, Brunet-Lecomte P, et al. Impact of trace elements and vitamin supplementation on immunity and infections in institutionalized elderly patients: A randomized controlled trial. MIN.VIT. AOX. Geriatric network, Arch Intern Med 1999;159:748–754.

86. Chandra RK. Excessive intake of zinc impairs immune responses. JAMA 1984;252:1443.

87. Prasad AS, Brewer GJ, Schoomaker EB, Rabbani P. Hypocupremia induced by zinc therapy in adults. JAMA 1978;240:2166–2168.

88. Ekmekcioglu C, Prohaska C, Pomazal K, Steffan I, Schernthaner G, Marktl W. Concentrations of seven trace elements in different hematological matrices in patients with type 2 diabetes as compared to healthy controls. Biol Trace Elem Res 2001;79:205–219.

89. Savarino L, Granchi D, Ciapetti G, Cenni E, Ravaglia G, Forti P, et al. Serum concentrations of zinc and selenium in elderly peiple:results in healthy nonagenarians/ centenarians. Exper Gerontol 2001;36:327–339.

90. Brown KM, Arthur JR. Selenium, selenoproteins and human health: A review. Public Health Nutr 2001;4:593–599.

91. Neve J. New approaches to assess selenium status and requirement. Nutr Rev 2000;58:363 369.

92. Beck MA, Kolbeck PC, Rohr LH, Shi Q, Morris VC, Levander OA. Amyocarditic coxsackievirus becomes myocarditic in selenium deficient mice. J Med Virol 1994;43:166–170.

93. Beck MA Nutritionally induced oxidative stress: effect on viral disease. Am J Clin Nutr 2000;71:1676S–1679S.

94. Beck MA, Nelson HK, Shi Q, Van Dael P, Schriffrin EJ, Blum S, et al. Selenium deficiency increases the pathology of an influenza virus infection. FASEB J 2001;10:1096.

95. Brawley OW, Parnes H. Prostate cancer prevention trials in the USA. Eur J Cancer 2000;36:1312–1315.

96. Goodman GE. Prevention of lung cancer. Crit Rev Oncol Hematol 2000;33:187–197.

97. Chavance, et al. Immunological and nutritional status among the elderly. Topics in aging research in europe 1984;1:231–237.

98. Meydani SN, Barklund MP, Liu S, Meydani M, Miller RA, Cannon JG, et al. Vitamin E supplementation enhances cell-mediated immunity in healthy elderly subjects. Am J Clin Nutr 1990;52:557–563.

99. Meydani SN, Meydani M, Rall LC, et al. Assessment of the safety of high-dose, short-term supplementation with vitamin E in healthy older adults. Am J Clin Nutr 1994;60:704–709.

100. Meydani SN, Meydani M, Blumberg JB, Leka LS, Siber G, Loszewski R, et al. Vitamin E supplementation and in vivo immune response in healthy elderly subjects. A randomized controlled trial. JAMA 1997;277:1380–1386.

101. Pallast EG, Schouten EG, de Waart FG, Fonk HC, Doekes G, von Blomberg BM, Kok FJ. Effect of 50- and 100-mg vitamin E supplements on cellular immune function in noninstitutionalized elderly persons. Am J Clin Nutr 1999;69:1273–1281.

102. Niki E, Noguchi N, Tsuchihashi H, Gotoh N. Interaction among vitamin C, vitamin E, and beta-carotene. Am J Clin Nutr 1995;62(6 suppl):13,22S–13,26S.

103. Kennes B, Dumont I, Brohee D, Hubert C, Neve P. Effect of vitamin C supplements on cell-mediated immunity in old people. Gerontology 1983;29:305–310.
104. Delafuente JC, Prendergast JM, Modigh A. Immunologic modulation by vitamin C in the elderly. Int J Immunopharmacol 1986;8:205–211.
105. Bogden JD, Bendich A, Kemp FW, Bruening KS, Shurnick JH, Denny T, et al. Daily micronutrient supplements enhance delayed-hypersensitivity skin test responses in older people. Am J Clin Nutr 1994; 60:437–447.
106. Chandra RK. Effect of vitamin and trace-element supplementation on immune responses and infection in elderly subjects. Lancet 1992;340:1124–1127.
107. Pike J, Chandra RK. Effect of vitamin and trace element supplementation on immune indices in healthy elderly. Int J Vitam Nutr Res 1995;65:117–121.
108. Walrand S, Moreau K, Caldefie F, Tridon A, Chassagne J, Portefaix G, et al. Specific and nonspecific immune response to fasting and refeeding differ in healthy young adult and elderly persons. Am J Clin Nutr 2001;74:670–678.
109. Chandra RK. Nutritional regulation of immunity and risk of infection in old age. Immunology 1989; 67:141–147.

31 Nutrition in Surgery, Trauma, and Sepsis

David A. Spain

1. INTRODUCTION

The geriatric segment is the fastest growing subset of the population. In addition, older adults are living much longer after retirement, and are remaining active in late life. The result has been a substantial increase in the number of elderly patients undergoing elective operations, including very complex procedures *(1,2)*. Cardiac and joint replacement operations are now commonly performed among patients in their 70s and 80s. In addition, the proportion of trauma patients age >65 yr admitted to the hospital is increasing along with the associated cost of their care *(3)*. In a 1990 study, the elderly represented 12% of the population, but accounted for >25% of discharges and total hospital costs related to trauma. It is estimated that the portion of trauma patients over the age of 65 will continue to grow to 40% of all admissions *(3)*.

Elderly trauma patients have an overall higher mortality rate when compared to younger patients, but they also tend to have more severe injuries *(4–6)*. Even when the severity of injury is taken into account, excess mortality is persistent *(6,7)*. This is true also for patients with minor injuries where mortality rates are higher after the age of 65 *(8)*. Elderly patients frequently have preexisting conditions, such as ischemic heart disease, chronic obstructive pulmonary disease, and diabetes, which significantly increase their risk of dying following trauma *(9)*. The diminished physiologic and metabolic reserve associated with the aging process contributes to the increased risk of mortality. This may be deleterious, as the elderly have decreased muscle mass and may have an exaggerated physiologic response to injury *(5)*, thus increasing demand on a limited system. However, for those patients who survive their initial injuries and are discharged from the hospital, the majority (60–85%) will return to their prior level of functioning *(10,11)*. This is true even for elderly patients with prolonged intensive care unit stays (ICU ≥ 3 wk) *(7)*. Therefore, most elderly patients who were functioning at a high level before injury and have potentially survivable injuries should be offered aggressive care in the ICU *(12)*.

From: *Handbook of Clinical Nutrition and Aging*
Edited by: C. W. Bales and C. S. Ritchie © Humana Press Inc., Totowa, NJ

2. NUTRITIONAL STATUS OF GERIATRIC SURGICAL PATIENTS AND OUTCOME

It has long been recognized that age alone is not a contraindication to elective surgery, even for complex operations such as open-heart surgery or aneurysm repair *(1,13)*. However, among elderly patients, preoperative malnutrition, usually defined as weight loss >10% or hypoalbuminemia, is strongly associated with an increased risk of postoperative complications *(14–19)*. The association between preoperative malnutrition and increased surgical risk has long been recognized *(20)*, but remains a common problem in surgical patients, especially if they require admission to the ICU *(21,22)*.

Among cardiac surgery patients, preoperative hypoalbuminemia increases the likelihood of postoperative organ dysfunction, infections, ICU stay and hospital death *(22)*. A serum albumin < 25 g/L or a body mass index (BMI) < 20 each independently predict increased mortality and mortality is highest in the group of patients with both *(14)*. In one of the largest studies of its kind, the National VA Surgical Risk Study prospectively evaluated over 54,000 surgical patients *(15)*. In a regression model, serum albumin was found to be the single best predictor of outcome. An albumin level >46 g/L was associated with a mortality of 1% and a morbidity of 10%, whereas patients with an albumin level <21 g/L had an increase in mortality to 29% and a morbidity of 65% *(15)*. Preoperative serum albumin level is a relatively low-cost and excellent tool to screen elderly patients at increased surgical risk, especially when combined with a history of weight loss. However, two crucial caveats remain. First, the value of hypoalbuminemia applies only to elective surgery. In the hospitalized patient, serum albumin levels are affected by so many factors (e.g., intravascular volume, acute illness, and infection) that its utility as a nutritional marker is severely limited in this patient population. Second, although hypoalbuminemia may portend a poorer outcome, it is unclear if efforts to correct this impacts the outcome in surgical patients.

The prevalence of malnutrition and/or hypoalbuminemia may vary widely depending on the surgical population. Hypoalbuminemia is present in 12–14% of elderly patients (age ≥75 yr) undergoing cardiac surgery and is a powerful predictor of perioperative complications *(18,22)*. Preoperative malnutrition, loosely defined as weight loss >10% or hypoalbuminemia, is present in 42% of older patients undergoing elective spinal fusion and was a significant independent predictor of complications *(17)*. Poor nutrition is common (approx 50%) among patients undergoing thoracic operations for either lung reduction (emphysema) or cancer *(16,23)* and malnutrition is an important predictor of the need for postoperative ventilation and mortality. Hypoalbuminemia may be present in anywhere from 15% to nearly 90% of elderly orthopedic patients and is strongly correlated with complications, length of postoperative stay and mortality (Table 1).

It is clear that elderly surgical patients frequently start off in a precarious situation. The metabolic response to operation or injury can be significant, especially if complications develop. These patients often have decreased reserves as evidenced by a low BMI and/or reduced lean body mass. This predisposes patients to complications, which increases the metabolic demands and sets up a viscous cycle. In addition, it may be difficult to find the opportunity to assess these patients. Elderly surgical patients are frequently admitted as emergencies and nutritional screening may not be practical. Most elective surgical patients are admitted to the hospital only postoperatively, where ability to interview the patient may be compromised. One solution is to have a dietitian call patients at home prior to

Table 1
Prevalence of Malnutrition in Elderly Orthopedic Patients and Impact on Outcomes

Patient type	% Malnourished	Measure	Outcome	Author
Hip fracture	–	Albumin	Increased mortality	Foster (57)
Arthroplasty	27	Albumin, TLC	5–7× wound infections	Green (58)
Hip fracture	18	Albumin, TLC	Increased LOS, mortality	Koval (59)
Arthroplasty	19	Albumin, TLC	Increased LOS, costs	Lavenia (60)
Femur fracture	31	BMI	No change	Maffulli (61)
Mixed	16	MNA	–	Murphy (62)
Hip fracture	58	Protein depletion	Increased LOS, complications	Patterson (63)
Hip fracture	89	Albumin	Increased LOS	Van Hoang (64)

LOS, length of stay; TLC, total lymphocyte count; BMI, body mass index; MNA, Mini-Nutritional Assessment.

admission to obtain a nutrition history (24). This has the potential to identify high-risk patients before admission for elective surgery and allow attempts at nutritional intervention.

3. METABOLIC RESPONSE TO INJURY OR OPERATION IN THE ELDERLY

In young, previously healthy patients, the metabolic response to injury is characterized by an increase in resting metabolic rate and catabolism of body proteins. Resting energy expenditure (REE) may increase by 30–50% in the first week following injury (4) and can increase by 80–100% for patients with burn injury. These generalizations are often applied to all trauma patients. However, the metabolic response of the injured elderly patient has only recently been examined. Unlike most young surgical patients, the elderly often have comorbidities that can affect metabolism and impact nutrition support. These include obesity, chronic obstructive pulmonary disease (COPD), hypo- or hyperthyroidism, Type II diabetes, and hyperlipidemia (1,9,25).

Peerless et al. (26) used continuous indirect calorimetry in the early postinjury period to assess the oxygen consumption and the metabolic response to resuscitation. Elderly patients, defined as age >65, had significantly lower oxygen consumption that did not change significantly with resuscitation. Yu et al. (27) found that critically ill surgical patients age 50–75 yr had a marked improvement in survival with efforts to increase oxygen delivery, but there was no benefit in those >75 yr of age. This might suggest a somewhat fixed metabolic response in the elderly patient and would be important to consider when developing a nutrition support regimen for an elderly patient.

Recently, Frankenfield et al. (4) investigated the influence of age on the metabolic response to injury in 21 trauma patients >60 yr of age and compared them to patients <60 yr. All of these patients had sustained multiple injuries and were on mechanical ventilation. At 6–7 d following injury, all patients underwent indirect calorimetry, bioelectric impedance plethysmography and assessment of nitrogen metabolism. Elderly patients had a modest reduction in resting metabolic rate and oxygen consumption (12%) following injury. However, in contrast to younger patients, there was no attenuation of

Table 2
Metabolic Response to Injury
in the Elderly Patient Compared to Younger Patients

Parameter	Elderly response
Fever	Less likely
SIRS*	Less likely
Resting energy expenditure	Less catabolic
Oxygen consumption	Lower
Hyperglycemia	More common
Nitrogen loss	Unchanged

*SIRS, Systemic Inflammatory Response Syndrome (at least two of the following: T° >38°C or <36°C, heart rate >90, leukocyte count >12,000/mL or <4000/mL and respiratory rate >20/min or mechanical ventilation) (65). Source: Frankenfeld et al. (4).

protein catabolism or nitrogen loss in the elderly (Table 2). Given the loss of lean body mass with aging, this would put the elderly patient population at risk for early protein–calorie malnutrition. In addition, metabolic complications of nutrition support (hyperglycemia and azotemia) were more common in the elderly even though patients with diabetes or preexisting renal dysfunction were excluded. In an earlier study, elderly patients were also found to have lower oxygen consumption and more frequent hyperglycemia (28). These studies indicate a decreased margin for error in the critically ill elderly patient and highlight the need to closely assess tolerance of nutrition support.

Elderly patients are also at high risk for euthyroid sick syndrome (ESS). This is an abnormality of thyroid function tests sometimes seen in critically ill patients, resulting from shunting of the conversion of thyroxine (T_4) to the inactive reverse T_3 (rT_3). This shunting is a result of the increased presence of stress hormones and is thought to represent a mechanism to control or downregulate the metabolic response. This can be differentiated from hypothyroidism by the normal levels of T4 seen in ESS (29). Although the clinical significance of ESS has been debated (30,31), it is very common among elderly patients requiring emergency operations (32). ESS is present preoperatively in >50% of elderly patients (age >70 yr) undergoing emergency procedure (32). The presence of ESS is associated with a more severe physiologic response, hypoalbuminemia, and higher stress hormone levels. Patients with ESS have longer lengths of stay (17 vs 12 d) and higher mortality (20% vs 0%). A serum albumin level on admission <35 g/L is strongly associated with ESS (32). It has been hypothesized that development of ESS may be related to selenium deficiency (33) and selenium supplementation normalizes T4 and rT3 levels in trauma patients (34). But it is unclear if ESS contributes to poorer outcomes or is simply another marker for the severity of illness. Regardless, hypoalbuminemia and altered thyroid function tests, especially in an elderly patient, should alert the clinician to a patient at high risk for postoperative complications and nutritional deterioration. Selenium supplementation should be considered in these patients.

The metabolic response to injury in the elderly may persist for a prolonged period of time, even following hospital discharge (35,36). Among patients sustaining hip fracture, resting energy expenditure is increased immediately after injury and remains elevated for up to 2 mo *(36)*. Thus, there may be no improvement in overall nutritional status despite what appears to be adequate energy intake.

4. NUTRITION SUPPORT IN GERIATRIC SURGICAL AND CRITICALLY ILL PATIENTS

Given the diminished reserves and the physiologic response to operation and injury, early nutrition support would seem vital for the elderly surgical or critically ill patient. Despite the aging of the surgical population and the prevalence of malnutrition among geriatric patients, the role of nutrition support in surgical or critically ill geriatric patients has received very little attention. Some supportive data has been generated through nutrition studies involving cancer patients, the majority of which are older (usually age >60 yr), although age has not been specifically evaluated. And recently, some interest has been generated in assessing the role of nutrition support among elderly patients sustaining hip fractures. This does provide some rational for nutrition support in elderly surgical and critically ill patients.

4.1. Surgical Oncology

Patients undergoing major oncologic resections may be at especially high-risk for nutritional deterioration in the postoperative period for several reasons. Many of these patients are malnourished preoperatively, which is associated with an increased risk of complications and mortality *(15,37–44)*. In a large study of nearly 400 patients, the VA Cooperative Study Group assessed the role of perioperative TPN in surgical having either following laparotomy or noncardiac thoracostomy *(43)*. Although this study was not exclusively for oncology patients, this was a common diagnosis. The authors of the study found that 7–15 d preoperative total parenteral nutrition (TPN) decreased complications. However, this benefit was only seen in severely malnourished patients as judged by the Subjective Global Assessment *(44)*. It seems likely that similar benefit should be seen with the preoperative use of enteral nutrition in malnourished patients *(45,46)*. Widespread use of preoperative TPN or enteral feedings in well-nourished patients is unlikely to provide benefit and may actually worsen outcome *(44,45,47)*. Elderly oncology patients are also at risk for preoperative compromise and further deterioration postoperatively resulting from altered swallowing or GI tract dysfunction. This needs to be assessed when planning these operations and consideration should be given to securing enteral access during the procedure.

Several studies among patients undergoing major, elective oncologic resections demonstrate benefit from perioperative nutrition support *(37–40,43,44)*. Most of these patients had either head and neck cancers or upper gastrointestinal tract tumors (esophagus, stomach, pancreas). The majority of these studies involved the use of immunonutrition formulas, which are enteral feedings that are supplemented mostly commonly with arginine, nucleotides (e.g., RNA) and omega-3 fatty acids, while some contain glutamine. The rationale for these various components is outlined in Table 3. Nutrition support was frequently initiated 5–7 d before the operation and continued in the postoperative period for an additional 5–7 d. Most of these studies demonstrate a decreased infection rate with an associated shorter length of stay and subsequent cost savings *(38,49,41)*. Although controversial and no studies have documented improved survival *(48,49)*, perioperative

Table 3
Components of Immunonutrition Formulas

Component	Rationale
Arginine	Increased macrophage cytotoxicity
	Increased specific cytolytic T-cell activity
	Increased cellular immunity
Nucleotides (RNA)	More rapid maturation of lymphocytes
Omega-3 fatty acids	Less bioactive PGE_2 and LTB_5
Glutamine	Trophic effect on enterocytes

PGE_2, prostaglandin E_2; LTB_5, leukotriene B_5.

immunonutrition would appear to be cost effective in geriatric surgical patients undergoing major oncologic resections.

The adage "if the gut works, use it" is widely quoted. A major benefit of these studies, as well as others involving trauma patients, is redefining what is a "working" gut. Braga et al. *(38)* started enteral feeding within 6 h in a group of patients with resection of neoplasms in the stomach, pancreas or colon, demonstrating that early postoperative enteral nutrition is feasible. Clearly, the old surgical dogma of waiting for bowel sounds or flatus, or even bowel movement, is no longer necessary. Currently, the major requirements to define a working gut are adequate perfusion and structural integrity. This awareness has led to more aggressive use of enteral nutrition and is one of the contributing factors in the decreasing reliance on TPN.

4.2. Hip Fracture

Perhaps the only elderly surgical population that has received any attention with regards to the role of nutrition support is patients with hip fractures. Malnutrition is common among these patients and has a significant negative impact on outcome (Table 1). In addition, the underlying malnutrition may actually predispose these patients to injury. This has led several investigators to use perioperative nutritional supplements in an effort to reduce complications in this group of patients.

In 1983, Bastow et al. *(50)* reported a randomized trial of supplementary tube feeding in thin or very thin elderly women with femoral neck fracture. Treated patients received enteral feeding delivered overnight by nasogastric tube and were allowed to eat during the day, while control patients received a standard diet. Nearly 20% of patients could not tolerate the feedings (nausea, distention, etc.), which is a common problem *(51)*. Nutritional supplementation was associated with improved anthropometric and plasma proteins measurement as well as shortened hospital stay. Mortality was less (8% vs 22%) but this did not reach statistical significance *(51)*. Almost identical results were observed in a subsequent study that used nightly feedings in a small group of elderly men (76 yr) with hip fractures *(52)*. At 6 mo postoperative, the mortality in the treatment groups was 0% when compared to 50% in the control group. Delmi et al. *(53)* also demonstrated an improvement in 6-mo mortality with postoperative supplementation (40% vs 74%).

Recently, Espaulella et al. *(54)* performed a double blind, randomized, placebo-controlled trial of nutritional supplementation in 171 patients with hip fracture, all age ≥70 yr. The supplement contained 20 g protein, 800 mg calcium, 25 IU vitamin D_3, and other vitamins and minerals. Although the treatment group had fewer total complications and shorter hospital stay, there was no difference in functional outcome or mortality at 6 mo. However, only 8% of patients were considered to be malnourished at the start of the trial, and 25% had poor consumption of the supplement *(54)*. Thus, a potential benefit may have been missed because of these factors.

A review of 15 randomized trials involving 1054 hip fracture patients found some support for oral protein and energy supplements in reducing morbidity but not mortality. Small study sizes, poor design and inadequate outcome assessment limited analysis of the data *(55)*. In addition, poor compliance and intolerance are common *(54,56)* and may limit effectiveness. Simply prescribing supplements without specific goals and assistance may not be sufficient *(56)*. Perioperative supplements are relatively inexpensive compared to the cost of postoperative complications and increased hospital stay. It would seem likely that sufficient delivery should decrease complication rates and shorten hospital stay. Perioperative oral supplements should represent a cost-effective and relatively safe method of decreasing complications in high-risk surgical patients.

5. SUMMARY

Despite the aging surgical population, very little attention has been paid to the role of nutrition support. All elderly geriatric patients should be screened preoperatively for malnutrition (weight loss, serum albumin, total lymphocyte count). A simple serum albumin level may be the easiest and least expensive screening tool in the ambulatory patient population. Patients being considered for elective operation with significant malnutrition (albumin < 2.5 mg/dL) should receive 7–10 d of preoperative nutrition supplementation, preferably by the enteral route. Patients scheduled for major oncologic resection should probably receive immunonutrition both preoperatively and during the early postoperative period. Immunonutrition may also be of benefit in the nonseptic, critically ill patient as well.

Older adult trauma patients and malnourished patients requiring emergency operation are at high-risk for nutritional deterioration and should have aggressive attempts made to gain enteral access and use the gastrointestinal tract. Unfortunately almost no specific data exists, making concrete recommendations difficult. Preexisting malnutrition and comorbidities often confound the metabolic response to operation and/or injury in the elderly. Indirect calorimetry and assessment of intolerance (i.e., hyperglycemia, azotemia, etc.) should be used liberally in the elderly surgical or critically ill patient to direct nutrition support.

6. RECOMMENDATIONS FOR CLINICIANS

1. Older adults should be screened for malnutrition, especially prior to elective surgery. Individuals with malnutrition or at a high risk for malnutrition should be referred to a nutritionist for further evaluation and intervention.
2. Given the relative decrease in proportion of lean body mass in older adults, careful attention should be paid to maintaining nitrogen balance and minimizing muscle breakdown.
3. Consider selenium supplementation for patients with euthyroid sick syndrome.
4. Consider preoperative nutrition supplementation in malnourished cancer patients scheduled for surgery.
5. Consider supplemental nocturnal feeding in hip fracture patients.

REFERENCES

1. Deiwick M, Tandler R, Mollhoff T, Kerber S, Rotker J, Roeder N, Scheld HH. Heart surgery in patients aged eighty years and above: Determinants of morbidity and mortality. Thorac Cardiovasc Surg 1997; 45:119–126.
2. Sundt TM, Bailey MS, Moon MR, Mendeloff EN, Huddleston CB, Pasque MK, et al. Quality of life after aortic valve replacement at the age >80 years. Circulation 2000;102:III70–III74.
3. MacKenzie EJ, Morris JA Jr, Smith GS, Fahey M. Acute hospital costs of trauma in the United States: Implications for regionalized systems of care. J Trauma 1990;30:1096–1101.
4. Frankenfield D, Cooney RN, Smith JS, Rowe WA. Age-related differences in the metabolic response to injury. J Trauma 2000;48:49–56.
5. Shabot MM, Johnson CL. Outcome from critical care in the "oldest old" trauma patients. J Trauma 1995; 39:254–259.
6. Young JS, Cephas GA, Blow O. Outcome and cost of trauma among the elderly: A real-life model of a single-payer reimbursement system. J Trauma 1998;45:800–804.
7. Miller RS, Patton M, Graham RM, Hollins D. Outcomes of trauma patients who survive prolonged lengths of stay in the intensive care unit. J Trauma 2000;48:229–234.
8. Morris JA Jr, MacKenzie EJ, Damiano AM, Bass SM. Mortality in trauma patients: The interaction between host factors and severity. J Trauma 1990;30:1476–1482.
9. Morris JA Jr, MacKenzie EJ, Edelstein SL. The effect of preexisting conditions on mortality in trauma patients. JAMA 1990;263:1942–1946.
10. Battistella FD, Din AM, Perez L. Trauma patients 75 years and older: Long-term follow-up results justify aggressive management. J Trauma 1998;44:618–623.
11. Carrillo EH, Richardson JD, Malias MA, Cryer HM, Miller FB. Long term outcome of blunt trauma care in the elderly. Surg Gynecol Obstet 1993;176:559–564.
12. Shapiro MB, Dechert RE, Colwell C, Bartlett RH, Rodriguez JL. Geriatric trauma: Aggressive intensive care unit management is justified. Am Surg 1994;60:695–698.
13. Ihaya A, Chiba Y, Kimura T, Morioka K, Uesaka T, Muraoka R. Abdominal aortic aneurysmectomy in the octogenarian. Ann Thorac Cardiovasc Surg 1998;4:247–250.
14. Engelman DT, Adams DH, Byrne JG, Aranki SF, Collins JJ Jr, Couper GS, et al. Impact of body mass index and albumin on morbidity and mortality after cardiac surgery. J Thorac Cardiovasc Surg 1999; 118:866–873.
15. Gibbs J, Cull W, Henderson W, Daley J, Hur K, Khuri SF. Preoperative serum albumin level as a predictor of operative mortality and morbidity: results from the National VA Surgical Risk Study. Arch Surg 1999;134:36–42.
16. Jagoe RT, Goodship TH, Gibson GJ. The influence of nutritional status on complications after operation for lung cancer. Ann Thorac Surg 2001;71:936–943.
17. Klein JD, Hey LA, Yu CS, Klein BB, Coufal FJ, Young EP, et al. Perioperative nutrition and postoperative complications in patients undergoing spinal surgery. Spine 1996;15:2676–2682.
18. Rich MW, Keller AJ, Schechtman KB, Marshall WG Jr, Kouchoukos NT. Increased complications and prolonged hospital stay in elderly cardiac surgical patients with low serum albumin. Am J Cardiol 1989; 63:714–718.
19. Seelig MH, Klingler PJ, Oldenburg WA. Simultaneous aortic surgery and malnutrition increase morbidity after revascularisation of the mesenteric arteries. Eur J Surg 2000;166:771–776.
20. Studley HO: Percentage of weight loss: A basic indicator of surgical risk in patients with chronic peptic ulcer. JAMA 1936;106:458–460.
21. Giner M, Laviano A, Meguid MM, Gleason JR. In 1995 a correlation between malnutrition and poor outcome in critically ill patients still exists. Nutrition 1996;12:23–29.
22. Rady MY, Ryan T, Starr NJ. Clinical characteristics of preoperative hypoalbuminemia predict outcome of cardiovascular surgery. J Parenter Enteral Nutr 1997;21:81–90.
23. Mazolewski P, Turner JF, Baker M, Kurtz T, Little AG. The impact of nutritional status on the outcome of lung volume reduction surgery: a prospective study. Chest 1999;116:693–696.
24. Schwartz DB, Gudzin D. Preadmission nutrition screening: Expanding hospital-based nutrition services by implementing earlier nutrition intervention. J Am Diet Assoc 2000;100:81–87.
25. Vasa FR, Molitch ME. Endocrine problems in the chronically ill critically ill patient. Clin Chest Med 2001;22:193–208.

26. Peerless JR, Epstein CD, Martin JE, Pinchak AC, Malangoni MA. Oxygen consumption in the early postinjury period: Use of continuous, on-line indirect calorimetry. Crit Care Med 2000;28:395–401.
27. Yu M, Burchell S, Hasaniya NW, Takanishi DM, Myers SA, Takiguchi SA. Relationship of mortality to increasing oxygen delivery in patients ≥ 50 yr of age: A prospective, randomized trial. Crit Care Med 1998;26:1011–1109.
28. Jeevanandam M, Petersen SR, Shamos RF. Protein and glucose fuel kinetics and hormonal changes in elderly trauma patients. Metabolism 1993;42:1255–1262.
29. Stanford GG. Endocrine problems. In: Surgical Critical Care. Weigelt JA, Lewis FR Jr (eds.), W.B. Saunders, Philadelphia, PA, 1996, pp. 397–410.
30. McIver B, Gorman CA. Euthyroid sick syndrome: an overview. Thyroid 1997;7:125–132.
31. Thrush DN, Austin D, Burdash N. Cardiopulmonary bypass temperature does not affect postoperative euthyroid sick syndrome? Chest 1995;108:1541–1545.
32. Girvent M, Maestro S, Hernandez R, Carajol I, Monne J, Sancho JJ, et al. Euthyroid sick syndrome, associated endocrine abnormalities, and outcome in elderly patients undergoing emergency operation. Surgery 1998;123:560–567.
33. Van Lente F, Daher R. Plasma selenium concentrations in patients with euthyroid sick syndrome. Clin Chem 1992;38:1885–1888.
34. Berger MM, Reymond MJ, Shenkin A, Rey F, Wardle C, Cayeux C, et al. Influence of selenium supplements on the post-traumatic alterations of the thyroid axis: A placebo-controlled trial. Intensive Care Med 2001;27:91–100.
35. Campillo B, Paillaud E, Bories PN, Noel M, Porquet D, Le Parco JC. Serum levels of insulin-like growth factor-1 in the three months following surgery for a hip fracture in elderly: relationship with nutritional status and inflammatory reaction. Clin Nutr 2000;19:349–354.
36. Paillaud E, Bories PN, Le Parco JC, Campillo B. Nutritional status and energy expenditure in elderly patients with recent hip fracture during a 2-month follow-up. Br J Nutr 2000;83:97–103.
37. Bozzetti F, Gavazzi C, Miceli R, Rossi N, Mariani L, Cozzaglio L, et al. Perioperative total parenteral nutrition in malnourished, gastrointestinal cancer patients: A randomized, clinical trial. J Parenter Enteral Nutr 2000;24:7–14.
38. Braga M, Gianotti L, Radaelli G, Vignali A, Mari G, Gentilini O, Di Carlo V. Perioperative immunonutrition in patients undergoing cancer surgery: results of a randomized double-blind phase 3 trial. Arch Surg 1999;134:428–433.
39. Daly JM, Lieberman MD, Goldfine J, Shou J, Weintraub F, Rosato E, Lavin P. Enteral nutrition with supplemental arginine, RNA, and omega-3 fatty acids in patients after operation: immunologic, metabolic, and clinical outcome. Surgery 1992;112:56–67.
40. Gianotti L, Braga M, Frei A, Greiner R, Di Carlo V. Health care resources consumed to treat postoperative infections: cost saving by perioperative immunonutrition. Shock 2000;14:325–330.
41. Senkal M, Zumtobel V, Bauer KH, Marpe B, Wolfram G, Frei A, et al. Outcome and cost-effectiveness of perioperative enteral immunonutrition in patients undergoing elective upper gastrointestinal tract surgery: A prospective randomized study. Arch Surg 1999;134:1309–1316.
42. Snyderman CH, Kachman K, Molseed L, Wagner R, D'Amico F, Bumpous J, Rueger R. Reduced postoperative infections with an immune-enhancing nutritional supplement. Laryngoscope 1999;109:915–921.
43. Perioperative total parenteral nutrition in surgical patients. The Veterans Affairs Total Parenteral Nutrition Cooperative Study Group. N Engl J Med 1991;325:525–532.
44. Rey-Ferro M, Castano R, Orozco O, Serna A, Moreno A. Nutritional and immunologic evaluation of patients with gastric cancer before and after surgery. Nutrition 1997;13:878–881.
45. McClave SA, Snider HL, Spain DA. Preoperative issues in clinical nutrition. Chest 1999;115:64S–70S.
46. Nourhashemi F, Andrieu S, Rauzy O, Ghisolfi A, Vellas B, Chumlea WC, Albarede JL. Nutritional support and aging in preoperative nutrition. Curr Opin Clin Nutr Metab Care 1999;2:87–92.
47. MacFie J, Woodcock NP, Palmer MD, Walker A, Townsend Mitchell CJ. Oral dietary supplements in pre- and postoperative surgical patients: a prospective and randomized clinical trial. Nutrition 2000;16:723–738.
48. Heslin MJ, Brennan MF. Advances in perioperative nutrition: Cancer. World J Surg 2000;24:1477–1485.
49. van Bokhorst-De Van Der Schueren MA, Quak JJ, von Blomberg-van der Flier BM, Kuik DJ, Langendoen SI, Snow GB, et al. Effect of perioperative nutrition, with and without arginine supplemen-

tation, on nutritional status, immune function, postoperative morbidity, and survival in severely malnourished head and neck cancer patients. Am J Clin Nutr 2001;73:323–332.

50. Bastow MD, Rawlings J, Allison SP. Benefits of supplementary tube feeding after fractured neck of femur: A randomised controlled trial. Br Med J 1983;287:1589–1592.

51. Hartgrink HH, Willie J, Konig P, Hermans J, Breslau PJ. Pressure sore and tube feeding in patients with a fracture of the hip: A randomized clinical trial. Clin Nutr 1998;17:287–292.

52. Sullivan DH, Nelson CL, Bopp MM, Puskarich-May CL, Walls RC. Nightly enteral nutrition support of elderly hip fracture patients: A phase I trial. J Am Coll Nutr 1998;17:155–161.

53. Delmi M, Rapin CH, Bengoa JM, Delmas PD, Vasey H, Bonjour JP. Dietary supplementation in elderly patients with fractured neck of the femur. Lancet 1990;335:1013–1016.

54. Espaulella J, Guyer H, Diaz-Escriu F, Mellado-Navas JA, Castells M, Pladevall M. Nutritional supplementation of elderly hip fracture patients. A randomized, double-blind, placebo-controlled trial. Age Ageing 2000;29:425–431.

55. Avenell A, Handoll HH. Nutritional supplementation for hip fracture aftercare in the elderly (Cochrane Review). Cochrane Database Syst Rev 2000;4:CD001880.

56. Lawson RM, Doshi MK, Ingoe LE, Colligan JM, Barton JR, Cobden I. Compliance of orthopaedic patients with oral nutritional supplementation. Clin Nutr 2000;19:171–175.

57. Foster MR, Heppenstall RB, Friedenberg ZB, Hozack WJ. A prospective assessment of nutritional status and complications in patients with fractures of the hip. J Orthop Trauma 1990;4:49–57.

58. Greene KA, Wilde AH, Stulberg BN. Preoperative nutritional status of total joint patients. Relationship to postoperative wound complications. J Arthroplasty 1991;6:321–325.

59. Koval KJ, Maurer SG, Su ET, Aharonoff GB, Zuckerman JD. The effects of nutritional status on outcome after hip fracture. J Orthop Trauma 1999;13:164–169.

60. Lavernia CJ, Sierra RJ, Baerga L. Nutritional parameters and short term outcome in arthroplasty. J Am Coll Nutr 1999;18:274–278.

61. Maffulli N, Dougall TW, Brown MT, Golden MH. Nutritional differences in patients with proximal femoral fractures. Age Ageing 1999;28:458–462.

62. Murphy MC, Brooks CN, New SA, Lumbers ML. The use of the Mini-Nutritional Assessment (MNA) tool in elderly orthopaedic patients. Eur J Clin Nutr 2000;54:555–562.

63. Patterson BM, Cornell CN, Carbone B, Levine B, Chapman D. Protein depletion and metabolic stress in elderly patients who have a fracture of the hip. J Bone Joint Surg Am 1992;74:251–260.

64. Van Hoang H, Silverstone FA, Leventer S, Wolf-Klein GP, Foley CJ. The effect of nutritional status on length of stay in elderly hip fracture patients. J Nutr Health Aging 1998;2:159–161.

65. American College of Chest Physicians: Society of Critical Care Medicine Consensus Conference. Definition for sepsis and organ failure and guidelines for the use of innovative therapies in sepsis. Crit Care Med 1992;20:864–867.

66. McClave SA. The effects of immune-enhancing diets (IEDs) on mortality, hospital length of stay, duration of mechanical ventilation, and other parameters. J Parenter Enteral Nutr 2001;25:S44–S49.

INDEX

About the Editors

Connie Watkins Bales is Associate Director for Education/Evaluation of the Geriatrics Research, Education and Clinical Center at the Durham VA Medical Center and Associate Research Professor of Geriatric Medicine at Duke University School of Medicine. Dr. Bales received her doctorate in Nutritional Sciences at the University of Tennessee–Knoxville and held an appointment in the Graduate Nutrition Division at the University of Texas–Austin before joining the faculty at Duke. Her research endeavors over the past two decades have focused on a variety of topics in geriatric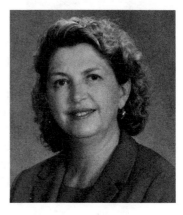
nutrition, and she has published extensively on nutrition and aging-related topics. Her current work focuses on energy balance and includes studies of nutritional frailty in the elderly, interaction of exercise with energy balance in overweight subjects, and effects of calorie restriction on the human aging process.

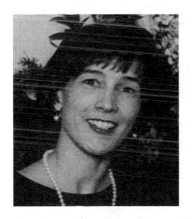
Christine Seel Ritchie is Associate Chief of Staff of Geriatrics and Extended Care at the Louisville VA Medical Center and Assistant Professor of Medicine at the University of Louisville. Dr. Ritchie received her medical degree at the University of North Carolina–Chapel Hill, and her Master's of Science in Public Health with emphasis on nutrition at the University of Alabama at Birmingham (UAB). After completing her internship, residency, and chief residency in internal medicine at UAB, she served as a fellow and then joined the faculty in Geriatric Medicine at UAB. She served as adjunct faculty at Boston University and lecturer at the Harvard University School of Dentistry. She most recently joined the faculty at the University of Louisville where she engages in nutrition-related research and serves as co-director of the Nutrition Curriculum for the University of Louisville School of Medicine. Her clinical practice includes care to frail, community-dwelling older adults, as well as to adults receiving end-of-life care.

About the Series Editor

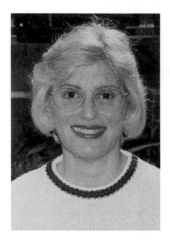

Dr. Adrianne Bendich is Clinical Director of Calcium Research at GlaxoSmithKline Consumer Healthcare, where she is responsible for leading the innovation and medical programs in support of TUMS and Os-Cal. Dr. Bendich has primary responsibility for the direction of GSK's support for the Women's Health Initiative intervention study. Prior to joining GlaxoSmithKline, Dr. Bendich was at Roche Vitamins Inc., and was involved with the groundbreaking clinical studies proving that folic acid-containing multivitamins significantly reduce major classes of birth defects. Dr. Bendich has co-authored more than 100 major clinical research studies in the area of preventive nutrition. Dr. Bendich is recognized as a leading authority on antioxidants, nutrition, immunity, and pregnancy outcomes, vitamin safety, and the cost-effectiveness of vitamin/mineral supplementation.

Dr. Bendich is the editor of nine books, including *Preventive Nutrition: The Comprehensive Guide for Health Professionals,* and is Series Editor of *Nutrition and Health* for Humana Press. She also serves as Associate Editor for *Nutrition: The International Journal of Applied and Basic Nutritional Sciences,* and Dr. Bendich is on the Editorial Board of the *Journal of Women's Health and Gender-Based Medicine,* as well as a member of the Board of Directors of the American College of Nutrition.

Dr. Bendich was the recipient of the Roche Research Award, a *Tribute to Women and Industry* Awardee, and a recipient of the Burroughs Wellcome Visiting Professorship in Basic Medical Sciences, 2000–2001. Dr. Bendich holds academic appointments as Adjunct Professor in the Department of Preventive Medicine and Community Health at UMDNJ, Institute of Nutrition, Columbia University P&S, and Adjunct Research Professor, Rutgers University, Newark Campus. She is listed in Who's Who in American Women.